Lecture Notes in Computer Science 1613

Edited by G. Goos, J. Hartmanis and J. van Leeuwen

Springer

Berlin
Heidelberg
New York
Barcelona
Hong Kong
London
Milan
Paris
Singapore
Tokyo

Attila Kuba   Martin Šámal
Andrew Todd-Pokropek (Eds.)

Information Processing in Medical Imaging

16th International Conference, IPMI'99
Visegrád, Hungary, June 28 – July 2, 1999
Proceedings

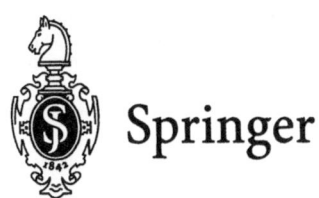 Springer

Series Editors

Gerhard Goos, Karlsruhe University, Germany
Juris Hartmanis, Cornell University, NY, USA
Jan van Leeuwen, Utrecht University, The Netherlands

Volume Editors

Attila Kuba
Department of Applied Informatics, József Attila University
Árpád tér 2., H-6720 Szeged, Hungary
E-mail: kuba@inf.u-szeged.hu

Martin Šámal
Institute of Nuclear Medicine, Charles University of Prague
Salmovska 3, CZ-120 00 Prague, Czech Republic
E-mail: samal@cesnet.cz

Andrew Todd-Pokropek
Department of Medical Physics, University College London
Gower Street, London WC1E 6BT, UK
E-mail: a.todd@ucl.ac.uk

Cataloging-in-Publication data applied for

Die Deutsche Bibliothek - CIP-Einheitsaufnahme

Information processing in medical imaging : 16th international conference ;
proceedings / IPMI '99, Visegrád, Hungary, June 28 - July 2, 1999. Attila Kuba
... (ed.). - Berlin ; Heidelberg ; New York ; Barcelona ; Hong Kong ; London ;
Milan ; Paris ; Singapore ; Tokyo : Springer, 1999
(Lecture notes in computer science ; Vol. 1613)
ISBN 3-540-66167-0

CR Subject Classification (1998): I.4, I.2.5-6, J.3

ISSN 0302-9743
ISBN 3-540-66167-0 Springer-Verlag Berlin Heidelberg New York

Typesetting: Camera-ready by author
SPIN: 10705157   06/3142 – 5 4 3 2 1 0   Printed on acid-free paper

Preface

The 1999 international conference on Information Processing in Medical Imaging (IPMI '99) was the sixteenth in the series of biennial meetings and followed the successful meeting in Poultney, Vermont, in 1997. This year, for the first time, the conference was held in central Europe, in the historical Hungarian town of Visegrád, one of the most beautiful spots not only on the Danube Bend but in all Hungary. The place has many historical connections, both national and international. The castle was once a royal palace of King Matthias. In the middle ages, the Hungarian, Czech, and Polish kings met here. Recently, after the summit meeting of reestablished democracies in the area, it became a symbol for the cooperation between central European countries as they approached the European Union. It was thus also symbolic to bring IPMI, in the year of the 30th anniversary of its foundation, to this place, and organize the meeting with the close cooperation of local and traditional western organizers.

It also provided a good opportunity to summarize briefly a history of IPMI for those who were new to the IPMI conference.

This year we received 82 full paper submissions from all over the world. Of these, 24 were accepted as oral presentations. These were divided into 6 sessions. In spite of our efforts, it was found to be impossible to make these sessions fully balanced and homogeneous. Therefore, the session titles express the leading themes of the respective sessions rather than provide a thorough description of all papers included in each of them.

The first session (traditionally) dealt with new imaging techniques. The topics here span from an analytical study of bioelasticity using ultrasound, to multipolar MEG, binary tomography, and navigated surgery. The second session concerned image processing in three-dimensional ultrasonography and dynamic PET. The third and the fifth sessions presented classic IPMI topics about image segmentation and registration. The papers on segmentation brought new ideas about hybrid geometric snake pedals, geodesic active contours, adaptive fuzzy segmentation, and segmentation of evolving processes in three dimensions. Papers on registration expanded both linear and non-linear approaches to elastic transformations and introduced hierarchical deformation models for 4-D cardiac SPECT data. The fourth session included a mixture of papers on segmentation and registration as applied to analysis of images of the brain cortex. The final (sixth) session dealt with feature detection and modelling. It included detection of masses in mammography, physiologically oriented models for functional MRI, comparison of MR and x-ray angiography, and a unified framework for atlas matching based on active appearance models. It was an explicit requirement of the IPMI Board, as well as the conviction of the organizers, to insist on a demonstration of medical applicability of all the image processing methods presented. We believe that all the selected papers fulfill this difficult but crucial criterion. The time alloted to oral presentations was 20 minutes plus 30 minutes for a (scheduled) discussion which, however, by IPMI tradition is virtually un-limited and depends on the importance of the problem, the clarity of the paper and the interest of the audience. In the proceedings, the space alloted to each oral presentation is 14 pages. It is a compromise between a need to provide the readers with sufficient details of the presentation and a requirement to keep the extent of the book to within 500 pages. The organizers regret that they could not accept the often justified requests of many authors to expand the space for their papers.

An additional 28 submissions were accepted as poster presentations. Ample time was given to the audience to meet the authors in front of their posters and to discuss the presentations in depth. In addition to short oral presentations, each of two poster sessions was concluded by a plenary discussion. In the proceedings, the space alloted to each poster presentation is 6 pages.

The poster presentations were divided into 2 sessions. The first dealt with var-ious methods of cardiovascular image analysis, modelling and analysis of shapes, and with the segmentation and detection of specific image structures. The sec-ond concerned reconstruction, measurement in medical images, registration, and image modelling. Although oral papers and plenary discussions form the tradi-tional basis of the IPMI meeting, the introduction of poster sessions further enlarged the space permitted for additional topics, for considering more specific applications, and for extended informal discussions.

The uniqueness of the IPMI meeting has been emphasized from various per-sonal viewpoints in the forewords of previous proceedings. It consists in a magic mixture of an interdisciplinary approach, informal communication, thorough dis-cussions, high scientific standards, the promotion of young researchers, and a friendly atmosphere. It is a great responsibility for the organizers to cultivate the IPMI tradition and sustain all its many flavours for the future. We sincerely wish IPMI many happy returns for its 30th birthday and wish it well, long into the 21th century.

March 1999

Attila Kuba
Martin Šámal
Andrew Todd-Pokropek

A brief history of the universe, the IPMI phenomenon (IPMI 1969-1999)

The big bang from the point of view of IPMI took place in late 1969. Some 20 odd (some of them very odd) researchers gathered together in Brussels for an ad hoc meeting on the use of computers in nuclear medicine, sponsored by a grant from Euroatom, obtained by our first 'president', François Erbsmann. The meeting was originally given the name Information Processing in Scintigraphy, and only Europeans participated. It is worth noting that at that time a computer with 4K of memory was considered respectable. By 1971, the expansion of this Universe had reached Hannover, under our second president, Eberhard Jahns, and by this time some grit from across the Atlantic had also been incorporated. From these first few seconds of the expanding IPMI universe, little (written) trace remains of the white heat of invention. The first meeting produced no written record, and the second proceedings only exist (but do exist) as an unpublished manuscript. One of the pieces of grit, present at the 2nd meeting, agreed to run the 3rd meeting in Boston (Cambridge), and so Steve Pizer (aided by Charlie Metz) permitted continuing expansion to North America. As a result of this, IPMI has been established of an oscillating universe with a period of 2 years with, at this interval, the centre of gravity switching between Europe and North America. We have considered further expansion to the far east, Australia, or South America, but have been prevented from doing so by the strong force effect (lack of money). A rare photograph exists of some of the participants at the Boston meeting, lounging on a lawn, not wearing very much, and observing attractive students go by. Ah, the universe was young then! By now, the ratio of North American contributions had reached 50%, a value which has been maintained. Although scintigraphy (nuclear medicine) was still the target application, tomographic reconstruction was considered important and a number of general image processing papers foreshadow a slow drift towards computer vision applications.

Two years later, in 1975, the meeting switched to Paris (Orsay) which I ran. The meeting was now scheduled for a total of 5 days, with one free afternoon, and another long lasting phenomenon was discovered, that of the IPMI football (soccer) match. Despite unwarranted complaints about bias in refereeing, this match has always been won by the European team, and it is hoped and anticipated that this strange effect will be preserved. We have also always had a few female scientists present at the IPMI meetings, but regrettably their charm has only been present in limited numbers. In Paris the IPMI universe reached the number of 100 participants, and a major aim of the meeting has been to try to limit total numbers to this order. IPMI has always permitted long presentations with effectively unlimited time for ensuing questions, and it has been a second major aim of IPMI to try to remove limits in total time to permit this disorder.

In 1977 we arrived in Nashville under the leadership of Randy Brill, and the title of the meeting now changed officially to Information Processing in Medical Imaging (IPMI). Many other clinical applications were now included, such as angiography, ultrasound, and CT, with a significant component of tomographic reconstruction. In 1979 we returned to (central) Paris, under the direction of Robert Di Paola, the first paper being about a relatively novel technique, magnetic resonance. The spin doctors have increased their influence at each successive meeting. The proceedings were published by INSERM. In 1981 we were laid back in California, activated by the acerbic wit of Michael Goris, but mainly thinking about nuclear medicine and ultrasound (and Californian fruit and wine). A major theme of the meeting was applications in cardiology

In 1983 we returned to Brussels, led by Frank Deconinck, and the first publication of the proceeding by a regular publisher was produced. All subsequent proceedings have been published, by Martinus Nijhoff, Plenum, Wiley, Kluwer, and for the majority, Springer. Papers such as 'Image analysis– topological methods' indicated new directions in scale space, and more substantial mathematical presentations. While evaluation continued to be an important topic, the meeting welcomed novel acquisition methods, here Impedance Tomography. In 1985 we passed to Washington and Steve Bacharach. While the scientific highlights of the meeting were significant, a couple of our Scottish participants yet again remain fondly in our memories as being those most responsible for the excellent social interactions always a feature of IPMI (here the infamous fire alarm incident).

We were received in The Netherlands in 1987 by Max Viergever and now bathed in the more abstract universe of general image processing (meta-models, multiresolution shape) whilst retaining our interest in reconstruction. One of our present chairmen gave his first paper expressing his deep angst with the title 'The reality and meaning of physiological factors'. As usual, the bar near our student accommodation remained open late in the night as the deeper notions of Information Processing were explored.

As a result of the tragic death of our first chairman, it was here that the François Erbsmann prize was established in recognition of his original intention, to aim the meeting towards promoting the work of young scientists (even if some of the lengthy questions and answer sessions do not always seem to reflect this). I should also sadly point out that we have also lost our 2nd chairman, Eberhard Jahns, as a result of a car accident. However, I am pleased to report that as far as we are aware, all the rest have so far survived (despite the ravages of time and of our Scottish colleagues).

Two years later we returned to California (1989), now as Berkeley ageing hippies (or at least some of us). MRI was now considered to warrant a whole session, segmentation even more, but image reconstruction was the major topic here. The quality of the papers had now reached a level where the competition to be included was such that then (and we hope now) authors reserved their best papers for this meeting, and braced themselves for the Spanish inquisition of the questions following their presentations. The final decade of the 20th century dawned for the IPMI universe in Wye in England, organised by Alan Colchester and Dave Hawkes (1991). The quality of the meeting seemed to have been maintained, as were the traditions. Multi-modality approaches appeared, MR was the dominant image type, and computer vision methods were emphasised. Posters were first introduced, but not published, at this meeting. A highlight was probably the sometimes violent philosophical discussions about whether an edge could actually exist. On the final day, after the football match, Nico Karsse-meijer was obliged to present his paper in plaster, having had his leg broken, illustrating yet again our tremendous dedication to science. From the embrace of the elegant pubs in Kent, 2 years later we stormed the mountains of Arizona, to be precise, Flagstaff, under the leadership of Harry Barrett (1993). The meeting continued its traditions, ranging from discussions of higher order differential structures to optical tomography. The arguments about segmentation continued, we were somewhat on edge and tetchy (a skeleton in our cupboard?), but the high point was reached by those climbing to the top of the nearby Humphrey's peak (3850m). The highlight of our next meeting, in Brest directed by Yves Bizais, was certainly the student celebration of their end of term where a group of them promenaded with loud drumming throughout the night. Fortunately, this did not worry everyone, as the student bar rarely closed before dawn. More posters were presented and now included in the proceedings. This excellent meeting was followed by that organised by Jim Duncan in Poultney, Vermont. The scientific quality was again considered to be excellent, and the surroundings beautiful. Neuroscience here clearly dominated other clinical applications. Despite this increasing interest in brains, somehow (again!) the Europeans won the football match. During the outing to a ski-resort a number of participants found refuge from the plague of insects, against instructions, by skiing down an icy ski-run (exceptionally open in June in a heat wave!). Jim Duncan as (to date) our last chairman has said how much he appreciated the cooperation and respect given to him by the enthusiastic participants at an IPMI meeting. At least he did not have to rescue any from jail as I have had to in the past.

I do not know what will be the highlights of the current meeting for which these proceedings represent the written trace. I hope that the scientific expansion of the meeting will continue, and that in the social context, we will also continue in the long tradition of IPMI to enjoy ourselves, have fun, and make many new friends. The proceedings of this meeting only reflects a small part of the value of the IPMI experience. The length of time allocated for questions and answers after presentations is an important part of the IPMI experiment, but unfortunately is not recorded (perhaps fortunately in some cases). A new 'Special Prize for Brilliance' has been suggested. The ability to discover and discuss new approaches in depth is just as important, which has always been the justification for limiting the total number of participants.

This brief and certainly biased history of the IPMI universe has not mentioned the first presentations of some very significant results, nor included the names of all the co-chairmen of the meetings, and especially the names of all the participants without whom the meetings could never have happened or been successful. Let us hope that the strange charm of the meeting will persist (where you can find a GUT in a TOE), with its ups and downs, strung together in theory, without loss of colourful traditions. Can this be maintained? This question is perhaps the big crunch (or is that the result of the next football match)?

March 1999   Andrew Todd-Pokropek

François Erbsmann Prize winners 1987–1997

1987 10th IPMI, Utrecht, NL:
John M. Gauch
Dept. of Computer Science, University of North Carolina, Chapel Hill, NC, USA
Gauch, J.M., Oliver, WR, Pizer, SM: Multiresolution shape descriptions and
their applications in medical imaging. In Information Processing in Medical
Imaging. Eds. de Graaf, CN, Viergever, MA, Plenum, New York (1988) 131-
149

1989 11th IPMI, Berkeley, CA, USA:
Arthur F. Gmitro
Dept. of Radiology, University of Arizona, Tucson, AZ, USA
Gmitro, A.F., Tresp, V., Chen, Y., Snell, R., Gindi, G.R.: Video-rate reconstruc-
tion of CT and MR images. In Information Processing in Medical Imaging. Eds.
D.A. Ortendahl, J. Llacer., Wiley-Liss. New York (1991) 197-210

1991 12th IPMI, Wye (Kent), UK:
H. Isil Bozma
Dept. of Electrical Engineering, Yale University, New Haven, CT, USA
Bozma, H.I., Duncan, J.S.: Model-based recognition of multiple deformable ob-
jects using a game-theoretic framework. In Information Processing in Medical
Imaging. Eds. Colchester, A.C.F., Hawkes, D.J., Springer, Berlin (1991) 358-372

1993 13th IPMI, Flagstaff, AZ, USA:
Jeffrey A. Fessler
Division of Nuclear Medicine, University of Michigan, Ann Arbor, MI, USA
Fessler, J.A.: Tomographic reconstruction using information-weighted spline
smoothing. In Information Processing in Medical Imaging. Eds. Barrett, H.H.,
Gmitro, A.F., Springer, Berlin (1993) 372-386

1995 14th IPMI, Brest, France:
Maurits K. Konings
Dept. of Radiology and Nuclear Medicine, University Hospital Utrecht, Utrecht,
The Netherlands
Konings, M.K., Mali, W.P.T.M., Viergever, M.A.: Design of a robust strategy to
measure intravascular electrical impedance. In Information Processing in Medical
Imaging. Eds. Bizais, Y., Barillot, C., Di Paola, R., Kluwer Academic, Dordrecht
(1995) 1-12

1997 15th IPMI, Poultney, VT, USA:
David Atkinson
UMDS, Radiological Sciences, Guy's Hospital, London, United Kingdom
Atkinson, D., Hill, D.L.G., Stoyle, P.N.R., Summers, P.E., Keevil, S.F.: An aut-
ofocus algorithm for the automatic correction of motion artifacts in MR im-
ages. In Information Processing in Medical Imaging. Eds. Duncan, J., Gindi, G..
Springer, Berlin (1997) 341-354

Conference Committee

Chair

Attila Kuba	József Attila University, Szeged, Hungary

Co-Chair

Martin Šámal	Charles University Prague, Czech Republic

Scientific Committee

Stephen Bacharach	National Institute of Health, USA
Christian Barillot	INRIA/CNRS, France
Harrison Barrett	University of Arizona, USA
Helmar Bergmann	University of Vienna, Austria
Yves Bizais	University of Bretagne Occidentale, France
Michael Brady	Oxford University, UK
Alan Colchester	University of Kent, UK
James Duncan	Yale University, USA
Guido Gerig	University of North Carolina, Chapel Hill, USA
David Hawkes	Guy's Hospital, London, UK
Karl Heinz Höhne	University of Hamburg, Germany
Gabor Herman	University of Pennsylvania, USA
Richard Leahy	University of Southern California, USA
Kyle Myers	Food and Drug Administration, USA
Stephen Pizer	University of North Carolina, Chapel Hill, USA
Jerry Prince	Johns Hopkins University, USA
Milan Šonka	University of Iowa, USA
Chris Taylor	University of Manchester, UK
Andrew Todd–Pokropek	University College London, UK,
	INSERM U494, France
Max Viergever	University of Utrecht, The Netherlands

Local Organising Committee

Marianna Dudásné Nagy
Csongor Halmai
László Martonossy
Antal Nagy
Kálmán Palágyi
Attila Tanács
(from József Attila University, Szeged, Hungary)

Acknowledgments

The XVIth IPMI conference would not have been possible without the efforts of many dedicated people. We are extremely grateful to all members of the scientific committee for their timely and careful reviewing of many manuscripts. Their expertise ensured the high scientific quality of the conference. We especially appreciate the invaluable advice and personal involvement of IPMI President J.S.Duncan and IPMI Board Member M.A.Viergever in the process of selecting the papers and finalising the scientific programme.

We thank all the researchers who submitted full-length manuscripts for consideration. Their work and interest is essential to permit the unique IPMI tradition to continue in the future. Almost all of the submitted papers were of very high quality and we regret that we had to turn down a significant number due to lack of space.

We would like to acknowledge in particular the help and support of the local organising committee

Finally, we most gratefully acknowledge and appreciate the financial support of the following organisations:

Institute of Informatics, József Attila University, Szeged, Hungary,

First Faculty of Medicine, Charles University, Prague, Czech Republic

Hungarian National Committee for Technological Development (OMFB),

Philips Medical Systems Nederland BV,

Czech Society of Nuclear Medicine, Czech Medical Association J.E. Purkyně,

Leapfrog Technology Ltd, London, UK.

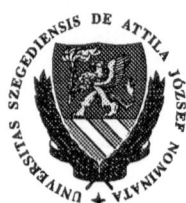  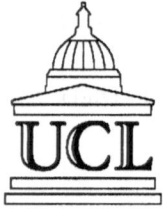

Table of Contents

New Imaging Techniques

3D Ultrasound and PET

Segmentation

Image Analysis of the Brain Cortex

Registration

Feature Detection and Modelling

Poster Session I

Cardiovascular Image Analysis

Shape Modeling and Analysis

Segmentation and Detection

Poster Session II

Measurement and Quantitative Image Analysis

Analysis of Image Sequences and Functional Imaging

Registration

Image Modeling

Analytical Study of Bioelasticity Ultrasound Systems

Michael F. Insana, Larry T. Cook, and Pawan Chaturvedi

Dept of Radiology, Univ of Kansas Med Center, Kansas City, KS 66160, USA
Insana@research.kumc.edu

Abstract. A framework is presented for designing and evaluating bioelasticity imaging systems.

1 Introduction

Manual palpation has been an essential technique for diagnosing disease since the time of the ancient Greeks. They found that by compressing the surface of the skin a stress field is created inside the elastic tissues of the body that can be sensed by the fingertips. Regions atop stiff objects like cancerous lesions produce a greater restoring force at the skin surface than do adjacent regions. Hence, abnormalities may be detected and, in some cases, identified and sized based on their elasticity. The clinical success of manual palpation is based on the high elasticity contrast that exists for many pathologies – orders of magnitude for some cancers [1] – producing intense stress fields that make it easy to detect surface lesions. Unfortunately those stress fields decay rapidly with distance from the lesion, so it is difficult to sense objects deep in the body.

Elasticity imaging is palpation by remote sensing. It is the name for a class of techniques used to visualize tissue stiffness with a sensitivity and spatial resolution much greater than manual palpation. Often local elastic properties are imaged using ultrasonic or magnetic resonance signals to track local movements in mechanically stimulated tissues [2,3,4,5]. We use ultrasound to track the motion produced during static compression [6,7,8]. Two sets of radio-frequency echo signals are recorded from a region in the body before and after applying a small compressive force. The two echo fields are compared using a series of correlation techniques to register the data and thereby estimate displacement in one, two, or three dimensions depending on the boundary conditions for motion and the dimensionality of the echo fields. Spatial derivatives of the displacement field are combined to estimate strain tensor components that we call *strain images*. If the stress field is approximately uniform, then strain is inversely proportional to elasticity, and strain images describe tissue stiffness directly. The key to elasticity imaging is precise displacement estimation at high spatial resolution.

Ostensibly the procedure for creating strain images is straightforward, but in practice achieving high-quality images requires great attention to detail. We must seek a careful balance between three experimental conditions: *high waveform coherence* and *accurate displacement estimation* are required for low noise

A. Kuba et al. (Eds.): IPMI'99, LNCS 1613, pp. 1–14, 1999.

and superior spatial resolution, and a *large applied compression* yields high strain contrast. Conditions resulting in high strain contrast often produce severe decorrelation noise, i.e. strain noise caused by the inability of the image formation algorithm to track motion when there is low coherence between pre- and post-compression echo fields. A balance is achieved by carefully selecting the applied stress, boundary conditions, ultrasonic system parameters, and signal processing, none of which are independent. Thus far, the designs of most elasticity imaging experiments are empirical. Comprehensive analyses provided by the time-delay estimation literature [9] are of limited value because, unlike most radar and sonar applications, ultrasound echo signals are stochastic and the spatially-spread scatterers move in three dimensions when tissue is deformed.

This paper briefly summarizes a maximum-likelihood (ML) strategy for ultrasonic strain image formation and outlines a new approach for evaluating experimental designs. The evaluation is based on the *Fourier crosstalk matrix* concept originated by Barrett and Gifford [10] for designing medical imaging systems. We describe two mathematical models of ultrasonic waveforms recorded from a deformed object. A continuous model leads to the ML approach to strain imaging. A discrete model leads to the crosstalk matrix. The paper concludes with applications of the crosstalk matrix to the evaluation of system design.

2   Continuous Waveform Model

Biological tissues are modeled as incompressible, viscoelastic materials containing randomly positioned point scatterers. The object function that describes the spatial distribution of scatterers is the acoustic impedance field, $z(\mathbf{x})$, a zero-mean, Gaussian random process. The three-space coordinate vector is $\mathbf{x} = (x_1, x_2, x_3)^t$, where $\mathbf{x}^t$ is the transpose of $\mathbf{x}$. A shift-invariant sensitivity function[1] $h(\mathbf{x})$ maps the object function $z(\mathbf{x})$ into the echo data $r(\mathbf{x})$ over a region of support $\mathcal{S}$ according to the convolution equation

$$r(\mathbf{x}) = \left[\int\!\!\int_{\mathcal{S}} d\mathbf{x}'\, h(\mathbf{x} - \mathbf{x}')\, z(\mathbf{x}') \right] + n_0(\mathbf{x})$$
$$= \bar{r}(\mathbf{x}) + n_0(\mathbf{x}) . \tag{1}$$

The additive noise process $n_0(\mathbf{x})$ is signal independent, zero-mean, band-pass white, and Gaussian with power spectral density G_n, i.e.,

$$E\{n_0^*(\mathbf{x})\, z(\mathbf{x})\} = 0 , \qquad E\{n_0(\mathbf{x})\} = 0 , \qquad E\{n_0^*(\mathbf{x})\, n_0(\mathbf{x}')\} = G_n\, \delta(\mathbf{x} - \mathbf{x}') ,$$

where $E\{fg\}$ is the expected value taken over all f and g. We assume a 2-D echo field from a linear array transducer. An echo field is a collection of waveforms

---

[1] Sensitivity functions combine the pulse-echo system response with two frequency-dependent functions that describe scattering and absorption in the medium. If the system response function is Gaussian, the Fourier transform of the sensitivity function, (6), is approximately Gaussian [11].

recorded from parallel transducer beams oriented along the coordinate axis x_1. Adjacent waveforms are arranged parallel to x_2. The scan plane is located at $(x_1, x_2, 0)$ (Fig. 1). Before compression (Fig. 1a), the object is scanned to record a *precompression* echo field defined by (1).

After compression (Figs. 1b and 1c), the same object region is re-scanned to find the *postcompression* echo field,

$$r_1(\mathbf{x}) = \left[\int_{\mathcal{S}} d\mathbf{x}' \, h(\mathbf{x} - \mathbf{x}') \, z(\mathbf{A}^{-1}\mathbf{x}' - \boldsymbol{\tau}_a) \right] + n_1(\mathbf{x})$$

$$= \bar{r}_1(\mathbf{x}) + n_1(\mathbf{x}) , \tag{2}$$

where the physical deformation of the object is reflected by a coordinate transformation of the object function $z(\mathbf{x})$. In modeling $r_1(\mathbf{x})$, we assume the movement of scatterers within all or part of the compressed object can be accurately described as an *affine transformation* [12] of the scatterer positional coordinates. Specifically, we use the material [13] or Lagrangian [14] description of motion: if $\tilde{\mathbf{x}}$ and $\mathbf{x}$ are the pre- and postcompression coordinate vectors, respectively, then $\mathbf{x}(\tilde{\mathbf{x}}) = \mathbf{A}(\tilde{\mathbf{x}} + \boldsymbol{\tau}_a)$, where $\mathbf{A}$ is a linear transformation matrix and $\boldsymbol{\tau}_a$ is a displacement vector. $\mathbf{A}^{-1}$ exists, its determinant $\det \mathbf{A}$ is approximately one, and it is straightforward to interpret $\mathbf{A}$ in terms of strain, s, when the applied compression is small.

3   Image Formation Algorithms

For example, the top surface of the object in Fig. 1a is uniformly displaced in Fig. 1b along the direction of the ultrasound beam axis, x_1, corresponding to an average downward displacement and scaling transformation of the object coordinates with non-zero components $A_{11} = 1 - s$ and $A_{22} = A_{33} = (1 - s)^{-1/2} \simeq 1 + s/2$. A finite-element algorithm (FEA) was used to compute the axial displacement field (Fig. 1d) and longitudinal strain (Fig. 1e). *Longitudinal* refers to the component of the strain tensor in the direction of the applied force [13], in this case along x_1, while *axial* is the direction parallel to the ultrasound beam axis, also along x_1 in this example. Bright areas in the two images indicate large displacements (in the frame of the moving transducer!) and large strains.

A second example is illustrated in Fig. 1c, depicting a nonuniform displacement of the object surface along x_1 at a shear angle $\beta = 5.7°$. The average deformation (Fig. 1g) is represented as a combination of displacement, scaling, and shearing with non-zero matrix elements A_{11}, A_{22}, and $A_{12} = \tan \beta$. Non-zero, off-diagonal elements of $\mathbf{A}$ indicate shearing and rotation.

Of course, the average transformation cannot adequately describe the complex deformation of a large region in elastically heterogeneous media. Notice there are variations in the strain field near the stiff inclusion and at the edges where the top and bottom surfaces were not allowed to slip. Consequently echo fields are partitioned into small regions, such as the triangular meshes in Fig. 1, and $\mathbf{A}$ and $\boldsymbol{\tau}_a$ are estimated for each region using companding [6] or warping with deformable mesh algorithms [15,16]. This particular tissue-like phantom was built [17] and scanned at 5 MHz [11] to produce the experimental strain image of the stiff inclusion shown as an insert in Fig. 1f.

Several image formation algorithms have been proposed to estimate strain under challenging experimental conditions. Most are based on least-squares techniques, e.g., block matching [4,6,8], deformable mesh [15,16] and filtered correlation [11,14]. The least-squares approach involves ML estimation through the use of a *wide-band ambiguity function*, Λ, which aims to determine all motion features simultaneously. In some cases, these estimators are efficient and unbiased [18]. An expression for the wide-band ambiguity function is

$$\Lambda(\mathbf{B}, \boldsymbol{\tau}_b) = \det \mathbf{B} \int_{-\infty}^{\infty} d\mathbf{x} \, r_1(\mathbf{x}) \, r_0^*(\mathbf{x}) \ , \quad \text{where} \quad r_0(\mathbf{x}) = r(\mathbf{B}^{-1}\mathbf{x} - \boldsymbol{\tau}_b) \ . \quad (3)$$

$\mathbf{B}$ and $\boldsymbol{\tau}_b$ are the linear transformation matrix and displacement vector *applied to the precompression echo field* $r(\mathbf{x})$ to match the physical deformation of the object as it is modeled using $\mathbf{A}$ and $\boldsymbol{\tau}_a$. Notice that (3) is a multi-dimensional representation of the correlation between $r_0(\mathbf{x})$ and $r_1(\mathbf{x})$ for various values of $\mathbf{B}$ and $\boldsymbol{\tau}_b$. With our current algorithm [16] and 2-D echo fields, $\mathbf{B}$ and $\boldsymbol{\tau}_b$ provide a total of six motion parameters. The algorithm computes Λ for the data within the triangular subregions of Fig. 1 and searches for a peak value, similar to the use of a cross correlator to estimate time delay. Parameter values at the peak become the estimates. In principle, an image formation algorithm based on the wide-band ambiguity function will achieve strain images with the lowest noise. In addition, joint estimates of $\mathbf{B}$ and $\boldsymbol{\tau}_b$ could determine the entire strain tensor resulting from the applied compression.

4   Definitions

Important familiar functions are stated below in the current notation.

Fourier-series coefficient estimates $\hat{R}_{jk}$ for the jth 2-D echo field and the kth spatial frequency are [19]

$$\hat{R}_{jk} = \frac{1}{S'} \int_S d\mathbf{x} \, r_j(\mathbf{x}) \, e^{-i2\pi \mathbf{u}_k^t \mathbf{x}} \qquad \text{for} \qquad j = 0, 1 \ . \qquad (4)$$

The wavevectors $\mathbf{u}_k$ define points on an infinite 2-D grid [20]. For convenience, the two integer indices required to define the grid are lumped into a single index $k = 1, \ldots, N$ that enumerates all N frequency points within S. S' , $\int_S d\mathbf{x}$ is the measure of S. The Fourier transform of $r_j(\mathbf{x})$ is related to the Fourier-series coefficients by the expression $R_j(\mathbf{u}) = \lim_{S' \to \infty} S' \, \hat{R}_{jk}$.

Applying the shift and scaling theorems [19], the forward Fourier transforms of $r_0(\mathbf{x})$ and $r_1(\mathbf{x})$ are, respectively,

$$\begin{aligned} R_0(\mathbf{u}) &= \mathcal{F}\{r_0(\mathbf{x})\} = \det \mathbf{B} \left[H(\mathbf{B}^t \mathbf{u}) \, Z(\mathbf{B}^t \mathbf{u}) + N_0(\mathbf{B}^t \mathbf{u}) \right] e^{-i2\pi \mathbf{u}^t \mathbf{B} \boldsymbol{\tau}_b} \quad \text{and} \\ R_1(\mathbf{u}) &= \mathcal{F}\{r_1(\mathbf{x})\} = \det \mathbf{A} \, H(\mathbf{u}) \, Z(\mathbf{A}^t \mathbf{u}) \, e^{-i2\pi \mathbf{u}^t \mathbf{A} \boldsymbol{\tau}_a} + N_1(\mathbf{u}) \ , \end{aligned} \qquad (5)$$

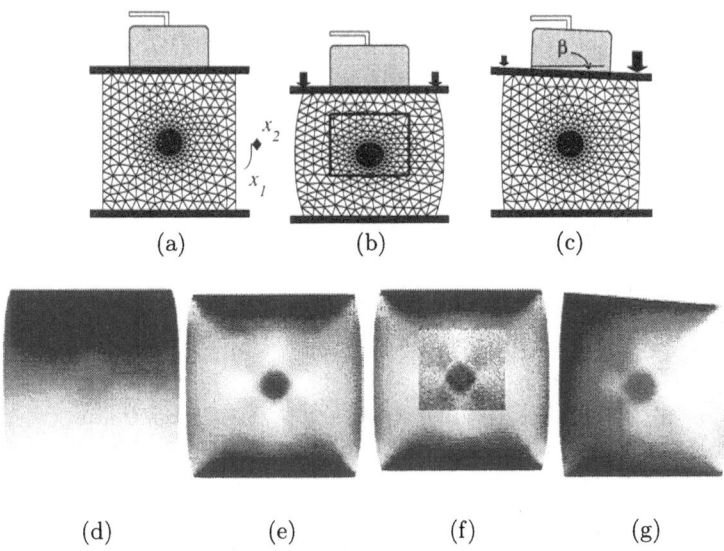

Fig. 1. Uniform compression (a,b) generates displacement (d) and strain (e) fields. Shear compression (c) produces (g). FEA simulations in (d-g); phantom image in (f)

where $Z(\mathbf{u}) = \mathcal{F}\{z(\mathbf{x})\}$, $N_j(\mathbf{u}) = \mathcal{F}\{n_j(\mathbf{x})\}$ and $\mathbf{u} = (u_1, u_2, u_3)^t$ is the continuous spatial-frequency vector corresponding to the spatial coordinate $\mathbf{x}$. Furthermore, we model the Fourier transform of the 2-D sensitivity function as

$$
\begin{aligned}
H(\mathbf{u}) \;=\; & \mathcal{F}\{h(\mathbf{x})\} \;=\; C_0 u_1^2 \exp\left(-\alpha(u_1)\right) \\
\times \; & \left[\exp\left(-2\pi^2(u_1 - u_0)^2 L_1^2\right) - \exp\left(-2\pi^2(u_1 + u_0)^2 L_1^2\right)\right] \exp\left(-2\pi^2 u_2^2 L_2^2\right) \quad (6)
\end{aligned}
$$

at carrier frequency u_0. L_1 and L_2 are pulse and beamwidth parameters, C_0 is a constant, and $\alpha(u_1)$ describes attenuation losses [11].

The cross power spectral densities for continuous and discrete frequencies are

$$
G_{r_0 r_1}(\mathbf{u}_k) = \mathcal{S}'^2 \, E\{\hat{R}_{0k}^* \hat{R}_{1k'}\} \xrightarrow[\mathcal{S}', N \to \infty]{} G_{r_0 r_1}(\mathbf{u}) = E\{R_0^*(\mathbf{u}) R_1(\mathbf{u})\} \;, \quad (7)
$$

the autospectral densities are $G_{r_0 r_0}(\mathbf{u}) = E\{|R_0(\mathbf{u})|^2\}$, $G_{r_1 r_1}(\mathbf{u}) = E\{|R_1(\mathbf{u})|^2\}$, and the magnitude squared coherence function is

$$
|\gamma_{r_0 r_1}(\mathbf{u})|^2 = \frac{|G_{r_0 r_1}(\mathbf{u})|^2}{G_{r_0 r_0}(\mathbf{u}) G_{r_1 r_1}(\mathbf{u})} \;, \quad (8)
$$

where $0 \leq |\gamma_{r_0 r_1}(\mathbf{u})|^2 \leq 1$ [21].

5   Maximum-Likelihood Estimation

Displacement. The ML estimator for displacement selects $\hat{\boldsymbol{\tau}}$ to maximize the value of the likelihood function $p(\hat{\mathbf{R}}|\boldsymbol{\theta})$ [22]. $\boldsymbol{\theta}$ is a vector of all deterministic parameters that affect the data, viz., the motion parameters $\mathbf{A}$, $\mathbf{B}$, $\boldsymbol{\tau}_a$, and $\boldsymbol{\tau}_b$ and waveform parameters $H(\mathbf{u})$, $G_{zz}(\mathbf{u})$, and $G_{nn}(\mathbf{u})$. Ignoring all terms independent of displacement, the log-likelihood function is [11]

$$\ln p(\hat{\mathbf{R}}|\boldsymbol{\theta}) \simeq \mathcal{S}' \int_{-\infty}^{\infty} d\mathbf{u} \ \mathrm{Re} \left\{ R_0^*(\mathbf{u}) R_1(\mathbf{u}) \ W^2(\mathbf{u}) \ e^{-i2\pi \mathbf{u}^t (\mathbf{A}\boldsymbol{\tau}_a - \mathbf{B}\boldsymbol{\tau}_b)} \right\} \ , \quad (9)$$

where $\mathrm{Re}\{\cdots\}$ is the real part of the argument and

$$W^2(\mathbf{u}_k) = \frac{|\gamma_{r_0 r_1}(\mathbf{u}_k)|}{\sqrt{G_{r_0 r_0}(\mathbf{u}_k) G_{r_1 r_1}(\mathbf{u}_k)} \ (1 - |\gamma_{r_0 r_1}(\mathbf{u}_k)|^2)}$$

is a frequency filter.

The ML strategy for displacement is defined by the generalized cross correlator [23] of (9). First, choose values for $\mathbf{B}$ and $\boldsymbol{\tau}_b$ that warp the precompression echo field to match the physical deformation defined by $\mathbf{A}$ and $\boldsymbol{\tau}_a$. Specifically, choose $\mathbf{B}\boldsymbol{\tau}_b = \mathbf{A}\boldsymbol{\tau}_a$ so that the value of the exponential factor in the brackets of (9) is one at all frequencies. Second, the ML estimator filters the pre- and the postcompression waveforms each with the function $W(\mathbf{u})$. Filtering increases the weight of the most coherent frequency components between r_0 and r_1 but only if the statistical properties of the waveform are known a priori. Third, the estimator cross correlates the filtered r_0 and r_1 and finds the displacement estimate $\hat{\boldsymbol{\tau}}$ at the peak cross correlation value. The main difference between the generalized cross correlator and the wide-band ambiguity function is that the former estimates parameters sequentially and the latter simultaneously.

Strain. The total displacement, $\boldsymbol{v}$, at each position in the deformed medium is given by the sum of the displacement applied during the echo field warp, $\boldsymbol{\tau}_b$, and that determined from the cross correlation measurement, $\hat{\boldsymbol{\tau}}$, i.e., $\boldsymbol{v} = \hat{\boldsymbol{\tau}} + \boldsymbol{\tau}_b$. The Eulerian strain tensor is [13]

$$\epsilon_{mn} = \frac{1}{2} \left[\frac{\partial v_n}{\partial x_m} + \frac{\partial v_m}{\partial x_n} \right] \ , \quad (10)$$

and the longitudinal strain measured along the axis of the sound beam is

$$s \ , \ \ \epsilon_{11} = \frac{\partial v_1}{\partial x_1} \ . \quad (11)$$

For imaging, strain is adequately approximated using difference formulas [3,4].

6   Variance Bounds

From the likelihood function of (9) and the strain estimate of (11), we computed the Cramér-Rao lower bound on strain variance for unbiased estimates to find [11]

$$\mathrm{var}(\hat{s}) \ \geq \ \frac{2(A_{12}^2 Y_1 + A_{22}^2 Y_2)}{T_1 \Delta T \ (A_{11} A_{22} - A_{12} A_{21})^2 \ Y_1 Y_2} \ . \quad (12)$$

where T_1 is the length of the data segment and ΔT is the distance between overlapping data segments. These experimental parameters are selected when using the difference equation to approximate the derivative in (11). ΔT is particularly significant since it determines the axial pixel size of the strain image. A_{mn} are components of the transformation matrix $\mathbf{A}$ and Y_1 and Y_2 are frequency integrals

$$Y_i \, , 2\mathcal{S}' \int_0^\infty d\mathbf{u} \, (2\pi u_i)^2 \, \frac{|\gamma_{r_0 r_1}(\mathbf{u})|^2}{(1 - |\gamma_{r_0 r_1}(\mathbf{u})|^2)} \quad .$$

Equation (12) describes how longitudinal strain errors are affected by motion in the plane – motion that includes scaling, shearing, and rotation.

We predicted strain errors from the variance bound of (12). These were compared with standard deviations of strain measurements obtained from a tissue-like phantom acquired under nearly ideal conditions [11] to assess estimation efficiency (Fig. 2). An elastically homogeneous material was uniformly compressed, as in Fig. 1b, while strain was measured in a small region near the center. Applied strains in excess of 1% generated significantly more error than that predicted because the predictions ignore the effects of echo-data sampling. The log-likelihood function was derived assuming a continuous waveform model with large object support. In reality, data are sampled at different rates along x_1 and x_2: typical sampling intervals for a linear array are $\Delta x_1 = 0.015$ mm and $\Delta x_2 = 0.180$ mm. So the predictions of (12) are not limited by the effects of aliasing or small data sets used to estimate displacement at high resolution. A continuous model led to error bounds, but to obtain a more realistic evaluation of elasticity system design, including the limitation of spatial resolution, we turn now to a discrete waveform model and an analysis of Fourier crosstalk.

7   Discrete Waveform Model

The process of imaging a continuous object $z(x)$ with a linear system characterized by the sensitivity function $h_m(x)$ to produce the mth discrete measurement sample r_m in noise n_m is represented by [24]

$$r_m = \left[\int_{-\infty}^\infty dx \, h_m(x) \, z(x) \right] \; + \; n_m$$
$$= \bar{r}_m \; + \; n_m \; . \tag{13}$$

M measurements are recorded from signals generated within the object support $\mathcal{S}$ such that $-(M-1)/2 \le m \le (M-1)/2$ where, for convenience, M is an odd integer. The discussion is limited to one spatial dimension for simplicity. The object function is exactly represented by the Fourier series [19]

$$z(x) = \sum_{\ell=-\infty}^\infty Z_\ell \, e^{i2\pi u_\ell x} \, \mathcal{S}(x) \; , \tag{14}$$

where Z_ℓ are Fourier coefficients and $e^{i2\pi u_\ell x}$ are Fourier basis functions. In our one-dimensional example, $S(x) = \mathrm{rect}(x/S')$ and $u_\ell = \ell/S'$. Integer indices m and ℓ indicate digitized waveform samples and frequencies, respectively.

Combining (13) and (14), the noise-free echo measurements are [20]

$$\bar{r}_m = \sum_{\ell=-\infty}^{\infty} \Psi_{m\ell}\, Z_\ell = (\boldsymbol{\Psi Z})_m \;, \qquad \text{where} \quad \Psi_{m\ell} = \int_S dx\, h_m(x)\, e^{i2\pi u_\ell x} \;. \quad (15)$$

$\Psi_{m\ell}$ are components of an $M \times \infty$ matrix whose rows are the Fourier transforms of the product of the sensitivity function and support function for each measurement. Equation (15) expresses the mth waveform sample as the sum over frequency of the $\Psi_{m\ell}$ components weighted by their respective Fourier coefficients. The object contributes to r_m through Z_ℓ, while the measurement process contributes to r_m through $\Psi_{m\ell}$.

Example: Ideal Ultrasonic Imaging System. Consider the perfect, linear, shift-invariant (LSI) system with sensitivity function

$$h_m(x) = \frac{1}{2\pi z_0} \frac{d^2}{dx^2}\, \delta(x - m\Delta x) \;.$$

For large support, (15) gives

$$\bar{r}_m = \sum_{\ell=-\infty}^{\infty} Z_\ell \left[\frac{1}{2\pi z_0} \int_{-\infty}^{\infty} dx\, \frac{d^2}{dx^2}\, \delta(x - m\Delta x)\, e^{i2\pi u_\ell x} \right]$$

$$= \frac{1}{2\pi z_0} \left(\frac{d^2 z(x)}{dx^2} \right)_{x=x_m} \;,$$

which is precisely the acoustic scattering function of the object, i.e., the second derivative of the relative impedance profile $z(x)/z_0$. Images from this ideal ultrasonic system reproduce the object function without distortion. We have assumed that the sampling interval satisfies the Nyquist criterion; specifically, if $Z_\ell = 0$ for $\ell \geq N$, then $\Delta x \leq S'/N$. The row (column) vectors of $\boldsymbol{\Psi}$ are orthogonal for the ideal system, and their components are second derivatives of the object basis functions.

To study displacement or strain, we must analyze the relationship between *two* ultrasonic echo fields. A discrete representation of those fields is

$$\bar{r}_{0m} = \sum_{\ell=-\infty}^{\infty} Z_\ell \left[B \int_S dx\, h_m(x)\, e^{i2\pi u_\ell x} \right] = \sum_{\ell=-\infty}^{\infty} \Psi_{0m\ell}\, Z_\ell \qquad \text{Warped Pre}$$

$$(16)$$

$$\bar{r}_{1m} = \sum_{\ell=-\infty}^{\infty} Z_\ell \left[\int_S dx'\, h_m(x')\, e^{i2\pi u_\ell \left(\frac{x'}{A} - \tau_a \right)} \right] = \sum_{\ell=-\infty}^{\infty} \Psi_{1m\ell}\, Z_\ell \;. \qquad \text{Post}$$

If the support is large compared with the range of motion, then the integrals over S before and after the coordinate transformation are approximately equal.

Equation (16) expresses an important symmetry: imaging a deformed object is mathematically equivalent to imaging the undeformed object with a deformed sensitivity function.

8   Crosstalk Matrix

Following the ML strategy of (9), we produce $\mathbf{r}_0$ by warping $\mathbf{r}$ to match the physical deformation in $\mathbf{r}_1$ (16). The echo fields are then filtered and cross correlated. A discrete form of the cross correlation function ϕ_q at lag index q for a particular $\bar{\mathbf{r}}_0$ and $\bar{\mathbf{r}}_1$ is

$$E\{\phi_q\}_{n|z} = \sum_{m=-(M-1)/2}^{(M-1)/2} \bar{r}_{0m}^* \, \bar{r}_{1(m+q)} = \sum_{\ell=1}^{\infty}\sum_{\ell'=1}^{\infty} Z_\ell \, Z_{\ell'} \, \beta_{q\ell\ell'} \, , \qquad (17)$$

where the ensemble average is over all noise realizations for a specific object, and

$$\beta_{q\ell\ell'} \, , \qquad \sum_{m=-(M-1)/2}^{(M-1)/2} \Psi_{0m\ell}^* \, \Psi_{1(m+q)\ell'} \qquad (18)$$

is the crosstalk matrix for ultrasonic displacement estimation. For an LSI system, $h_m(x) = h(x - m\Delta x)$. Hence, a general form of the crosstalk matrix is

$$\beta_{q\ell\ell'} = \sum_{m=-(M-1)/2}^{(M-1)/2} \left[B \, H^*(u_\ell) e^{-i2\pi u_\ell \frac{m\Delta x}{B}} \right] \left[H\left(\frac{u_{\ell'}}{A}\right) e^{i2\pi u_{\ell'}\left(\frac{(m+q)\Delta x}{A} - \tau_a\right)} \right]$$

$$= \left[B \, H^*(u_\ell) \, H\left(\frac{u_{\ell'}}{A}\right) \right] \left[e^{-i2\pi u_{\ell'}\left(\tau_a - \frac{q\Delta x}{A}\right)} \right] \left[M \frac{\operatorname{sinc} M \left(\frac{u_\ell}{B} - \frac{u_{\ell'}}{A}\right)\Delta x}{\operatorname{sinc}\left(\frac{u_\ell}{B} - \frac{u_{\ell'}}{A}\right)\Delta x} \right] (19)$$

Frequencies u_ℓ refer to the warped precompression data while $u_{\ell'}$ refer to the postcompression data. We used the Dirichlet kernel in the expression above:

$$\sum_{m=-(M-1)/2}^{(M-1)/2} e^{i2\pi my} = M \frac{\operatorname{sinc} My}{\operatorname{sinc} y} \, , \qquad \text{where} \quad \operatorname{sinc} x \, , \, \frac{\sin \pi x}{\pi x} \, .$$

The crosstalk matrix predicts the coherence between $\mathbf{r}_0$ and $\mathbf{r}_1$ for an experiment independent of the object, and therefore provides the comparison we require for evaluating alternative experimental designs. In general, the matrix is complex with three indices: ℓ and ℓ' are over frequency and q is over space.

The first factor on the right-hand side (19) is a band-pass filter; the diagonal elements of the matrix, $\beta_{\ell\ell}$, are the system transfer function that defines the sensitivity and spatial resolution of the ultrasound system *for estimating displacement*.

The second factor in (19) is the phase shift corresponding to the object displacement. When the correlation lag $q\Delta x$ equals the scaled translation of the object $A\tau_a$, displacement estimates are accurate, the second factor is unity, and the crosstalk matrix is real. As with the Cramér-Rao bound, we assume $q\Delta x = A\tau_a$ to focus on the two frequency dimensions of the crosstalk matrix, $\beta_{\ell\ell'} = \beta_{q\ell\ell'}|_{q=A\tau_a/\Delta x}$. The most important use of the second factor is to describe the effects of estimating a discrete displacement value $q\Delta x/A$ when in fact the true displacement τ_a is continuous.

The third factor in (19) is the crosstalk between Fourier components of $\mathbf{r}_0$ and $\mathbf{r}_1$. Under-sampling and incomplete warping generate non-zero off-diagonal components that indicate energy from frequency channels in $\mathbf{r}_0$ is not being placed into the same frequency channels in $\mathbf{r}_1$. Increased crosstalk is exactly what is meant by a loss of waveform coherence.

9 Examples of Strain Imaging

Using $\beta_{\ell\ell'}$, the Gaussian system response function of (6), and applying the ML strategy of (9), we can predict realistic consequences for strain noise of using sampled ultrasonic waveforms. Figures 3 and 4 illustrate β for a typical 5 MHz linear array configuration when there is no object deformation. Figure 3 illustrates the crosstalk matrix along the axis of the ultrasound beam x_1, where the echo field consists of a set of band-pass signals whose spectra are peaked at ± 5 MHz. Figure 4 is an image of the crosstalk matrix along the axis x_2 that is perpendicular to the beam axis, where the echo field consists of base-band signals peaked at 0 MHz.[2] Figures 5 and 6 are analogous to 3 and 4 except a 5% scaling deformation was applied to the former along x_1. Each quadrant of Figs. 3 and 5 is a copy of the others except for polarity. Off-diagonal components for band-pass signals (Figs. 3 and 5) are not crosstalk. These are cross terms from the correlation at $u_\ell = -u_{\ell'} = \pm 5$ MHz.

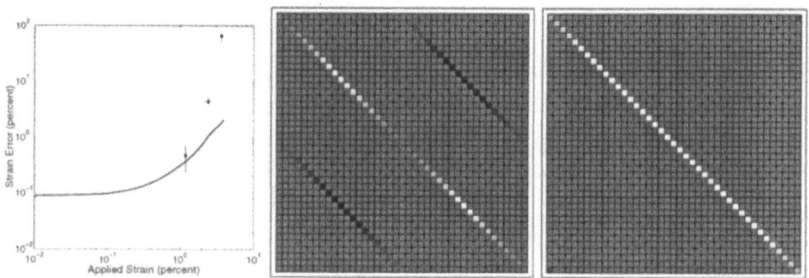

Fig. 2. Strain errors: pre-
dicted and measured ($\bullet$)   **Fig. 3.**   Axial   crosstalk
matrix, no deformation   **Fig. 4.** Lateral crosstalk
matrix, no deformation

---

[2] Bandwidth was extended to facilitate clearer comparisons between Figs. 4 and 6.

The 41×41 element matrices depicted in these figures include 20 negative frequencies, 20 positive frequencies, and $u_\ell = u_{\ell'} = 0$ at the center. System parameters were selected to represent broad-band pulsed transmission with a 5 MHz carrier frequency from a Gaussian-weighted aperture. Waveforms were sampled at the Nyquist rate. Examining any quadrant of the band-pass matrix (Fig. 3) or the entire base-band matrix (Fig. 4) we find no crosstalk (non-zero, off-diagonal elements) because the ultrasound data are adequately sampled and there only rigid-body translation. This highly-coherent system is limited only by bandwidth and additive noise. Sensitivity is low only for motion of small scattering structures detectable at the highest spatial frequencies.

Figures 5 and 6 show $\mathrm{Re}\{\beta_{\ell\ell'}\}$ for the same measurement system but with uncompensated deformation: $A_{11} = 0.95$, $A_{22} = 1.05$, $A_{12} = A_{21} = 0$ and $\mathbf{B} = \mathbf{I}$. The effect of axial compression on the axial crosstalk matrix (Fig. 5) is to "rotate" the matrix patterns *counterclockwise* about the origin. Rotation is a consequence of the third factor in (19). Hence the greatest loss of coherence, i.e., the most energy removed from the diagonal, occurs at the high frequencies. The concomitant lateral expansion is seen in the lateral crosstalk matrix (Fig. 8) as a *clockwise* rotation of the patterns about the origin. Deformation creates low-amplitude crosstalk that appears as ringing in Figs. 5 and 6 from the loss of matrix orthogonality. Normally, patterns along any row or column are given by the ratio of sinc functions in (19). With a constant sampling interval, the frequency components are naturally orthogonal since the harmonic frequencies occur at zeros of the sinc function. In summary, the crosstalk matrix shows us that uncompensated deformation reduces waveform coherence by (a) misplacing information along the matrix diagonal, (b) disturbing frequency component orthogonality, and (c) aliasing signal components just beyond the Nyquist frequency (see upper-right and lower-left corners of Fig. 6). Crosstalk is eliminated by accurate warping, viz., $\mathbf{A}\tau_a = \mathbf{B}\tau_b$.

The diagonal of the crosstalk matrix may be used to quantify spatial resolution for displacement estimates. We plotted diagonal components of the axial crosstalk matrix in Fig. 7 for 0%, 2.5%, and 5% axial compression. The plots show that deformation reduces the effective bandwidth for displacement estimation and that high spatial frequencies are preferentially lost. Warping, however, only partially restores the lost resolution. The full matrix shows the location of energy missing from the diagonal.

While the crosstalk matrix reveals many aspects of strain imaging physics, it is convenient to develop a scalar quantity that summarizes design performance. We propose the trace of the crosstalk matrix divided by its L_2 norm as that figure of merit:

$$\mathcal{B} \; , \; \frac{\mathrm{tr}\,\beta}{\|\beta\|_2} \; = \; \left(\sum_\ell \beta_{\ell\ell} \right) \left(\sum_{\ell,\ell'} \beta_{\ell\ell'}^2 \right)^{-1/2} . \tag{20}$$

We computed (20) for the longitudinal strain images shown in Fig. 8 to see if $\mathcal{B}$ correlates with visual impressions of image quality. Each echo field was simu-

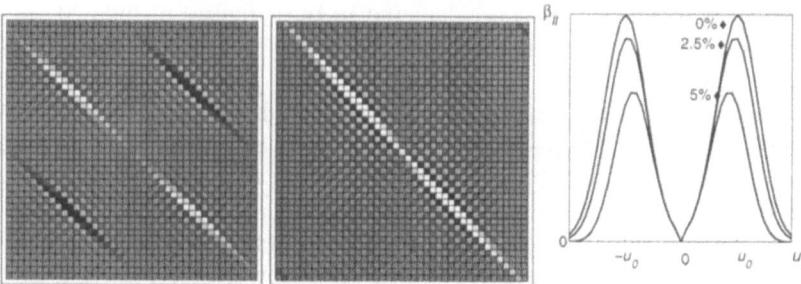

Fig. 5. Axial crosstalk, **Fig. 6.** Lateral crosstalk, **Fig. 7.** Crosstalk matrix
5% axial compression   5% axial compression   diagonals for three com-
                                                  pressions

lated by combining an ultrasound waveform simulator with a FEA as described
previously [7]. Relative to the tissue-like background, the bright circles are soft
and the dark circles are hard. The object was "scanned" with linear array trans-
ducers having different point spread functions (psfs) whose envelopes are shown
enlarged near the upper right corner. Along x_1 the same Gaussian pulse length
was applied for all, but the aperture function varied giving different psfs along x_2.
We used a rectangular aperture in Figs. 8a-c with the corresponding f-numbers
f/1.5, f/3.0, and f/4.5. In Fig. 8d, the f/3.0 aperture of 8b was apodized using
a Hanning function weighting to supress side-lobes at the expense of the main
lobe width.

The object was scanned, compressed 3%, and rescanned, as in Fig. 1b, to
generate the strain images of Fig. 8. Noise was greatest in Fig. 8c, which had the
most weakly focused beam, and least in Fig. 8a, which had the most strongly
focused beam. Axial shear occurring near the inclusions reduces waveform coherence more for wide beams than narrow. The rank order of $\mathcal{B}$, shown in Fig. 8,
tracks the visual impression of image quality and such quantitative measures as
mean-square error. Consequently, the quickly-computed $\mathcal{B}$ correctly predicted
that decorrelation noise is minimized with the most focused beams. Figure 8 is
a realistic simulation describing how the crosstalk matrix enables designers to
explore the physics of strain imaging and provide summary measures of design
quality.

10   Summary

The ML estimator for displacement is consistent with the well-known generalized cross correlator for time-delay estimation [23]. Another implementation
is the wide-band ambiguity function [18], which estimates all motion parameters simultaneously. Comparisons of measured variances with the Cramér-Rao
lower bound showed that our implementation of the ML estimator using sampled
waveforms was not efficient for compressions greater than 1% (Fig. 2). A discrete waveform model was developed to formulate the Fourier crosstalk matrix

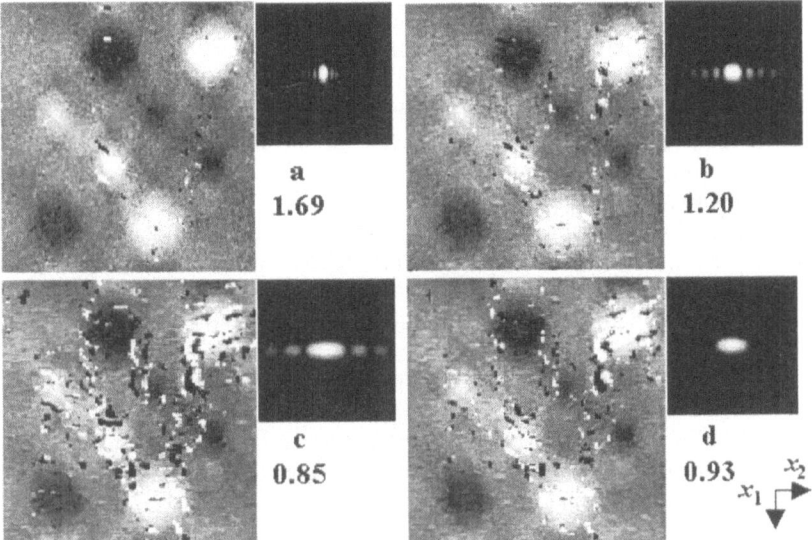

Fig. 8. Simulated strain images for different ultrasonic point spread functions shown at upper right. Four stiff (dark) and soft (bright) targets are included. Values of $\mathcal{B}$, (20), are shown

for ultrasonic strain imaging using sampled waveforms, and thus obtain a realistic means for evaluating experimental system designs from first principles. The crosstalk matrix was found to provide important new insights into experimental design, e.g., the diagonal of the matrix evaluated at the true displacement value is a rigorous measure of spatial resolution for displacement and strain estimation.

Acknowledgements

This work was supported in part by NSF BES-9708221 and NIH R01 DK43007.

References

1. Sarvazyan, A., Skovoroda, A., Emelianov, S., Fowlkes, J., Pipe, J., Adler, R., Buxton, R., Carson, P.L.: Biophysical bases of elasticity imaging. In Acoustical Imaging **21** (1995) 223-240 NewYork:Plenum Press
2. Lerner, R., Huang, S., Parker, K.: Sonoelasticity images derived from ultrasound signals in mechanically vibrated tissues. Ultrasound Med. Biol. **16** (1990) 231-239
3. Céspedes, I., Ophir, J., Ponnekanti, H., Yazdi, Y., Li, X.: Elastography: elasticity imaging using ultrasound with application to muscle and breast in vivo. Ultrasonic Imaging **15** (1993) 73-88
4. O'Donnell, M., Skovoroda, A., Shapo, B., Emelianov, S.: Internal displacement and strain imaging using ultrasonic speckle tracking. IEEE Trans. Ultrason. Ferroelec. Freq. Contr. **41** (1994) 314-325

5. Muthupillai, R., Lomas, D., Rossman, P., Greenleaf, J., Manduca, A., Ehman, R.: Magnetic resonance elastography by direct visualization of propagating acoustic strain waves. Science **269** (1995) 1854-1857

6. Chaturvedi, P., Insana, M.F., Hall, T.J.: 2-D companding for noise reduction in strain imaging. IEEE Trans. Ultrason. Ferroelec. Freq. Contr. **45** (1998) 179-191

7. Chaturvedi, P., Insana, M.F., Hall, T.J.: Testing the limitations of 2-D companding for strain imaging using phantoms. IEEE Trans. Ultrason. Ferroelec. Freq. Contr. **45** (1998) 1022-1031

8. Insana, M.F., Chaturvedi, P., Hall, T.J., Bilgen, M.: 3-D companding using linear arrays for improved strain imaging. Proc. IEEE Ultrason. Symp. **97CH36118** (1997) 1435-1438

9. Carter, G.C.: Coherence and Time Delay Estimation. Piscataway, NJ: IEEE Press (1993)

10. Barrett, H.H., Gifford, H.: Cone-beam tomography with discrete data sets. Phys. Med. Biol. **39** (1994) 451-476

11. Insana, M.F., Cook, L.T., Bilgen, M., Chaturvedi, P.: Maximum-likelihood approach to strain imaging using ultrasound. J. Acoust. Soc. Am. (1999) (submitted)

12. Wolberg, G.: Digital Image Warping. Los Alamitos, CA: IEEE Computer Society Press (1990)

13. Fung, Y.: A First Course in Continuum Mechanics. Englewood Cliffs: Prentice Hall 3/e (1994)

14. Maurice, R.L., Bertrand, M.: Lagrangian speckle model and tissue motion estimation – theory. IEEE Trans. Med. Imag. (1999) (submitted)

15. Yeung, F., Levinson, S.F., Fu, D., Parker, K.J.: Feature-adaptive motion tracking of ultrasound image sequences using a deformable mesh. IEEE Trans. Med. Imag. (1999) (in press)

16. Zhu, Y., Chaturvedi, P., Insana, M.F.: Strain imaging with a deformable mesh. Ultrasonic Imaging (1999) (submitted)

17. Hall, T.J., Bilgen, M., Insana, M.F., Krouskop, T.A.: Phantom materials for elastography. IEEE Trans. Ultrason. Ferroelec. Freq. Contr. **44** (1997) 1355-1365

18. Jin, Q., Wong, K.M., Luo, Z-Q.: The estimation of time delay and Doppler stretch of wideband signals. IEEE Trans. Sig. Proc. **43** (1995) 904-916

19. Papoulis, A.: The Fourier Integral and its Applications. New York: McGraw-Hill (1962)

20. Barrett, H.H., Denny, J.L, Wagner, R.F., Myers, K.J.: Objective assessment of image quality II: Fisher information, Fourier crosstalk and figures of merit for task performance. J. Opt. Soc. Am. A **12** (1995) 834-852

21. Carter, G.C., Knapp, C.H., Nuttall, A.H.: Estimation of the magnitude-squared coherence function via overlapped fast Fourier transform processing. IEEE Trans Audio and Electroacoustics **21** (1973) 337-344

22. Kay, S.M.: Fundamentals of Statistical Signal Processing: Estimation Theory. Englewood Cliffs, NJ: PTR Prentice Hall (1993) Chapters 7 and 15

23. Knapp, C.H., Carter, G.C.: The generalized correlation method for estimation of time delay. IEEE Trans. Acoust., Speech, Signal Processing **24** (1976) 320-327

24. Barrett, H.H., Aarsvold, J.N., Roney, T.J.: Null functions and eigenfunctions: tools for the analysis of imaging systems. In Progress in Clinical and Biological Research **363** (1991) 211-226.

MEG Source Imaging Using Multipolar Expansions

John C. Mosher[1], Richard M. Leahy[2], David W. Shattuck[2],
and Sylvain Baillet[2]

[1] Los Alamos National Laboratory, MS D454
Los Alamos, New Mexico USA 87545
mosher@LANL.Gov
[2] Signal and Image Processing Institute
University of Southern California
Los Angeles, California USA 90089-2564
{leahy, shattuck, silvin}@sipi.usc.edu

Abstract. We describe the use of truncated multipolar expansions for producing dynamic images of cortical neural activation from measurements of the magnetoencephalogram. We use a signal-subspace method to find the locations of a set of multipolar sources, each of which represents a region of activity in the cerebral cortex. Our method builds up an estimate of the sources in a recursive manner, i.e. we first search for point current dipoles, then magnetic dipoles, and finally first order multipoles. The dynamic behavior of these sources is then computed using a linear fit to the spatiotemporal data. The final step in the procedure is to map each of the multipolar sources into an equivalent distributed source on the cortical surface. The method is demonstrated through a Monte Carlo simulation.

1 Introduction

Magnetoencephalography (MEG) data are measurements of the magnetic fields produced by neural current sources within the brain. The problem of estimating these sources is highly ill-posed due to the inherent ambiguities in the associated quasistatic electromagnetic inverse problem, the limited number of spatial measurements and significant noise levels. To overcome these problems, constraints can be placed on the location and form of the current sources. Mapping studies using direct electrical measurements, fMRI and PET reveal discrete focal areas of strong activation within the cortex that are associated with specific cognitive, sensory and motor activities. Consequently, a plausible model for the current generators in an event related study consists of a number of focal cortical regions each of which has an associated time course [12]. The MEG inverse problem requires estimation of the spatial and temporal characteristics of these sources.

There are two major classes of methods for solving the MEG inverse problem which we will refer to as "imaging" and "model based." The imaging methods typically constrain sources to a tessellated representation of the cortex, assume

A. Kuba et al. (Eds.): IPMI'99, LNCS 1613, pp. 15–28, 1999.

an elemental current source in each area element, and solve the linear inverse problem that relates these current sources to the measured magnetic field. Accurate tessellations of the cortex require on the order of 10^5 elements. Since the maximum number of MEG sensors in the current generation of whole head MEG system is approximately 300, the problem is highly underdetermined. By using regularized linear methods based on minimizing a weighted L_2-norm on the image, we can produce unique stable solutions [11,14]. Unfortunately, these methods tend to produce very smooth solutions that are inconsistent with the focal model described above. Many nonlinear algorithms have been proposed that attempt to avoid this oversmoothing problem. While they have met with some success, the cost functions required to achieve more focal solutions are usually highly nonconvex and computation times can be very high, e.g. [1,11].

The model-based methods assume a specific parametric form for the sources. By far the most widely used models in MEG are multiple current dipoles [4,9,12]. These assume that the neural sources are relatively small in number and each sufficiently focal that they can be represented by a few equivalent current dipoles with unknown locations and orientations. Parametric methods can be extended to model the temporal correlation expected in the solutions through fitting the multiple dipole model to the entire data set and estimating the time course for each estimated dipole location. As with the nonlinear imaging methods, the cost functions are nonconvex. Signal subspace based methods such as MUSIC or RAP-MUSIC [7,8,9] can be used to rapidly locate the sources in a sequential fashion and avoid the problem of trapping in local minima.

The equivalent current dipole model is directly interpretable as a current element restricted to the cortical surface. As discussed in [10], the dipole may also represent locally distributed sources that are not necessarily restricted to a single point. However, one of the perceived key limitations is that these distributed sources may not be adequately represented by the dipole model. This problem was one of the prime motivations for the development of the imaging approaches. An alternative solution is to remain within the model-based framework but to broaden the model to allow parametric representations of distributed sources. The multipolar expansion provides a natural framework for generating these models. The multipolar expansions are formed using a Taylor series representation of the magnetic field equations. If the expansion point is chosen near the center of a distributed source, then the contribution of higher order terms will drop off rapidly as the distance from the source to the sensor increases. Using this framework we expand the set of sources to include magnetic dipoles and first order multipoles. These sources are able to represent the field from a distributed source more accurately than is the current dipole. While the idea of using multipolar expansions in MEG source modeling is not new, the approach has generally seen only limited used in magnetocardiography, e.g. [6,15].

The parameters of the estimated higher-order multipolar terms are not easily related to the actual physiological processes that produce the MEG signals. We describe here a two-stage procedure in which we first estimate the locations and parameters of the multiple multipoles, then relate each of the multipoles to equivalent cortical sources. The method described here for estimating the location and moment parameters of these multipolar representations is an extension of the RAP-MUSIC method developed in [8] for localizing current dipoles. The algorithm recursively builds a model for the current source configuration by first testing for the presence of point current dipoles, then magnetic dipoles, and finally first order multipoles. In this way the model order and complexity is gradually increased until the combined estimated sources adequately explain the data.

In the cortical re-mapping stage, we find regions of cortex in the vicinity of the parametric source on which we fit current distributions consistent with the fields associated with each estimated multipole. The final result is then a dynamic image of current activity mapped onto a tessellated representation of the cortex which reveals the time varying behavior at the various locations on the cerebral cortex activated during a particular experiment.

2   Multipolar Source Modeling

2.1   Multipolar Expansions

The relationship between the measured magnetic field and the current sources is determined by the quasistatic form of Maxwell's equations. In the special case in which the head is modeled as a set of concentric nested spheres, each with uniform and isotropic conductivity, there is a simple integral equation that relates the external magnetic field to the current sources. We use this result to derive the multipolar expansion. We include details only for the case where measurements are made of the radial component of the magnetic field. They extend directly both to the case of non-radial magnetic field measurements and to measureme   collected using an EEG syste

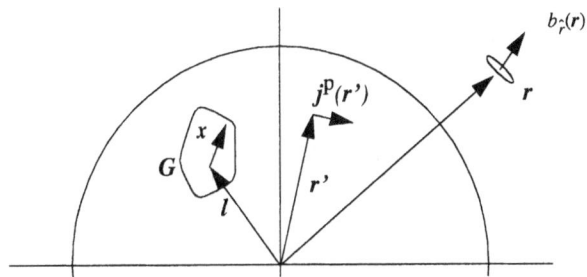

Fig. 1. Primary neural activity of current density $j^p(r')$ at location r' inside a closed conducting volume generates an external magnetic field at location r as detected by a magnetometer with radial orientation r/r, to yield the scalar magnetic measurement $b_r(r)$. We develop a multipolar expansion for sources in a small region, G, using a Taylor series for local displacement x

A truncated multipolar expansion will be used to represent the measured magnetic field for the case of a current source restricted to a relatively small volume, G as illustrated in Fig. 1. As the extent of the source grows, more terms are required in the expansion to adequately represent the external magnetic field. In the following we will develop expressions for the special cases of (i) point sources that are exactly represented as *point current dipoles*, (ii) highly focal sources that can be represented by a *magnetic dipole model*, and (iii) locally distributed sources that can be represented by a *first-order multipole model*.

The external magnetic field is generated by the sum of the *primary neural activity*, designated by the current density vector $j^p(r')$, and the *volume* or *return currents* resulting from the electric field produced by the current source. It is the primary currents that are the sources of interest in MEG inverse problems [4]. The contribution of the volume currents to the external field must be accounted for but the currents themselves are of little interest. In the special case treated here of radial measurements for sources confined to a spherical volume, the volume currents do not contribute to the measured field, and the radial component $b_r(r)$ of the magnetic field $b(r)$ at location r is given by direct extension of the well known Biot-Savart equation:

$$b_r(r) \equiv \frac{r}{r} \cdot b(r) = \frac{r}{r} \cdot \frac{\mu_0}{4\pi} \int_G \frac{r' \times j^p(r')}{d(r,r')^3} dr' = \frac{r}{r} \cdot \frac{\mu_0}{4\pi} \int_G \frac{M(r')}{d(r,r')^3} dr', \quad (1)$$

where $d(r,r') = r - r'$ is the distance vector between the two arguments, $d(r,r') = \|r - r'\|$ the corresponding scalar distance, and G is any volume containing the source. For the final equality, we define the *magnetic moment density* or *magnetization* as $M(r') = r' \times j^p(r')$ (e.g., [5](eq. 5.53)).

The multipolar representation is found using the Taylor series expansion of a scalar function

$$\psi(r + x) = \sum_{n=0}^{\infty} (x \cdot \nabla)^n \psi(r)/n!, \quad (2)$$

applied to the distance $d(r,r')$, where ∇ represents the gradient with respect to r. Using the equalities $\nabla r = I$ (where I is the identity matrix), $\nabla r^n = \nabla(r \cdot r)^{n/2} = nr^{n-2}r$, and $\nabla d(r,r')^n = -\nabla' d(r,r')^n = nd(r,r')^{n-2}d(r,r')$ (where ∇' is w.r.t. the primed variable), yields the expansion about r':

$$d(r, r' + x)^{-3} = d(r, r')^{-3} + 3d(r, r')^{-5}(x \cdot d(r, r')) + \dots. \quad (3)$$

To produce the multipolar expansion, we use (3) to expand (1) about r_l, the centroid of the region to which the primary source is confined (cf. [6] (eq. 9.3.18)):

$$b_r(r) = \frac{\mu_0}{4\pi} \frac{r}{r\|r - r_l\|^3} \cdot$$
$$\int_G \left(M(r_l + x) + \frac{3M(r_l + x)}{\|r - r_l\|^2} x \cdot (r - r_l) + \dots \right) dx. \quad (4)$$

If $\|x\| \ll \|r - r_l\|$, then we may generally neglect the higher order terms. From Fig. 1 we can see that this inequality is equivalent to the extent of the distributed source being much smaller than the distance from the source to the sensor. We now consider the three types of sources that will be used to represent regions of increasing size in our model of cortical activation.

Point Current Dipole: We consider first the case where the current source is confined to a single point, i.e. $j^p(r') = \delta(r' - r_l)q$ where q is the current dipole moment and δ is the Dirac delta functional. Substitution into (4) produces the result

$$b_r(r) = \frac{\mu_0}{4\pi} \frac{r \times r_l}{rd(r, r_l)^3} \cdot q, \tag{5}$$

since all terms but the first are identically zero. This is the standard current dipole model that is widely used in the MEG and EEG literature. The source is characterized by the location r_l and moment q.

Magnetic Dipole: We now consider the effect of allowing the extent of the source to grow so that it can no longer be represented using a delta function. We let the extent of the source be sufficiently small that the second and higher order terms are negligible, and we rewrite the first term of (4) as

$$b_r(r) \cong \frac{\mu_0}{4\pi} \left(\frac{r}{rd(r, r_l)^3} \cdot \int_G M(r_l + x)dx \right) = \frac{\mu_0}{4\pi} \frac{r}{rd(r, r_l)^3} \cdot m, \tag{6}$$

where we define m to be the *magnetic dipole* moment

$$m = \int_G (r_l + x) \times j^p(r_l + x)dx. \tag{7}$$

Thus we can characterize the magnetic dipole with the moment vector m and location r_l. In (7) we can define $q(r_l) = \int_G j^p(r_l + x)dx$ to be the equivalent current dipole moment and $\tilde{m}(r_l) = \int_G x \times j^p(r_l+x)dx$ to be the local magnetic dipole moment, i.e. a local "spin" of the source about a central point. We can therefore express the magnetic moment as $m(r_l) = r_l \times q(r_l) + \tilde{m}(r_l)$, and the magnetic dipole includes the equivalent current dipole as the special case.

First-Order Multipole: Now we consider the final case where the source is sufficiently large that the first two terms in the Taylor series should be included. In this case we can rewrite (4) as

$$b_r(r) \cong \frac{\mu_0}{4\pi} \frac{r}{rd(r, r_l)^3} \cdot \left(m + \frac{3(Q(r_l) \cdot d(r, r_l))}{d(r, r_l)^2} \right), \tag{8}$$

where $Q(r_l)$ is the *magnetic quadrupolar* term defined as the matrix formed from the tensor product

$$Q(r_l) \equiv \int_G M(r_l + x)x dx. \tag{9}$$

We can rewrite (8) using the Kronecker product $a \otimes b$, defined as the concatenation of the product of each element of a with the vector b, and the operator $\text{vec}(A)$, defined as the concatenation of the columns of a matrix into a vector:

$$b_r(r) \cong \frac{\mu_0}{4\pi} \left(\frac{r}{rd(r, r_l)^3} \cdot m + \frac{3(d(r, r_l) \otimes r)}{rd(r, r_l)^5} \cdot \text{vec}(Q(r_l)) \right). \qquad (10)$$

We therefore characterize the first-order multipole using the combination of the magnetic dipole moment vector m, the nine magnetic quadrupolar terms in $Q(r_l)$, and the location r_l.

We could obviously continue to expand the multipolar series to higher-order terms. In theory, focal sources could exist such that the leading terms of the expansion integrate to zero, leaving only the higher-order terms. In practice, however, our assumption that the primary activity is modeled as elemental dipoles restricted to the cortex minimizes our need to consider these higher terms. The spatial distance from the cortex to the sensors, the relative smoothness of the cortical surface, and the relatively high noise levels suppress these higher-order moments in relatively focal regions of activation.

2.2 The Forward Problem

The multipolar development above includes three models of assumed increasing spatial extent, each of which produces a radial magnetic field measurement which is a nonlinear function of the location (i.e. the center of expansion for the Taylor series) and a linear function of its moments. In the inverse problem, both the linear and nonlinear terms are assumed unknown. The decomposition into linear and nonlinear components for the current dipole model has previously been used to simplify nonlinear least squares fitting [9] and localization using signal subspace methods such as MUSIC [7,8]. Since the magnetic dipole and first order multipole are similarly decomposed, these methods can be directly extended to include searches for distributed non-dipolar sources. Furthermore, as noted above, the expansions included here can be readily extended to the case of non-radial MEG and EEG measurements for the spherical head models.

The radial magnetic field can be represented for each of the three types of source as the inner product of a *gain* vector and the vector of linear parameters, $b(r) = g(r, r_l) \cdot l$. The separation of nonlinear and linear parameters are clearly shown in (5), (6), and (10). We assume an MEG array of m sensors sampling the magnetic field of the source. By concatenating these measurements into a vector, we can represent the "forward field" of the source as

$$\left[b(r_1) \ldots b(r_m) \right]^T = \left[g(r_1, r_l), \ldots, g(r_m, r_l) \right]^T l = G(r_l)l \qquad (11)$$

where $G(r_l)$ is the "gain matrix" which accounts for all possible orientations of the source at r_l [9]. The forward model for an arbitrary combination of sources can be found by linear superposition. To extend the forward model to include temporal variations, we adopt the assumption that there are a finite combination of sources that are active. The solution of the inverse involves estimating the location, moment parameters and time courses of each of these sources.

It is possible for two sources to be synchronous. For example, bilateral activation in sensory or auditory cortex could be represented by two synchronous focal dipoles, one in each hemisphere. To account for this possibility in the subspace methods described below, we adopt an *independent topography model* [7] in which each topography consists of one or more elementary sources, all of which have identical time courses. For a *p-source topography* sampled over m sensors and n time instances, we may express the resulting $m \times n$ spatiotemporal data matrix as

$$
\begin{bmatrix} b(\boldsymbol{r}_1, t_1) & \cdots & b(\boldsymbol{r}_1, t_n) \\ \vdots & \ddots & \vdots \\ b(\boldsymbol{r}_m, t_1) & \cdots & b(\boldsymbol{r}_m, t_n) \end{bmatrix} = \begin{bmatrix} \boldsymbol{G}(\boldsymbol{r}_{l_1}), & \cdots, & \boldsymbol{G}(\boldsymbol{r}_{l_p}) \end{bmatrix} \begin{bmatrix} l_1(t_1) & \cdots & l_1(t_n) \\ \vdots & \ddots & \vdots \\ l_p(t_1) & \cdots & l_p(t_n) \end{bmatrix} \quad (12)
$$

where $l_j(t_k)$ represents the linear parameters for the jth source sampled at the kth time instance. Since all of these sources have the same time course, the matrix of linear parameters is rank one and may be decomposed using an SVD into the outer product of a single pair of singular vectors $\boldsymbol{u}$ and $\boldsymbol{v}$ scaled by the singular value σ,

$$
\boldsymbol{u}\sigma\boldsymbol{v}^T = \begin{bmatrix} l_1(t_1) & \cdots & l_1(t_n) \\ \vdots & \ddots & \vdots \\ l_p(t_1) & \cdots & l_p(t_n) \end{bmatrix}. \quad (13)
$$

Defining the scalar time series of this independent topography to be $\boldsymbol{s} = \sigma\boldsymbol{v}$, we may rewrite (12) as

$$
\begin{bmatrix} \boldsymbol{G}(\boldsymbol{r}_{l_1}) & \cdots & \boldsymbol{G}(\boldsymbol{r}_{l_p}) \end{bmatrix} \boldsymbol{u} \begin{bmatrix} s(t_1), & \cdots, & s(t_n) \end{bmatrix} = \boldsymbol{a}(\rho_1, \boldsymbol{u}_1)\boldsymbol{s}^T. \quad (14)
$$

The p-source topography vector is a function of the set ρ_1 of p source locations, $\rho_1 = \{\boldsymbol{r}_{l_i}\}$, $i = 1, \dots, p$ and the unit norm vector $\boldsymbol{u}_1$ from (13). The vector $\boldsymbol{u}_1$ may be viewed as a generalization of an "orientation" vector by concatenating all of the linear source parameters and scaling by its length,

$$
\boldsymbol{u}_l \equiv \begin{bmatrix} \boldsymbol{l}_1^T, \dots, \boldsymbol{l}_p^T \end{bmatrix}^T \Big/ \left\| \begin{bmatrix} \boldsymbol{l}_1^T, \dots, \boldsymbol{l}_p^T \end{bmatrix} \right\|. \quad (15)
$$

To complete the full model for the observed MEG data we simply concatenate the r independent topographies that make up the complete source and add noise:

$$
\boldsymbol{F} = \boldsymbol{A}(\rho, \boldsymbol{u})\boldsymbol{S}^T + \boldsymbol{N} = \begin{bmatrix} \boldsymbol{a}(\rho_1, \boldsymbol{u}_1), & \dots, & \boldsymbol{a}(\rho_r, \boldsymbol{u}_r) \end{bmatrix} \begin{bmatrix} \boldsymbol{s}_1^T \\ \vdots \\ \boldsymbol{s}_r^T \end{bmatrix} + \boldsymbol{N}, \quad (16)
$$

where each $m \times 1$ column vector $\boldsymbol{a}(\rho_i, \boldsymbol{u}_i) \equiv \boldsymbol{G}(\rho_i)\boldsymbol{u}_i$ represents the ith independent topography corresponding to the ith time series $\boldsymbol{s}_i$. The set ρ comprises the r sets of source locations $\{\rho_i\}$ and the set $\boldsymbol{u}$ the corresponding topography orientations $\{\boldsymbol{u}_i\}$. Each topography may comprise one or more multipolar sources, but only a single time series. By our definition of independent topographies, the matrix of time series $\boldsymbol{S}$ is rank r, and the matrix of topographies $\boldsymbol{A}$ is assumed to be unambiguous and also of rank r. The matrix $\boldsymbol{N}$ represents additive random noise, which we will assume to be spatially and temporally white with zero mean and variance σ_e^2.

2.3   Signal Subspace

Under the assumption that the signal is uncorrelated with the noise, the autocorrelation matrix for the $m \times n$ spatiotemporal data in (16) is

$$R = E\{FF^T\} = A(S^T S)A^T + n\sigma_e^2 I. \tag{17}$$

The autocorrelation matrix can expressed using an eigendecomposition as:

$$R = [\boldsymbol{\Phi}_s | \boldsymbol{\Phi}_e] \begin{bmatrix} \boldsymbol{\Lambda}_s & 0 \\ 0 & \boldsymbol{\Lambda}_e \end{bmatrix} [\boldsymbol{\Phi}_s | \boldsymbol{\Phi}_e]^T \tag{18}$$

where the diagonal matrix $\boldsymbol{\Lambda}_s = \boldsymbol{\Lambda} + n\sigma_e^2 I$ represents the r largest "signal plus noise" eigenvalues and their corresponding eigenvectors form the matrix $\boldsymbol{\Phi}_s$. The diagonal matrix $\boldsymbol{\Lambda}_e = n\sigma_e^2 I$ represents the smallest "noise" eigenvalues and their corresponding eigenvectors form the matrix $\boldsymbol{\Phi}_e$.

We refer to $\boldsymbol{\Phi}_s$ as spanning the *signal subspace* and to $\boldsymbol{\Phi}_e$ as spanning the *noise-only subspace*. In practice, we estimate the signal $\boldsymbol{\Phi}_s$ and noise $\boldsymbol{\Phi}_e$ subspace basis vectors by a eigendecomposition of the outer product $\boldsymbol{FF}^T$ or an SVD of $\boldsymbol{F}$. We denote the estimate of $\boldsymbol{\Phi}_s$ as $\hat{\boldsymbol{\Phi}}_s$.

3   Source Localization

3.1   RAP-MUSIC

The RAP-MUSIC algorithm is described in detail in [8]. Here we briefly review the method and describe its application in combination with the multipolar models developed above. The first source is found at the location which produces the global maximum of the metric

$$\rho_1 = \arg \max(subcorr(\boldsymbol{G}(\rho), \hat{\boldsymbol{\Phi}}_s)_1). \tag{19}$$

The function $subcorr(\cdot)$ represents the "subspace correlations" between the two matrices. The subspace correlations are the ordered set of cosines of the principal angles as defined in [3]. The first subspace correlation, $subcorr(\cdot)_1$, corresponds to the cosine of the smallest principal angle and will be unity if the two matrices have at least a one-dimensional subspace in common. If we define $\boldsymbol{U_G}$ to be the orthogonal matrix spanning the same space as $G(\rho)$, then the square of the subspace correlations are found as the eigenvalues of the matrix

$$U_G^T \hat{\Phi}_s \hat{\Phi}_s^T U_G. \tag{20}$$

By maximizing the first subspace correlation in (19), we identify the source location and corresponding gain matrix that has the smallest principal angle with respect to the signal subspace. Since we only need to search over the location parameter, a nearly exhaustive search over a relatively dense three-dimensional grid within the brain volume can be performed relatively quickly for any of the three source models of the previous section. For the case of synchronous sources, the dimensionality of the search increases by at least a factor of two and the computational cost rises dramatically, but the procedure nonetheless proceeds directly.

To complete the first independent topography model, we need the corresponding source orientation vector, which is a simple linear transformation of the eigenvector of (20) corresponding to the maximum eigenvalue [3,7]. The resulting estimates yield the first estimated independent topography, $a(\hat{\rho}_1, \hat{u}_1) = G(\hat{\rho}_1)\hat{u}_1$.

For each of the remaining $k = 1, 2, \ldots, r$ RAP-MUSIC recursions, the nonlinear source location parameters are found as

$$\hat{\rho}_k = \arg\max \left(subcorr \left(\Pi_{\hat{A}_{k-1}}^{\perp} G(\rho), \Pi_{\hat{A}_{k-1}}^{\perp} \hat{\Phi}_s \right)_1 \right) \tag{21}$$

where $\hat{A}_{k-1} = [a(\hat{\rho}_1, \hat{u}_1), \ldots, a(\hat{\rho}_{k-1}, \hat{u}_{k-1})]$ represents the composite independent topography matrix, and the projection operator $\Pi_{\hat{A}_{k-1}}^{\perp}$ is computed as

$$\Pi_{\hat{A}_{k-1}}^{\perp} = I - \hat{A}_{k-1} \hat{A}_{k-1}^{\dagger} \tag{22}$$

where $\hat{A}_{k-1}^{\dagger} \equiv (\hat{A}_{k-1}^T \hat{A}_{k-1})^{-1} \hat{A}_{k-1}^T$ is the pseudoinverse of $\hat{A}_{k-1}$. Through this recursion, we sequentially remove the components of the signal subspace that can be explained by the sources that have already been found. We then search the remaining signal subspace for additional sources.

At each iteration the source location set ρ in (21) may represent one or more multipolar sources. To find the simplest sources consistent with the data, we begin the search with the current dipole model, then progress through the magnetic and first-order multipole models. The decision to increase the complexity of the model is based on a minimum correlation threshold. In this paper, we will restrict the search to one-source models only, halting the recursion when the first-order multipole maximum subspace correlation drops too low. Examples of different correlation thresholds are given in the Monte Carlo simulations in the next section. Extensions to multiple synchronous dipolar sources are discussed in [7], with obvious extensions to multiple multipolar sources.

With all sources in the data identified and their independent topographies represented in the final topography matrix $\hat{A}_r$, estimates of the corresponding time series are readily found as $\hat{S} = (\hat{A}_r^T \hat{A}_r)^{-1} \hat{A}_r^T F$ or in some regularized form thereof.

3.2 Mapping Parametric Sources onto Cerebral Cortex

The linear parameters of the multipolar model computed using the RAP-MUSIC search are estimates of the moments formed by integrating the primary current sources as defined in (1). When the sources are confined to cortex, which we can represent as a continuous surface, the moments are generated as integrals over a surface patch containing the sources. For the single-source topographies considered here, we assume that each source represents the activation of a single contiguous cortical patch. The final step in our parametric imaging method is then to relate the multipolar moments back to a plausible distribution on the cortical surface which consists of a set of patches of activation consistent with the estimated moments. Fitting the moments to sources on the cortex involves estimation of both the surface patch and the current distribution on that patch. As with the original MEG inverse problem, the solutions are ambiguous. However, under the assumption that each surface patch is contiguous and in the vicinity of the estimated multipole, the degree of ambiguity is greatly reduced.

To perform the final stage of the multipolar imaging method we use a finely tesselated cortical surface extracted from an MRI volume. In fitting the multipolar sources to the cortex, we allow a current element at the vertex of each triangular patch on the surface, with an orientation derived as a weighted sum of the triangular normals adjacent to the vertex. To fit a specific multipolar source with topography $a(\rho_i, u_i)$ to the cortical surface, we begin by creating a list of candidate locations on the cortex in the vicinity of the source location. For each candidate point, we test the subspace correlation between the point and the topography. If the point with the highest correlation meets a minimum threshold (e.g. 98%), we designate it as the corresponding re-mapped cortical source for that topography and halt. Otherwise, we add adjacent points to each of the candidate points to form small distributed patches and continue to swell each candidate point until we find a patch that meets the threshold.

This approach will generate a patch of minimal size consistent with the identified topography. We may continue to swell the patch and find additional possible sources consistent with the topography, a consequence of the ambiguity in the inverse problem rather than a specific limitation of the method described. Currently we grow the patch by adding a ring of triangles around the elements already in the patch. A more sophisticated approach based on testing a number of possible candidates to add to each patch may prove more robust. Alternatively, we could adopt a stochastic model for the mapping between the estimated multipolar parameters and the corresponding cortical activation. This approach could readily incorporate the activation models described in our previous work on Bayesian MEG imaging [11].

4 Monte Carlo Simulations

In the first simulation we used the tesselated human cortex shown in Fig. 2 which contains approximately 230,000 triangles. Radial magnetic fields sensors and a spherical forward model were used in the generation of the simulated

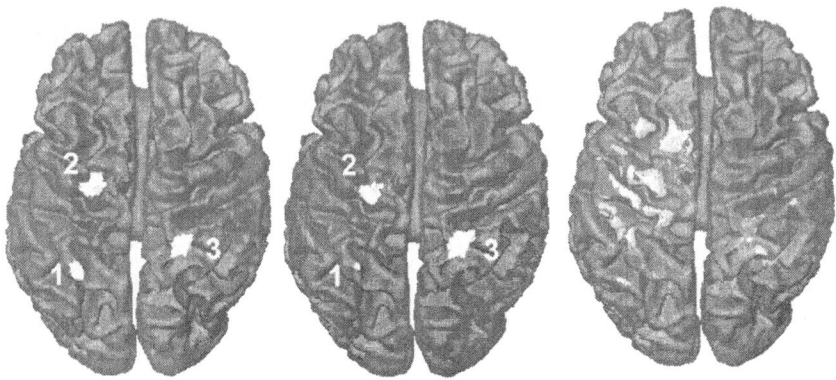

Fig. 2. (a) The ground truth for the simulation study showing mappings of the three sources onto the cortical surface; (b) Reconstruction of the cortical activity using the multipolar method; (c) Reconstruction of the data from time $t = 10$ using a regularized minimum L_2 norm method

data and in the inverse method. Three distributed sources were created on the cortical surface, also shown in Fig. 2. The three sources were given overlapping independent time courses as shown in Fig. 3. The forward magnetic field was measured by a simulated array of 104 magnetometers spaced approximately uniformly on the upper hemisphere at a radius of 12 cm. Zero mean Gaussian white noise was added to the sensor data at a ratio of 100:1 signal to noise variance.

Although analysis of the singular value spectrum of this high SNR data clearly revealed a rank of three, we overspecified the rank to ten to demonstrate robustness to selecting too great a rank. We set the acceptance threshold for correlation at 98%. The RAP-MUSIC algorithm was first run with the simplest of the source topographies, the current dipole (5), for which a maximum correlation of 99.9% was found. On the second recursion, the correlation with the dipole model dropped below the threshold of 98%. We therefore increased the complexity of the model to the magnetic dipole (6) and achieved a correlation of 98.3%. The third recursion was below the threshold for the magnetic dipole, so we increased the model to a first-order multipole (10) to obtain a correlation of 99.9%. On the fourth recursion, the correlation plummeted to 62% for the multipole and the recursion was halted at three sources. The three topographies found were then used in a least-squares fit to determine the time series of the three sources, Fig. 3.

We mapped the three topographies into the minimal cortical source regions, also shown in Fig. 2. For comparison we also include a regularized minimum L_2-norm solution fitted at one of the intermediate time slices, for which the spatial distribution and time series are also shown in Fig. 2 and Fig. 3. We see that although the re-mapped topographies obtained using the multipolar method are not identical to the "ground truth" they are indeed similar. In comparison,

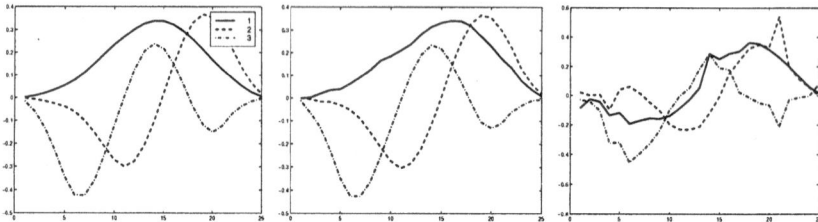

Fig. 3. Time courses for the three sources (a) ground truth; (b) time courses estimated using the multipolar method; (c) time courses averaged over each of the true activation areas computed from the minimum norm solutions. In this high SNR example, the time series reconstruction in (b) is nearly perfect, while (c) exhibits high noise sensitivity

the minimum norm solution exhibits substantial source blurring due to the low resolution of the linear inverse methods.

As discussed above, the multipolar source center is assumed to be near the distributed cortical source. We tested this assumption in a Monte Carlo simulation of 10,800 distributed sources over a range of noise levels. We also tested the effects of the correlation threshold parameter used in the RAP-MUSIC algorithm to accept a model. Each source was centered randomly on the upper half of the brain surface in Fig. 2. With a 50% probability, each source was either a "monophasic" contiguous patch of 200 mm^2 or a "biphasic" patch of two 200 mm^2 patches centered about 8 mm apart (about 50% overlap) and of opposite polarity. Each Monte Carlo realization simulated three such sources with overlapping non-orthogonal time series. No attempt was made to force the three sources to be widely separated, so that source overlaps were possible in any single realization. A hemispherical array of 138 magnetometers was simulated a few centimeters above the cortical surface. Although the true signal subspace rank was three, we intentionally selected a larger rank of five for each realization.

Twelve cases of SNR and correlation threshold were tested, with 300 Monte Carlo realizations per case, for a total number of 10,800 sources. For each simulated source, we determined the geometric centroid of the patch. We then computed the distance from this centroid to the multipolar source location nearest to the source as an indication of the accuracy of the estimate. However, we note that the multipole that gives the best fit to a particular distributed cortical source does not necessarily lie *on* the cortex.

The global statistics presented in Table 1 show that the current dipolar locations are in general closer to the patch centroids than the non-dipolar locations. The 20 dB SNR case represents a mostly noiseless signal to allow observations of the modeling effects. Even though the sources were spatially large, the majority of the monophasic and some of the biphasic sources were modeled quite well as dipoles, even at the 99% correlation level. The first-order multipole model accounted for the remainder. The 3 dB SNR case represents a rather severe case of 67% signal variance to 33% noise variance. At 99% correlation, most sources

Table 1. Monte Carlo Study. SNR is ten times the log base-ten of the ratio of the total signal variance to the total noise variance, both values measured at the array of sensors. Correlation threshold is the minimum subspace correlation value for the model to be accepted. The first row summarizes the results over all trials for a total of 10,800 sources localized. Each additional row represents a different Monte Carlo trial of 300 realizations and 900 sources. The sources are described in the text. The mean and standard deviation (in mm) for the solution distances are given for the ECD model and the non-ECD (magnetic dipoles and first-order multipoles combined). The final column gives the number not localized at the given threshold.

SNR (dB)	Correlation Threshold	Number of ECDs	Mean, Std.Dev	Non-ECDs	Mean, Std.Dev	Missing Sources
ALL	ALL	6659	(5.34, 4.56)	2977	(7.06, 5.98)	1164
3	0.94	643	(6.51, 5.38)	183	(6.05, 5.81)	74
3	0.96	565	(5.69, 4.03)	215	(6.28, 6.58)	120
3	0.98	378	(5.17, 3.88)	282	(7.25, 6.59)	240
3	0.99	65	(6.32, 3.98)	220	(14.58, 8.37)	615
10	0.94	698	(6.35, 5.81)	198	(4.85, 6.70)	4
10	0.96	641	(5.68, 4.86)	254	(4.43, 5.55)	5
10	0.98	575	(4.47, 3.15)	302	(4.20, 3.41)	23
10	0.99	489	(3.99, 2.86)	332	(4.41, 3.57)	79
20	0.94	737	(6.03, 5.60)	163	(4.99, 6.72)	0
20	0.96	702	(4.97, 4.17)	198	(4.73, 5.27)	0
20	0.98	625	(4.69, 3.94)	275	(3.96, 3.56)	0
20	0.99	541	(4.26, 3.38)	355	(3.96, 2.97)	4

are lost in the noise, but at the lower correlation thresholds we see the majority of sources still detected quite well as either dipoles or multipoles. Although we intentionally set too large a rank for the signal subspace, we also note the important fact that no spurious sources were found, i.e. we never saw more than three sources. As we might expect, the effect of lowering the correlation threshold is to allow more sources to be detected, but at the cost of greater mean distance between the source locations and the patch centroids.

5 Conclusion

We have described an algorithm for computing estimates of cortical current activity from MEG data. The method exploits the low dimensionality of parametric multipolar models to estimate the locations of equivalent representations of the current sources. These representations are then mapped onto a tessellated representation of the cortical surface resulting in a spatiotemporal estimate of cortical activity. Monte Carlo simulations indicate that the potential of this method to extend the parametric approach to the representation of more distributed sources. The resulting images avoid the very low resolution encountered using minimum norm methods and the high computational costs of the other nonlinear imaging methods. Planned studies include experimental phantoms and human studies of self paced and visually cued motor activation.

Acknowledgements: This work was supported in part by the National Institute of Mental Health Grant RO1-MH53213 and the Los Alamos National Laboratory, operated by the University of California for the United States Department of Energy under contract W-7405-ENG-36. S.B. is a laureate of the Lavoisier research fellowship from the French Ministry of Foreign Affairs.

References

1. Baillet, S., Garnero, L.: A Bayesian approach to introducing anatomo-functional priors in the EEG/MEG inverse problem. IEEE Trans. Biomed. Eng., **44** (1997) 374–385
2. Dale, A.M., Sereno, M.I.: Improved localization of cortical activity by combining EEG and MEG with MRI cortical surface reconstruction: a linear approach. J. Cog. NeuroSci., **5** (1993) 162–176
3. Golub G.H., Van Loan, C.F.: Matrix Computations, Second Edition. Johns Hopkins University Press, (1984).
4. Hämäläinen, M., Hari, R., Ilmoniemi, R.J., Knuutila, J., Lounasmaa, O.V.: Magnetoencephalography-theory, instrumentation, and applications of noninvasive studies of the working human brain. Rev. Mod. Phys., **65** (1993) 413–497
5. Jackson, J.D.: Classical Electrodynamics, Second Edition. John Wiley and Sons, New York, (1975).
6. Katila, T., Karp, P.: Magnetocardiography: Morphology and multipole presentations. In: Williamson, S.J., Romani, G.-L., Kaufman, L., Modena, I. (eds.): Biomagnetism, An Interdisciplinary Approach. Plenum, New York (1983) 237–263
7. Mosher, J.C., Leahy., R.M.: Recursive music: A framework for EEG and MEG-source localization. IEEE Trans. Biomed. Eng., **45** (1998) 1342–1354
8. Mosher, J.C., Leahy., R.M.: Source localization using recursively applied and projected (RAP) MUSIC. IEEE Trans. Signal Proc., **47** (1999) 332–340.
9. Mosher, J.C., Lewis, P.S., Leahy, R.M.: Multiple dipole modeling and localization from spatio-temporal MEG data. IEEE Trans. Biomed. Eng., **39** (1992) 541–557
10. de Munck, J.C., van Dijk B.W., Spekreijse H.: Mathematical dipoles are adequate to describe realistic generators of human brain activity. IEEE Trans. on Biomedical Engineering, **35** (1988) 960–966
11. Phillips, J.W., Leahy, R.M., Mosher, J.C.: MEG-based imaging of focal neuronal current sources. IEEE Trans. on Medical Imaging, **16** (1997) 338–348
12. Scherg, M., von Cramon, D.: Two bilateral sources of the late AEP as identified by a spatiotemporal dipole model. Electroenceph. and Clin. Neurophys., **62** (1985) 32–44
13. R.O. Schmidt.: Multiple emitter location and signal parameter estimation. IEEE Trans. on Ant. and Prop., **AP-34** (1986) 276–280
14. Wang, J. Z., Williamson, S. J., Kaufman, L.: Magnetic source images determined by a lead-field analysis: The unique minimum-norm least-squares estimation. IEEE Trans. Biomed. Eng., **39** (1992) 665–675.
15. Wikswo, J.P.: Biomagnetic sources and their models, In: Williamson, S.J., Hoke, M., Stroink G., Kotani M. (eds.): Advances in Biomagnetism. Plenum, New York (1989).

Binary Tomography for Triplane Cardiography

Bruno M. Carvalho[1], Gabor T. Herman[1], Samuel Matej[1],
Claudia Salzberg[1], and Eilat Vardi[2]

[1] University of Pennsylvania, Department of Radiology, Medical Image Processing
Group, Blockley Hall, Fourth Floor, 423 Guardian Drive, Philadelphia, PA
19104-6021, USA
{carvalho, gabor, matej, claudia}@mipg.upenn.edu
[2] Technion - Technical Institute of Israel, P.O. Box 41, Haifa 32000, Israel
seilat@techst02.technion.ac.il

Abstract. The problem of reconstructing a binary image (usually an
image in the plane and not necessarily on a Cartesian grid) from a few
projections translates into the problem of solving a system of equations
which is very underdetermined and leads in general to a large class of
solutions. It is desirable to limit the class of possible solutions, by using
appropriate prior information, to only those which are reasonably typical
of the class of images which contains the unknown image that we wish to
reconstruct. One may indeed pose the following hypothesis: if the image
is a typical member of a class of images having a certain distribution,
then by using this information we can limit the class of possible solutions to only those which are close to the given unknown image. This
hypothesis is experimentally validated for the specific case of a class of
binary images representing cardiac cross-sections, where the probability
of the occurrence of a particular image of the class is determined by a
Gibbs distribution and reconstruction is to be done from the three noisy
projections.

1 Introduction

The subject matter of this paper is the recovery of binary images from their
projections. A binary image is a rectangular array of pixels, each one of which
is either black or white. In the case of cardiac angiography, we can represent a
section through the heart as a binary image in which white is assigned to those
pixels which contain contrast material. A projection of a binary image is defined
as a data set, which for every line (in a set of parallel lines, each of which goes
through the center of every pixel which it intersects at all) tells us, at least
approximately, how many white pixels are intersected by that line. According
to this definition there can be only four projections: one horizontal, one vertical
and two diagonal. There exist more general definitions of projections in the
literature [1], but it is typical for many applications that only a few projections
are available [2,3].

The problem of *binary tomography* is the recovery of a binary image from
its projections. This problem can be represented by a system of equations which

A. Kuba et al. (Eds.): IPMI'99, LNCS 1613, pp. 29–41, 1999.

is very underdetermined and leads typically to a large class of solutions. It is desirable to reduce the class of possible solutions to only those which are reasonably "close" to the (unknown) image which gave rise to the measurement data. Appropriate prior information on the image may be useful for this task [4]. In addition to the inherent information in binary tomography that there are only two possible values, *Gibbs priors* [5,6] describing the local behavior/character of the image can also provide useful information. We pose the hypothesis that, for certain *Gibbs distributions*, knowledge that the image is a random element from the distribution is sufficient for limiting the class of possible solutions to only those which are close to the (unknown) image which gave rise to the measurement data.

Binary images can be described in many applications by the following simplified characterization: a set of *objects* - "white" regions - are located in a "black" background. (We adopt the convention that 1 represents white and 0 represents black.) This can be easily translated into Gibbs distributions by using a set of configurations of neighboring image elements and assigning a value (which is an indicator of the likelihood of occurrence) to each of these configurations.

One type of test presented in this paper is motivated by the task of reconstructing semiconductor surface layers from a few projections. Fishburn *et al.* [3] designed three test phantoms for assessing the suitability of binary tomography for that task. These phantoms have been recently used in the binary tomography literature by the several other researchers (see, e.g., [1]). The common experience reported by these researchers is that knowing the horizontal, vertical and one diagonal projection is not sufficient for exact recovery of such phantoms. However, it is shown in [7] that an algorithm, which makes use of an appropriate Gibbs prior, correctly recovers the test phantoms of [3] from three projections.

The following section introduces Gibbs distributions and discusses their definition using a look-up table. A reconstruction algorithm based on two given perfect projections and a Gibbs prior is presented in the third section, where it is also illustrated for the phantoms of [3] that the algorithm (while achieving its mathematical aim) fails to recover the original object. Since three projections are sufficient to recover these test phantoms based on semiconductor surface layers, it appears possible that three projections would also be sufficient for the recovery of cardiac cross-sections. An algorithm to do this is presented in Section 4; this algorithm does not assume that the projections are noiseless. Its performance is investigated in Section 5, where the influence of noise is also demonstrated. The final section presents our conclusions.

2   Gibbs Distributions Associated with Binary Images

Local properties of a given binary image ω defined on H pixels (each pixel is indexed by an integer h, $1 \leq h \leq H$, and $\omega(h)$ is either black or white) can be characterized by a Gibbs distribution of the form

$$\Pi(\omega) = \frac{1}{Z} e^{\beta \sum_{h=1}^{H} I_h(\omega)} , \tag{1}$$

where $\Pi(\omega)$ is the probability of occurrence of the image ω, Z is the normalizing factor (which insures that Π is a probability density function; i.e. that the sum of $\Pi(\omega)$ over all possible binary images is 1), β is a parameter defining the "peakedness" of the Gibbs distribution (this is one of the parameters controlling the appearance of the typical images), and $I_h(\omega)$ is the "local energy function" for the pixel indexed by h, $1 \leq h \leq H$. The local energy function is defined in such a way that it encourages certain local configurations, such as uniform white or black clusters of pixels and configurations forming edges or corners. Each of these configurations can be encouraged to a different extent by assigning to them a specific value. In this paper we have adopted the convention that the local energy function at a pixel depends only on its own color and those of its eight neighbors. Thus, the color of a particular pixel influences the value of the local energy function of only itself and its eight neighbors.

Appropriate definition of the local energy function plays an important role in successful image recovery. The definition should reflect the characteristics of a typical image of the particular application area. There are many possible ways of defining the local energy function. One of them is to use a look-up table which contains a value for each possible configuration. (In our case, there are 512 possible configurations.) Given an ensemble of typical images for a particular application (a training set), the look-up table can be created by counting the number of times each particular configuration appears in the images. Then the $I_h(\omega)$ of (1) is defined as $\ln(q+1)$, where q is the value in the look-up table of the local configuration in the image ω at the pixel h. The usefulness of the resulting prior depends on the size of the training set (the larger, the better) and on how representative the images in the training set are for the application area.

3 Biplane Tomography: Preliminary Experiments

Ryser showed in the 1950's [8] that if one matrix of 0's and 1's has the same row and column sums as another such matrix then the first matrix can be transformed into the second by a finite sequence of simple switching operations each of which changes two 1's to 0's and two 0's to 1's and leaves the row and column sums unaltered. This can be regarded as a result of binary tomography, since matrices of 0's and 1's can be viewed as binary images; two matrices that have the same row and column sums correspond to two binary images which have the same horizontal and vertical projections. We refer to such images as being *tomographically equivalent*. The simple switching operation described above will be referred to as a *rectangular 4-switch*.

Let $\mathcal{C}$ be any tomographic equivalence class of binary images. Consider the graph whose vertices are in $1 - 1$ correspondence with the binary images in $\mathcal{C}$, in which two vertices are adjacent if and only if the image corresponding to one vertex can be obtained from the image corresponding to the other by a single rectangular 4-switch. We will call this the *Ryser graph* of the tomographic equivalence class $\mathcal{C}$.

The Ryser graph is a finite graph since each tomographic equivalence class is finite. In view of Ryser's result [8], the Ryser graph is connected.

We now give an application of the Ryser graph. Let $\mathcal{P}$ be the set of all binary images. Consider the following problem: Given a binary image $\omega \in \mathcal{P}$, find an image in ω's tomographic equivalence class for which $\Pi(\omega)$ of (1) has a relatively high value. (Ideally, we would like to find an image that maximizes $\Pi(\omega)$, but we do not expect to always achieve this.)

Kong and Herman [9] describe (two versions of) an iterative stochastic algorithm to do this. The algorithm is a typical instance of a class of algorithms known in the literature as Metropolis algorithms [10]. Since such algorithms are often time consuming, [9] devotes a considerable amount of space to the achievement of a relatively efficient implementation. The essential idea is to first find a single binary image which satisfies the two given projections and then iteratively investigate the effect on $\Pi(\omega)$ of making a random rectangular 4-switch.

Roughly speaking, a single step in the Metropolis procedure starts with "randomly picking" a possible rectangular 4-switch for the current image ω_1. Let ω_2 be the image that is obtained by performing this rectangular 4-switch on ω_1. Let p be the ratio of $\Pi(\omega_2)$ to $\Pi(\omega_1)$. The single step of the iterative procedure is completed by replacing ω_1 by ω_2 if p is greater than 1, and replacing ω_1 by ω_2 with probability p (and hence retaining ω_1 with probability $1 - p$) if p is less than 1. As explained in [9], properties of Ryser graphs and of the Metropolis algorithms guarantee that the procedure just described will produce images ω with relatively high values of $\Pi(\omega)$; for a precise statement (as well as for a discussion of implementational concerns), see [9].

In order to test out our ideas on reconstructions from two projections, we implemented the algorithms described in [9] and applied them to the binary images in [3] representing semiconductor surface layers. (For these experiments, the lookup-table was created using the three phantoms of [3].) For all three phantoms (these are shown on the left of Figs. 1, 2 and 3, respectively), the algorithms of [9] performed "too well" in the sense that the reconstructed images (these are shown on the right of Figs. 1, 2 and 3, respectively) have a higher value of $\Pi(\omega)$ than the originals. One might say after looking at these figures that the reconstructions are versions of the original binary images in which the boundaries have been smoothed.

As a result of these preliminary experiments combined with the fact that all three phantoms of [3] were perfectly recovered when Gibbs priors were combined with three perfect projections [7], we decided to investigate the efficacy of triplane rather than biplane cardio-angiography.

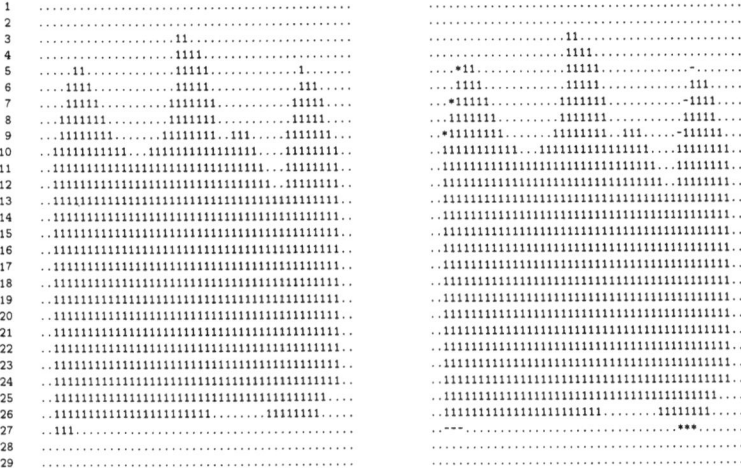

Fig. 1. Phantom 1 (left) and its reconstruction (right) based on Ryser graphs and a Metropolis algorithm from perfect horizontal and vertical projections; . and 1 represent the values zero and 1 (respectively) in the phantom and at correctly reconstructed locations; - and * represent incorrectly reconstructed values of zero and one (respectively); the total number of incorrectly reconstructed pixels is 12

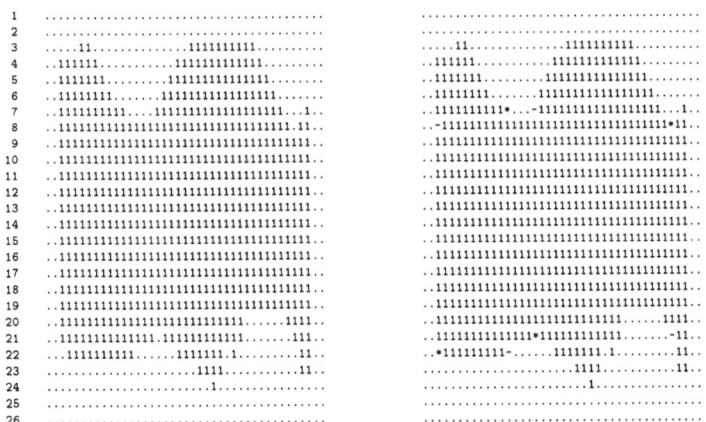

Fig. 2. Phantom 2 (left) and its reconstruction (right) based on Ryser graphs and a Metropolis algorithm from perfect horizontal and vertical projections; . and 1 represent the values zero and 1 (respectively) in the phantom and at correctly reconstructed locations; - and * represent incorrectly reconstructed values of zero and one (respectively); the total number of incorrectly reconstructed pixels is 8

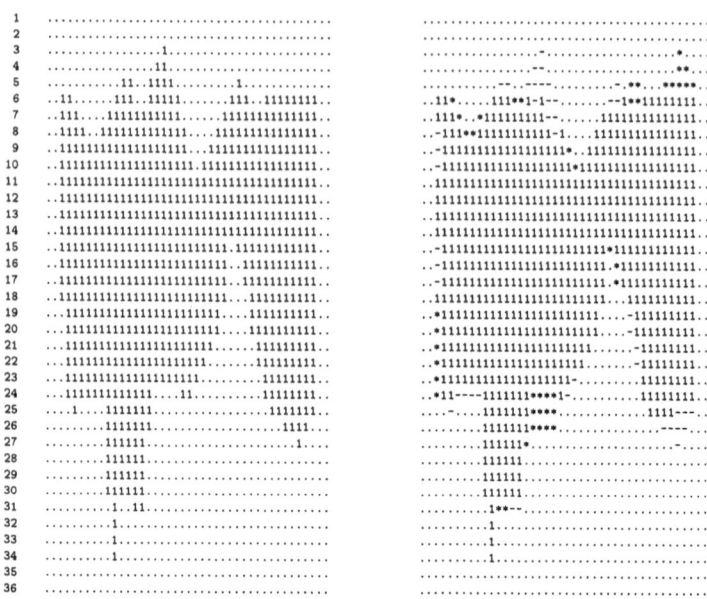

Fig. 3. Phantom 3 (left) and its reconstruction (right) based on Ryser graphs and a Metropolis algorithm from perfect horizontal and vertical projections; . and 1 represent the values zero and 1 (respectively) in the phantom and at correctly reconstructed locations; - and * represent incorrectly reconstructed values of zero and one (respectively); the total number of incorrectly reconstructed pixels is 90

4 A Reconstruction Algorithm for Three Noisy Projections

Assume that our data consist of estimates of three (horizontal, vertical and one diagonal) projections of an image, which we believe to be a random sample from a known Gibbs distribution. Then a reconstruction algorithm should find an image which is not only consistent with the data, but which is also a typical sample from the known Gibbs distribution. We use a modified Metropolis algorithm in which the search for a likely image is altered to take also into account the effect of replacing ω_1 by ω_2 on the consistency with the given projection data. Roughly speaking, if the data inconsistency is increased or decreased, then the change is discouraged or encouraged, respectively. The relative influence of the data inconsistency is controlled by a parameter α $(\alpha \geq 0)$.

To be exact, the Metropolis algorithm is modified as follows. First, since it may no longer be possible to find a binary image which satisfies our (noisy) projection data exactly, we do not attempt to start the iterative process with such an image. (In the experiments which are reported below, the initial image is always totally black.) Second, in the iterative step, the current image ω_1 is changed into ω_2 by randomly picking a single pixel h_1 and changing its color. The role of p is replaced by

$$p' = e^{\beta(\{\sum_{h \in N(h_1)}[I_h(\omega_2) - I_h(\omega_1)]\} - \alpha\{F_{h_1}(\omega_2) - F_{h_1}(\omega_1)\})}, \qquad (2)$$

where $N(h_1)$ is the set of at most nine pixels consisting of h_1 and its neighbors and

$$F_{h_1}(\omega) = |d_{h_1}(\omega) - m_{h_1}|, \qquad (3)$$

$$d_{h_1}(\omega) = \sum_{i=1}^{3} d_{h_1}^i(\omega), \qquad (4)$$

$$m_{h_1} = \sum_{i=1}^{3} m_{h_1}^i, \qquad (5)$$

where $d_{h_1}^i(\omega)$ is the number of white pixels in image ω on the line going in the direction i through the pixel h_1 and $m_{h_1}^i$ is the value of the corresponding item in the given projection data. Finally, ω_2 may, or may not, replace ω_1 as determined by the Metropolis principle with p' defined as in (2). To be exact, ω_1 is replaced by ω_2 if p' is greater than 1 and ω_1 is replaced by ω_2 with probability p' (and hence ω_1 is retained with probability $1 - p'$) if p' is less than 1.

Such a procedure is guided preferentially towards images which have relatively large probability, as defined by (1), and are at the same time not too inconsistent with the projection data. The procedure is run for a "long time" (see below) and at its termination we select as its output that image from the sequence produced by it which has the maximum probability (1).

5   Triplane Tomography: Application to Cardiac Angiography

For this application, we have identified a statistical ensemble of mathematically described images based on cardiac cross-sectional images in [11]. These images all consisted of three geometrical objects (an ellipse representing the left ventricle, a circle representing the left atrium and the difference between two circular sectors representing the right ventricle) of statistically variable size, shape and location. By assigning white to every pixel whose center is inside one of these objects (and black to every other pixel) each mathematically described image gives rise to a binary image; we refer to such binary images as "phantoms". (The reason why the binary assumption is justified is that the intended application is *subtraction* angiography in which the projection data are obtained by subtracting a pre-injection x-ray picture from a post-injection x-ray picture; the difference is the

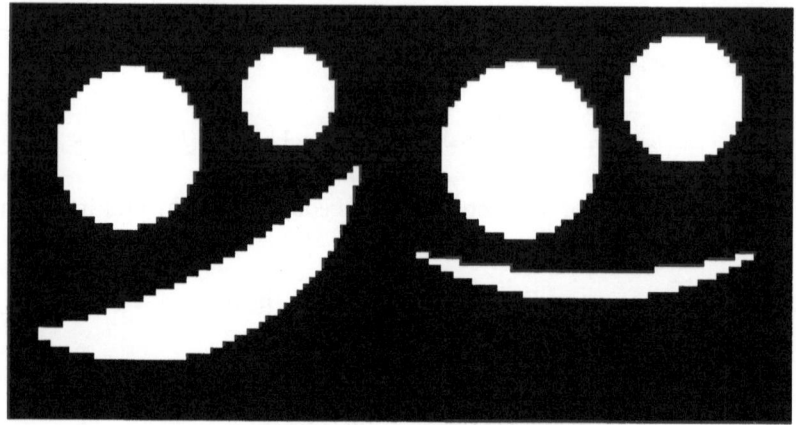

Fig. 4. Two of the 10 phantoms from the training set

projection data of the image containing either the injected contrast material or nothing.)

Ten phantoms were randomly generated to create our training set. (Two of these are shown in Fig. 4.) Based on them, we collected the Gibbs prior information, by simply counting the occurrences of each possible configuration of a 3×3 window over all the images of our training set. This produces a look-up table, and hence a Gibbs distribution, as explained in Section 2.

The phantoms were defined on the square grid with height and width equal to 63 pixels. Thus, in our experiments, we have H=3,969. The phantoms and the raysums were generated using the software SNARK93 [12] and the pixel size used was $1mm$, producing $63mm \times 63mm$ images. Using SNARK93, we added noise to the raysums generation, producing raysums corrupted by an additive noise of mean 0.0 and standard deviations (σ) equal to 0.0 (noiseless case), 0.5 and 1.0. Since SNARK93 generates the projection data based on the geometrically described objects, even the "noiseless" data are only approximations of the projections of binary images of the discretized phantoms.

In our experimental study we investigated the actual benefit of prior information for cardiac cross-sectional binary image reconstruction. Our testing set consisted of 10 phantoms (from the same ensemble as the training set, but statistically independent), and for each phantom and each noise level (0.0, 0.5 and 1.0) three projections were generated; horizontal ($\leftarrow$), vertical ($\downarrow$) and diagonal ($\nearrow$). Since the image size was 63×63, for each phantom and noise level we produced 63 horizontal, 63 vertical and 125 diagonal raysums, adding to a total of 251 raysums. The algorithm received as input the raysums generated by SNARK93 and values for α and β in (2). The values of α and β for the noiseless case were selected based on the Gibbs prior (look-up table), that was generated by scanning the images of the training set and counting the pixel configurations on a 3×3 window. Using this knowledge, we selected $\alpha = 23.0$ and $\beta = 0.1$ for the experiments using noiseless raysums. The selected α and β values balance

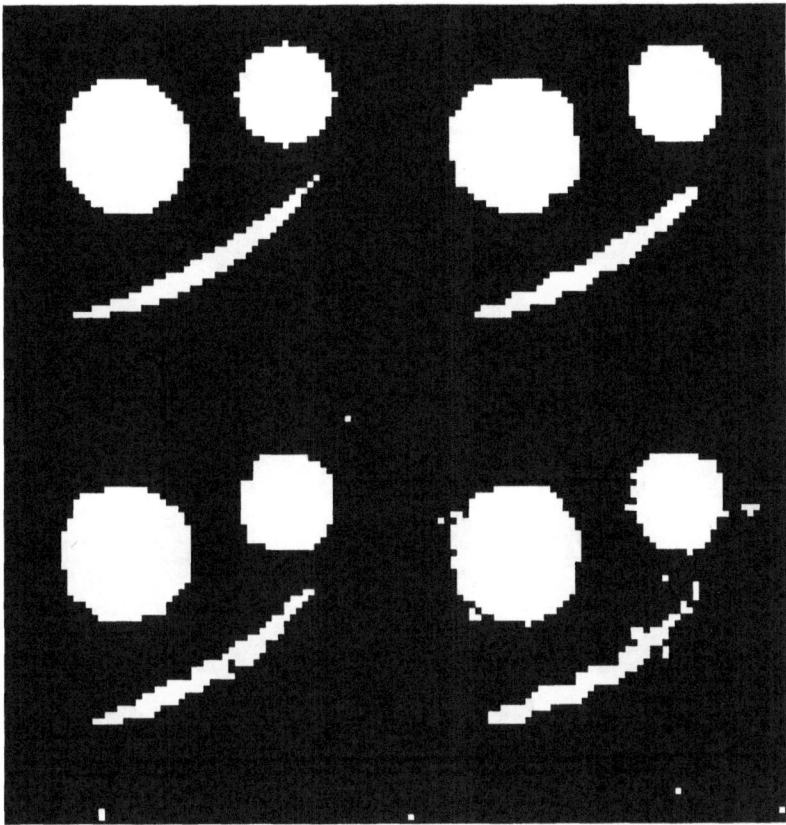

Fig. 5. A phantom (upper left corner) and its reconstructions using noiseless raysums (upper right corner) and raysums with additive noise of mean 0 and standard deviation (σ) of 0.5 (lower left corner) and 1.0 (lower right corner)

the contribution of the raysums and the Gibbs prior to the image reconstruction. Since, in the other cases, some noise was introduced into the raysums generation, we selected smaller α values, $\alpha = 18.4$ for $\sigma = 0.5$ and $\alpha = 13.8$ for $\sigma = 1.0$ (reflecting change in our confidence level on the raysums), while maintaining $\beta = 0.1$ for both cases.

For any binary image we define its *energy* as the sum of the local energy function over all pixels; i.e., $\sum_{h=1}^{H} I_h(w)$. In all experiments, the program outputs the image with the highest energy after 50,000 cycles (excluding the first 5,000 cycles, during which the totally black starting image could still have an influence on the image energy). In each cycle the algorithm randomly visits 3,969 pixels in the image and performs the modified Metropolis step as defined in Section 4. Using the phantom and the output image, we computed their energy difference, the number of pixels for which the output has a different color from the phantom and the total difference of their projections. Another quality measurement

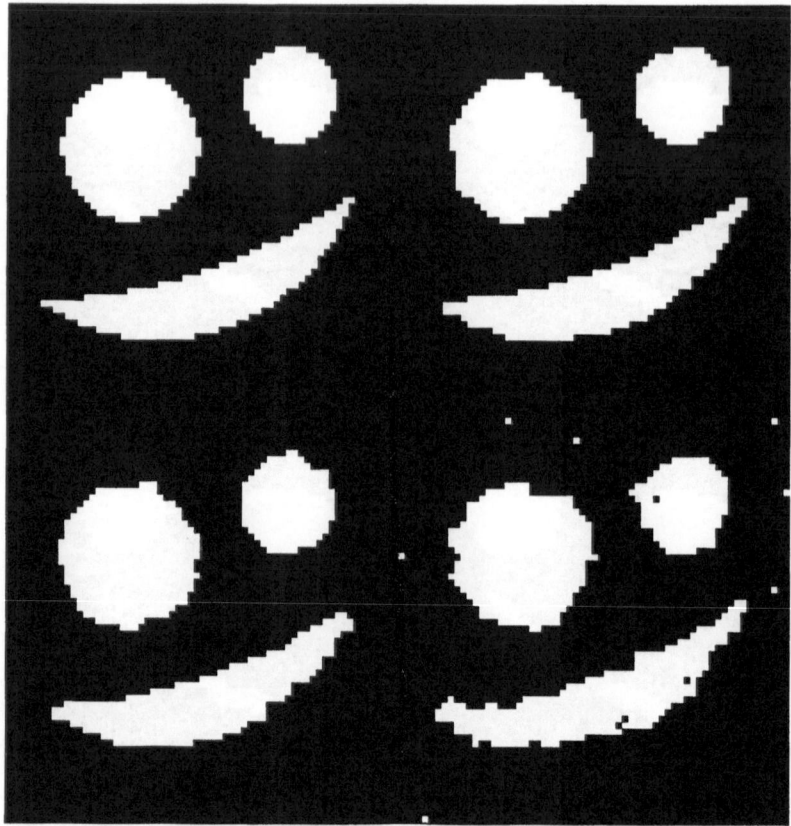

Fig. 6. A phantom (upper left corner) and its reconstructions using noiseless raysums (upper right corner) and raysums with additive noise of mean 0 and standard deviation (σ) of 0.5 (lower left corner) and 1.0 (lower right corner)

used was the absolute difference (measured in pixels) of the areas of the objects representing the right ventricle, left ventricle and left atrium, in the phantom and in the reconstruction. In a reconstruction an "object" is defined as a component (a maximally connected subset) of the set of white pixels under 8-adjacency (two pixels are 8-adjacent if they share a corner or an edge). Two examples of a phantom (phantoms number 3 and 7) and the corresponding reconstructions using the raysums generated with the three different noise levels are shown in Figs. 5 and 6. (In this initial work we concentrated on investigating the possibility of accurate reconstructions from triplane data and paid no attention to the efficiency of implementation. Because of this the total computer time for the 50,000 cycles is 5 hours on an Sun ultra 10 300MHz.)

As can be seen in Table 1, all ten phantoms were reconstructed successfully for all three noise-levels. The table shows the results for the ten phantoms of the testing set with the three different noise levels for each one. The energy

Table 1. Table reporting the phantom numbers and energy values (Energy), and the energy difference (DEnr, where DEnr = Enr$_{phantom}$ - Enr$_{reconstruction}$), pixel difference (DPi) and projection difference (DPr) for reconstructions using raysums corrupted by three different noise levels ($\sigma = 0.0, 0.5$ and 1.0). The energy difference average is computed using the sum of the absolute values of the energy differences and all values in the last row (Avg) are calculated by averaging the ten individual values in the same column. (Negative values of DEnr indicate that the energy of the reconstruction is higher than that of the phantom)

Phantom		σ=0.0			σ=0.5			σ=1.0		
Num	Energy	DEnr	DPi	DPr	DEnr	DPi	DPr	DEnr	DPi	DPr
1	36480.53	-45.43	35	23	-11.40	54	42	596.05	98	82
2	36087.34	-50.89	60	24	-54.48	79	60	442.01	157	157
3	36986.62	-220.74	51	27	-27.03	60	61	662.92	105	106
4	37427.52	-77.94	72	23	-34.01	96	46	421.38	94	88
5	36344.12	-32.58	39	24	149.69	68	49	556.40	128	95
6	36171.59	16.10	44	26	148.82	80	55	682.61	127	84
7	36414.56	-30.55	41	31	32.81	61	40	751.89	141	97
8	36905.06	-97.57	49	24	-62.91	64	46	705.68	104	100
9	36273.46	-56.87	59	20	155.52	109	51	532.50	165	91
10	36064.98	-40.43	60	26	84.34	77	46	507.49	118	89
Avg	36515.58	-63.18	51	25	38.13	75	50	585.97	124	99

difference (DEnr) was computed as DEnr = Enr$_{phantom}$ - Enr$_{reconstruction}$, the pixel difference (DPi) reports the number of pixels that were different between the phantom and the reconstruction, and the projection difference (DPr) reports the sum of the absolute differences between the data (phantom raysums) and the projection sums for the reconstructed image. The total number of pixels and projections were equal to 3,969 and 251, respectively. The last row of Table 1 reports the average (Avg) of the absolute energy differences, pixel differences and projection differences for the ten phantoms. The averages pixel differences (DPi) and projection differences (DPr) were rounded to the nearest integer. The average percentages of misclassified pixels are 1.3% (if σ=0.0), 1.9% (if σ=0.5) and 3.1% (if σ=1.0).

The numbers reported for the phantoms in Table 2 refer to the total number of pixels in the three objects, while the numbers under LA, LV and RV report the absolute difference of the areas measured for the three objects in the phantom and reconstructions. The area difference averages (DA) reported in Table 2 contains information about all ten phantoms (rounded to the nearest integer). The average percentage errors in the areas are 1.0% (if σ=0.0), 1.3% (if σ=0.5) and 2.6% (if σ=1.0).

Since the choices of the α and β in (2) and the "measurement model" expressed in (3)-(5) are somewhat arbitrary, we have looked into the possibility of improving on our results by a more careful choice of these. To date we have not

Table 2. Table reporting the areas for the three objects (left atrium, left ventricle and right ventricle) in the phantoms and the absolute difference between the the object areas in the phantom and in the reconstructions using raysums corrupted by three different noise levels ($\sigma = 0.0, 0.5$ and 1.0). The last row reports the average of such differences (DA) for each object over all phantoms rounded to the nearest integer

Phantom				$\sigma=0.0$			$\sigma=0.5$			$\sigma=1.0$		
Num	LA	LV	RV	LA	LV	RV	LA	LV	RV	LA	LV	RV
1	293	441	170	0	1	8	0	2	4	11	8	3
2	213	539	238	7	1	1	7	3	4	8	2	16
3	197	355	119	0	1	0	2	5	8	5	9	11
4	109	439	101	2	2	1	1	2	0	2	3	11
5	97	527	358	3	4	2	3	1	4	7	3	2
6	177	469	382	1	1	2	3	10	3	10	3	4
7	177	389	367	2	7	2	5	2	0	5	1	2
8	177	349	255	10	1	1	8	2	3	18	7	3
9	185	583	218	1	2	0	4	5	12	1	5	15
10	225	515	349	3	2	3	0	1	0	2	11	7
DA	182	452	258	3	2	2	3	3	4	7	5	7

succeeded to do this; other models we tried did not improve upon the results resported in Tables 1 and 2.

6   Conclusions

We have shown how Gibbs priors can be defined and used in binary reconstruction problems. Experimental tests were done for the case when data are known for two or three projections. An algorithm based on the Ryser graph and the Metropolis algorithm was tested and it was found that two views were not sufficient to determine the object even if the data are noiseless and the Gibbs prior is based on the very pictures to be reconstructed. On the other hand, in the case of three views, our results indicate that a similar approach could be useful in triplane cardiac angiography even in the presence of noise in the data.

A modified Metropolis algorithm based on the known Gibbs prior proved to provide a good tool to move the reconstruction process towards the correct solution when the projection data by themselves are not sufficient to find such a solution. Our experiments suggest that if an algorithm is able to maximize the Gibbs probability subject to consistency with the data, then it is likely to be able to (nearly) recover a random image from the Gibbs distribution. This supports our hypothesis posed in the introduction, namely that if an image is a typical member of a class of images having a certain Gibbs distribution, then by using this information we can usually limit the class of possible solutions to only those which are close to the (unknown) image which gave rise to the measurement data.

Acknowledgements

This work was supported by the National Science Foundation Grant DMS-9612077, by the National Institutes of Health Grants HL-28438 and CA-54356 and by CAPES-BRASILIA-BRAZIL.

References

1. Herman, G.T., Kuba, A. (eds.): Special Issue on Discrete Tomography. Int. J. Imaging Syst. and Technol. **9** No. 2/3 (1998)
2. Chang, S.-K., Chow, C. K.: The Reconstruction of Three-Dimensional Objects from Two Orthogonal Projections and its Application to Cardiac Cineangiography. IEEE Trans. on Computers **22** (1973) 18-28
3. Fishburn, P., Schwander, P., Shepp, L., Vanderbei, R.J.: The Discrete Radon Transform and its Approximate Inversion via Linear Programming. Discrete Applied Mathematics **75** (1997) 39-61
4. Chan, M.T., Herman, G.T., Levitan, E.: A Bayesian Approach to PET Reconstruction Using Image-Modeling Gibbs Priors: Implementation and Comparison. IEEE Trans. Nucl. Sci. **44** (1997) 1347-1354
5. Winkler, G.: Image Analysis, Random Fields and Dynamic Monte Carlo Methods. Springer-Verlag, Berlin Heidelberg New York (1995)
6. Levitan, E., Chan, M., Herman, G.T.: Image-Modeling Gibbs Priors. Graph. Models Image Proc. **57** (1995) 117-130
7. Matej, S., Vardi, A., Herman, G.T., Vardi, E.: Binary Tomography Using Gibbs Priors. In Herman, G.T., Kuba, A. (eds.): Discrete Tomography: Foundations, Algorithms and Applications. Birkhauser, Boston Cambridge (to appear)
8. Ryser, H.J.: Combinatorial Properties of Matrices of Zeros and Ones. Can. J. Mathematics **9** (1957) 371-377
9. Kong, T.Y., Herman, G.T.: Tomographic Equivalence and Switching Operations. In Herman, G.T., Kuba, A. (eds.): Discrete Tomography: Foundations, Algorithms and Applications. Birkhauser, Boston Cambridge (to appear)
10. Metropolis, N., Rosenbluth, A.W., Rosenbluth, M.N., Teller, A.H., Teller, E.: Equations of State Calculations by Fast Computing Machines. J. Chem. Phys. **21**, (1953) 1087-1092
11. Ritman, E.L., Robb, R.A., Harris, L.D.: Imaging Physiological Functions. Praeger, New York (1985)
12. Browne, J.A., Herman, G.T., Odhner, D.: SNARK93: A Programming System for Image Reconstruction from Projections. Technical Report No. **198**. Medical Image Processing Group, Department of Radiology, University of Pennsylvania, Philadelphia (1993)

Real Time 3D Brain Shift Compensation

Oskar M. Škrinjar[1] and James S. Duncan[1,2]

Departments of Electrical Engineering[1] and Diagnostic Radiology[2],
Yale University, New Haven, CT 06520-8042, USA
oskar.skrinjar@yale.edu

Abstract. Surgical navigation systems are used intraoperatively to provide the surgeon with a display of preoperative and intraoperative data
in the same coordinate system and help her or him guide the surgery.
However, these systems are subject to inaccuracy caused by intraoperative brain movement (brain shift) since commercial systems in use today
typically assume that the intracranial structures are rigid. Experiments
show brain shifts up to several millimeters, making it the cause of the
dominant error in the system. We propose an image-based brain shift
compensation system based on an intraoperatively guided deformable
model. We have recorded a set of brain surface points during the surgery
and used them to guide and/or validate the model predictions. Initial
results show that this system limits the error between its brain surface
prediction and real brain surfaces to within 0.5 mm, which is a significant improvement over the systems that are based on the rigid brain
assumption, that in this case would have an error of 3 mm or greater.

1 Introduction

The use of surgical navigation systems has become a standard way to assist
the neurosurgeon in navigating within the intraoperative environment, planning
and guiding the surgery. One of the most important features of these systems is
the ability to relate the position of the surgical instruments to the features in
the preoperative images. Ideally, they should provide a 3D display of the neuroanatomical structures of interest and include visualization of surgical instruments within the same frame. In order to be reliably used, the surgical navigation
system should be as precise as possible, preferably to within the voxel size of the
used dataset (see [4]). Most of the current systems use preoperatively-acquired
3D data and register it to the patient coordinate system (see [3,4,5]). However,
they assume that the brain and other intracranial structures are rigid and fixed
relative to the skull. The preoperative data is registered to the patient coordinate
system at the beginning of the surgery. While this can be done with a precision
to within 1 mm at the initial moment (see [4]), since the brain deforms over time,
the accuracy of the system deteriorates. The median brain shift of points on the
brain surface was estimated to range from 0.3 mm to 7.4 mm (see [1]). It is clear
that the system based on the rigid brain assumption cannot achieve a precision
better than a few millimeters at the outer structures. Since the deeper brain

A. Kuba et al. (Eds.): IPMI'99, LNCS 1613, pp. 42–55, 1999.

structures deform less than the outer ones, the error is the largest at the cortical surface. The brain deforms even more after interventions, e.g. post-resections. Furthermore, the average brain shift for cases in which hematoma or tumors were removed was reported to be 9.5 mm and 7.9 mm, respectively (see [2]). In such cases the error is even larger.

In our research we are mainly concerned with (but not limited to) issues surrounding epilepsy surgery. To quantitatively investigate such a case we have recorded six points on the exposed brain surface approximately every ten minutes during the surgery starting when the dura was opened. The mean shift in the direction perpendicular to the brain surface was about 3 mm. The initial and final set of points displayed over the rigid (initial) brain surface are shown in Fig. 1. This result clearly shows the need for a high quality intraoperative 3D acquisition system and/or a method for estimating brain shift. The tradeoffs among different approaches to these problems are discussed later in the paper. The approach we have taken is to use a biomechanically-based deformable model

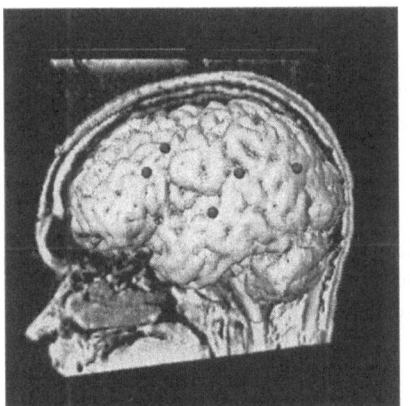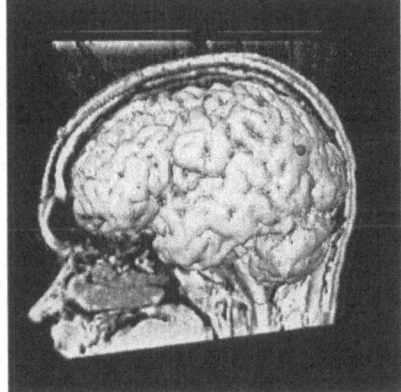

Fig. 1. Intraoperatively recorded points on the brain surface at the beginning of the surgery are shown at left, while their positions one hour later relative to the non-deformed (initial) brain surface are shown at right. Gravity is perpendicular to the sagittal plane. The points moved in the direction of gravity and they are hidden under the brain surface (only one of the points is still visible in the figure at right). Since the brain deformed (in the direction of the gravity vector) the surface points moved relative to the original (initial) brain surface

that incorporates the effects of gravity and can be driven by intraoperative measurements. Currently, we have performed only partial validation of the deformation results, since a full human in-vivo 3D validation is practically difficult with current technology. With this system, 3D estimation of the brain shift can be performed in real-time, i.e. faster or equal to the real brain deformation, and for this reason can be used in an actual operating room (OR) application. This project is a continuation of our endeavors to overcome the brain shift problem in surgical navigation, initialized by our modeling efforts reported in [6]. This work extends the model, puts the model in touch with real data and discusses our plans for a complete brain shift compensated surgical navigation system. We also note relevant work in soft tissue deformation (see [2,7,8,9,10,11]).

2   System Overview

Our approach to brain shift compensation is to deform an intraoperatively-guided model and use the model data during the surgery to display (deformed according to the current model state) preoperative data. Therefore we propose an image based brain shift compensation system made up of several components: segmentation, mesh generation, a model, registration of the model to the intraoperative environment, driving and guiding the model, and displaying the deformed data.

The first step is segmentation of the brain tissue and the skull since they are the two most important parts of the model. For brain tissue extraction we have adopted the automatic segmentation algorithm suggested in [12], enhanced with a few pre- and post-processing steps. Eventually, the skull segmentation will be done from CT scans, and then it will be registered with the initial MRI data. However, for this preliminary effort, we approximate the inner skull surface segmentation using dilation and erosion operators applied to the previously segmented brain tissue. An output is shown in Fig. 2. It is important to have the inner skull surface available for the model since it defines the boundary conditions. Clearly, the brain is bounded by the skull and it cannot go outside it. When a gravitational force is applied to the brain, slightly globally, but non-rigidly, it shifts downward, and from the bottom and sides it is resisted by the inner skull surface. Therefore, the largest deformation is on the top of the brain.

For object surface rendering we have used an improved version of the algorithm suggested in [13]. Some of the surfaces produced by this algorithm can be seen in Figs. 1, 4 and 6.

In order to display and use brain surface points a correspondence between the patient and MRI dataset coordinate systems has to be established. We used a set of markers placed on the patient's skin. In the OR, the marker coordinates were recorded using a mechanical localizer [16]. In addition the markers were manually localized in the MRI dataset. Next, a robust point matching algorithm for resolving the correspondence and finding the optimal transformation between the two sets was applied. It is important to notice that for various reasons, the surgeon is not always able to touch all of the markers. Therefore one of the two sets could contain outliers. Our point matching algorithm covers such cases in an automatic fashion. The result of the matching between the two sets of markers

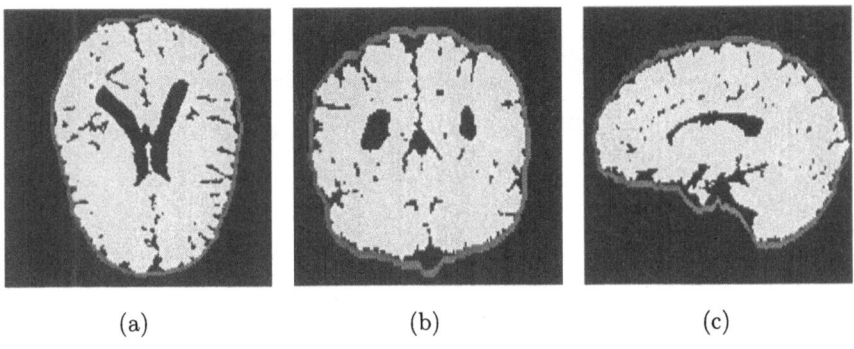

(a)   (b)   (c)

Fig. 2. An output of the inner skull surface segmentation algorithm in three orthogonal slices: **(a)** axial, **(b)** coronal and **(c)** sagittal. The brain tissue is colored white, inner skull surface gray and CSF black

is shown in Fig. 3. The same mechanical localizer is used to record the points on the brain surface during the surgery. Once the correspondence was established, the brain surface points were transformed to the MRI coordinate system.

The next step is to generate the model mesh from the segmented brain tissue. Here we use prism ("brick") elements, having 8 nodes at the vertex positions. The output of our mesh generator is shown in Fig. 4. The mesh does not capture all of the fine details of the segmentation output, since this mesh density allows for reasonable performance (in terms of errors). A much finer mesh that would capture all brain geometric details (i.e. all sulcal structures) would have too many nodes and would slow down computation, not achieving a significant improvement in performance. Once the current node positions are known, any information obtained prior to surgery can be deformed according to the model interpolation functions (the trilinear back interpolation used for this purpose is explained in the next section). Currently, we use the model to deform the MRI gray scale image slices (three orthogonal slices) using texture maps and the outer brain surface, but it can as easily be used to deform additional CT, functional MRI, MRA or any other volumetric preoperatively-acquired data with update speed limited only by the graphics capabilities of the display engine.

3   Model

3.1   Brain Tissue Modeling

According to our findings and findings of other groups (see [1,2]) brain shift is a relatively small deformation and a slow process. This fact facilitates our approach to brain tissue modeling. As we move in these directions we also note relevant work in soft tissue deformation (see [2,7,8,9,10,11]). Here, we employ a linear stress-strain relation, which is a good approximation for small tissue displacements. The model consists of a set of discrete interconnected nodes each representing a small part of the brain tissue. Nodes have masses depending

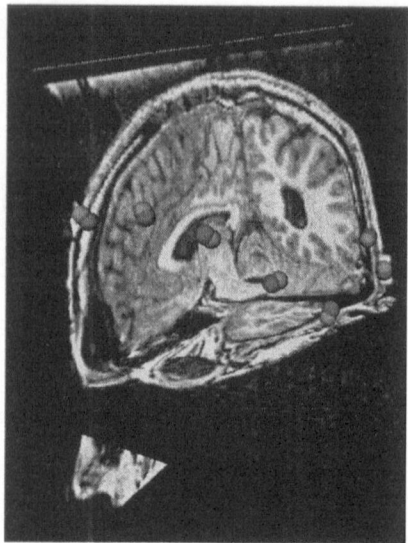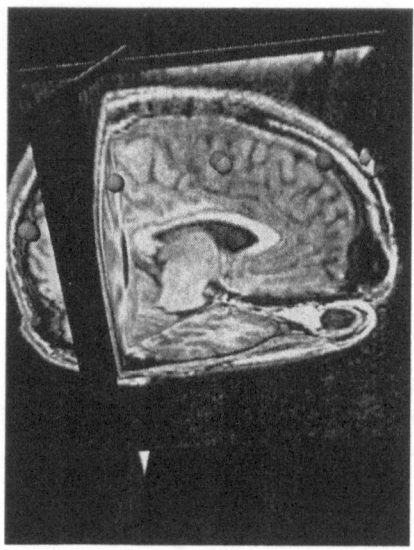

Fig. 3. The lighter points are the marker positions obtained from the MRI dataset, while the darker ones are the markers touched by the surgeon in the OR. These two figures show the marker sets after the correspondence has been established. There are 12 markers, but in this case, the surgeon managed to touch only 10 of them. Our correspondence algorithm handles the outlier problem as well

on the size of the volume they represent and on the local tissue density. Each connection is modeled as a parallel connection of a linear spring and dashpot, known as the Kelvin solid model (see [14]). As for the nodes, the connection parameters can depend on their position in the brain. The Kelvin solid model is a model for a visco-elastic material subject to slow and small deformations, which is exactly the case with brain shift. It is also a rather simple approach, which is a desirable property since the model deformation should be computed in real time, i.e. faster or at least at the speed of the brain deformation, since it must be utilized (e.g. displayed) during the surgery. The constitutive relation for the Kelvin solid model is

$$\sigma = q_0 \epsilon + q_1 \dot{\epsilon}, \qquad (1)$$

where σ is stress and ϵ strain, while q_0 and q_1 are local parameters. The dotted variables represent the time derivatives, e.g. $\dot{\epsilon} = \frac{d}{dt}\epsilon$.

The equation (1) can me rewritten in the following way. If two nodes are at positions r_1 and r_2, have velocities v_1 and v_2, and are connected in the above fashion, then the force acting on the first node is

$$f_{inner}(r_1, r_2, v_1, v_2) = [k_s(\|r_2 - r_1\| - r_{12}) - k_d(v_2 - v_1)n_{21}]\, n_{21}, \qquad (2)$$

where k_s is the stiffness coefficient, k_d is the damping coefficient and r_{12} is the rest length of the spring connecting the two nodes. In a general case they can

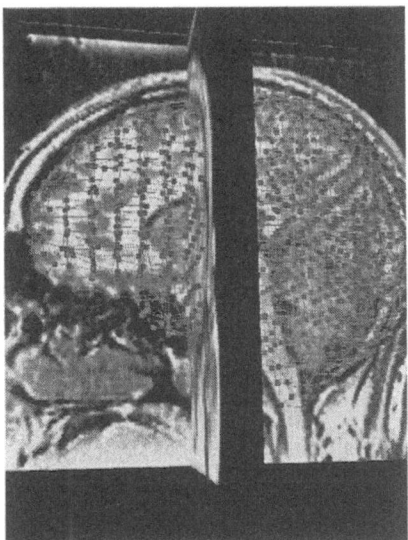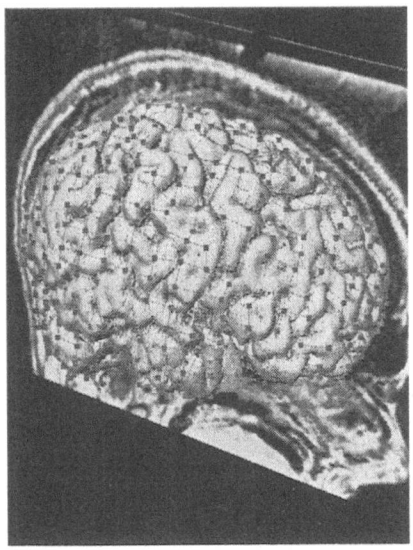

Fig. 4. The mesh generator output. The left figure shows the mesh, while the right one shows the mesh and the outer brain surface

vary from connection to connection depending on the local material properties. n_{21} is the unit vector from r_1 to r_2. Note that the same force acts on the other node but in the opposite direction.

3.2   Modeling the Brain — Skull Interaction

The brain–skull interaction as modeled in our initial efforts in [6], is a highly nonlinear function, and significantly slows down the adaptive step-size numerical integration. The consequence was that the steady-state for this previous 3D model was reached in approximately four hours, which is much slower than the real brain deformation, and therefore the model cannot be used for display updating during the surgery. A coarse approximation could be to make the outer brain surface nodes rigid in the bottom part of the brain (bottom with respect to gravity) as used in [11]. However, we think that having the brain–skull interaction contributes to the total precision of the system.

For this reason we now use an alternate approach. Prior to the simulation, the skull and brain tissue have to be segmented. Ideally, the MRI scan would be used for brain tissue segmentation, and CT scan for skull segmentation, but for the aforementioned reason we have used the procedure explained in the previous section to extract the inner skull surface. The brain–skull interaction is not directly incorporated in the model equations, but rather incorporated via the numerical integration, through a contact algorithm. As the model evolves over time, when a node enters the skull area, it is returned to its previous position (to its position from the previous step in the numerical integration). This prevents nodes from entering the skull, but permits them to come arbitrarily close to it (more precisely, close up to the precision set in the numerical integration) and can move along the skull surface if pulled by forces that are not perpendicular to the skull surface. Effectively, nodes can move freely unless they reach the skull, in which case they can move only in the direction tangential to the skull surface. This behavior is identical to the one achieved by the brain–skull interaction suggested in [6], but it is much faster to simulate. As a result, the 3D model now needs about 10 minutes to reach the steady state, which is faster than the actual brain deformation (which is approximately half an hour). Thus, this model can potentially be used during the surgery, which is our eventual goal.

3.3   The Model Equations

Newton's Second Law for each node j in the model gives

$$m^j a^j = m^j g + \sum_{i=1}^{n^j} f_{inner}{}^j_{s^j_i},$$
(3)

where m^j is the node's mass, a^j is its acceleration, $f_{inner}{}^j_{s^j_i}$ is the interaction between nodes j and s^j_i defined by (2) and g is the gravity acceleration, while $\{s^j_1, s^j_2, \dots, s^j_{n^j}\}$ is the set of the neighboring nodes of the node j. Equation (3) represents a system of second order nonlinear ordinary differential equations.

One can define the state variables to be $x_{2j-1} = r^j$ and $x_{2j} = v^j$ for $j = 1, \dots, N$, where N is the number of the brain model nodes. Obviously, $\dot{x}_{2j-1} = x_{2j}$. The expression for $\dot{x}_{2j}$ follows directly from (3), since $\dot{x}_{2j} = \frac{d}{dt} x_{2j} = a^j$. It depends only on state variables but not on their time derivatives. Now it is clear that (3) can be rewritten in the compact state-space form $\dot{\mathcal{X}} = f(\mathcal{X})$, where $\mathcal{X}$ is the vector of the state variables and $\dot{\mathcal{X}} = \frac{d}{dt} \mathcal{X}$. It is assumed that the brain starts deforming from a rest position, i.e. $v^j(t = 0) = 0$ for all j. The initial node positions $r^j(t = 0)$ were obtained from the preoperative images, as discussed in the previous section.

The system in state-space form is suitable for numerical integration (see [15]). In this case the fourth order Runge-Kutta method with adaptive stepsize was employed. The brain–skull interaction is implicitly included in the numerical integration as explained in the previous section.

3.4   Interpolation

The output of the numerical integration is the set of model nodes over time. One usually wants to display deformed gray scale data (e.g. from preoperative MRI) using texture maps, brain structure surfaces or any other preoperative data. For this purpose we have employed trilinear interpolation.

The texture map (we use texture maps to display three orthogonal slices in the MRI datasets) deformation and the brain surface deformation are principally different procedures. In the case of the texture map deformation for a given voxel position in the current frame, one should find the element ("brick") it belongs to, find the voxel local coordinates in the element, and then find the voxel position in the original (initial) model state, using the same local coordinates in the corresponding initial element. Since the corresponding initial position is generally not exactly at a voxel center we perform an interpolation among the neighboring voxels. This procedure is referred to as back interpolation. The brain surface deformation is a reverse process. For a given point in the initial state, one should find out the element it falls in and the corresponding local coordinates and then, using the same local coordinates find the new (deformed) coordinates in the same element in the current frame.

The trilinear interpolation, i.e. the dependence between the global x, y and z coordinates and local element α, β and γ coordinates is given by the following equation:

$$\begin{aligned}
x &= (c_1^x + c_2^x \alpha)(c_3^x + c_4^x \beta)(c_5^x + c_6^x \gamma), \\
y &= (c_1^y + c_2^y \alpha)(c_3^y + c_4^y \beta)(c_5^y + c_6^y \gamma), \\
z &= (c_1^z + c_2^z \alpha)(c_3^z + c_4^z \beta)(c_5^z + c_6^z \gamma).
\end{aligned} \tag{4}$$

The equation (4) can be expressed using matrix notation in the following way,

$$\begin{bmatrix} x \\ y \\ z \end{bmatrix} = A_{3,8} \begin{bmatrix} 1 \ \alpha \ \beta \ \gamma \ \alpha\beta \ \alpha\gamma \ \beta\gamma \ \alpha\beta\gamma \end{bmatrix}^T. \tag{5}$$

It is obvious that the function is nonlinear, but it is linear with respect to any single local coordinate (e.g. it is linear with respect to γ). Therefore it is called a trilinear function. To be strict, this function should be called a "tri-affine function" but it is commonly referred to as being trilinear. The 24 elements of the matrix A are uniquely determined from the fact that the local coordinates take either 0 or 1 at the eight element vertex positions. It is easy to show that this interpolation provides C_0 continuity.

One can directly compute the global coordinates for given local coordinates using (5). However, it is not simple to solve (5) for α, β and γ (the solution expressions are huge). For this reason we have used an iterative search method to determine local coordinates for given global coordinates. The method converges very fast, i.e achieves the given precision (0.1 mm) in several iterations.

An example of texture map deformation is given in Fig. 5. The increase in the gap between the skull and brain at the top is small (approximately 3 mm - check Table 1 in the next section for the maximal surface movement value). The MRI dataset is a 256 by 256 by 124 T1 weighted sequence (1 mm by 1 mm by 1.5 mm).

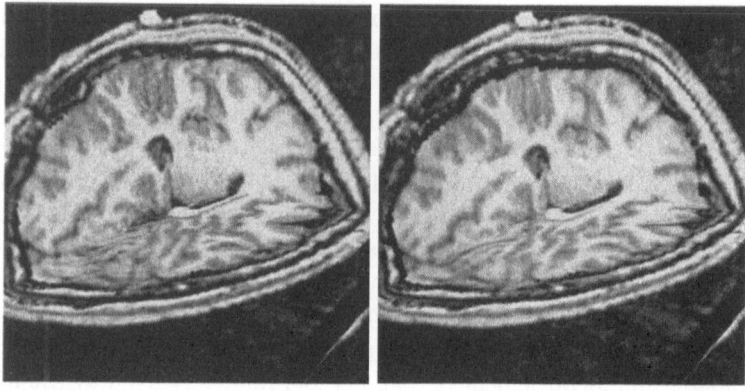

Fig. 5. The texture map deformation. The left figure shows the initial state while the right shows the final state. Note the increase in the gap between the skull and brain at the top

4   Parameter Estimation

The global problem in modeling, especially in modeling heterogeneous materials, is reliable model parameter setup and estimation. The approach we have employed here is to use intraoperative measurements to estimate model parameters.

Although our model allows for local parameter control, we still assume a homogeneous model for two reasons. First, it is very difficult to estimate the brain tissue parameters locally and second, there are contradictory reports in the literature regarding white and gray stiffness properties. Even in the case of a homogeneous model there are two parameters to be estimated: stiffness coefficient k_s and damping coefficient k_d in (2).

For parameter estimation we have used so called off-line parameter estimation, where the whole sequence of the recorded (and registered) brain surface "time" points was used. Practice shows that the steady state does not depend on the choice of the damping coefficient, but only on the stiffness coefficient. The damping coefficient determines how fast the steady state will be reached, while the stiffness coefficient determines the final shape of the brain.

For this reason we use the steady state to estimate the stiffness coefficient. An approximate value for this coefficient is initially assumed, the model is driven to the steady state and signed average distance over all six of the recorded points to the model surface is computed. Based on the signed average distance a new stiffness coefficient is chosen, and the procedure is repeated until the final average signed error was small enough (we required it to be smaller than 0.5 mm).

Once the stiffness coefficient is determined, the damping coefficient is determined in a similar fashion, but this time reducing the average signed distance in the transient period.

The Table 1 shows the average distance between the rigid (initial) gray/CSF brain surface and recorded brain surface points over time (i.e. during the operation) in row "surface movement". In addition, row "model error" contains the average error between the model prediction of the gray/CSF brain surface and the recorded brain surface points over time. This table contains data for a single patient undergoing epileptic (implant) surgery. The surgeon touched six points (measured their positions with the mechanical arm) every 7 minutes (on average).

Table 1. Average brain surface movement and model error

time[min:sec]	0:00	7:40	14:40	19:40	24:40	34:52	49:00	max
surface movement [mm]	0.34	1.38	2.21	2.30	2.74	3.24	3.29	3.29
model error [mm]	0.34	0.45	0.30	0.13	0.20	0.32	0.04	0.45

One can see that the distance between the initial gray/CSF brain surface and the recorded brain surface points increases over time reaching 3.29 mm. The model with optimal parameters (determined in the off-line way) has maximal error of 0.45 mm over time. Clearly, the use of the model has done a reasonable job of estimating the brain shift near the brain surface (where the error is the greatest).

However, the off-line parameter estimation cannot be used in OR applications, since at each moment only the current and previous measurements are available, not all the measurements over time. The parameters would need to be estimated using the available intraoperative data. An idea for on-line parameter estimation is to start with reasonable initial parameters, based on previous experiments (say, on other patients), and then to adjust the parameters according to the error between the model prediction and the measurements. At the moment, the intraoperative measurements we have are too sparse and noisy to allow for on-line parameter estimation. Refer to the Discussion section for our future work plans including on-line parameter estimation.

5   Intraoperative Model Guidance

In addition to designing a reasonable model, and estimating model parameters in an optimal sense, one can guide the model by intraoperative data. The idea is to readjust the model at the time points when the intraoperative measurements are available, and in between to let the model deform on its own. The model tries to predict the node positions at the moment of new measurements, new measurements are used to readjust the model, and so on. The denser the intraoperative data are both in space and time the smaller the error between the model and real brain.

We have employed such an approach using the model parameters estimated as described above. The results are given in the Table 2 (this table also contains data for a single patient). It is clear that performance has improved over the case of non-data-guided model. The maximal error in the case of guided model is 0.20 mm (not taking into the account the initial state), but over time it is even smaller because of the feedback-like guidance. The error does not approach zero over time due to noise in data.

Table 2. Average brain surface movement and model errors

time[min:sec]	0:00	7:40	14:40	19:40	24:40	34:52	49:00	max
surface movement [mm]	0.34	1.38	2.21	2.30	2.74	3.24	3.29	3.29
non-guided model error [mm]	0.34	0.45	0.30	0.13	0.20	0.32	0.04	0.45
guided model error [mm]	0.34	0.20	0.05	0.01	0.03	0.08	0.02	0.20

The last two rows represent the same type of error as the model error in Table 1, but for non-guided and guided models. One should be aware that the errors reported in Table 2 for guided model are very small since the six recorded brain surface points are used to guide the model, and then the error is computed with respect to them. A more realistic error estimation is given in the next section. However, in an OR application one should use all available intraoperative data to guide the model.

The results of the brain deformation modeling are shown in the Fig. 6. The brain model is deformed by taking into account the measurements (points), and the surface of the brain is computed according to the current model state. One can see that the surface (prediction) matches the points (measurements).

5.1 Validation

To completely validate the model reliability one would need to obtain a dense time sequence of 3D brain datasets using intra-operative sensing, and then compare the model predictions to the actual deformations. This can be done by using intraoperative MRI, or maybe an intraoperative CT or ultrasound scanner. Since at this point we have brain surface points recorded over time as the only intra-operative data, we used two of the points to guide the model and compared the model predictions to the rest four points. The results are given in the Table 3.

Table 3. Average brain surface movement and model error

time[min:sec]	0:00	7:40	14:40	19:40	24:40	34:52	49:00	max
surface movement [mm]	0.34	1.38	2.21	2.30	2.74	3.24	3.29	3.29
validated model error [mm]	0.34	0.12	0.38	0.44	0.35	0.49	0.14	0.49

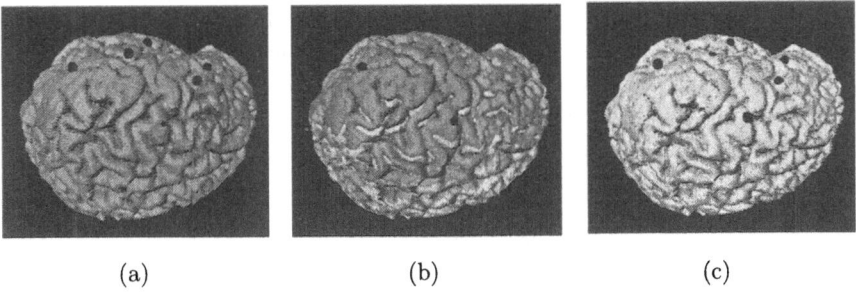

$$(a) \qquad\qquad (b) \qquad\qquad (c)$$

Fig. 6. The results of the model deformation: (**a**) represents the recorded points at initial time with the initial brain surface. The points are on the brain surface, (**b**) represents the final brain surface points with initial brain surface (darker) and final brain surface (lighter). One can see that the brain surface points moved inside the original brain. This is due to the effect of gravity that pulled the brain downwards, (**c**) represents the final brain surface points and final brain surface. The points are again on the brain surface. The final brain surface is obtained from the final model state, i.e. it is a prediction of the surface, while the final points are the measurements on the brain surface when the brain settled down (after approximately one hour from the moment when the dura was opened). The prediction (surface) matches the measurements (points)

As before the last row represents the error defined in the same way as the model error in Table 1, but in this case for the validated model (validated by the four left points - first two were used for model guidance). This partial validation suggests that the use of our model reduces the error caused by the brain shift, i.e. the difference between the current brain and the current model state is smaller than the difference between the current brain and the initial brain.

6   Discussion

The main contribution of the model we have suggested is the ability to signif-icantly reduce the error in real time[1]. The model has 2088 nodes, 11733 con-nections and 1521 elements (bricks) and it takes typically less than 10 minutes on an Octane SGI workstation (R10000 250 MHz processor) to reach the steady

---

[1] By real time we mean the following. The brain deforms with certain speed (it takes about 30 minutes to assume a steady state). At the other hand it takes certain time to simulate the brain deformation on a computer, i.e. to deform the model. However, at say 8 minutes after opening the dura (8 minutes of the actual, surgical time) the corresponding model state (the state that corresponds to the 8th minute of the actual time) has already been computed and stored in the memory, and can be used for displaying (deformed) surfaces, texture maps or whatever is needed. Thus, the simulation of the brain deformation is computed faster than the actual brain deformation, i.e. in real time. If this is not the case, i.e, if the simulation of brain takes more time than the actual brain deformation, then the model cannot be used during the surgery (in real time) for displaying the deformed surfaces and datasets.

state. This is significant improvement compared to our previous model (see [6]). For these reasons it can be used in a real time application as a part of surgical navigation system. Once the model deformation is computed, any preoperative data, including but not limited to brain structure surfaces, slice texture maps of MRI, fMRI, CT or MRA data can be deformed accordingly. In other words, knowing the model state (the deformed mesh) at certain time (t_0), and knowing the initial model state, and preoperative say fMRI dataset, one can directly calculate the corresponding deformed fMRI data (at time t_0).

As noted above, an alternative is to use an intraoperative MRI system (see [3,4]). They certainly have their own advantages, but they are expensive, restrict surgical access to the patient, prevent usage of metal surgical tools and their spatial resolution is typically not as high as that of preoperative MRI. However, a combination of a deformable model and intraoperative MRI and/or CT would probably provide a surgical navigation system with a means to handle a variety of deformations potentially including those due to tissue removal with an acceptable precision.

To successfully model the brain deformation one needs to take into account not only the soft tissue mechanics, but also neuro-anatomical knowledge. For instance, our neurosurgical colleagues observe that it appears that the cerebellum does not deform due to toughness of tentorium. If this assumption is valid, this part of brain does not need to be modeled, and the deformable part of the volume is reduced, causing the performance (both in precision and speed) to be enhanced.

Our future work is eventually aimed at on-line parameter estimation, richer intraoperative data acquisition, including intraoperative (portable) CT imaging, CSF modeling and non-homogeneous brain tissue modeling.

Acknowledgements

We are thankful to Dr. Dennis Spencer and Kevin McCarthy from Department of Neurosurgery, Yale School of Medicine, for collaboration, useful discussions and for providing us with data.

References

1. Hill, D., Maurer, C., Wang, M., Maciunas, R., Barwise, J., Fitzpatrick, M.: Estimation of Intraoperative Brain Surface Movement. CVRMed–MRCAS'97, Grenoble, France (1997) 449–458
2. Bucholz, R., Yeh, D., Trobaugh, J., McDurmont, L., Sturm, C., Baumann, C., Henderson, J., Levy, A., Kessman, P.: The Correction of Stereotactic Inaccuracy Caused by Brain Shift Using an Intraoperative Ultrasound Device. CVRMed–MRCAS'97, Grenoble, France (1997) 459–466
3. Grimson, W.E.L., Ettinger, G.J., White, S.J., Gleason, P.L., Lozano–Perez, T., Wells III, W.M., Kikinis, R.: Evaluating and Validating an Automated Registration System for Enhanced Reality Visualization in Surgery.

4. Grimson, W.E.L., Ettinger, G.J., White, S.J., Gleason, P.L., Lozano-Perez, T., Wells III, W.M., Kikinis, R.: An Automatic Registration Method for Frameless Stereotaxy, Image Guided Surgery, and Enhanced Reality Visualization. IEEE Transactions on Medical Imaging **15** (1996) 129–140

5. Peters, T., Davey, B., Munger, P., Comeau, R., Evans, A., Olivier, A.: Three-Dimensional Multimodal Image-Guidance for Neurosurgery. IEEE Transactions on Medical Imaging **15** (1996) 121–128

6. Škrinjar, O., Spencer, D., Duncan, J.: Brain Shift Modeling for Use in Neurosurgery. Proceedings of MICCAI'98, Chambridge MA (1998) 641–649

7. Shi, P., Sinusas, A. J., Constable, R.T., Duncan, J.S.: Volumetric Deformation Analysis Using Mechanics-Based Data Fusion: Applications in Cardiac Motion Recovery. International Journal of Computer Vision, Kluwer, submitted.

8. Duncan, J., Shi, P., Constable, R.T., Sinusas, A.: Physical and Geometrical Modeling for Image-Based Recovery of Left Ventricular Deformation. Progress in Biophysics and Molecular Biology, in press.

9. Edwards, P.J., Hill D.L.G., Little, J.A., Hawkes, D.J.: Deformation for Image Guided Interventions Using a Three Component Tissue Model. 15th International Conference, Proceedings of IPMI'97 (1997) 218–231

10. Gibson, S., Samosky, J., Mor, A., Fyock, C., Grimson, E., Kanade, T., Kikinis, R., Lauer, H, McKenzie, N., Nakajima, S., Ohkami, H., Osborne, R. Sawada, A.: Simulating Arthroscopic Knee Surgery Using Volumetric Object Representations, Real-Time Volume Rendering and Haptic Feedback. CVRMed-MRCAS'97, Grenoble, France (1997) 369–378

11. Miga, M., Paulse, K., Kennedy, F., Hoopes, J., Hartov, A., Roberts, D.: Initial In-Vivo Analysis of 3D Heterogeneous Brain Computations for Model-Updated Image-Guided Neurosurgery., Proceedings of MICCAI'98, Chambridge MA (1998) 743–752

12. Stokking R.: Integrated Visualizaton of Functional and Anatomical Brain Images. PhD Thesis, University Utrecht, 1998

13. Gibson, S.: Constrained Elastic Surface Nets: Generating Smooth Surface from Binary Segmented Data. Proceedings of MICCAI'98, Chambridge MA (1998) 888–898

14. Pamidi, M.R., Advani, S.H.: Nonlinear Constitutive Relations for Human Brain Tissue. Journal of Bio–Mechanical Engineering **100** (1978) 44–48

15. Press, W.H., Teukolsky, S.A., Vettrling, W.T., Flannery, B.P.: Numerical Recipes in C. 2nd Edition, Camridge University Press, 1992.

16. Operation of the Mayfield^R Acciss^{TM} Stereotactic Workstation, QUICK REFERENCE, OMI^R Surgical Products, March 1997

Computer Assisted Human Follicle Analysis for Fertility Prospects with 3D Ultrasound

Bart M. ter Haar Romeny[1], Bart Titulaer[1], Stiliyan Kalitzin[1],
Gabriëlle Scheffer[2], Frank Broekmans[2], Joes Staal[1], and Egbert te Velde[2]

[1] Image Sciences Institute, Utrecht University,
PO Box 85500, NL–3508 GA Utrecht, The Netherlands
B.terHaarRomeny@isi.uu.nl
[2] Division of Obstetrics and Gynaecology, Subdivision for Reproductive Medicine,
University Hospital Utrecht, The Netherlands
F.Broekmans@dog.azu.nl

Abstract. Knowledge about the status of the female reproductive system is important for fertility problems and age-related family planning. The volume of these fertility requests in our emancipated society is steadily increasing. Intravaginal 3D ultrasound imaging of the follicles in the ovary gives important information about the ovarian aging, i.e. number of follicles, size, position and response to hormonal stimulation. Manual analysis of the many follicles is laborious and error–prone. We present a multiscale analysis to automatically detect and quantify the number and shape of the patient's follicles. Robust estimation of the centres of the follicles in the speckled echographic images is done by calculating so-called winding number of the intensity singularity, i.e. the path integral of the angular increment of the direction of the gradient vector over a closed neighbourhood around the point. The principal edges on 200–500 intensity traces radiating from the detected singularity points are calculated by a multiscale edge focussing technique on 1D winding numbers. They are fitted with 3D spherical harmonic functions, from which the volume and shape parameters are derived.

1 Introduction

Changes in societal behaviour have led to postponement of childbearing in most developed countries. In the Netherlands the mean age at which a woman gives birth to her first child has now risen to 30 years. As female fecundity decreases with advancing age an increasing number of couples is faced with unexpected difficulties in conceiving. It is estimated that approximately 15,000 couples visit infertility clinics in the Netherlands annually. For some 70% of these couples, age-related fecundity decline may play a role and a further increase is to be expected.

The decline in the number of follicles containing oocytes from the ovary and a decrease in the quality of these oocytes are the main causes of the decline in female fecundity. This loss in functional capacity of the ovary is more rapid in some women. Identification of women with advanced loss in ovarian function has been quite difficult so far. Recent research has shown that the number of visible

A. Kuba et al. (Eds.): IPMI'99, LNCS 1613, pp. 56–69, 1999.

follicles, assessed by ultrasound in a group of women, is correlated with proven fertility [3,4,18]. Based on this observation, ultrasound-based follicle counts are being developed as a 'test' for reproductive age. This enables us to recognise infertile women with exhausted reproductive capacity and advise them to refrain from further diagnosis and treatment. Likewise, recognition of especially younger infertile women with advanced loss of follicles will lead to prompt referral for the application of assisted reproduction techniques. In our modern emancipating society, questions are being raised related to the planning tension between career and family: when I am young, what is the status of my reproductive system; can I safely postpone childbearing and first pursue a career? When I get older, until what age am I still likely to be able to conceive spontaneously? It is known that the decrease in number of follicles is bi–exponential, and accelerates after the age of 37 [4,18] (Fig. 1). Furthermore, the risk of damage to the ovary during chemo– or radiotherapy is another reason to predict the age when the follicular storage is depleted.

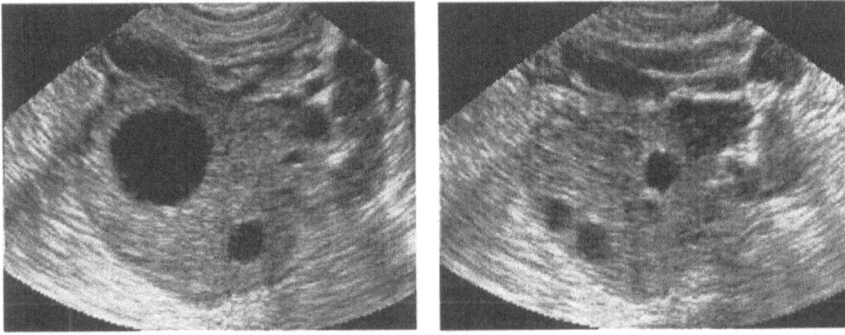

Fig. 1. Two 2D slices from a 3D ultrasound image of a normal 23 year old volunteer. The follicles are clearly visible as dark hypo-echogenic circular areas in the ovary, which is visible as a slightly darker background in the central part of the images. Typical diameters of follicles are 2–8 mm, in a 2–4 cm diameter slightly ellipsoidal ovarian capsule

For a large–scale evaluation of these application areas, high quality and automated information about the ovarian anatomy, especially of the follicles, is needed. 3D ultrasound turns out to be an practical and cost effective acquisition mode. Manual counting and measuring all the follicles by inspecting the 2D slices from a 3D dataset is tedious and time consuming, and often inaccurate. Automated analysis reports have been few and only in 2D [15,16,21,22]. Ultrasound data are characterised by interference noise, a wide range of often-occurring artefacts, and low contrasts. So robust and noise resistant methods must be developed to find the follicle centres and contours. Often follicles are not spherical, particularly when they are touching each other, making Hough transform methods less suitable [16]. This paper describes a new scale-space based method to detect and delineate the follicles automatically and accurately in 3D ultrasound. The paper focuses on the multiscale detection methods. A clinical paper describing the patient studies in detail is in preparation.

2   Ovarian Anatomy

The decline of human quota of oocytes begins before birth when ovarian aging begins. At birth some million follicle are present, the number falling continuously during childhood and adulthood until a few hundreds to thousands remain at the age of about 50 [18]. During the total reproductive lifespan only a few hundred will reach full maturation and ovulation. The left and right ovaries are thumb size structures, containing the collection of follicles. Follicles are round or oval structures embedded in the tissue of the ovarian stroma. The wall of the follicles comprises hormone-producing cells that are responsible for the production of fluid that is contained by the follicle wall and are filled with liquid. In transvaginal ultrasound they appear as clear low echoic spheres (Fig. 1). A prime indicator for ovarian aging is the number of antral follicles exceeding a certain size, their relative position in the ovary, and their responsiveness (expressed in growth rate) to hormonal stimulation [7]. This last measurement typically requires multiple periodic measurements, i.e. daily measurements over 3–5 consecutive days.

3   3D Ultrasound

2D vaginosonography can only yield sagittal and frontal sections of the lesser pelvis; 3D volume scanning, however, visualises all three perpendicular planes simultaneously on a monitor screen. The 3D ultrasound system (Combison 5600, Kretz Technik AG, Medicor, Austria / Korea) can be equipped with a 12 MHz transvaginal 3D probe of 2.2 cm diameter, focal distance of 2–10 cm. The system is capable of a full 3D image acquisition in about 2 seconds. From the pyramidal volumetric dataset a Cartesian dataset is extracted with equidistant voxels by interpolation. Sonographically, follicles with diameters of 3 mm and above can be detected reliably. 3D ultrasound has some important advantages over 2D imaging. Volume measurements using 2D ultrasound methods have been found to be much less accurate than 3D ultrasound methods for irregularly shaped objects [17]. It is a step towards interactive follicle puncturing [5]. To prevent as much as possible the appearance of vessels just outside the ovary and to restrain the field of view to the ovary proper, the operator, guided by 3 simultaneous orthogonal multiplanar reformatted views, performs a 3D cut–off of the total volume (maximum size 256^3 voxels). Typical resulting datasets are $180 \times 180 \times 150$ voxels (1 byte/voxel intensity range).

4   Detection of Follicle Centres by 3D Topological Winding Numbers

The key clinical question is the automatic counting of the number of antral follicles and their size distribution as the indicator for fertility from noisy datasets. From Gaussian scale–space theory we know that the extraction of (invariant) differential structural information like edges and curvature needs to be done with regularised differential operators, i.e. Gaussian derivative kernels [6]. The centre of a hypo–echoic follicle is characterised as a singularity of the luminance field; here the intensity (of the observed, thus multiscale, blurred image) reaches a minimum. A singularity is defined as a point where the intensity gradient vanishes. The local isophote curvature reaches infinity, due to the vanishing of the gradient. Singular points are important topological structural descriptors of images, especially when their behaviour is studied as a function of scale. They are used in the next step after local features detection, as important nodes in a perceptual grouping process, when the multiscale context of pixels needs to be taken into account.

The detection of singular points can conveniently be done by studying the so–called winding numbers. From the theory of vector fields [13] important theorems exist (Stoke's and Gauss') giving the relation between something happening in a volume and just on its surface, i.e. we can detect the singularities by measurements *around* the singularity. To explain the notion, we start in 2D. Image intensity is denoted by ξ, the gradient is denoted in index notation by ξ_i, where indices always run over the dimensions: $\xi_i = \{\partial \xi/\partial x, \partial \xi/\partial y\}$. The winding number ν is defined as the number of times the image gradient vector rotates over 2π when we walk around the point: i.e. we integrate over a closed path, indicated by ∂W, the increments of angle the vector ξ_i is making:

$$\nu = \oint_W \xi_i d\xi_j \epsilon^{ij}.$$

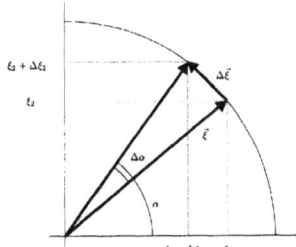

Fig. 2. Small rotation a vector along the contour of the closed path around the point of study

From Fig. 4 we see:

$$\tan \alpha = \frac{\xi_2}{\xi_1}, \qquad \tan(\alpha + \Delta\alpha) = \frac{\xi_2 + \Delta\xi_2}{\xi_1 + \Delta\xi_1}.$$

We expand the left– and right–hand side of the last equation in a Taylor series up to first order in α and ξ_1, respectively. For the left–hand side we obtain

$$\tan(\alpha + \Delta\alpha) = \tan \alpha + \frac{1}{\cos^2 \alpha} \Delta\alpha + O(\Delta\alpha^2)$$

and for the right hand side we obtain

$$\frac{\xi_2 + \Delta\xi_2}{\xi_1 + \Delta\xi_1} = \frac{\xi_2 + \Delta\xi_2}{\xi_1} - \frac{\xi_2 + \Delta\xi_2}{\xi_1^2}\Delta\xi_1 + O(\Delta\xi_1^2)$$

$$= \frac{\xi_2}{\xi_1} + \frac{\xi_1\Delta\xi_2 - \xi_2\Delta\xi_1}{\xi_1^2} + O(\Delta\xi_1^2).$$

Taking the limit $\Delta\alpha \to 0$ and using the expression for $\tan\alpha$ we get

$$d\alpha = \frac{\xi_1 d\xi_2 - \xi_2 d\xi_1}{\xi_1^2 + \xi_2^2}.$$

In our case we consider a unit gradient vector, so $\xi_1^2 + \xi_2^2 = 1$, and using subscript notation we obtain $d\alpha = \xi_i d\xi_j \varepsilon^{ij}$, where ε^{ij} is the antisymmetric tensor $\{\{0, -1\}, \{1, 0\}\}$.

The rotation is always an integer number times 2π (in 2D), which gives interesting robustness through rounding. In 3 dimensions we calculate the space angle of the gradient $\xi_i d\xi_j \wedge d\xi_k$, where we recognise the gradient ξ_i and a directed infinitesimal surface element $d\xi_j \wedge d\xi_k$. This is a so–called wedge ($\wedge$) product (see e.g. [13]). We integrate these surface elements now over the closed surface around our point of study, and see how often a full space angle of 4π is reached. This is then the 3D–winding number.

In practice, in 3D it is calculated as follows: we investigate the 26 voxels around a specific voxel. The form is defined in 3D as

$$\Phi = \xi_i d\xi_j \wedge d\xi_k \varepsilon^{ijk} = \xi_i \partial_l \xi_j \partial_m \xi_k dx^l \wedge dx^m \varepsilon^{ijk}.$$

Indices in pairs are summed over the dimensions, which process is called contraction of indices (the summing symbol in front of the equation is routinely left out: the so–called Einstein convention). Performing the contraction of indices on l and m gives

$$\Phi = \varepsilon^{ijk}\xi_i \ (\ (\partial_x\xi_j\partial_y\xi_k - \partial_y\xi_j\partial_x\xi_k)dx \wedge dy$$
$$+ (\partial_y\xi_j\partial_z\xi_k - \partial_z\xi_j\partial_y\xi_k)dy \wedge dz$$
$$+ (\partial_z\xi_j\partial_x\xi_k - \partial_x\xi_j\partial_z\xi_k)dz \wedge dx \ ).$$

This expression has to be evaluated for all voxels of our closed surface. We can do this e.g. for the 6 planes of the surrounding cube. On the surface $z =$ constant the previous equation reduces to

$$\Phi = \varepsilon^{ijk}\xi_i((\partial_x\xi_j\partial_y\xi_k - \partial_y\xi_j\partial_x\xi_k)dx \wedge dy.$$

Performing the contraction on the indices i, j and k gives

$$\Phi = 2\xi_x(\partial_x\xi_y\partial_y\xi_z - \partial_x\xi_z\partial_y\xi_y)$$
$$+ 2\xi_y(\partial_y\xi_x\partial_y\xi_z - \partial_x\xi_x\partial_y\xi_z)$$
$$+ 2\xi_z(\partial_x\xi_x\partial_y\xi_y - \partial_x\xi_y\partial_y\xi_z).$$

The gradient vector elements $\xi_i = \xi_x, \xi_y, \xi_z = \partial\xi/dx, \partial\xi/dy, \partial\xi/dz$ can be calculated e.g. by neighbour subtraction, as can be done in a similar way for the derivatives of the gradient field, e.g. $\partial_x\xi_y = \partial\xi_y/dx$. The single pixel steps dx and dy are unity.

The general theory comes from homotopy theory, where so–called topological homotopy class numbers are defined [9,10,11]. In d dimensions we again see how these reflect the behaviour of the intensity gradient ξ_i in a close neighbourhood ∂W around a given point. So, the d–dimensional homotopy class number ν of an image pixel over the surface ∂W of the small environment W around the point is defined as follows:

$$\nu = \oint_{\partial W} \xi_{i_1} d\xi_{i_2} \wedge d\xi_{i_3} \ldots d\xi_{i_d} \varepsilon^{i_1 i_2 \ldots i_d}.$$

There are no singularities on ∂W. For *regular* points, i.e. when no singularity is present in W, the winding number is zero, as we see from the Stokes' theorem:

$$\Phi = \xi_{i_1} d\xi_{i_2} \wedge d\xi_{i_3} \ldots d\xi_{i_d} \varepsilon^{i_1 i_2 \ldots i_d}, \qquad Stokes: \oint_{\partial W} \Phi = \oint_W d\Phi \equiv 0,$$

where the fact that the $(d-1)$–form Φ is a closed form was used. So, as most of our datapoints are regular, we detect singularities very robustly as integer values embedded in a space of zeros.

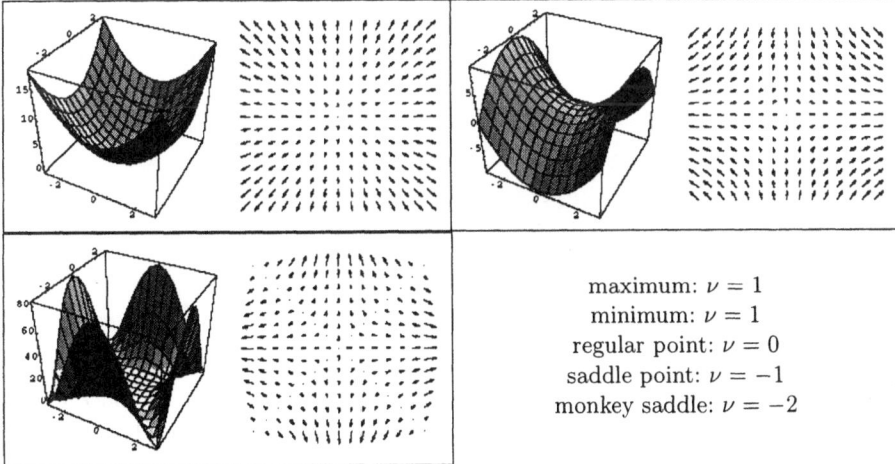

maximum: $\nu = 1$
minimum: $\nu = 1$
regular point: $\nu = 0$
saddle point: $\nu = -1$
monkey saddle: $\nu = -2$

Fig. 3. The direction of the gradient as a vectorfield for a minimum (upper left), saddlepoint (upper right) and monkeysaddle (lower left) in a 2D spatial intensity distribution. The number of full rotations of the gradient vector tracing a path around a point is the *winding number* ν, here indicated as multiples of one full rotation 2π of the gradient vector. All regular points give rise to $\nu = 0$. The centre of a follicle is a singular point in 3D, i.e. a minimum with $\nu = 1$

The winding number has nice properties:

- Within the closed contour there is a conservation of winding number; when we enclose a saddlepoint and a minimum, we measure the sum of the winding numbers (they sum to zero in this case as we are close to their annihilation);
- The winding number is independent of the shape of ∂W, it is a topological entity;
- The winding number only takes integer values as multiples of the full rotation angle; even when the numerical addition of angles does not sum up to precisely an integer value, we may rightly round off to the nearest integer;
- The winding number is a scaled notion, the neighbourhood defines the scale;
- The behaviour over scale of winding numbers generates a treelike structure which shows typical annihilations, creations and collisions, from which much can be learned about the 'deep structure' of images;
- The winding number is very easy to compute, in any dimension;
- The winding number is a robust characterisation of the singular points in the image: small deformations have a small effect.

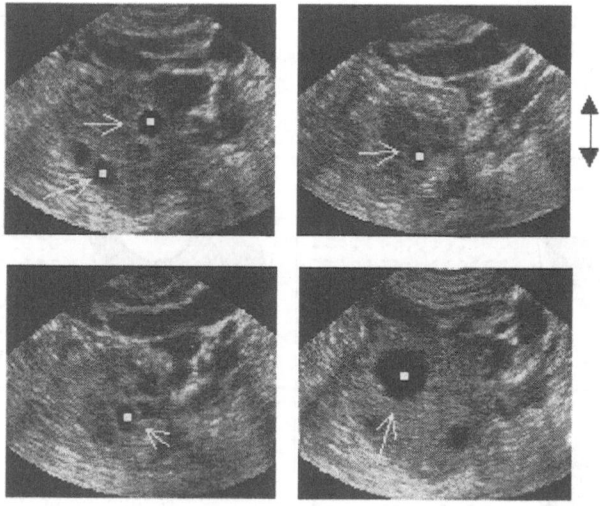

Fig. 4. 2D echographic slices from the 3D dataset. Follicles appear as black circles (yellow (white) arrows). Detected follicle centres are marked yellow (white), oversized for clarity. Length arrow: 1 cm

In 1D the homotopy class number boils down to the difference of the sign of the signals second derivative taken from the left and from the right. We will use the 'edge focusing' multiscale behaviour of this 1D number in the sequel for the characterisation of multiple points on the surface of the follicle. The theory of homotopy numbers can easily be extended to subdimensional manifolds (strings, surfaces) in higher dimensions and for other vectorfields, such as the frames spanned by the eigenvectors of the Hessian, or any other well defined vectorfield [9].

5   The Detection of Follicle Centres and Boundary Points by 3D and 2D Topological Numbers

The winding number in 3D is computed by adding the increments in orientation angle of the gradient vector when moving the gradient over a closed surface around the point of study, e.g. along the 6, 8 or 26 neighbouring pixels. Because we need detection of the minima of extended structures, i.e. the follicles, which are much larger then the noise grains of the raw data, we need to move to a higher scale of analysis (i.e. blur). We perform the following steps for the automatic detection of the follicles:

– isotropic blurring of the 3D ultrasound data, and the establishment of an optimal scale in the sense of minimising the number of false-positives; a too small scale gives too many minima, a too large scale too few;
– calculation of 3D winding numbers as estimators for the follicle centres; this gives their number and spatial distribution;
– generation of 200–500 radial rays in a homogeneous orientation distribution from these centres and determine the most pronounced 1D intensity edge along the ray by its 'lifetime' over scale;
– fit spherical harmonics functions to some order to the detected endpoints in order to get an analytical description of the shape of the follicle; from this the volume can easily be calculated, and statistics on shape.

In Fig. 4 we show a typical result for a patient dataset; the detected winding numbers are indicated as yellow (white) dots, indicated by arrows. The winding numbers do not show up in all follicles because only the slices through the follicle centres are shown. From the winding number locations, 200–500 rays (1D profiles) are drawn in all directions, and a maximum length of 32 pixels. The search for the most prominent contrast step along the rays is done by edge focusing of the 1D winding number over scales 0 to 2 pixels in increments of 0.1.

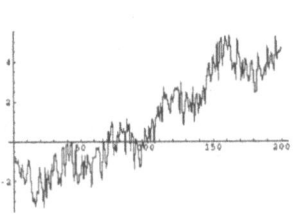
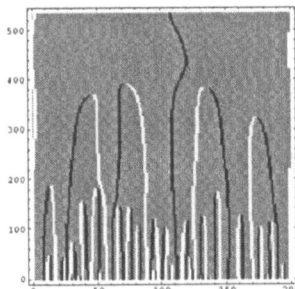

Fig. 5. Hierarchical multiscale edge detection. Left: noisy 1D intensity profile Right: sign of the second derivative (subtraction of neighbours) as a function of scale. Scale (vertical axis) ranging from 1 to 5 pixel units. The sign of the second derivative (black −, white +) is plotted as a function of scale. Note the closure of the extrema (causality in a linear scale-space)

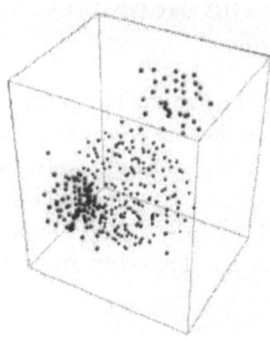 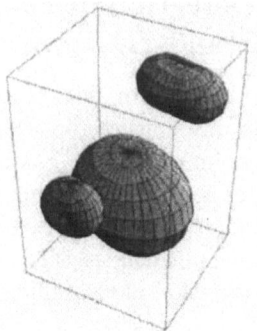

Fig. 6. Left: 3D scatterplot of the detected edgepoints of three bovine ovary follicles. Right: the corresponding fitted spherical harmonics. Note the irregular shape of the follicles

Figure 5 shows an example where seemingly no edge is present but where at high scale one edge emerges despite the noise, which is traced down to the lowest scale. The longest lifetime is taken as a measure of importance of the edge, indicating a follicle boundary point. When more edges survive at $\sigma = 2$ pixels we decided to take the edge at $\sigma = 2$ pixels which is closest to the centre of the follicle. The detected edgepoints are then fitted with 3D spherical harmonic functions $Y_l^m(\Theta, \phi)$ using *Mathematica*[TM1]. Spherical harmonics are orthogonal functions with respect to integration over the surface of the unit sphere, and form a natural basis for the description of (in our case convex) 3D shape. The advantages of spherical harmonics are the wide range of shapes that can be modelled, giving explicit knowledge about the deviation from a pure spherical shape, and that the volume of the follicle can easily be calculated by analytical integration.

Figure 6 shows a set of detected points, and the corresponding 3D fit by spherical harmonics. The method was tested on artificial data: 3 spherical test follicles with diameters of 3, 6 and 12 pixels (intensity 0) in a 643 pixel cube (background intensity 1) with additive and uncorrelated Gaussian noise of $\sigma = 0.1, 0.25, 0.5$ and 1.0 intensity unit. Figure 1 shows a plane with some of the 225 edgepoints detected by edge focusing for the largest follicle in the noisy test dataset ($\sigma = 0.25$) and a blurring scale of 6 pixels. The detection works well, and the average radii were correct within a half a pixel for all tests. The detection of follicle minima from the 3D US data by 3D winding numbers is scale-dependent and we need multiple scales. Some follicles are only detected at small scales, other at large scales.

---

[1] *Mathematica* commands to generate the spherical harmonics to 4th order and do the fitting:
```
fitset = Table[SphericalHarmonicY[l,m,Θ,φ],{m,-l,l,1},{l,0,4}];
fitted[Θ,φ] = Fit[data,fitset,{Θ,φ}];
ParametricPlot3D[fitted[Θ,φ]{Cos[Θ],Sin[Θ] Cos[φ],Sin[Θ] Sin[φ]},
  {Θ,0,π},{φ,0,π}];
```

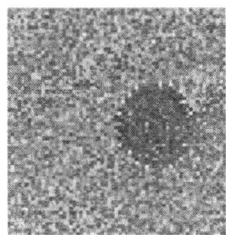

Fig. 7. Edgepoints are successfully detected on the surface of the follicle in the noisy testset. Background intensity 1, follicle intensity 0. Additive uncorrelated Gaussian noise: $\sigma = 0.25$. Blurring scale 6 pixels. Image resolution 64^2 pixels. The detected edgepoints are indicated as dots on the ultrasound image

Figure 1 shows the detected number for blurring scales 3, 4, 6 and 10 pixels. At $\sigma = 3$ pixels, many minima are detected, but also many false positives. At scale $\sigma = 4$ pixels (without scale $\sigma = 3$ pixels) only one minimum is missed. At $\sigma = 6$ pixels we have little errors, but also few new detections. At $\sigma = 10$ pixels we have no errors, we only detect the large follicle(s). These cannot be seen at smaller scales, due to the impossibility to detect minima at a small scale in a homogeneous region of a follicle (i.e. the follicle is large relative to the size of the operator). This leads to the conclusion that two scales suffice: $\sigma = 3$ and $\sigma = 10$ cover the detection range well for the 3D US datasets. Processing times for typical datasets ($150 \times 150 \times 150$ pixels) take about 1 minute per scale on a 300 MHz Pentium II PC.

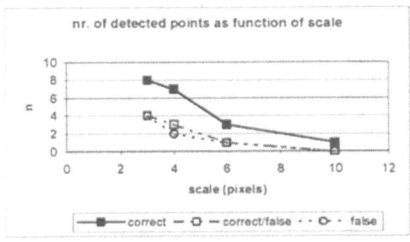

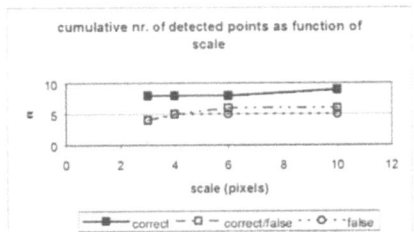

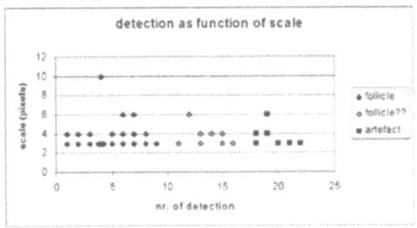

Fig. 8. Upper left: number of detected points as a function of scale. Upper right: cumulated number of detected points. Lower left: Diagram of detected follicles in bovine ovary II as a function of the blurring scale (vertical scale, in pixels)

False positive winding numbers also generated 225 edgepoints which should be discarded. If such a winding number emerged as a noise minimum, the set of edgepoints can be tested for roundness i.e. discriminated by the large variance of the detected radii length, or a test can be done on the (low) intensity of the internal pixels of the pseudo-follicle. This turned out to be very difficult due to the great variability in echo amplitude output. If the false winding number is due to another structure (vessel, another follicle) the shape derived from the edgepoint fit may discriminate. We have not performed this test yet. However, if the data is cut off in such a way as only to include the ovary, such detections are unlikely to occur. We employed this strategy as much as possible, because it is a fairly easy task to restrict the Cartesian volume to the ovarian space after scanning.

The algorithm was implemented in a universal image analysis program written in Borland C++ (Image Explorer by van Ginneken and Staal (ISI)).

6   Validation of the Detection Procedures with Bovine Ovaries

To calibrate the full range of steps of the automatic detection procedure, two fresh bovine ovaries with multiple follicles of widely different diameters were used as test objects. The thumbsize ovaries were subsequently:

- scanned with 3D–US, immersed in physiological salt solution and with the 3D ultrasound probe at the same typical object–probe distance (2–4 cm) as applied on female patients; three subsequent acquisitions with different probe positions;
- scanned with high resolution FSE (fast spin–echo pulse sequence) MRI: slice thickness 0.5 mm, non–overlapping, in–plane pixelsize 100×100 μ, TR = 20 ms, TE = 75 ms; (An example 2D slice from the 3D MRI is given in Fig. 4.)
- sliced with a microtome, embedded in CMC (carboxymethylcellulose) and after freezing (-30 to -35 $^{\circ}$C), into anatomical coupes of 25 micron thickness. Image resolution 1528×1146 at 100–micron intervals with a digital camera (300 images, no histological staining).

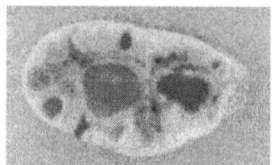 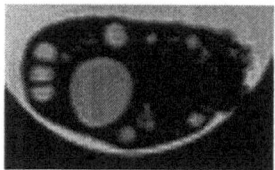 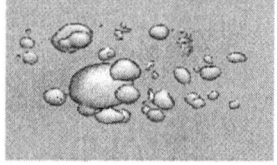

Fig. 9. Calibration of the automated method with two bovine ovaries. Left: Anatomical coupe. Middle: Coronal MRI, FSE. Right: 3D surface rendering of the follicles from the MRI acquisition shows their spatial relationship. Segmentation by thresholding

We analysed the 3D–US data with scales $\sigma = 3, 4, 6$ and 10 pixels. The cumulated number of pixels detected as a function of scale for the first bovine ovary is indicated in Fig. 9 (left). For $\sigma = 3$ we find 11 follicles detected, when also scale $\sigma = 4$ is included, we find 12. Adding $\sigma = 6$ we find 13, and adding $\sigma = 10$ no extra follicle is added. If we start from a slightly higher scale, i.e. $\sigma = 4$, we see in Fig. 9 (right) that only 5 follicles are detected, then adding $\sigma = 3$ gives 12 detected. Only scales $\sigma = 4$ and $\sigma = 6$ gives 7 detected follicles, and only scales $\sigma = 3$ and 6 gives 13 detected. The conclusion here is that two scales suffice: $\sigma = 3$ and $\sigma = 10$. If computing time is no penalty, $\sigma = 6$ could be added.

The images from MRI and anatomical slices were analysed with standard image visualisation and measurement tools. The 3D-ultrasound data were acquired three times individually. The method of winding numbers introduces negligible dislocation of the minima despite the wide range of blurring scales, as can be seen in Table 1 where the x, y, z co–ordinates, the distances between the minima and the volumes of the three largest follicles of each acquisition is given. The average diameters (over 3 perpendicular directions) of the test follicles were measured after identification of the follicles in the corresponding 3D ultrasound datasets. The volume measured from the MRI and anatomical data are estimated from the average diameters and assuming a spherical shape.

Table 1. x, y, z co–ordinates in pixels of the centres of the three largest follicles, from three individual 3D ultrasound acquisitions (v00, v01 and v44) of bovine ovary I. Independent measurements. Note the accurate correspondence in the calculated distances between the winding number points, indicating independence of scale-dependent dislocation. The difference in volume from the spherical harmonics fit was about 4% for the two larger, and 10% for the smallest follicle. The three methods of volume measuring compare very favourably

Follicle #	x centre	y centre	z centre	distance to neighbour (pixels)	volume from spherical harmonics (mm^3)	volume from MRI	volume from anatomy
v00	99	51	35	25.4	259.7	250.0	262.1
	93	28	44	45.0	28.4	27.0	29.8
	113	55	74	41.6	56.2	54.9	59.3
v01	33	41	66	25.3	242.3		
	47	22	75	44.5	34.0		
	64	49	44	38.9	54.7		
v44	72	49	84	25.4	239.7		
	69	28	70	45.2	28.4		
	32	51	82	40.1	59.3		

7   Patient Data

This study focuses on the methodology to automatically count and analyse the follicles from the 3D-ultrasound data, and only limited patient studies have been carried out so far. The follicle count results on 10 patients are shown in Table 2. Each dataset was cut off to include only the ovary immediately after scanning by an experienced echographer, and automatic and human expert counts were compared. We are currently finalising a clinical PC-based system with a user-friendly user–interface. In a next phase of the study the accuracy and efficacy of the method will be evaluated on a large patient group.

8   Conclusion and Discussion

The automatic detection of follicles from 3D ultrasound data is not an easy task, given the strong noise characteristics of the ultrasound signal, the size and contrast of the follicles and the follicle looking like structures in and at the

Table 2. Performance of the algorithm compared with a human expert. Number of follicles found. Data for 6 patients. The datasets are cut off to contain only the ovary. Scales used: $\sigma = 3.6, 4.8, 7.2$ and 12 pixels

Patient #	manual	Computer	Patient #	Manual	computer
1	17	15	4	14	9
2	10	8	5	9	7
3	7	5	6	9	7

immediate neighbourhood of the ovary. Clinically, the most important parameter is the number of follicles. Still, with the introduction of multiscale topological and edge focusing methods we are able to extract the follicles automatically with 95% accuracy. Good cut-off to leave only the ovary region in the resulting 3D datacube by the operator immediately after scanning is an important step to higher score.

We exploit knowledge about the convex shape of the follicles by means of spherical harmonics function fitting. This can be exploited in other ways, such as by a Hough transform, parametrically deformable contours [23] or scale–space primal sketch blobs, each over a range of scales. Our approach however enables a much better accuracy of shape description than e.g. a 5 parameter Hough transform for ellipsoidal shapes [15,16]. The approach is computationally efficient, with just sign differences over 1D signals. The method can now be applied in a larger scale clinical setting, which is scheduled as a next phase of the project.

Acknowledgments. We like to thank Jan Doorn and Gerda van Wieringen of the Dept. of Functional Anatomy, Utrecht University, for the anatomical preparations and digital images of the bovine ovaries, Bram van Ginneken for the effective PC program *Image Explorer* enabling fast implementation. The support of the Foundation for Neural Networks and the Dutch Foundation for Applied Sciences is greatly acknowledged.

References

1. Block, E.: Quantitative Morphological Investigations of the Follicular System in Women. Variations at Different Ages. Acta Anat. **14** (1952) 108-123
2. Broekmans, F.J., Scheffer, G.J., Dorland, M., Blankenstein, M.A., de Jong, F.H., te Velde, E.R.: "Ovarian Reserve Tests in Infertility and in Normal Fertile Women", Maturitas, in press.
3. Chang, M.Y., Chang, C.H., Chiu, T.H., Hsieh, T.T., Soong, Y.K.: The Antral Follicle Count Predicts the Outcome of Pregnancy in a Controlled Ovarian Hyperstimulation/Intrauterine Insemination Program. J. Assisted Reprod. Genet. **15** (1998) 12-17
4. Faddy, M.J., Gosden, R.G., Gougeon, A., Richardsen, S.J., Nelson, J.F.: Accelerated Disappearance of Ovarian Follicles in Mid-Life: Implications for Forecasting Menopause. Human Reproduction. **7** (1992) 1342-1346
5. Feichtinger, W.: Follicle Aspiration with Interactive Three-Dimensional Digital Imaging (Voluson): a Step toward Realtime Puncturing under Three-Dimensional Ultrasound Control. Fertil. Steril. Aug **70** (1998) 374-377

6. Florack, L.M.J., ter Haar Romeny, B.M., Koenderink, J.J., Viergever, M.A.: Scale and the Differential Structure of Images, Image and Vis, Comp. **10** (1992) 376-388
7. Gore, M.A., Nayudu, P.L., Vlaisavljevic, V., Thomas, N.: Prediction of Ovarian Cycle Outcome by Follicular Characteristics, Stage I, Human Reproduction **10** (1995) 2313-2319
8. ter Haar Romeny, B.M., Florack, L.M.J., Koenderink, J.J., Viergever, M.A.: Scale-Space: Its Natural Operators and Differential Invariants, Colchester, A. C. F. and Hawkes, D. J. (Eds.), Proc. Information Processing in Medical Imaging, Lecture Notes in Computer Science **511**, Springer Verlag, Berlin (1991) 239-255
9. Kalitzin, S.: Topological Numbers and Singularities in Scalar Images. Scale-Space Evolution Properties. In: Gaussian Scale-Space Theory, Eds.: J. Sporring, M. Nielsen, L. Florack, P. Johansen, Kluwer Academic Publishers (1997) 181-189
10. Kalitzin, S., ter Haar Romeny, B.M., Viergever, M.A.: On Topological Deep-Structure Segmentation. In: Proc. Intern. Conf. on Image processing, Santa Barbara, CA (1997) 863-866,
11. Kalitzin, S., ter Haar Romeny, B.M., Salden, A.H., Nacken, P.F.M., Viergever, M.A.: Topological Numbers and Singularities in Scalar Images: Scale-Space Evolution Properties. J. of Math. Imaging and Vision **7** (1998), In press.
12. Kemeter, P., Feichtinger, W.: Ultrasound Monitoring of Follicle Growth in IVF. Wien Med. Wochenschr. **141** (1991) 9-13
13. Marsden, J.E., Tromba, A.J.: "Vector Calculus", W.H. Freeman and Company, New York, 4th edition (1996)
14. Peluso, J.J., Damien, M., Nulsen, J.C., Luciano, A.A.: Identification of Follicles with Fertilizable Oocytes by Sequential Ultrasound Measurements during Follicular Development. J. In Vitro Fert. Embryo. Transf. **7** (1990) 304-309
15. Potocnik, B., Zazula, D, and Korze, D.: Automated Computer-Assisted Detection of Follicles in Ultrasound Images of Ovary, Proceedings CBMS 97, Maribor, Slovenia, 11- 13 June 1997, pp. 16-21. And in: J. Med. Syst. **21** (1997) 445-57
16. Potocnik, B., Zazula D., and Solina, F.: Classical Image Processing vs. Computer Vision Techniques in Automated Computer-Assisted Detection of Follicles in Ultrasound Images of Ovary, Proceedings IPA 97, Dublin, Ireland (1997) 551-555,
17. Riccabona, M., Nelson, T.R., Pretorius, D.H.: Three-Dimensional Ultrasound: Accuracy of Distance and Volume Measurements. Ultrasound Obstet. Gynecol. **7** (1996) 429-434
18. Richardsen, S.J., Senikas, V., Nelson, J.F.: Follicular Depletion during the Menopausal Transition: Evidence for Accelerated Loss and Ultimate Exhaustion. J. Clin. Endocrinol. Metab. **65** (1987) 1231-1237
19. Robinson, R., Chakraborty, A., Johnson, M., Reuss, M.L., Duncan, J.: Segmentation of Ovarian Follicles using Geometric Properties, Texture Descriptions and Boundary Information, SPIE **2710** (1996) 321-330
20. Ruess, M.L., Kline, J., Santos, R., Levin, B., Timor-Tritsch, I.: Age and the Ovarian Follicle Pool Assessed with Transvaginal Ultrasonography. Am. J. Obstet. Gynecol. **174** (1996) 624-627
21. Sarty, G.E., Sonka, M., Liang, W., Pierson, R.A.: The Development of an Automatic Follicle Isolation Tool for Ovarian Ultrasonographic Images, Proc. SPIE Medical Imaging: Image Processing (1997) 822-829
22. Sarty, G.E., Liang, W., Sonka, M., Pierson, R.A.: Semi-automated Segmentation of Ovarian Follicular Ultrasound Images using a Knowledge-based Algorithm. Ultrasound Med. Biol. **24** (1998) 27-42
23. Staib, L.H., Duncan, J.S.: Boundary Finding with Parametrically Deformable Models, IEEE Tr. PAMI **14** (1992) 1061-1075

Volume Measurement in Sequential Freehand 3-D Ultrasound

Graham Treece[1], Richard Prager[1], Andrew Gee[1], and Laurence Berman[2]

[1] Department of Engineering, University of Cambridge, Trumpington Street,
Cambridge, UK, CB2 1PZ,
{gmt11, rwp, ahg}@eng.cam.ac.uk
[2] Department of Radiology, University of Cambridge, Addenbrooke's Hospital,
Cambridge, UK, CB2 2QQ,
lb@radiol.cam.ac.uk

Abstract. It has previously been demonstrated that using 3-D rather than 2-D ultrasound can increase the accuracy of volume measurements. Unfortunately, the time required to produce them is also increased. While *freehand* 3-D ultrasound allows complete freedom of movement during scanning, the resulting B-scans are generally resampled onto a low resolution, regular voxel array before subsequent processing — increasing the time even further. In contrast, *sequential* freehand 3-D ultrasound does not require a voxel array, and hence both the data resolution and the processing times are improved. Such a system is presented here, incorporating three novel algorithms, each operating directly on non-parallel B-scans. Volume is measured using *Cubic planimetry*, which requires fewer planes than step-section planimetry for a given accuracy. *Maximal disc guided interpolation* can be used to interpolate non-parallel cross-sections. *Regularised marching tetrahedra* can then be used to provide a regular triangulation of the zero iso-surface of the interpolated data. The first of these algorithms is presented in detail in this paper.

1 Introduction

There has been much research in the last two decades on systems which allow the construction and visualisation of three dimensional (3-D) images from medical ultrasound data. One of the more compelling applications where 3-D ultrasound can provide a real benefit is in the accurate measurement of volume. This is important in several anatomical areas, for instance the heart [7], foetus [5], placenta [8], kidney [6], prostate [1], bladder and eye [11]. Measurements have traditionally been made with 2-D ultrasound, but it is generally accepted that 3-D ultrasound can provide much greater accuracy.

Freehand 3-D ultrasound allows the clinician unrestricted movement of the ultrasound probe. The ultrasound images (B-scans) are digitised and stored in a computer. In addition, the position and orientation of the probe is measured and recorded with each B-scan. The various 3-D ultrasound systems are reviewed in [5]. One of the disadvantages of freehand scanning is that the recorded B-scans

A. Kuba et al. (Eds.): IPMI'99, LNCS 1613, pp. 70–83, 1999.

are not parallel — this makes processing of the data more complex, hence most systems interpolate this data to a regular 3-D voxel array, or *cuberille*. However, this can take considerable time and generate potentially misleading artifacts.

By contrast, in *sequential* freehand 3-D ultrasound, the original B-scan data, and the order of acquisition of the B-scans, are maintained throughout the subsequent processing. This reduces the time from scanning to display, at a cost of a slight increase in processing time for *each* display. Moreover, any sequential method which does not require human interaction[1] has the potential to be performed *during scanning*, greatly decreasing the residual (post scanning) processing time.

It has already been demonstrated that re-slice displays (i.e. 2-D displays in new orientations) and panoramic displays (i.e. 2-D displays with extended coverage) can be performed efficiently by sequential methods [14]. Resampling is only performed once, rather than once to the cuberille and once again to the viewing plane, which leads to increased quality displays. This paper demonstrates that volume measurements and organ surfaces can also be efficiently estimated in a sequential manner. Segmentation remains the most complex and time consuming step in this process. In view of this, the proposed algorithms are designed for *sparse cross-sections*, to limit the time spent segmenting, in *non-parallel planes*, so the segmentation can be performed in the original B-scans (which do not suffer from interpolation artifacts). Reducing total organ volume measurement time is particularly important in a clinical setting.

2 Volume Measurement Using Ultrasound

2.1 Sequential Volume Measurement from Scan Plane Data

Volume measurement using conventional 2-D ultrasound is achieved by approximating the organ of interest as an ellipsoid, or some other simple shape, and estimating the main dimensions from appropriate B-scans. A correction is then made to the result, dependent on the organ, the age and sex of the patient and other factors. There are many formulations for the resulting equations [8,16].

Ellipsoid formulae are easy to use, but they make geometrical assumptions about the shape of a given organ, leading to errors in the volume measurement which can be greater than 20%. *Planimetry* is an alternative approach, made possible with 3-D ultrasound, in which object cross-sections are outlined on each scan plane, and the volume is calculated from the cross-sectional areas and plane positions. The most common implementation of this is step-section planimetry, which assumes that the cross-sections are parallel.

There are numerous reports which indicate that step-section planimetry is much more accurate than ellipsoid or other geometrical formulae [1,13,15]. In one exception, planimetry was compared with 16 equations for measuring prostatic volume and $\frac{\pi}{6}(transverse\ diameter)^2(anteroposterior\ diameter)$ was found to be

---

[1] All the algorithms presented here are fully automatic, save segmentation.

marginally more accurate [16]. However, planimetry has recently been shown to have much better intra- and inter-observer variability [17].

Freehand 3-D ultrasound does not generate data on parallel planes. Volume measurement is most often achieved by interpolating to form a cuberille, then segmenting the entire cuberille, resulting in a set of parallel cross-sections whose volume can be measured using step-section planimetry. This is equivalent to counting the voxels inside the object.

There are two alternatives to this approach, which do not require the creation of a cuberille, and hence can in general be performed sequentially. The first is an extension of planimetry developed by Watanabe [20] to non-parallel, and even overlapping, cross-sections, which has been used to determine the volume of the prostate [2]. The second, and more common, is to estimate the surface directly from the cross-sections, then calculate the volume of this surface.

2.2   Volume Measurement from Surface Reconstructions

Surface estimation is generally achieved by triangulation between neighbouring cross-sections. Such techniques have been developed for *parallel* cross-sections, but can usually be adapted for slightly non-parallel cases. Even for parallel cases, estimating the surface in a robust manner is difficult, which is evident from the wealth of related literature.

Once the surface of an object has been estimated, the volume can be calculated by several different methods, dependent on surface representation.

Tetrahedral Volume. If the surface has been estimated by forming tetrahedra, the volume can be calculated from the sum of the volumes of these tetrahedra. Alternatively, the polyhedral approximation formula developed in [4] can be used. This is based on tetrahedral volume, but formulated in terms of the points making up the object cross-section on each plane. Although this appears to allow volume calculation from cross-sections without triangulation, in fact a simple triangulation is assumed in the algorithm which will only be correct for simple shapes. This technique is used, for instance, in [7].

Cylindrical/Pyramidal Volume. If the scanning pattern is rotational, parts of cross-sections can be connected with the mid-point of the rotation to form pyramidal or cylindrical part sections, from which the volume can be calculated. This technique has been used for the eye [11]. Moritz also applied it to freehand scans by re-sampling these scans in a rotational pattern and then calculating the volume from the new cross-sections [12].

Volume from Triangulation. Hughes has suggested two ways of measuring the volume directly from a triangulated surface. 'Ray Tracing' involves projecting rays from a 2-D grid through the object, and calculating the volume from the length of the part of each ray contained by the object [9]. Alternatively, a discrete version of Gauss' theorem can be adapted to calculate the volume component for each individual triangle such that the sum of these components is equivalent to the object volume [10].

Comparisons of some of the various freehand volume measurement techniques have been performed [9] — it is clear that any of the non-geometrical methods are to be preferred over the ellipsoid equations [7]. There are two areas that warrant further research, in the context of sequential volume measurement. Firstly, it is suggested in the literature [2,20] that using a cubic interpolant would increase the accuracy of the, already flexible, non-parallel planimetry technique. However, this has never previously been reported. Secondly, a sequential surface estimation algorithm is required which can handle cross-sections with the same complex topology and arbitrary orientation as this planimetry technique.

3   A Sequential Volume Measurement System

A fast and accurate volume measurement system has been incorporated into Stradx[2] [14]. Stradx is a flexible *sequential* freehand 3-D ultrasound tool which can be used to grab ultrasound video images and orientation information and display these in various ways, including re-slicing and panoramic displays, without creating a cuberille. The volume measurement system includes three novel algorithms for estimating volume, interpolating segmented data and triangulating the iso-surface of this data, all from the original freehand B-scans. The first of these algorithms, for estimating volume, is presented in detail in Sect. 4.

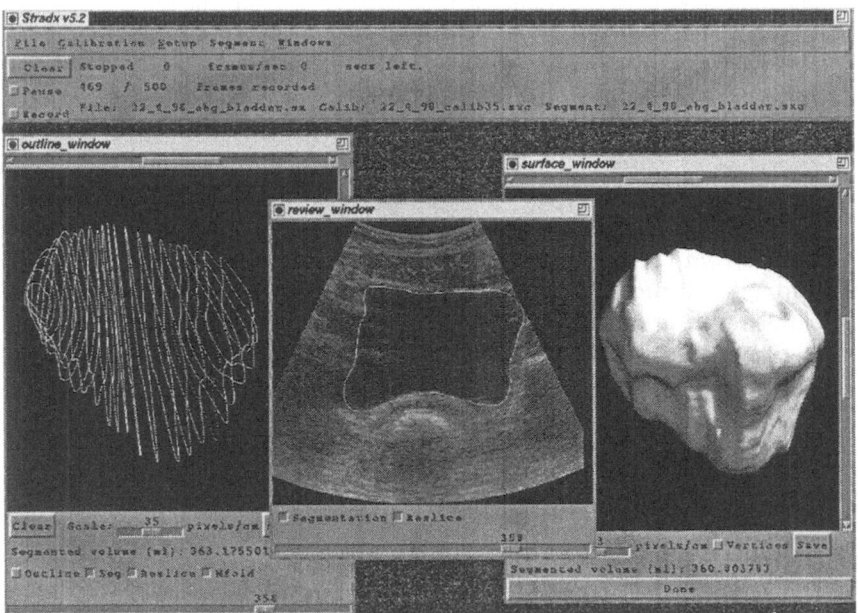

Fig. 1. Stradx v5.2 interface

---

[2] http://svr-www.eng.cam.ac.uk/~rwp/stradx/.

Figure 1 is an example of the interface provided for this purpose. The steps in the volume estimation are as follows.

Manual segmentation. This is performed by the clinician on a subset of the original B-scans, using a mouse (the **review_window** in Fig. 1). Although many automatic segmentation algorithms have been investigated, none are flexible enough to be used for generic ultrasound data in a manner which is faster than manual segmentation. This is no surprise — often the clinician will draw a cross-section through apparently featureless data, guided only be their prior knowledge of the organ shape and a 3-D reconstruction they have in their head. Semi-automatic segmentation methods which *do* use prior models are generally difficult to use, because it is hard to make the model both flexible enough to be used in different circumstances and detailed enough to be helpful.

Real-time display of cross-sections. The cross-sections are displayed in 3-D wire-frame format as they are drawn (the **outline_window** in Fig. 1). This provides feedback on both the shape and the spacing of the cross-sections, allowing the clinician to concentrate on the more complicated areas.

Real-time volume estimate. As the cross-sections are completed, a real-time volume estimate is calculated using *cubic planimetry* (the volume in the **outline_window** of Fig. 1), described in more detail in Sect. 4.

Surface estimation and display. Estimation and display of the object surface is useful for giving the clinician confidence in the segmentation. In order to achieve this, a distance field is calculated from the cross-sections, and an iso-surface triangulation algorithm used to extract the zero surface of this field (the **surface_window** of Fig. 1). This is a more robust method than triangulating the cross-sections directly. The distance field is calculated from the non-parallel cross-sections using *maximal disc guided shape based interpolation*, described in [19], which is a fast, simple method that can handle complex cross-sections. The iso-surface is triangulated using *regularised marching tetrahedra*, described in [18], another fast method which generates triangles with good aspect ratios.

Secondary volume estimate from surface. The volume of the triangulated surface can be calculated by a variant of Gauss' theorem [9] (the volume in the **surface_window** of Fig. 1). Although this is less accurate than the cubic planimetry volume [19], similarity between the volume estimates gives confidence in the cubic planimetry volume.

4 Cubic Planimetry

4.1 Volume from Arbitrarily Oriented Planes

The equation for the volume v of any object defined from sequential cross-sections is given by Watanabe [20] as

$$v = \left| \int_L \boldsymbol{s} \cdot d\boldsymbol{\omega} \right| \tag{1}$$

where $\boldsymbol{\omega}$ is the position vector of the centroid of the cross-sectional surface S whose vector area is given by $\boldsymbol{s}$, and L is the path of $\boldsymbol{\omega}$ as the object is scanned. Equation (1) can be evaluated discretely by approximating the integral using the trapezoidal rule between each pair of slices, which gives

$$v = \left| \sum_{i=2}^{N} \frac{1}{2} \left(\boldsymbol{s}_i + \boldsymbol{s}_{i-1} \right) \cdot \left(\boldsymbol{\omega}_i - \boldsymbol{\omega}_{i-1} \right) \right| \tag{2}$$

where N cross-sections have vector areas $\boldsymbol{s}_1, \ldots, \boldsymbol{s}_N$ and centroids $\boldsymbol{\omega}_1, \ldots, \boldsymbol{\omega}_N$. This approximation is equivalent to assuming that the surface area projected onto a plane normal to the path of the centroids, L, varies linearly from one slice to the next. This is clearly true for objects whose cross-sectional area does not vary, e.g. prisms, and in this case (2) is the exact solution. Paraboloids also have this property. However, objects which are either more concave or more convex than a paraboloid will not be correctly approximated by this equation. For example, the volume of a cone will be overestimated, and that of a sphere or an ellipsoid will be underestimated. The error increases as the number of scan planes reduces.

Equation (2) can easily be implemented on a computer once the cross-sections have been determined and the areas and centroids calculated. In practice, the first step is by far the most time consuming, typically taking half a minute or so for each cross-section for manual segmentation. Once this has been done, the calculation of the volume is trivially fast in comparison (a few milliseconds).

Clearly, some form of cubic rather than trapezoidal interpolation would increase the accuracy of the volume estimate and eliminate the bias towards paraboloids or prisms. It has been argued [2] that the small increase in accuracy this would represent does not justify the additional complexity that would be required. However, two points can be made in defence of this approach. Firstly, the additional complexity is completely transparent to the user — once the algorithm has been implemented, the user performs precisely the same operations (i.e. outlining of the cross-sections) in both cases. Secondly, the reduction in the number of cross-sections required for an accurate volume estimation with cubic planimetry is very welcome, since segmentation is the time consuming step in the process. We present results to demonstrate this advantage in Sect. 5.

4.2   2-D Representation of the Problem

Interestingly, the whole problem can be reduced to finding the area of a carefully constructed 2-D graph which represents a combination of the original 3-D object with the scanning pattern. The equivalence between the 3-D and 2-D representations is shown in Fig. 2.

The area enclosed within the dashed and solid lines in the 2-D representation is equivalent to the volume which would be calculated by Watanabe's trapezoidal equation from the 3-D representation. This can be easily proved by considering the 2-D representation to have a nominal thickness of 1 unit, and then applying

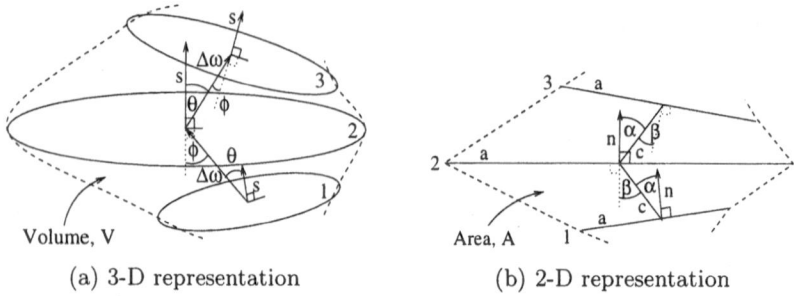

(a) 3-D representation   (b) 2-D representation

Fig. 2. 3-D and 2-D representation equivalence. i) The length of a 2-D line, a, is equivalent to the area of the cross-section, $|s|$. ii) The length of the line, c, is equal to the magnitude of the vector, $|\Delta\omega|$. iii) The angle, α, between the line c joining the centres of each line a and the normal to those lines is equal to the angle, θ, between the vector area s and the vector $\Delta\omega$ joining the centroids of each area. iv) Similarly, the angle, β, is equal to the angle, ϕ

(2) to calculate the area

$$
A = \left| \sum_{i=2}^{N} \frac{1}{2} (a_i \hat{n}_i + a_{i-1}\hat{n}_{i-1}) \cdot (c_{i-1}) \right|
$$

$$
= \left| \sum_{i=2}^{N} \frac{|c_{i-1}|}{2} (a_i \hat{n}_i \cdot \hat{c}_{i-1} + a_{i-1}\hat{n}_{i-1} \cdot \hat{c}_{i-1}) \right|
$$

$$
= \left| \sum_{i=2}^{N} \frac{|c_{i-1}|}{2} (a_i \cos\beta + a_{i-1}\cos\alpha) \right|. \tag{3}
$$

Equation (2) can be similarly re-written as

$$
v = \left| \sum_{i=2}^{N} \frac{|\Delta\omega_{i-1}|}{2} (|s_i|\cos\phi + |s_{i-1}|\cos\theta) \right| \tag{4}
$$

If the variables in (3) and (4) are equated for all values of i, then $A \equiv v$. There is, however, significant redundancy in this conversion. Firstly, only the multiple of the lengths of the lines a and c is used, and hence an arbitrary scale factor can be multiplied into one, so long as it is divided from the other. This has the effect of stretching or shrinking the 2-D graph, but has no bearing on the volume calculation. Secondly, only the cosine of the angles α and β are used, hence they can be arbitrarily positive or negative. The effect of this choice is demonstrated in Fig. 3.

Although the choice of angles has no effect on the volume calculated by the trapezoidal method, it clearly does affect how well the 2-D representation matches the original 3-D representation. Cubic interpolation involves the use of information from several sequential slices and, therefore, an additional heuristic rule is required to ensure that the angles α and β are chosen correctly.

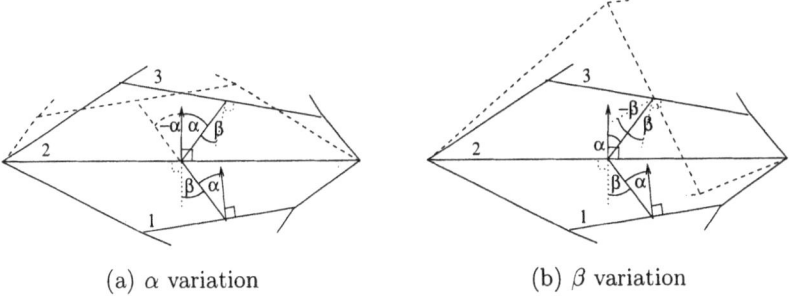

(a) α variation   (b) β variation

Fig. 3. Choice of angles for 2-D representation

For each choice of angle α between the line joining centroids c_i and the area representation a_i, the angle which c_i makes with c_{i-1} is also calculated. The value of α is then chosen for which this calculated angle is closest to the 3-D version (i.e. the angle which $\Delta\omega_i$ makes with $\Delta\omega_{i-1}$). A similar rule is employed for the angle β, using the area normals rather than the lines joining the centroids as the reference.

The result of this entire process is shown for an ellipsoid in Fig. 4. The ellipsoid was sliced with a scanning pattern which varied in position, azimuth, elevation and roll. The resulting 2-D graph retains some of the shape of the ellipsoid but also reflects the way in which it was scanned.

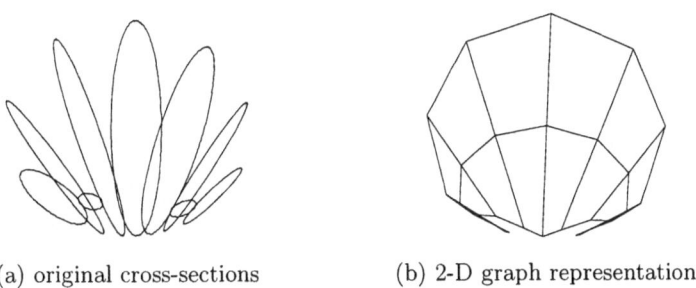

(a) original cross-sections   (b) 2-D graph representation

Fig. 4. Freehand scanned ellipsoid in 3-D and 2-D representations

4.3   Cubic Interpolation of 2-D Representation

If instead of joining the end points of the lines a with straight lines, a smooth curve is fitted between them, then the area enclosed by these curves should represent a more accurate measure of the volume of the original object. The curves must at least be cubic, since we would like to have continuity in at least the first derivative (i.e. the curves are smooth at the joints). They must also be defined parametrically, since we expect them to have multiple values in both x and y directions.

The smoothest possible curve could be obtained by fitting an appropriate function through all the end-points simultaneously. However, this sort of global optimisation is in general costly to compute, which would violate one of the motivations for improving the volume calculation, namely that the increase in processing time is negligible. A less optimal but faster solution can be found by using parametric cubic splines. We require a spline which *interpolates* the control points, i.e. the resulting curve passes through the points which are used to define it. This can be achieved with a spline introduced by Catmull and Rom [3], which uses four sequential control points (in our case the end points of the lines a), fitting a curve between the middle two of these points.

The first and last curve segments are necessarily a special case, since only three points can be used to fit the curve. There are a variety of ways of handling this, which can all be implemented by inventing an additional control point. If this is chosen to be the same as the second to last point, the effect is to place a null gradient constraint at the end point, which results in a rate of change of gradient of zero. Figure 5 shows the curve for the same situation as in Fig. 4, together with the actual curve which results from scanning in smaller steps.

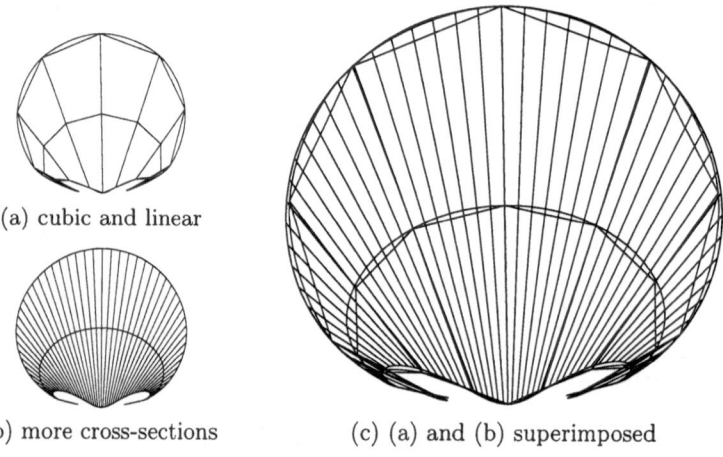

(a) cubic and linear

(b) more cross-sections   (c) (a) and (b) superimposed

Fig. 5. Cubic and linear interpolations compared with actual 2-D graph for a scanned ellipsoid. The actual volume is 2.009. (a) the linear planimetry volume is 1.857 (92.4%), and cubic volume is 1.989 (99.0%). (b) using linear planimetry with more cross-sections gives 2.008 (99.9%)

Once the curves joining the end points of the lines a have been defined, the area enclosed by them can be calculated directly from the parametric coefficients of each curve. This calculation is based on the application of (1), and is given in Appendix A.

5   Results

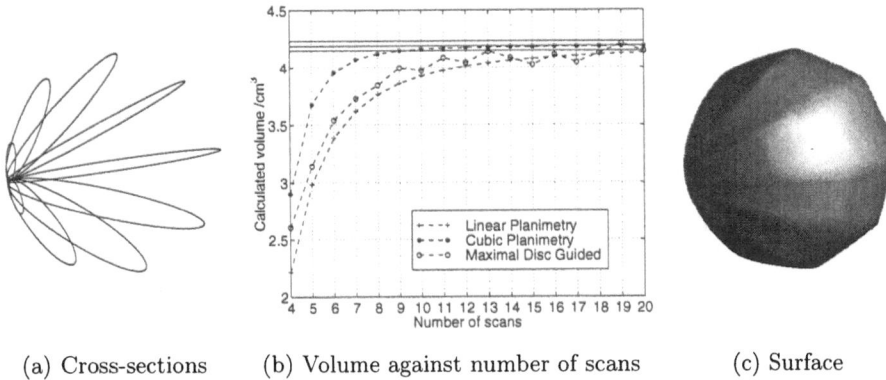

(a) Cross-sections   (b) Volume against number of scans   (c) Surface

Fig. 6. Results: Sphere, scanned using a fanning action

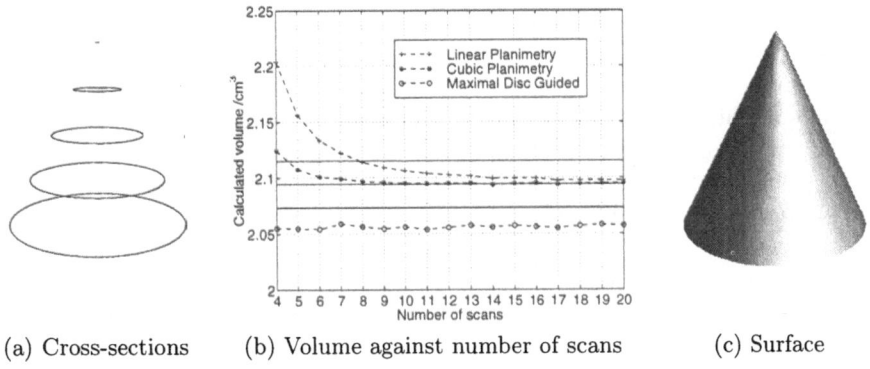

(a) Cross-sections   (b) Volume against number of scans   (c) Surface

Fig. 7. Results: Cone, scanned using a linear sweep

In order to verify the accuracy of the volume measurement algorithm, a computer simulation was constructed in which mathematical objects could be 'scanned' with freehand sweep patterns, and pre-segmented cross-sections generated. The results of this process are shown for a sphere, a cone and a 'baseball glove' shape in Figs. 6, 7 and 8 (a more thorough investigation is reported in [19]). The number of scans was varied in each case from 4 to 20, keeping the first and last scans fixed. The graphs show the volume measurements, using linear and cubic planimetry, and from a surface estimated with maximal disc guided

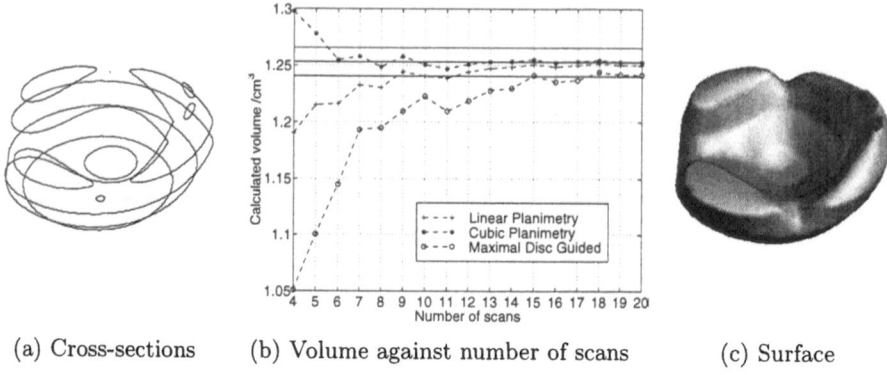

(a) Cross-sections   (b) Volume against number of scans   (c) Surface

Fig. 8. Results: Glove shape, scanned using a linear sweep

interpolation. Solid horizontal lines indicate the actual volume and a margin of ±1%. Cross-sections and surfaces are displayed for the minimum number of scans for which the cubic planimetry volume was within this margin.

It is clear from these graphs that the cubic planimetry volume converges much faster than the alternative volume measurements — very few cross-sections are required to give an accuracy better than ±1%. This is the case both for complex shapes and freehand scanning patterns. In addition, maximal disc guided interpolation creates surfaces from these cross-sections which are good approximations of the actual shapes.

In order to validate *in vivo* volume measurements, the actual volume must be known. This can be done for the human bladder, by measuring the amount of voiding. The input to the bladder is difficult to measure, but can be estimated from sequential volume measurements in periods with no voiding. The bladder wall is very well defined by ultrasound, and is therefore easier to segment than, for instance, the kidney.

Ten scans were performed of an initially full bladder, in pairs, with partial voiding between each pair. The bladder was completely voided after the eighth scan. The scans were performed in fast sequence, the output being collected for later measurement, in order to limit the amount of bladder filling during the experiment. The output was then measured using a 20ml or 60ml graded syringe (dependent on the volume) to an accuracy of approximately 1ml. The stored ultrasound B-scans were then segmented, using 15 to 20 cross-sections per examination: Figure 9(a) shows an example of this. Volumes calculated from these cross-sections using cubic planimetry are tabulated in Table 1.

The amount of bladder filling was estimated in three stages. Firstly, the linear rate of filling was calculated, for each pair of scans, from the volume measurements. Secondly, cubic splines were used to interpolate these values and give a continuous bladder filling rate. Thirdly, this function was integrated, to give the estimated amount by which the bladder had filled at any point during the experiment. This information was used to estimate the actual bladder volume

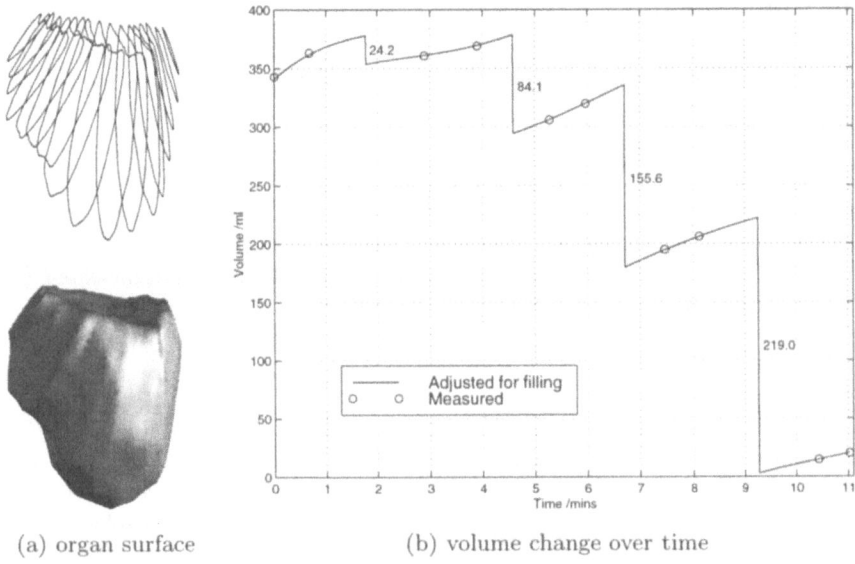

(a) organ surface   (b) volume change over time

Fig. 9. Results: Human bladder. The bladder was partially voided four times during the examination. Two sets of scans were recorded between each partial voiding. The data is tabulated in Table 1

at any point in time. The resulting curve is shown in Fig. 9(b), along with the estimated amount of voiding from this curve.

Table 1. Results: Human bladder. **Fill** is the estimated rate at which the bladder was filling. **Diff** is the calculated difference in volumes, adjusted for bladder filling, and **Void** is the actual measured output. The interpolated volume and difference are shown graphically in Fig. 9(b)

Time, m:s	00:00	00:40	02:54	03:54	05:17	05:58	07:28	08:07	10:26	11:02
Volume, ml	342.7	363.4	360.9	369.2	306.0	319.8	194.8	206.2	14.7	20.3
Fill, ml/min	30.7		8.3		20.0		17.5		9.3	
Diff, ml		24.2		84.1		155.6		219.0		
Void, ml		25		74		156		234		
Error, %		1.6		6.8		0.1		3.2		

The errors in Table 1 are calculated for the *actual volume measurements,* rather than the amount of voiding. The amount of voiding is a complicated function of the volume measurements, due to the adjustments for bladder fill rate. Since it is essentially a measure of difference, the actual volume errors are assumed to *add* to give the voiding error, hence these errors are approximated to be half the voiding error.

6   Conclusions

Cubic planimetry allows accurate measurement of volume with sequential free-hand 3-D ultrasound. None of the algorithms presented place any restrictions on the scanning pattern, and they do not require the construction of a cuberille. Volumes can be measured to $\pm 1\%$ in simulation and $\pm 7\%$ *in vivo*, with typically only 10–20 cross-sections. The entire process, including scanning and manual segmentation of the organ of interest, can be completed in only 5–10 minutes. This makes the system both a practical and accurate method of measuring organ volume using ultrasound in a clinical setting.

References

1. Aarnink, R.G., de la Rosette, J.J.M.C.H., Debruyne, F.M.J., Wijkstra, H.: Reproducibility of prostate volume measurements from transrectal ultrasonography by an automated and a manual technique. British Journal of Urology **78** (1996) 219–223
2. Basset, O., Gimenez, G., Mestas, J.L., Cathignol, D., Devonec, M.: Volume measurement by ultrasonic transverse or sagittal cross-sectional scanning. Ultrasound in Medicine and Biology **17** (1991) 291–296
3. Catmull, E., Rom, R.: A class of local interpolating splines. Computer Aided Geometric Design (Barnhill R., Risenfeld, R. eds.), Academic Press, San Francisco (1974) 317–326
4. Cook, L.T., Cook, P.N., Lee, K.R., Batnitzky, S., Wong, B.Y.S., Fritz, S.L., Ophir, J., Dwyer III, S.J., Bigongiari, L.R., Templeton, A.W.: An algorithm for volume estimation based on polyhedral approximation. IEEE Transactions on Biomedical Engineering **27** (1980) 493–500
5. Fenster, A., Downey, D.B.: 3-D ultrasound imaging: A review. IEEE Engineering in Medicine and Biology (1996) 41–51
6. Gilja, O.H., Smievoll, A.I., Thune, N., Matre, K., Hausken, T., Ødegaard, S., Berstad, A.: In vivo comparison of 3D ultrasonography and magnetic resonance imaging in volume estimation of human kidneys. Ultrasound in Medicine and Biology **21** (1995) 25–32
7. Gopal, A.S., Schnellbaecher, M.J., Shen, Z., Akinboboye, O.O., Sapin, P.M., King, D.L.: Freehand three-dimensional echocardiography for measurement of left ventricular mass: *In Vivo* anatomic validation using explanted human hearts. Journal of the American College of Cardiology **30** (1997) 802–810
8. Howe, D., Wheeler, T., Perring, S.: Measurement of placental volume with real-time ultrasound in mid-pregnancy. Journal Clinical Ultrasound **22** (1994) 77–83
9. Hughes, S.W., D'Arcy, T.J., Maxwell, D.J., Chiu, W., Milner, A., Saunders, J.E., Sheppard, R.J.: Volume estimation from multiplanar 2D ultrasound images using a remote electromagnetic position and orientation sensor. Ultrasound in Medicine and Biology **22** (1996) 561–572
10. Hughes, S.W., D'Arcy, T.J., Maxwell, D.J., Saunders, J.E., Ruff, C.F., Chiu, W.S.C., Sheppard, R.J.: Application of a new discreet form of Gauss' theorum for measuring volume. Physics in Medicine and Biology **41** (1996) 1809–1821
11. Jensen, P.K., Hansen, M.K.: Ultrasonographic, three-dimensional scanning for determination of intraocular tumor volume. Acta Ophthalmologica **69** (1991) 178–186

12. Moritz, W.E., Pearlman, A.S., McCabe, D.H., Medema, D.K., Ainsworth, M.E., Boles, M.S.: An ultrasonic technique for imaging the ventricle in three dimensions and calculating its volume. IEEE Transactions on Biomedical Engineering **30** (1983) 482–492

13. Nathan, M.S., Seenivasagam, K., Mei, Q., Wickham, J.E.A., Miller, R.A.: Transrectal ultrasonography: why are estimates of prostate volume and dimension so inaccurate? British Journal of Urology **77** (1996) 401–407

14. Prager, R.W., Gee, A.H., Berman, L.: Stradx: real-time acquisition and visualisation of freehand 3D ultrasound. Medical Image Analysis (in press)

15. Rahmouni, A., Yang, A., Tempany, C.M.C., Frenkel, T., Epstein, J., Walsh, P., Leichner, P.K., Ricci, C., Zerhouni, E.: Accuracy of In-Vivo assessment of prostatic volume by MRI and transrectal ultrasonography. Journal of Computer Assisted Tomography **16** (1992) 935–940

16. Terris, M.K., Stamey, T.A.: Determination of prostate volume by transrectal ultrasound. The Journal of Urology **145** (1991) 984–987

17. Tong, S., Cardinal, H.N., McLoughlin, R.F., Downey, D.B., Fenster, A.: Intra– and inter–observer variability and reliability of prostate volume measurement via two-dimensional and three-dimensional ultrasound imaging. Ultrasound in Medicine and Biology **24** (1998) 673–681

18. Treece, G.M., Prager, R.W., Gee, A.H.: Regularised marching tetrahedra: improved iso-surface extraction. Tech. Report CUED/F-INFENG/TR 333, Cambridge University Engineering Dept, September 1998

19. Treece, G.M., Prager, R.W., Gee, A.H., Berman, L.: Fast surface and volume estimation from non-parallel cross-sections, for freehand 3-D ultrasound. Medical Image Analysis (in press)

20. Watanabe, Y.: A method for volume estimation by using vector areas and centroids of serial cross sections. IEEE Transactions on Biomedical Engineering **29** (1982) 202–205

A   Area from Parametric Cubic Splines

Given two curves, each defined parametrically:

$$\begin{bmatrix} x_i(t)\ y_i(t) \end{bmatrix} = \begin{bmatrix} t^3\ t^2\ t\ 1 \end{bmatrix} \begin{bmatrix} x_{i3}\ y_{i3} \\ x_{i2}\ y_{i2} \\ x_{i1}\ y_{i1} \\ x_{i0}\ y_{i0} \end{bmatrix} \quad \text{where} \quad 0 \le t \le 1.$$

If each curve is connected to the other by two straight lines joining the points, $t = 0$ and $t = 1$, the enclosed area can be calculated from the application of (1):

$$A = \left| \int_{t=0}^{1} s \cdot d\omega \right| \tag{5}$$

where s is a vector normal to the line joining the curves at the same value of t, and ω is the position of the centre of that line:

$$s(t) = \begin{bmatrix} y_1(t) - y_2(t)\ x_2(t) - x_1(t) \end{bmatrix} \tag{6}$$

$$d\omega(t) = \frac{1}{2} \begin{bmatrix} dx_1(t) + dx_2(t)\ dy_1(t) + dy_2(t) \end{bmatrix}. \tag{7}$$

Automated Identification and Measurement of Objects via Populations of Medial Primitives, with Application to Real Time 3D Echocardiography

George D. Stetten[1,2] and Stephen M. Pizer[1]

[1] Medical Image Display and Analysis Group, UNC, Chapel Hill
`george@stetten.com, smp@cs.unc.edu`
[2] NSF/ERC for Emerging Cardiovascular Technologies, Duke University

Abstract. We suggest that identification and measurement of objects in 3D images can be automatic, rapid and stable, based on the statistical properties of populations of medial primitives sought throughout the image space. These properties include scale, orientation, endness, and medial dimensionality. The property of medial dimensionality differentiates the sphere, the cylinder, and the slab, with intermediate dimensionality also possible. Endness results at the cap of a cylinder or the edge of a slab. The values of these medial properties at just a few locations provide an intuitive and robust model for complex shape. For example, the left ventricle during systole can be described as a large cylinder with an apical cap at one end, a slab–like mitral valve at the other (closed during systole), and appropriate interrelations among components in terms of their scale, orientation, and location. We demonstrate our method on simple geometric test objects, and show it capable of automatically identifying the left ventricle and measuring its volume *in vivo* using Real–Time 3D echocardiography.

1 Introduction

The lineage of the medial approach may be traced to the medial axis (otherwise known as symmetric axis or skeleton) introduced on binary images by Blum and developed by Nagel, Nackman, and others [1–3]. Pizer has extended the medial axis to gray–scale images producing a graded measure called *medialness*, which links the aperture of the boundary measurement to the radius of the medial axis to produce what has been labeled a *core*, a locus in a space of position, radius, and associated orientations [4, 5] Methods involving these continuous loci of medial primitives have proven particularly robust against noise and variation in target shape [6]. Determining locations with high medialness and relating them to a core has been accomplished by analyzing the geometry of loci resulting from ridge extraction [7]. Models including discrete loci of medial primitives have also provided the framework for a class of active shape models known as *Deformable Shape Loci* [8].

A. Kuba et al. (Eds.): IPMI'99, LNCS 1613, pp. 84–97, 1999.

The objective of the work reported here is to build on these ideas to produce a method for analyzing the shape of the heart in Real Time 3D ultrasound, a new imaging modality that uses a matrix array of transducer elements to scan the moving heart in 3D at more than 20 frames/second [9]. The approach to analyzing this data aims to extract the scale, orientation and dimensionality (shape type) of sections of cardiac anatomy by statistical analysis of populations of medial primitives. In particular, the primitives are identified by first searching for individual boundary points throughout the image in an initial sweep, and then by matching pairs of boundary points to form what are called *core atoms*. Core atoms tend to cluster along a medial ridge and allow for statistical analysis of the core and its underlying figure. Core atoms have already been developed for analysis of 2D shape [10] and are generalized here to 3D. The analysis is also extended to spatially sampled populations of core atoms. This research is part of a Ph.D. dissertation which covers many aspects in greater detail [11].

2 What is a Core Atom?

A *core atom* is defined as two boundary points b_1 and b_2 that satisfy particular requirements (described in detail below) guaranteeing that the boundaries face each other. A core atom can be represented by a single vector $c_{1,2}$ from the first boundary point to the second. The core atom is said to be "located" at a *center point* midway between the boundary points (see Fig. 1). The *medialness* at the center point is high because the *boundariness* at both boundary points is high and because the boundary normals face each other. Core atoms carry orientation, width and position, providing the ability for populations of core atoms to be analyzed in these terms.

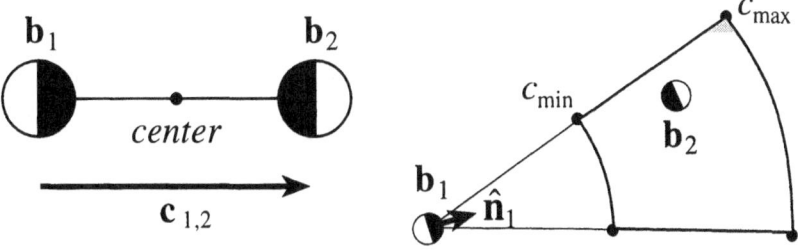

Fig. 1. A core atom consists of two boundary points that face each other across an acceptable distance, and a center point at which the core atom is said to be located. The search area (gray) for boundary point b_2 determined by boundary normal $\hat{n}_1$

Unlike medial models where *object angle* (half the angle between lines from the center point to each respective boundary point) is permitted to vary, the object angle of a core atom is fixed at 90°. Core atoms thus follow in the tradition of Brady [12] . As in Brady, the underlying figure is not required to have parallel boundaries. In the experiments presented below, boundariness is based on a Difference of Gaussian (DOG) measurement of intensity gradient, accomplished by repeated application of a binomial kernel. The number of applications determines the aperture of the boundariness detector, and is generally proportional to the size of the core atom. Further constraints are placed on the levels of intensity along the gradient direction. Other forms of boundariness, such as those based on texture analysis, could also be used for core atoms, provided an orientation is established for each boundary point.

Boundariness vectors are sampled on a rectilinear grid, and their magnitude compared to a threshold to select a population of boundary points b_i at locations x_i with orientations $\hat{n}_i$ ("$\hat{v}$" denotes normalization, $\hat{v} \equiv v/\|v\|$). The strength inherent to the statistics of populations is meant to counteract the weakness of thresholding. Core atoms are created from this population by finding pairs of candidate boundary points that satisfy the following three criteria:

1. The magnitude of the core atom vector $c_{1,2}$, i.e., the distance from one boundary point to the other, must be between c_{min} and c_{max}.

$$c_{1,2} = x_2 - x_1 \quad c_{min} \leq \|c_{1,2}\| < c_{max}. \tag{1}$$

   The core atom vector can be oriented either way since the order of the boundary points is arbitrary.

2. The boundary points must have sufficient face–to–faceness defined as

$$F(b_1, b_2) = f_1 \cdot f_2 \quad f_1 = \hat{c}_{1,2} \cdot \hat{n}_1 \quad f_2 = \hat{c}_{2,1} \cdot \hat{n}_2. \tag{2}$$

   Since f_1 and f_2 are normalized to lie between +1 and -1, their product F must also lie between +1 and -1. Values for F near +1 occur when the boundaries face towards (or away from) each other across the distance between them. A threshold for acceptable face–to–faceness is set within some error ϵ_f such that $F(b_1, b_2) > 1 - \epsilon_f$.

3. Assuming $F(b_1, b_2) > 0$, it follows that f_1 and f_2 are both positive, or both negative. The sign of f_1 (or f_2) is called the *polarity*. The appropriate polarity is either + or - depending on whether the expected target is lighter or darker than the background.

Although at first glance the search for pairs of boundary points appears to be $O(n^2)$, hashing individual boundary points beforehand by location yields a large reduction in computation time. The search area for b_2 is limited to a solid sector surrounding the orientation $\hat{n}_1$ of the *first* boundary point, and to a range between c_{min} and c_{max}. The width of the sector depends on ϵ_f (see Fig. 1).

3 Three Basic Configurations: Sphere, Cylinder, and Slab

Observe that collections of core atoms can group in three basic ways corresponding to the fundamental geometric shapes shown Fig. 2. The surfaces are shown in dark gray with the corresponding cores shown in light gray. Beneath each object is the population of core atoms that would be expected to form with such objects, the core atoms being depicted as simple line segments.

The sphere generates a "Koosh ball" like cloud of core atoms with spherical symmetry, with the core atom centers clustered at the center of the sphere. The cylinder generates a "spokes–of–a–wheel" arrangement with radial symmetry along the axis of the cylinder, and the core atom centers clustered along the axis of the cylinder. The slab results in a "bed–of–nails" configuration across the slab, with core atom centers clustered in the mid–plane of the slab. It is reassuring to find that the cores of these basic objects are the point, the line, and the plane. As shown in Fig. 2, a system of shape–specific coordinate axes, namely $\hat{a}_1$, $\hat{a}_2$, and $\hat{a}_3$, can be assigned in each case, although not all the axes are unique given the symmetries involved. For example, in the slab, $\hat{a}_1$ and $\hat{a}_2$ can rotate freely about $\hat{a}_3$. Such a set of coordinate axes can be found for any population of core atoms using eigenanalysis, as will be shown below. Furthermore, the extent to which a core atom population resembles one of the three basic configurations depends on the corresponding eigenvalues.

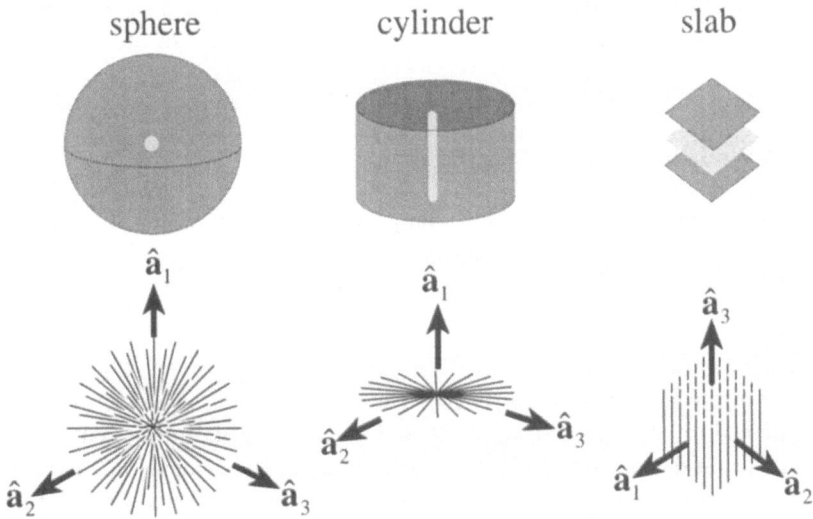

Fig. 2. Fundamental shapes (dark gray), corresponding cores (light gray), core atom populations (line segments) and eigenvectors $\hat{a}_1$, $\hat{a}_2$ and $\hat{a}_3$

Given a population of m core atoms c_i, $i = 1, 2, 3, \ldots m$, the analysis of a core atom population begins by separating each core atom vector c_i into its magnitude

c_i and its orientation $\hat{c}_i$. We ignore, for the moment, the location of the core atom. The analysis of magnitude c_i over a population of core atoms is straightforward, yielding a mean and standard deviation for the measurement of width in the underlying figure. The orientation $\hat{c}_i$ of core atoms in a population lends itself to eigenanalysis, yielding measures of dimensionality and overall orientation for the population. We develop the eigenanalysis here in n dimensions, although for the remainder of the paper n will be 3.

Given the population of m vectors in n dimensions, we find an n–dimensional vector $\hat{a}_1$ that is most orthogonal to that population as a whole by minimizing the sum of squares of the dot product between $\hat{a}$ and each individual $\hat{c}_i$.

$$\hat{a}_1 = \arg\min_{\hat{a}} \frac{1}{m} \sum_{i=1}^{m} (\hat{a} \cdot \hat{c}_i)^2 = \arg\min_{\hat{a}} (\hat{a}^T C \hat{a}) \quad \text{where} \quad C = \frac{1}{m} \sum_{i=1}^{m} \hat{c}_i \hat{c}_i^T. \quad (3)$$

The C matrix is positive definite, symmetric, and has a unit trace. Therefore, its eigenvalues are positive and sum to 1, and its eigenvectors are orthogonal. If the eigenvalues of C are sorted $\lambda_1 \leq \lambda_2 \leq \ldots \leq \lambda_n$, the corresponding eigenvectors $\hat{a}_1 \ldots \hat{a}_n$ are the axes of a coordinate system in which $\hat{a}_1$ is the most orthogonal to the population $\hat{c}_i$ as a whole. For example, it would be the axis of the cylinder in Fig. 2. Furthermore, the eigenanalyis guarantees that $\hat{a}_2$ is the most orthogonal to the population $\hat{c}_i$ among those directions that are already orthogonal to $\hat{a}_1$. This process can be repeated until $\hat{a}_n$ remains the *least* orthogonal to the population $\hat{c}_i$, representing a form of *average* orientation for $\hat{c}_i$.

4   The Lambda Triangle

Returning now specifically to 3D, the previous analysis yields three eigenvalues which describe the dimensionality of the core.

$$\lambda_i \geq 0 \quad \lambda_1 + \lambda_2 + \lambda_3 = 1. \quad (4)$$

An eigenvalue of zero means that the corresponding eigenvector is perfectly orthogonal to every core atom $\hat{c}_i$. Such is the case for $\hat{a}_1$ in the cylinder, and for both $\hat{a}_1$ and $\hat{a}_2$ in the slab. In the sphere none of the eigenvectors is completely orthogonal to the core atom population. Given the symmetries of the three basic shapes, the eigenvalues shown in Fig. 3 result.

Since λ_3 is dependent on the other two, the system may be viewed as having only two independent variables, λ_1 and λ_2. Because of constraints already mentioned, possible values for λ_1 and λ_2 are limited by $\lambda_1 \leq \lambda_2$ and $\lambda_2 \leq (1 - \lambda_1)/2$ which define a triangular domain we call the *lambda triangle* (Fig. 3).

The vertices of the lambda triangle correspond to the three basic shapes in Fig. 2, with all possible eigenvalues falling within the triangle. A rather crude simplification of dimensionality is possible by dividing the triangle into three

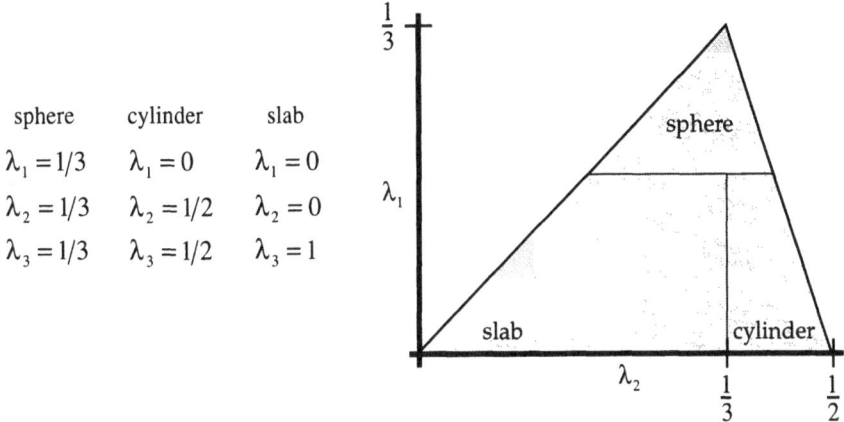

sphere	cylinder	slab
$\lambda_1 = 1/3$	$\lambda_1 = 0$	$\lambda_1 = 0$
$\lambda_2 = 1/3$	$\lambda_2 = 1/2$	$\lambda_2 = 0$
$\lambda_3 = 1/3$	$\lambda_3 = 1/2$	$\lambda_3 = 1$

Fig. 3. The lambda triangle defines the domain of possible eigenvalues

compartments to provide an integer description of dimensionality. Arbitrary thresholds of $\lambda_1 = 0.2$ and $\lambda_2 = 1/3$ will be used to divide the triangle into such areas of integer dimensionality to clarify our experimental results. However, it should be remembered that the underlying dimensionality is not an integer or even a single scalar, but rather two independent scalars, λ_1 and λ_2 whose values are constrained by the lambda triangle.

5   Spatial Sampling in the Corona

We now return to the question of core atom location, which we have so far ignored. To incorporate location into the analysis of core atoms, we sort them into bins on a regular 3D lattice by the location of their center points. Thus each bin represents a spatial sampling of medialness. The number of core atoms in a sample volume can be thought of as the *medial density* at that location.

How do we choose an appropriate size for the sample volume? As we shall see, the local distribution of core atoms can have a significant cross section, and the density within that distribution may not be uniform. To preserve resolution, the sample volume needs to be smaller than the typical cross section of a core atom cloud. When a core is sampled off–center, it will demonstrate a distortion in its dimensionality. For example, the zero–dimensional core at the center of a sphere will appear to be one–dimensional (cylindrical) when sampled off center, as shown in Fig. 4. The vector from the theoretical core (center of the sphere) to the center of the density in the sample volume is called the *displacement vector* p (See Fig. 4C). The core atom population within a sample volume may not contain the entire thickness of the core, but rather a sub–sampling of the core called a *coronal density*. We can generally expect, in fact, to be sampling coronal densities. It would be helpful to know where, in a given cloud around the core, a sample was collected, but that presupposes knowledge about the overall distribution of core atoms which we may not have.

We can, at least, predict certain relationships to exist between the distribution of core atoms over the entire core and that of a sample volume displaced from the center of the core. The displaced sample of core atoms will be flattened in a plane orthogonal to p, and thus develop orthogonality to that direction. This can be seen in Fig. 4, where the spherical distribution of core atoms in 4B has been flattened into a cylindrical distribution in 4C. The same effect can be seen in the case of the cylinder in Fig. 5, where, displaced off the central axis of the cylinder by p, the population of core atoms becomes slab–like and orthogonal to p. One expects the displacement vector to be one of the eigenvectors at the closest point on the theoretical core, because (1) the displacement vector will be orthogonal to the core at that point, and (2) the normal to the core is always one of its eigenvectors. In 3D, the medial manifold can have at most 2 dimensions and thus will always have such a normal.

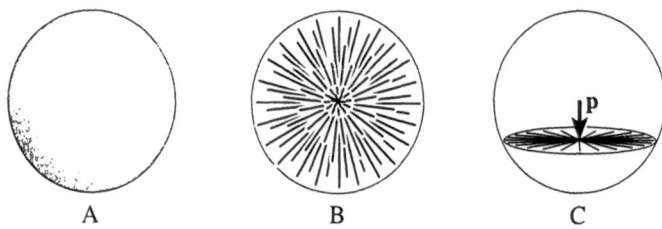

Fig. 4. A. sphere. B. all core atoms C. cylindrical coronal density displaced by p

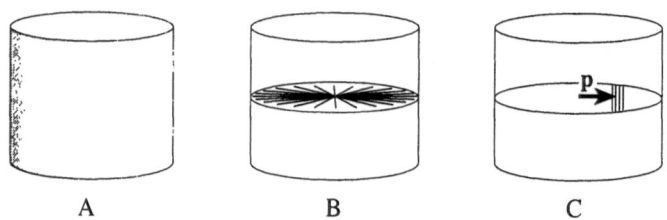

Fig. 5. A. cylinder. B. all core atoms C. slab–like coronal density displaced by p

Figs. 4 and 5 suggest that the displacement vector p could somehow be used to compensate for the dimensional distortion in the corona. However, an isolated density that is, for example, cylindrical cannot know whether it represents the true center of a cylinder or simply the corona of a sphere. The results of the eigenanalysis for each density may be used in a Hough–like fashion simultaneously to vote for its own dimensionality and center of mass, and for possible densities whose corona it may inhabit. The voting takes place within ellipsoids around each density. The axes of each ellipsoid are long in directions orthogonal to the core atom population in its density. Thus the ellipsoid can be expected to extend in the p direction, orthogonal to the core atoms.

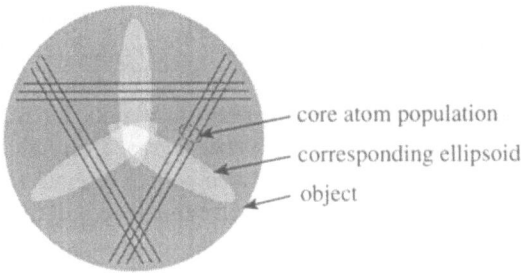

Fig. 6. Ellipsoids of three coronal core atom densities coalescing at the true center

Fig. 6 demonstrates this concept. A circular cross–section through an object is shown with three coronal densities (each containing 3 core atoms) displaced from the center. An ellipsoid is associated with each density, with the major axis of each ellipsoid along the eigenvector most orthogonal to the corresponding core atoms. The three ellipsoids intersect at the center the circle. The figure can be interpreted as the cross–section of a sphere with the populations of core atoms being cylindrical (seen in cross–section) and the ellipsoids intersecting at the center of the sphere (as in Fig. 4). Alternatively it can be interpreted as the cross–section of a cylinder with the populations of core atoms being slab–like and the ellipsoids intersecting along the axis of the cylinder (as in Fig. 5). There are various ways to construct such ellipsoids. We have chosen the following heuristic for its simplicity. The axes of each ellipsoid are the eigenvectors of its density's C matrix. The lengths a_i of the axes are related to the eigenvalues λ_i as follows:

$$a_1 = \gamma \bar{c}, \ a_2 = \frac{\alpha_2}{\alpha_1} a_1, \ a_3 = \frac{\alpha_3}{\alpha_1} a_1 \ \text{ where } \ \alpha_i = 1 - \lambda_i, \ \gamma = \frac{1}{2}. \qquad (5)$$

The scalar distance $\bar{c}$ is the mean diameter of the core atoms in the density, and the dimensionless number γ relates $\bar{c}$ to the size of the ellipsoid, determining how many neighbors will be reached. The ellipsoids make it possible to cluster the core atoms for a given cloud, in effect to coalesce the corona. Each sample volume (the *votee*) receives votes from all the neighboring sample volumes whose ellipsoids overlap it. The votes from those ellipsoids are assigned a strength v, where $v = m \cdot exp(-d_e{}^2)$, m being the number of core atoms in the voting density, and d_e the ellipsoidal distance

$$d_e = \sqrt{\sum_{i=1}^{3} \left(\frac{\hat{a}_i \cdot d}{a_i} \right)^2}. \tag{6}$$

from the center of the voter ellipsoid to the votee, d being the vector from the voter to the votee. Votes are constructed to contain information about the voter, including its C matrix which may simply be summed (scaled by v) for an eigenanalysis of the entire constituent core atom population of a particular candidate. Thus are formed what we call *superdensities*, clusters of core atoms that no longer suffer from coronal distortion. The center of mass for the constituent core atom population of a superdensity will tend to be at the true core, rather than in the corona.

6   Tests with Parametric Objects

To validate these methods, we applied them to three parametric test objects with simple geometries: a sphere, a torus, and a spherical shell. The torus is basically a cylinder of varied and known orientation, and the spherical shell is likewise a slab of varied and known orientation. (The sphere is simply itself.)

Eigenanalysis of the coronal densities collected in a rectilinear lattice of sample volumes yielded the following results. Fig. 7 shows all densities containing greater than 1% of the entire core atom population plotted on the lambda triangle. The sphere shows two groups of densities, one near the top (sphere) vertex of the triangle and another near the right (cylinder) vertex, consistent with the dimensional effects of the corona predicted in Fig. 4. The torus, which is locally a cylinder, shows clustering near the right (cylinder) vertex, with some spreading towards the left (slab) consistent with the dimensional effects of the corona predicted in Fig. 5. The spherical shell, which is locally a slab, shows tight clustering at the left (slab) vertex consistent with the observation that core atoms in a slab are collinear with p and therefore will not develop significant orthogonality.

Unfortunately, Fig. 7 does not contain spatial information about the sampled densities. The spatial distribution of densities for the test objects is shown Fig. 8. Each sample volume whose density contains more than 1% of the total core atoms is shown as a thin–lined symbol. The simple partition of the lambda triangle in Fig. 3 is used to decide between three possible symbols: a slab is represented as a single line, a cylinder as a cross, and a sphere as 3 intersecting axes. The length of the thin lines is constant, chosen for clarity in each test object. The orientation of the thin lines indicates the predominant direction(s) of core atoms in each density, i.e. across the slab, or orthogonal to the axis of the cylinder, keeping in mind that perfect spheres have no predominant orientation and perfect cylinders allow arbitrary rotation around the axis.

As expected the sphere shows cylindrical densities in its corona oriented towards the center. Further out from the center a few slabs–like densities reflect simply the paucity of core atoms in those sample volumes. Near the center one

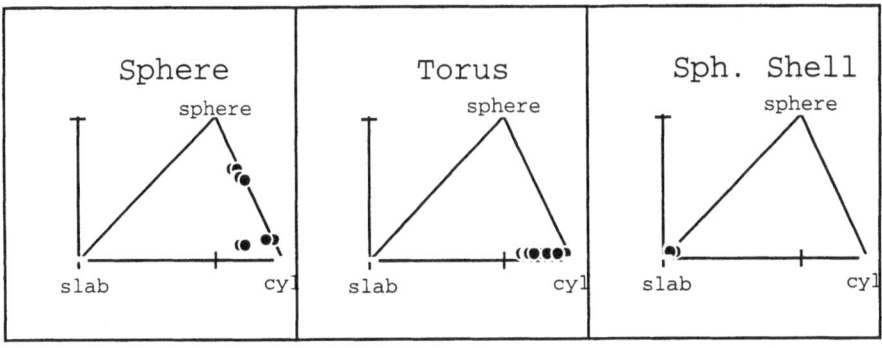

Fig. 7. Distribution of densities on lambda triangles, for parametric test objects

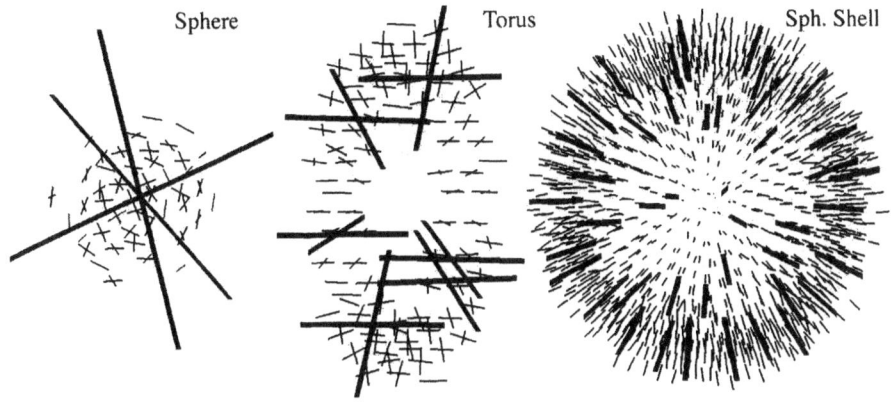

Fig. 8. Densities and superdensities for parametric objects

true spherical density (a small 3–axis symbol) may be discerned. The thick–lined symbols show the results of ellipsoidal voting, i.e., they represent superdensities. To prevent a cluttered illustration, superdensities are limited to non–overlapping constituencies. They are represented by thick lines in a manner similar to the densities, except the length of the axes now corresponds to the actual mean scale of the constituent core atoms. Thus the thick–lined 3–axis cross indicates the actual diameter of the spherical object. For the sphere there is only one predominant winning superdensity, with virtually every core atom in its constituency. The torus shows cylindrical densities properly oriented but dispersed throughout the corona. At the outer regions of the corona a few slab–like densities are visible. The superdensities, by contrast, are centered on the circular mid–line of the torus. The spherical shell shows only slab–like densities, which coalesce with ellipsoidal voting into slab–like superdensities. The orientation of both are across the local slab. Ellipsoidal voting is seen to perform another function, that of connecting densities that share a core along the mid–plane of a slab or the axis of a cylinder.

7   Endness

Some attention must be paid to cases where a cylinder ends at a hemispherical cap, or a slab ends at a hemicylindrical edge. The property of endness has been described by Clary, et al. [13] . Endness as viewed from the core atom perspective is illustrated in Fig. 9A and 9B. To detect endness, densities of core atoms are used as starting points. Once a local cylinder has been established, boundary points are sought along the axis of the cylinder in either direction as evidence of a cap. Similarly, once a local slab has been found, boundary points indicating an edge can be sought. Mathematics for this is derived elsewhere [11].

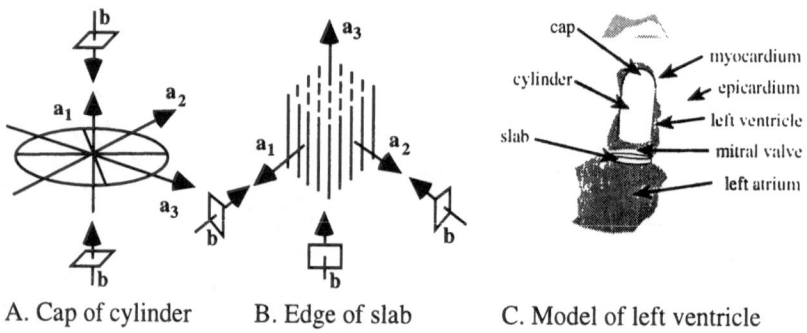

A. Cap of cylinder   B. Edge of slab   C. Model of left ventricle

Fig. 9. Endness, manifested as a cap on a cylinder (A) and the edge of a slab (B)

8   Identifying and Measuring the Cardiac Left Ventricle

We now turn to a useful clinical application, the automated determination of left ventricular volume using Real Time 3D (RT3D) echocardiography. RT3D is a new imaging modality that electronically scans a volume in 3D using a matrix array instead of the conventional linear array. RT3D is described in detail elsewhere [9] , but its primary novelty is the ability to capture a single cardiac cycle at 22 frames/second, which no other available imaging modality can accomplish.

RT3D images of an *in vivo* human heart present a significant challenge to image analysis techniques, including high noise, low resolution, path dependence, and a non–rectilinear data space. These problems are addressed elsewhere [11] , but the suggestion that the statistical nature of our method yields robustness is severely tested in its application to RT3D echocardiography.

We now expand on the example from the abstract: The left ventricle during systole is basically a large cylinder with an apical cap at one end, and a slab–like mitral valve at the other (we limit ourselves here to apical scans, and to times when the mitral valve is closed). The model is shown in Fig. 9C. To identify the cylinder in the image data, core atoms of an appropriate range of diameters

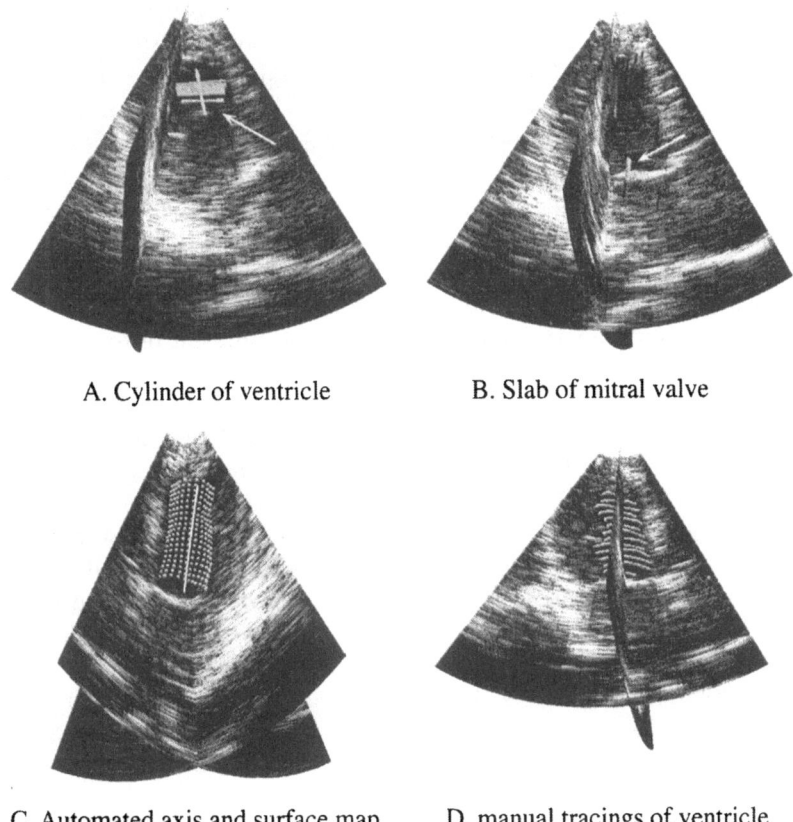

A. Cylinder of ventricle   B. Slab of mitral valve

C. Automated axis and surface map   D. manual tracings of ventricle

Fig. 10. Real Time 3D ultrasound with automated and manual identification of LV

were collected in sample volumes on a regular lattice, and ellipsoidal voting was applied. An example of the resulting superdensities is displayed in Fig. 10A. Crosses are shown in the cylindrical chamber of the ventricle. Due to the preselection of core atoms by scale, no other significant densities of core atoms were found.

Next, the mitral valve was sought, by limiting the formation of core atoms to an appropriately smaller scale, and to orientations nearly perpendicular to the transducer. As shown in Fig. 10B, the strongest superdensities (short vertical line segments) were clustered around the center of the mitral valve, although weaker false targets were detected in the myocardium. To eliminate these false targets, a criterion was established for the formation of appropriate pairs of superdensities, in the spirit of core atoms. Only slab–like densities appropriately located and oriented with respect to cylindrical densities were accepted. These pairs were allowed to vote for their constituent superdensities, and the mean location of the winning superdensities used to establish a single mitral valve location and a single LV cylinder location. The vector between these two locations was used to establish a cone for expected boundary points at the apex of the LV, and the mean distance to the resulting boundary points used to determine the location of the apical cap along that vector. Thus an axis between the apex and the mitral valve was established. Given this axis, LV volume was estimated by collecting boundary points around the axis. Only boundaries that faced the axis were accepted. The boundary points were organized into bins using cylindrical coordinates, in other words, disks along the axis and sectors within each disk. An average radius from the axis was established for the boundary points in each bin, creating a *surface map* of the endocardial surface. Fig. 10C shows such a surface map (dots) and the underlying axis. The problem of empty bins was avoided by convolving the surface map with a binomial kernel in 2D until each bin had some contribution to its average radius. Volumes were then calculated by summing over all sectors. The entire procedure including identification and volume measurement of the LV was automated, and required approximately 15 seconds on a 200 MHz Silicon Graphics O2 computer.

The automated volumes were compared to manual tracings performed on a stack of flat slices orthogonal to a manually–placed axis (see Fig. 10D). This axis employed the same anatomical end–points (the ventricular apex and the center of the mitral valve) as the axis determined automatically above. The volumes and locations of the end–points were compared to those determined automatically. Results are shown in Fig. 11. They are very encouraging, particularly for the automated placement of the axis end points, which had an RMS error of approximately 1 cm. Volume calculations introduced additional errors of their own, but were still reasonable for ultrasound. Only four cases have been tried, and all are shown. The method worked in all cases.

9   Conclusions

We have described a new method for identifying anatomical structures using fundamental properties of shape extracted statistically from populations of medial primitives, and have demonstrated its feasibility by applying it under challenging conditions. Further studies are presently underway to establish reliability over a range of data. Future directions include introducing greater specificity and adaptability in the boundary thresholding, incorporating more than 2 nodes into the model, introducing variability into the model to reflect normal variation and pathologic anatomy, extending the method to the spatio–temporal domain, and applying it to visualization.

Acknowledgments

Whitaker Biomedical Engineering grant, NSF grant CDR8622201, NIH grants 1K08HL03220, P01CA47982, HL46242, data from Volumetrics, Durham, NC.

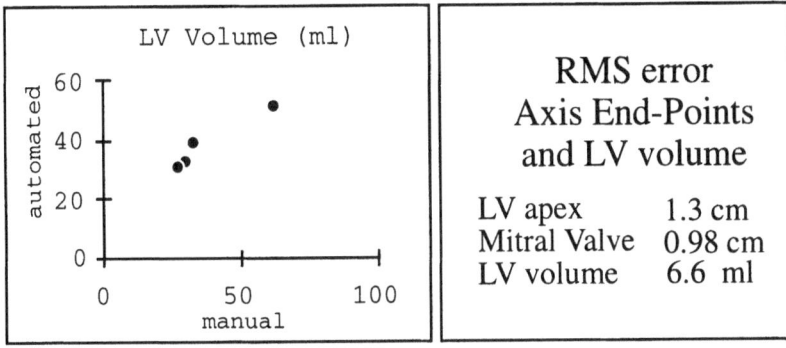

Fig. 11. Volume measurement and axis end–point location, manual vs. automatic

References

1. Blum, H and Nagel, R.N.: Shape description using weighted symmetric axis features. Pattern Recognition **10** (1978) 167-180
2. Nackman, L.R.: Curvature relations in 3D symmetric axes, CVGIP **20** (1982) 43-57
3. Nackman, L.R., and Pizer, S.M.: Three-Dimensional shape description using the symmetric axis transform I:Theory. IEEE Trans. PAMI **2** (1985) 187-202
4. Burbeck, C.A., and Pizer, S.M.: Object representation by cores: Identifying and representing primitive spatial regions. Vision Research **35** (1995) 1917-1930
5. Pizer, S.M., Eberly, D.H., Morse, B.S., and Fritsch, D.S.:Zoom invariant vision of figural shape: the mathematics of cores. Computer Vision and Image Understanding **69** (1998) 55-71
6. Morse, B.S., Pizer, S.M., Puff, D.T., and Gu, C.: Zoom-Invariant vision of figural shape: Effect on cores of image disturbances. Computer Vision and Image Understanding **69** (1998) 72-86
7. Furst, J.D., and Pizer, S.M.:Marching Cores: A method for extracting cores from 3D medical images. Proceedings of the Workshop on Mathematical Methods in Biomedical Image Analysis, San Francisco, CA, June 1996.
8. Fritsch, D., Pizer, S.M., Yu, L., Johnson, V., and Chaney, E.: Segmentation of Medical Image Objects Using Deformable Shape Loci. Information Processing in Medical Imaging, Poultney, Vermont (1997)
9. Stetten, G., Ota, T., Ohazama, C., Fleishman, C., Castelucci, J., Oxaal, J., Kisslo, J., and Ramm, O.T.v.: Real-Time 3D Ultrasound: A New Look at the Heart. J. Cardiovasc. Diagnosis and Proc. **15** (1998) 73-84
10. Stetten, G., Landesman, R., and Pizer, S.M.: Core-Atoms and the spectra of scale, (Technical Report TR97-006, UNC Dept. Computer Science. SPIE Medical Imaging Conference (1997)
11. Stetten, G.: Automated Identification and Measurement of Cardiac Anatomy Via Analysis of Medial Primitives. Ph.D. Dissertation, Stephen Pizer, advisor, UNC Chapel Hill, (expected, 1999).
12. Brady, M.: Criteria for representations of shape. New York, Academic Press (1983)
13. Clary, G.J., Pizer, S.M., Fritsch, D.S., and Perry, J.R.: Left ventricular wall motion tracking via deformable shape loci. CAR International Symposium and Exhibition, Amsterdam (1997)

Continuous Time Dynamic PET Imaging Using List Mode Data

Thomas E. Nichols[1], Jinyi Qi[2], and Richard M. Leahy[2]

[1] Department of Statistics, Carnegie Mellon University, Pittsburgh, PA 15213-3890, USA
nicholst@stat.cmu.edu

[2] Signal & Image Processing Institute, University of Southern California, Los Angeles, CA 90089-2564, USA
{jqi, leahy}@sipi.usc.edu

Abstract. We describe a method for computing a continuous time estimate of dynamic changes in tracer density using list mode PET data. The tracer density in each voxel is modeled as an inhomogeneous Poisson process whose rate function can be represented using a cubic B-spline basis. An estimate of these rate functions is obtained by maximizing the likelihood of the arrival times of each detected photon pair over the control vertices of the spline. By resorting the list mode data into a standard sinogram plus a "timogram" that retains the arrival times of each of the events, we are able to perform efficient computation that exploits the symmetry inherent in the ordered sinogram. The maximum likelihood estimator uses quadratic temporal and spatial smoothness penalties and an additional penalty term to enforce non-negativity. Corrections for scatter and randoms are described and the results of studies using simulated and human data are included.

1 Introduction

Dynamic PET imaging usually involves the collection of a series of frames of sinogram data over contiguous time intervals that can range in duration from 10 seconds to over 20 minutes. Data from each of the frames is independently reconstructed to form a set of images. These images can then be used to estimate physiological parameters [8]. This approach involves selection of the set of acquisition times, where one must choose between collecting longer scans with good counting statistics but poor temporal resolution, or shorter scans that are noisy but preserve temporal resolution. List mode data acquisition avoids this problem by allowing frame durations to be determined after acquisition. Alternatively, the problem of temporal binning can be avoided entirely by directly using the arrival times in the list mode data to estimate a dynamic image.

Snyder [23] developed a list mode maximum likelihood (ML) method for estimation of dynamic PET images using inhomogeneous Poisson processes. Each voxel has an associated time-varying tracer density that is modeled using basis functions that are based on assumptions about the physiological processes generating the data, e.g. blood activity curves convolved with a basis of exponentials.

A. Kuba et al. (Eds.): IPMI'99, LNCS 1613, pp. 98–111, 1999.

The observed list mode PET data are then inhomogeneous Poisson processes whose rate functions are linear combinations of the dynamic voxel tracer densities. Here we follow a similar approach but instead work with rate functions formed as a linear combination of known basis functions. Not only does the linearity of the model lend itself to efficient computation of the estimates, but also we can better represent the dynamic activity seen in experimental data that is not well modeled by the more restrictive physiological models.

A second advantage of using list mode data arises in cases where the number of detected photon pairs in a particular study is far less than the total number of detector pairs. This is often the case in modern 3D PET systems which can have in excess of 10^8 sinogram elements in a single frame. To reduce this number to manageable proportions, the data are often rebinned by adding nearby elements together. Alternatively, the raw list mode data case be stored and the need for rebinning is avoided. Barrett *et al.* [1,18] describe a list mode maximum likelihood method for estimation of a temporally stationary image. While this method will often reduce storage costs and avoid the need for rebinning, the random spatial ordering of the detected events in the list mode data does not lend itself to fast forward and backprojection and exploitation of the many symmetries in 3D projection matrices [10,19]. To avoid this problem we use a hybrid combination of the standard sinogram and list mode formats that allows the reconstruction algorithm to exploit the same matrix symmetries used in our static imaging work [19]. All events in a dynamic study are collected into a single standard sinogram; this is then augmented by a "timogram" which contains the arrival times of each event stored so that they are indexed using the values in the associated sinogram.

In this paper we present a method for reconstructing a continuous time estimate of a dynamic PET image using list mode data and the theory of inhomogeneous Poisson processes. A general B-spline model is used to represent the dynamic activity in each voxel so that the dynamic image is parameterized by a sequence of control vertex "images" where the control vertices are the coefficients for the spline basis. Tomographic projections of these control vertices produce the control vertices for the rate functions of the inhomogeneous Poisson processes representing coincidence detections between each detector pair. A maximum likelihood estimate of the control vertices for each voxel can then be computed using the standard likelihood function for inhomogeneous Poisson processes [21,22]. The final result is a temporally continuous representation of the PET image that utilizes the temporal resolution of list mode data.

Our parameterization of the inhomogeneous Poisson rate function is applicable to any linear combination of basis functions. This form encompasses the parametric imaging work of Matthews [14], Snyder [21] and mixture models of O'Sullivan [17]. We also note that Ollinger [16] used list mode data to reconstruct rate functions as histograms with adaptive bin-widths; our work could be viewed as a continuous-time extension of this. For this paper we consider only cubic B-splines. The key advantage of B-splines are that they have systematic compact support. In particular, for any point on a cubic spline only 4 basis functions are nonzero. Also, simple closed forms exist for all derivatives and integrals of a polynomial spline.

Since inhomogeneous Poisson rate functions are unnormalized densities, we note that the density estimation literature using splines is closely related to our work (e.g. [24,6]). The standard methods involve exponentiated splines or squared splines. While these implicitly constrain the rate function to be positive, they cannot be represented with a linear basis. As there are substantial computational savings to having a common basis for all voxels and projections, we did not pursue these approaches.

The paper is organized as follows. We describe the model and maximum likelihood method in Sections 2 and 3, respectively. Methods for selecting the spline knot points and methods for randoms and scatter correction are included in Section 4. Computational considerations including resorting data into a timogram format and the details of the algorithm used for computing the ML estimate are given in Section 5. In Section 6 we demonstrate the performance of the method with some preliminary simulation and experimental results.

2   Dynamic Modeling Using Inhomogeneous Poisson Processes

We model the positron emissions from each voxel in the volume as an inhomogeneous Poisson process. The rate function for the voxel represents, to within a scalar calibration factor, the time varying PET tracer density. We parameterize the rate functions using a cubic B-spline basis:

$$\eta_j(t) = \sum_\ell w_{j\ell} B_\ell(t), \; \eta_j(t) \geq 0 \, \forall t,$$

where $\eta_j(\cdot)$ is the rate function for voxel j, $w_{j\ell}$ is the ℓth basis weight (control vertex) for voxel j, and $B_\ell(t)$ is the ℓth spline basis function. The problem of reconstructing the dynamic PET image is then reduced to estimating the control vertices for each voxel.

We denote by p_{ij} the probability of detecting at detector pair i a photon pair produced by emission of a positron from voxel j. The probabilities p_{ij} are identical to those used in static PET imaging. Here we use the factored matrix forms developed in [19]. Assuming that the detection probabilities are independent and time invariant, it follows that coincidence detection at detector pair i is also an inhomogeneous Poisson process with rate function

$$\lambda_i(t) = \sum_j p_{ij} \sum_\ell w_{j\ell} B_\ell(t) = \sum_\ell \left(\sum_j p_{ij} w_{j\ell} \right) B_\ell(t) \tag{1}$$

where the right-most term demonstrates that the rate functions for the data are also B-splines.

The Poisson process observed at the detectors is corrupted by random and scatter components that can also be modeled as inhomogeneous Poisson processes. Combining the three components, we have the model:

$$\lambda_i^*(t) = \lambda_i(t) + r_i(t) + s_i(t)$$

where $r_i(\cdot)$ and $s_i(\cdot)$ are the randoms and scatter rate functions for detector pair i and $\lambda_i^*(t)$ is the rate function for the process actually observed at detector pair i. In estimating the rate function parameters $w_{j\ell}$ we will assume that the rate functions for the random and scatter components have been determined through a calibration procedure and can be treated as known processes.

For a Poisson process with rate function $\lambda(t)$, with N events observed from time T_0 to T_1 and event arrival times $a_1, \ldots, a_k, \ldots, a_N$, the likelihood function is [22]

$$P(a_1, \ldots, a_k, \ldots, a_N | \lambda(t)) = \left(\prod_{k=1}^{N} \lambda(a_k) \right) \exp \left\{ - \int_{T_0}^{T_1} \lambda(u) du \right\}. \quad (2)$$

For $N = 0$, the product is defined as unity.

For the set of independent events recorded in the list mode data the log likelihood is therefore given by

$$L(\mathcal{D}|W) = \sum_i \sum_k \log \lambda_i^*(a_{ik}) - \sum_i \int \lambda_i^*(u) du, \text{ s.t. } \lambda_i^*(t) \geq 0 \forall t. \quad (3)$$

where $\mathcal{D}$ denotes the list mode data and W the set of parameters for the rate functions. We represent the data as $\mathcal{D} = (\boldsymbol{x}, \boldsymbol{a}_1, \ldots, \boldsymbol{a}_i, \ldots, \boldsymbol{a}_I)$, where $\boldsymbol{x} = (x_1, \ldots, x_i, \ldots, x_I)$ are the sinogram count data, and $\boldsymbol{a}_i = (a_{i1}, \ldots, a_{ik}, \ldots, a_{ix_i})$, the set of x_i event arrival times at detector pair i. For the B-spline basis, $W = (w_{j\ell} | \ell = 1, \ldots, L, j = 1, \ldots, J)$ are the set of basis coefficients. While $\boldsymbol{x}$ is a function of $\boldsymbol{a}$ and hence redundant, we use the sinogram counts to index the arrival times, as described in section 5.1.

3   Penalized Maximum Likelihood Estimation

We estimate the image control vertex values that define our dynamic image using penalized maximum likelihood. The objective function of the statistical model is modified with three regularizing terms

$$L^*(\mathcal{D}|W) = L(W|\mathcal{D}) - \alpha\rho(W) - \beta\phi(W) - \gamma\nu(W). \quad (4)$$

The terms $\rho(W)$ and $\phi(W)$ regularize temporal and spatial roughness, respectively; $\nu(W)$ penalizes negativity of the image rate functions; α, β and γ are the tuning parameters. We now describe each of these terms.

We employ a temporal smoothing term to control the roughness of the spline rate functions [3]. The form of the roughness penalty is the integrated squared curvature. For voxel j this is

$$\int \left\{ \frac{\partial^2}{\partial u^2} \eta_j(u) \right\}^2 du.$$

Fortunately, for cubic splines this quantity has a simple expression, a quadratic form of the control vertices ([3], pg. 238). We denote the symmetric, banded matrix of this quadratic form Q. Thus the temporal roughness penalty is given by

$$\rho(\mathcal{W}) = \sum_j \sum_{\ell_1} \sum_{\ell_2} w_{j\ell_1} Q_{\ell_1 \ell_2} w_{j\ell_2}.$$

We regularize the estimates of the control vertices using a spatial smoothing function equivalent to the pair-wise quadratic penalty used previously in penalized ML [4] and Bayesian estimation [19] of static PET images:

$$\phi(\mathcal{W}) = \sum_\ell \sum_j \sum_{j' \in \mathcal{N}_j, j' > j} \kappa_{jj'} (w_{j\ell} - w_{j'\ell})^2.$$

where $\mathcal{N}_j$ denotes a set of neighbors of voxel j and $\kappa_{jj'}$ is the reciprocal of the Euclidean distance between voxel j and j'. Other possible choices of the penalty function include the discrete approximation of the thin plate spline bending energy [12] or a non-quadratic edge preserving function such as that described in [5].

We now justify applying the same regularization to the control vertices as has previously been applied to images. First, the spline basis is the same for all voxels, so the control vertices have the same meaning for all voxels. Second, each member of the spline basis has limited support so that the effect of spatial smoothing is localized in time. Lastly, the B-spline basis we use is well conditioned [3], meaning that small changes in the control vertices produce small changes in the spline function. Hence if we expect two rate functions to be similar, then it is sufficient to constrain their control vertices to be similar.

The optimization method must account for the non-negativity of the image rate functions $\eta_j(t)$. We use unconstrained optimization with a penalty function [13]. The problem is complicated somewhat in that the control vertices themselves are not necessarily non-negative; instead we need to ensure that the corresponding spline does not become negative. The local extrema of a cubic spline have a closed form, so we initially tried to penalizing negative local minima. This approach complicated the gradient and Hessian and made their evaluation prohibitively slow.

Instead we simply penalize negative values computed at a finite number of time points. The vector z contains the locations at which we enforce positivity. It is constructed by uniformly spacing d_z points in each inter-knot interval. Any elements of z for which the spline is negative are penalized with the square of the spline value, resulting in the penalty:

$$\nu(\mathcal{W}) = \sum_j \sum_m \min \left(0, \sum_\ell w_{j\ell} B_\ell(z_m) \right)^2.$$

This approach does not necessarily ensure that the spline is non-negative everywhere. However, we have found that when used in combination with the temporal roughness penalty, the resulting estimates do not become negative, except possibly in the intervals just preceding a large increase in activity.

It is straightforward to show that each of the four terms in the penalized likelihood (4) have negative semi-definite Hessian matrices. Their null spaces only intersect at the zero vector. Therefore, the objective function is strictly concave and has a unique global maximum which can be found by a gradient-based search algorithm.

4 Calibration Procedures

4.1 Selection of Knot Spacing

Before proceeding to the estimation we must decide on the spacing between knots in the B-spline basis. A cubic B-spline basis is defined by knot locations, $u = (u_1, \ldots, u_{L+4})$, where $L \geq 4$ is the number of basis elements and the first and last 4 knots are identical, to allow discontinuity at the end points. Uniformly spaced knots will not be efficient for most tracer studies since early changes in concentration have much greater magnitude than those later in the study. While we do not attempt to adaptively place the knots, in a modest attempt to optimize knot placement, we use the head curve to define knots that produce approximately equal arc lengths, as suggested in [3]. The head curve is a temporal histogram using all of the list mode data and it serves as an estimate of the average rate function. Once the knot locations are determined, the actual basis functions are computed using the recurrence relations as described in [2,3].

4.2 Randoms and Scatter Rate Functions

To apply the penalized likelihood estimation procedure described above, we should first apply calibration procedures to account for the presence of scattered and random events in the list mode data. We note that the simple randoms subtraction method that is used in static imaging is not applicable to list mode data. While neither randoms or scatter are included in the preliminary results presented here, they are described for completeness and will be essential in extracting accurate quantitative dynamic information from our results.

The randoms rate varies approximately as the square of the true coincidence rate. We can model the randoms rate for each detector pair using an inhomogeneous Poisson process:

$$r_i(t) = \sum_{\ell} \gamma_{i\ell} B_\ell(t),$$

where $\gamma_{i\ell}$, $\ell = 1, \ldots, L$ are the control vertices for the randoms component in the ith line of response (LOR). The list mode data produced on the ECAT HR+ (CTI Systems, Knoxville Tennessee) contains both prompt (on-time) and delayed events. We can use the delayed events to compute an ML estimate of these control vertices. The number of counts per LOR in the delayed events is typically quite small so that these estimates would probably exhibit high variance. However, after scaling for variations in individual detector sensitivities, there is a high degree of spatial smoothness in the mean randoms sinogram [15]. Consequently we can use a penalized ML estimate in which substantial spatial smoothing is used to regularize the estimator. By choosing the knot spacing for the randoms rate functions to be at the same locations as for the image rate functions, the separate treatment of randoms in the estimation algorithm below produces little increase in the computational cost.

The spatio-temporal scatter distribution is a function of both the dynamic tracer distribution and the object. We assume no interaction between the temporal and spatial distribution and scale a fixed spatial scatter estimate over time. While this is a rather crude approximation, we anticipate that it will be reasonably accurate due to the very smooth nature of the scatter contribution to the sinogram. However, for certain ligand studies of the brain, where the tracer eventually binds solely to subcortical structures, this approximation may perform poorly.

Integrating the coincidence detections over time yields a sinogram from which we estimate the spatial scatter distribution using the simulation method in [25]. Let S_i denote the estimated scatter contribution at the ith LOR. Next we calculate a least-squares spline estimate of the head curve using the same B-spline basis of the dynamic study; we normalize this spline to integrate to unity. Denote this estimate as $h(t) = \sum_\ell h_\ell B_\ell(t)$ where h_ℓ are the control vertices of the head curve spline fit. The estimated scatter rate function is then

$$s_i(t) = S_i h(t) = S_i \sum_\ell h_\ell B_\ell(t).$$

Note that when computing S_i and $h(t)$ we subtract the delayed events from the prompts to correct for randoms.

5   Computational Considerations and Image Estimation

5.1   The "Timogram"

The raw list mode data is in a form that is inconvenient for computing the gradient of the penalized likelihood function. The list mode events arrive in random spatial order and hence require random rather than sequential access to the control vertices that define the rate functions in the sinogram domain. We have therefore developed a means to store list mode data in sinogram form while preserving the temporal information. This is achieved using a single standard sinogram that contains all detected events augmented by a second file listing the arrival times of all events sorted in projection order. We call this second file the "timogram". The timogram simply consists of the arrival times of each event. The sinogram is required to indicate how many arrival times to read for each bin. The resulting pair of files can be substantially smaller than either the original list mode data file or the set of sinograms that would be stored in a conventional dynamic study. We note that Ollinger [16] also resorted list mode data prior to reconstruction, though his format did not completely eliminate the random spatial order.

ECAT HR+ list mode data consists of a sequence of 4-byte event words, each either a coincident event or a timing event. The coincident events record the sinogram bin, optional gating information, and are identified as "prompt" or "delay". The timing events are inserted in the list mode stream every 1 millisecond, and they also record time with a 27 bit integer. By re-encoding the arrival time of each coincidence event using 16 bits, we can retain a temporal resolution of 256ms and a maximum acquisition time of 4.6 hours. Using this format we need only 2 bytes per event in the timogram. Thus we can discard all of the timing events in the list mode data and save a factor of two in the space required to store the remaining coincidence arrival times. The space savings from discarding the timing events are significant. For example, in a 90 minute scan, the timing events take more space than a 3D sinogram set and hence the raw list mode data will always take more space than the sinogram-timogram, even if no coincidences are detected!

The sinogram-timogram format will also be more space efficient than a multi-frame sinogram when the space required to store the event arrival times in the timogram is less than the 2nd through nth sinograms. For example, an 11 frame acquisition is 10 frames larger ($\sim$ 200MB larger) than a sinogram-timogram with no events; only after 200MB-worth of events, or 100 million counts are stored will the sinogram-timogram be less space efficient.

The sinogram-timogram format could be made even more compact by storing inter-arrival times and then performing entropy-based compression [9]. The motivation for this is that LOR's with high activity will tend to have short inter-arrival times, hence will have many high bits consistently zero, a property that compression can exploit.

5.2 Preconditioned Conjugate Gradient Based Reconstruction

A preconditioned conjugate-gradient method was used to maximize the objective function. The particular method closely follows our previous work on static reconstructions [15,19], so we only describe the method briefly here. We use the following preconditioned Polak-Ribiere form of the conjugate gradient method.

$$\mathcal{W}^{(n+1)} = \mathcal{W}^{(n)} + \alpha^{(n)} s^{(n)}$$
$$s^{(n)} = d^{(n)} + \beta^{(n-1)} s^{(n-1)}$$
$$d^{(n)} = C^{(n)} g^{(n)}$$
$$\beta^{(n-1)} = \frac{(g^{(n)} - g^{(n-1)})' d^{(n)}}{g^{(n-1)'} d^{(n-1)}}$$

where $g^{(n)}$ is the gradient vector of the penalized likelihood (4) at $\mathcal{W} = \mathcal{W}^{(n)}$, $C^{(n)}$ is a preconditioner, and the step size $\alpha^{(n)}$ is found using a Newton-Raphson line search.

In this study $C^{(n)}$ was chosen analogously to the static PET reconstruction [20] as

$$C^{(n)} = \text{diag}\left\{\frac{|w_{j\ell}^{(n)}| + \delta}{\sum_i p_{ij}}\right\},$$

where δ is a small positive number to ensure that $C^{(n)}$ is positive definite. Here we set δ equal to $0.01\max_{jl}\{w_{j\ell}^{(n)}\}$.

The algorithm was initialized with a constant image for which the forward projected rate function matches the average rate of the data after subtracting scatters and randoms. The search vector is initialized by setting $s^{(0)} = d^{(0)}$. At each iteration we test whether the search vector is an ascent direction, i.e $g^{(n)'}s^{(n)} > 0$. If not, then we reinitialize the PCG algorithm with $s^{(n)} = d^{(n)}$.

The logarithm in the likelihood function requires that the line search in (5) is performed with the hard constraint that the forward projected rate function at any arrival time is non-negative, i.e.

$$\lambda_i(a_{ik}) \geq 0, \quad \forall i, k.$$

The negativity penalty in (4) is soft allowing small negative values. The hard constraint can be satisfied by limiting the step size in the update step of the conjugate gradient algorithm. To minimize the effect of this constraint on the convergence rate, we use a bent, rather than truncated, line search [11].

6   Simulation Studies and Performance Evaluation

6.1   Simulation Study

We evaluated our method with simulated and real data. We simulated a blood flow data set using a single slice of the Hoffman brain phantom. We evaluated the simulated data on the basis of instantaneous rate accuracy as described below. The real data consisted of one 2D subset of a 10 minute 3D ^{15}O-water list mode brain study. Our subjective evaluations focused on tissues that are known to have distinctly different dynamics with this tracer.

The simulated data was a simplified model of the dynamics of a bolus injection of ^{15}O-water using tissue time activity curves generated by the Kety autoradiographic model ([7], Figure 3B). We chose two extreme curves, one corresponding to very high blood flow, one to very low blood flow. White matter voxels were assigned to have low blood flow, gray matter voxels to have high blood flow. We used an 11 element B-spline basis with support from 0 to 140 seconds; the spacing of the knot locations were determined by equally spacing 7 points along a medium blood flow curve. We used 7 negativity penalty points (d_z) in each knot interval. Approximately 5 million counts were generated for this data set.

As a preliminary evaluation we computed the mean squared error (MSE) between the true source and the instantaneous rate estimate at three times, $t =$

10, 23 and 60 seconds. We compared this MSE to that obtained by estimating the instantaneous rate with a static sinogram based on events arriving in the interval $[t - d/2, t + d/2]$, for $d = 1$, 2, 4, 10, and 20 seconds. In both cases the MSE's are based on one realization, the mean taken over voxels. While this comparison of instantaneous rate accuracy could be regarded as an unfair since the static data has no information on the nonstationarity of the tracer distribution, it is comparable to existing methods. We did not attempt to match the spatial smoothness (bias) of the two methods; for each d, the static data sets were reconstructed with an ML estimate ($\beta = 0$) with 25 iterations.

Figure 1 shows the results of the blood flow simulation for 120 iterations. The rate functions for six voxels are shown in top left; there is generally good agreement between true and estimated functions. The plot of instantaneous mean squared error is shown top right. The spline estimates (horizontal lines) have appreciably lower MSE than all static estimates with frame durations less than 10 seconds. Note that of the 20 second static estimates, the one with largest MSE occurs at $t = 23$ seconds, corresponding to the mode of the high-flow curve. This is expected since averaging across greater durations from the mode will bias the static estimate downward; at the other time points the rate function is approximately linear and there will be less bias in the static estimate.

6.2 Human Study

For the real data we used a 15 element B-spline basis with support over the whole acquisition duration, 0 to 600 seconds; knot spacing was determined by approximate equal spacing of 11 points along the head curve; again $d_z = 7$. The subject was injected with a 5 mCi ($\sim$ 200 MBq) bolus of ^{15}O-water approximately 30 seconds after the start of 3D data acquisition. To create the 2D data set we rebinned data from eight ring pairs into a single dataset with about 400,000 counts, using only the prompt events.

Figure 2 shows the results of the human study after 40 iterations. A three panel image shows the tracer distribution at 20, 60 and 120 seconds post injection. At 20 seconds the carotid arteries are visible, especially the right one; at 60 seconds the water has perfused the brain and surrounding tissue and the carotids are sill visible; at 120 seconds the carotids are indistinguishable from background tissue though the brain still has increased activity. This differing temporal character is clear from the plot of selected voxels. The carotid artery shows a sharply peaked distribution, while brain tissue rises later and more smoothly; the sinus region has much lower flow though it's rate function shows a similar character to that of the brain tissue.

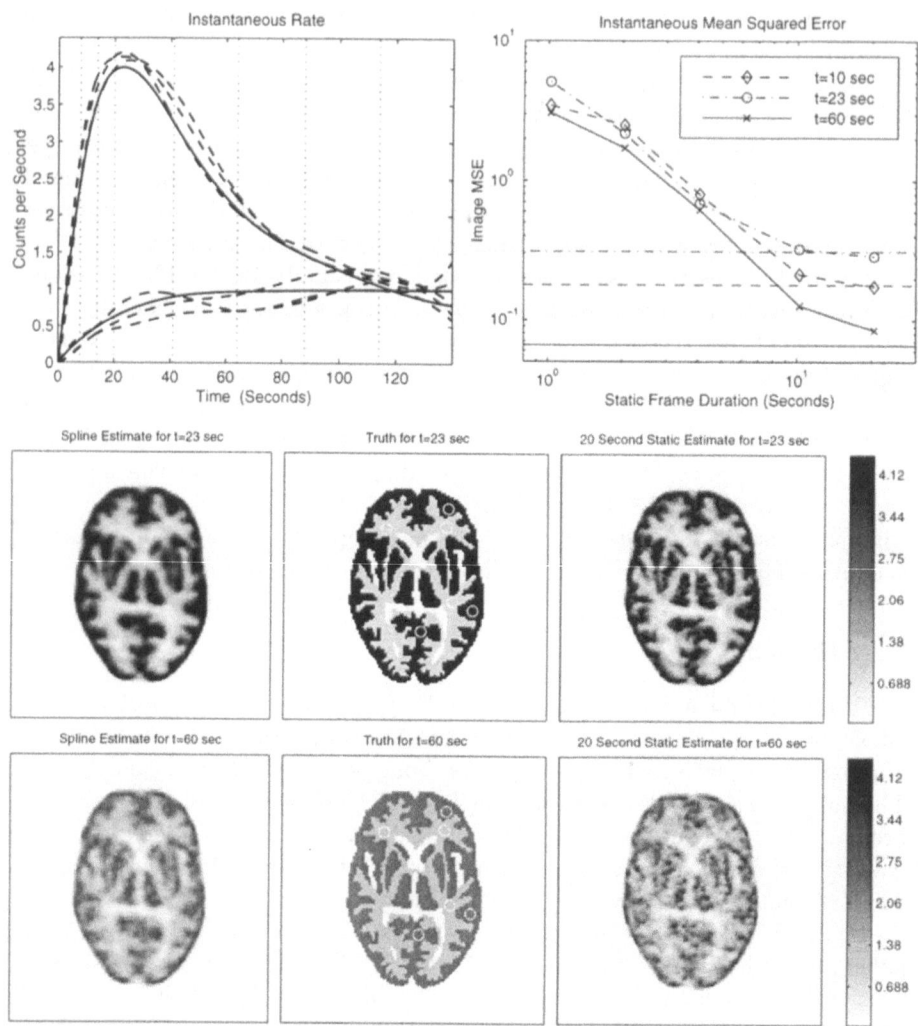

Fig. 1. This figure shows the results of the blood flow simulation. The top left plot shows the estimated (*dashed*) and true (*solid*) rate functions; the vertical lines (*dotted*) indicate knot locations. The top right plot shows the mean squared error over the image for estimating the instantaneous rate at 3 time points; the horizontal lines are for the spline estimate, the decreasing curves show mean squared error for the static estimates of different frame lengths. The bottom two rows show instantaneous rate images; the top row is for $t=23$ seconds, the bottom row for $t=60$ seconds. The left column is the spline estimate, the center column is the truth and the right column is the estimate from the longest static acquisition; the truth images have circles noting the location of the voxels plotted top left

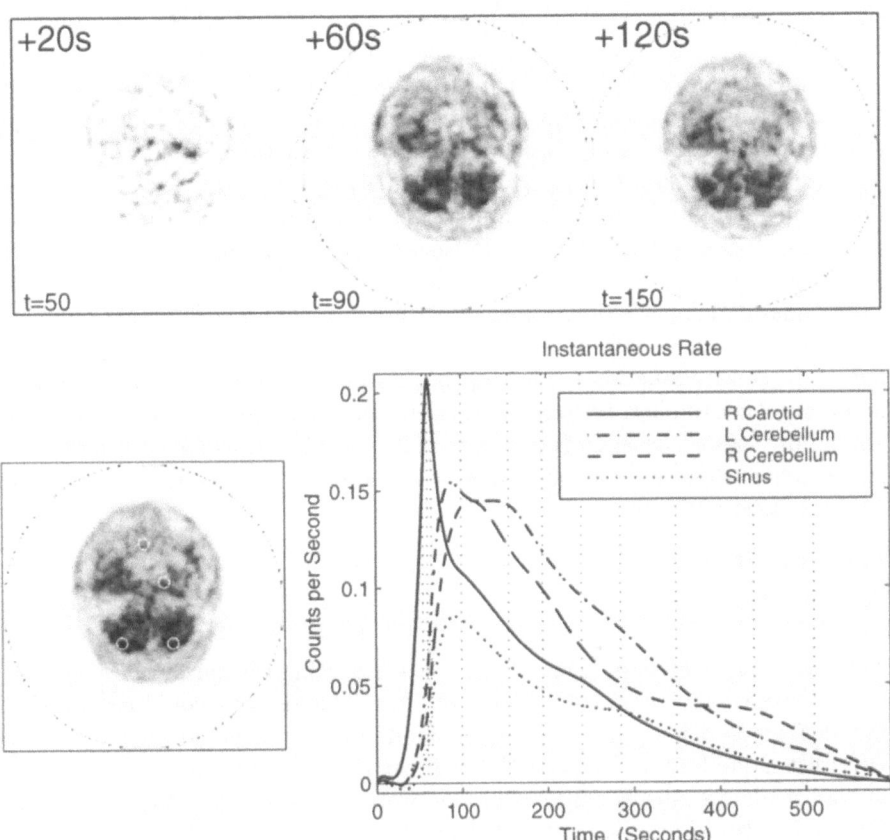

Fig. 2. This figure shows the result of our method using real data. The top row shows a sequence of instantaneous rate images for 20, 60 and 120 seconds post-injection. (Injection occurred at $t \approx 30$ seconds). The early arrival and fast clearance of the tracer in the carotid artery is apparent, as the carotid is visible in the left and center images, but not in the right. The bottom right shows the estimated rate functions for 4 individual voxels; the vertical dotted lines are the knot-locations. The image on left is the total counts image; circles indicate the location of the 4 voxels plotted; the bilateral circles mark the right and left cerebellum, the circle outside of brain tissue is the sinus and the other circle is the right carotid artery

7   Discussion and Conclusions

We have presented preliminary results on estimating continuous time dynamic PET images from list mode PET data. We modeled the dynamic tracer density as an inhomogeneous Poisson process and parameterized the rate functions with a B-spline basis. We introduced the timogram as a means to compactly represent the temporal information of list mode data. The B-spline basis and the timogram's spatial ordering both contribute to an efficient implementation that makes the creation of continuous time reconstructions feasible.

We have presented basic performance analysis with arbitrarily chosen tuning parameters for spatial and temporal regularization. While these results are encouraging in general, Monte Carlo simulations are needed to assess bias and variance in ROI's and in the image at different parameter values.

Estimating images of physiological parameters is a possible extension of this work. This could be accomplished either through embedding the physiological model in the rate function (as in [16]) or estimating parameters with the spline functions. The standard to compare these results to would be estimates from the temporally binned data. In fact, temporally binned data could also be applied in this inhomogeneous Poisson framework, as there is a counterpart to equation (2) for binned data [22].

Acknowledgments

This work was conducted while T.E.N. was a visiting scholar at the University of Southern California in the summer of 1998. The authors would like to thank David Townsend for providing the list mode data and for information on the HR+ list mode format. We also thank Peter Bloomfield for generously sharing his list mode decoder source code. This work was supported by the National Cancer Institute under grant R01 CA59794.

References

1. Barrett, H.H., White, T., Parra, L.C.: List-mode likelihood. Journal of the Optical Society of America, **14** (1997) 2914–2923
2. Bartels, R.H., Beatty, J.C., Barsky, B.A.: An introduction to splines for use in computer graphics and geometric modeling. M. Kaufmann Publishers, Los Altos, CA (1986)
3. de Boor, C.: A Practical Guide to Splines. Vol. 27 of Applied Mathematical Sciences. Springer-Verlag, New York (1978)
4. Fessler, J.A.: Penalized weighted least-squares image reconstruction for PET. IEEE Transactions on Medical Imaging **13** (1994) 290–300
5. Geman, S., McClure, D.E.: Statistical methods for tomographic image reconstruction. In Proceedings of The 46th Session of The ISI, Bulletin of The ISI **52** (1987)
6. Gu, C., Qiu, C.: Smoothing spline density estimation: Theory. The Annals of Statistics **21** (1993) 217–234

7. Herscovitch, P., Markham, J., Raichle, M.E.: Brain blood flow measured with intravenious $H_2\,^{15}O$. I. Theory and error analysis. Journal of Nuclear Medicine **24** (1983) 782–789

8. Huang, S.C., Phelps, M.E.: Principles of Tracer Kinetic Modeling in Posistron Emission Tomography and Autoradiography. In: Positron Emission Tomography and Autoradiography. Principles and Applications for the Brain and Heart. Raven Press, New York (1986)

9. Huffman, D.A.: A method for the construction of minimum-redundancy codes. Proceedings of the Institute of Radio Engineers **40** (1952) 1098–1101

10. Johnson, C., Yan, Y., Carson, R., Martino, R., Daube-Witherspoon, M.: A system for the 3D reconstruction of retracted-septa PET data using the EM algorithm. IEEE Transactions on Nuclear Science **42** (1995) 1223–1227

11. Kaufman, L.: Maximum likelihood, least squares, and penalized least squares for PET. IEEE Transactions on Medical Imaging **12** (1993) 200–214

12. Lee, S.-J., Rangarajan, A., Gindi, G.: Bayesian image reconstruction in SPECT using higher order mechanical models as priors. IEEE Transactions on Medical Imaging **14** (1995) 669–680

13. Luenberger, D.: Linear and nonlinear programming. Addison-Wesley, Reading, Mass (1989)

14. Matthews, J., Bailey, D., Price, P., Cunningham, V.: The direct calculation of parametric images from dynamic PET data using maximum-likelihood iterative reconstruction. Physics in Medicine and Biology **42** (1997) 1155–1173

15. Mumcuoglu, E.U., Leahy, R., Cherry, S.R., Zhou, Z.: Fast gradient-based methods for Bayesian reconstruction of transmission and emission PET images. IEEE Transactions on Medical Imaging **13** (1994) 687–701

16. Ollinger, J.M.: Algorithms for parameter estimation in dynamic tracer studies using postiron emission tomography. PhD thesis, Washington University School of Medicine, St. Louis, MO (1986)

17. O'Sullivan, F. Image radiotracer model parameters in PET: A mixture analysis approach. IEEE Transactions on Medical Imaging **12** (1993) 399–412

18. Parra, L., Barrett, H.H.: List-mode likelihood: EM algorithm and image quality estimation demonstrated on 2D PET. IEEE Transactions on Medical Imaging **17** (1998) 228–235

19. Qi, J., Leahy, R.M., Cherry, S.R., Chatziioannou, A., Farquhar, T.H.: High resolution 3D bayesian image reconstruction using the microPET small animal scanner. Physics in Medicine and Biology **43** (1998) 1001–1013

20. Qi, J., Leahy, R.M., Hsu, C., Farquhar, T.H., Cherry, S.R.: Fully 3D Bayesian image reconstruction for ECAT EXACT HR+. IEEE Transactions on Nuclear Science **45** (1998) 1096–1103

21. Snyder, D.: Parameter estimation for dynamic studies in emission-tomography systems having list-mode data. IEEE Transactions on Nuclear Science **31** (1984) 925–931

22. Snyder, D., Miller, M.: Random Point processes in time and space, 2nd edition. Springer-Verlag, New York (1991)

23. Snyder, D.L.: Utilizing side information in emission tomography. IEEE Transactions on Nuclear Science **31** (1984) 533–537

24. Wahba, G.: Interpolating spline methods for density estimation. I: Equi-spaced knots. The Annals of Statistics **3** (1975) 30–48

25. Watson, C.C., Newport, D., Casey, M.E., deKemp, R.A., Beanlands, R.S., Schmand, M.: Evaluation of simulation based scatter correction for 3D PET cardiac imaging. IEEE Transactions on Nuclear Science **44** (1997) 90–97

Hybrid Geometric Active Models for Shape Recovery in Medical Images

Yanlin Guo[1] and Baba C. Vemuri[2]

[1] Sarnoff Corporation,
CN5300, Princeton, NJ 08530
email: yguo@sarnoff.com

[2] Department of Computer & Information Sciences & Engr.,
University of Florida, Gainesville, FL 32611
email: vemuri@cise.ufl.edu

Abstract. In this paper, we propose extensions to a powerful geometric shape modeling scheme introduced in [14]. The extension allows the model to automatically cope with topological changes and for the first time, introduces the concept of a global shape into geometric/geodesic snake models. The ability to characterize global shape of an object using very few parameters facilitates shape learning and recognition. In this new modeling scheme, object shapes are represented using a parameterized function – called the generator – which accounts for the global shape of an object and the pedal curve/surface of this global shape with respect to a geometric snake to represent any local detail. Traditionally, pedal curves/surfaces are defined as the loci of the feet of perpendiculars to the tangents of the generator from a fixed point called the pedal point. We introduce physics-based control for shaping these geometric models by using distinct pedal points – lying on a snake – for each point on the generator. The model dubbed as a "snake pedal" allows for interactive manipulation via forces applied to the snake. Automatic topological changes of the model may be achieved by implementing the geometric active contour in a level-set framework. We demonstrate the applicability of this modeling scheme via examples of shape estimation from a variety of medical image data.

1 Introduction

Extracting shapes of anatomical structures from medical image data is a challenging problem in Medical Image Analysis and has been the focus of research of numerous researchers in the medical imaging community over the past several years. Since the inception of active contours/surfaces a.k.a. snakes, in the vision/graphics community by Kass *et al.* [5], these elastically deformable contours/surfaces have been widely used for a variety of applications including Medical Image Analysis where it has facilitated boundary detection and representation, motion tracking etc. of anatomical structures of interest. The classical approach to object shape recovery using the snakes is based on deforming an initial configuration of the snake represented by a position vector $\mathcal{P}_0$ towards the

A. Kuba et al. (Eds.): IPMI'99, LNCS 1613, pp. 112–125, 1999.
© Springer-Verlag Berlin Heidelberg 1999

boundary of the shape being detected by minimizing a functional that can be regarded as the bending energy stored in a thin flexible beam/rod or a stretchable string subject to loading. There are several problems associated with this approach, such as initialization, the automatic specification of the physical or elasticity parameters etc. Moreover, this energy model requires that the topology of the shape to be estimated be known a priori. Several researchers have addressed these issues in detail and some of them are open research issues to date.

A viable alternative to the snakes model was proposed by Malladi *et al.* [8] and Caselles *et al.* [1]. These models are based on the theory of curve evolution and geometric flows. Automatic changes in topology can be handled in a natural way in this modeling technique, by implementing the curve evolution using the level-set embedding schemes. A generalization of this model was later proposed simultaneously by Caselles et. al., [2] and Kichenassamy et. al., [6]. The generalization also known as the *geometric active contours* showed the link between the Kass et. al., [5] snakes and the *geometric active contours* a.k.a. *geodesic/geometric snakes*. For details on the theory of curve/surface evolution and its level-set implementation, we refer the reader to [1,8,9,2,6,12,13,15]. Geoemtric active contours and its variants are quite successful in recovering shapes from medical as well as non medical images. They do not suffer from the initialization problems, do not have too many user specified parameters and can handle arbitrary topologies in an elegant manner. One might ask, what then is lacking in these models? Firstly, there is no way to characterize the global shape of an object or anatomical structure, which is a useful property to have in describing shape for identification purposes. Secondly, it is not easy to incorporate prior shape information. In this paper, we will address these problems and propose a novel modeling scheme along with efficient numerical techniques for use in shape recovery from image data.

1.1 Overview of the Hybrid Geometric Active Contour Model

In many Medical Imaging applications such as shape recognition, characterizing the global shape of an object is crucial. Traditional geometric active contour/surface models do not possess the capability to characterize the global shape of an object. In this paper, we introduce a novel concept of a global/core model into the PDE-based curve evolution framework by embedding the snake pedal model into a level-set framework. Instead of characterizing a shape boundary by the position of every point on the boundary, our proposed model, referred to as the hybrid geometric active model, now describes a shape as a combination of a global/core shape such as an ellipse, super-ellipse, etc. and a variable offset defined with respect to the global shape. The variable offsets are controlled by this global shape and an evolving curve — the controlling snake in the snake pedal model. For the model to recover the object boundary, we introduce a reliable and efficient numerical method which consist of a global plus local shape estimation technique in the model fitting. We use the Levenberg-Marquardt (LM) for estimating the global shape and a combination of up-wind and minmod finite difference schemes in a level-set framework for estimating the local shape. The hybrid geometric active contour/surface model retains all the advantages of traditional geometric active models (for example, topology change, ability to model complex geometries and amenability to stable numerical implementation) and has the added ability/advantage of being able to compactly represent global shape of an object. Augmentating the curve evolution framework with a global shape/core will be very useful in shape learning/recognition and image indexing applications.

1.2   Organization of the Paper

In Section 2.1 we briefly discuss the snake pedal model introduced in [14] and then present the novel hybrid geometric active models in Section 2.2. The numerical issues of the model fitting process will be discussed in Section 2.3, followed by the implementation results in Section 3.

2   Hybrid Geometric Active Model

In this section we will first briefly review the snake pedal model – introduced in [14] – with the aid of 3D model fitting examples. We will then present the hybrid geometric active model which is obtained by replacing the snake in the snake pedal with a geometric/geodesic snake implemented in a level-set framework.

2.1   The Snake Pedal Model

Let α be a planar curve, the **pedal curve** [3] of α is defined as the locus of points on the foot **f** of the perpendicular from a fixed point **p** called the **pedal point** to a variable tangent of α. Let β be the pedal curve of α with respect

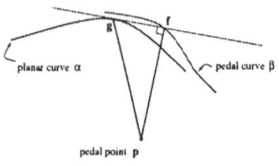

Fig. 1. **f** is on the pedal curve of α with respect to the pedal point **p**

to the pedal point **p**, and let $\alpha(t) = \mathbf{g}, \beta(t) = \mathbf{f}$, as shown in the Fig. 1. The projection of $\alpha(t) - \mathbf{p}$ in the direction $J\alpha'(t)$ must be $\beta(t) - \mathbf{p}$, where $\alpha'(t)$ is the tangent line of the plane curve $\alpha(t)$, $J : \Re^2 \longrightarrow \Re^2$ is a linear map given by $J(p_1, p_2) = (-p_2, p_1)$. J can be geometrically interpreted as a rotation by $\pi/2$ in a counterclockwise direction. We can thus define a pedal curve as follows [3]:

Definition 1. *The* **pedal curve** *of a regular curve* $\alpha : (c, d) \longrightarrow \Re^2$ *with respect to a fixed (pedal) point* $\mathbf{p} \in \Re^2$ *is given by*

$$\mathbf{pedal}[\mathbf{p}, \alpha](t) = \mathbf{p} + \frac{(\alpha(t) - \mathbf{p}) \cdot J\alpha'(t)}{\|J\alpha'(t)\|^2} J\alpha'(t). \tag{1}$$

In Fig. 2, we present examples depicting the pedal curves of an ellipse for different positions of the pedal point (shown by a bold dot). Note that the pedal curve is capable of exhibiting local as well as a global deformations and the location of the local deformation is in the locality of the pedal point. By moving the position of the pedal point, it is possible to synthesize a variety of local deformations as depicted in the Fig. 2. The curve $\alpha(t)$ will be referred to as the **generator** for the pedal curve $\beta(t)$ and process of generating a pedal curve will be referred to as the **pedaling operation**.

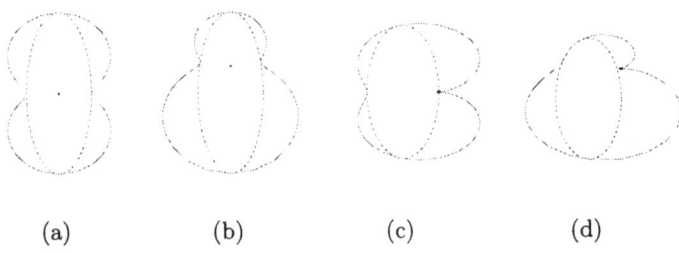

(a)   (b)   (c)   (d)

Fig. 2. Examples of pedal curves of an ellipse for different pedal point positions. Pedal points are shown by a dot in each case

More general shapes may be synthesized by letting the pedal point be different for each point of the generator. We can let the pedal points be specified by another curve $\mathbf{p}(t)$ represented by a standard snake [5] and then apply the **pedaling operation** to each point on the generator $\alpha_i = \alpha(t_i)$ with respect to corresponding pedal point $\mathbf{p}_i = \mathbf{p}(t_i)$. The generator can be either a parameterized or an implicit function representing a curve. The pedaling operation generates a new curve that we dub a **snake pedal** $\mathbf{x}(t)$ as shown in Fig. 3. If the generator is an ellipse as shown in Fig. 3 (a), we can represent it in a parametric form by

$$\alpha(t) = \begin{bmatrix} cos\theta & sin\theta \\ -sin\theta & cos\theta \end{bmatrix} \begin{bmatrix} a_1 \ cost \\ a_2 \ sint \end{bmatrix} + \begin{bmatrix} m_1 \\ m_2 \end{bmatrix} \tag{2}$$

where a_1, a_2 are aspect ratio parameters, θ is the rotation angle between the intrinsic (material) coordinates and inertial coordinates, $\mathbf{m} = (m_1, m_2)^T$ is the centroid of the generator in the world coordinates. We collect the generator parameters into the global parameter vector $\mathbf{q} = (a, b, \theta, m_1, m_2)^T$.

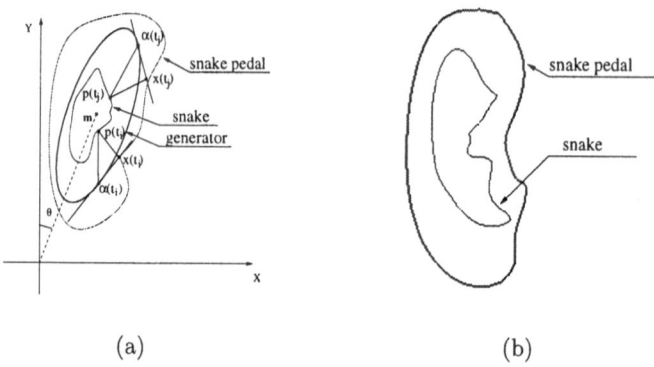

(a)   (b)

Fig. 3. (a) The process of generating a snake pedal with an ellipse generator. (b) "snake pedal" controlled by the snake using an ellipse generator

In Fig. 4(a)-(b) we depict some examples of snake pedals, curves generated using snakes and an ellipse as the generator. Note the variety of local deformations that can be generated using this modeling technique. We remind the reader that the snake pedal itself is a geometric model and that it is not *directly* responsive to the application of external forces unlike the standard snake models [5].

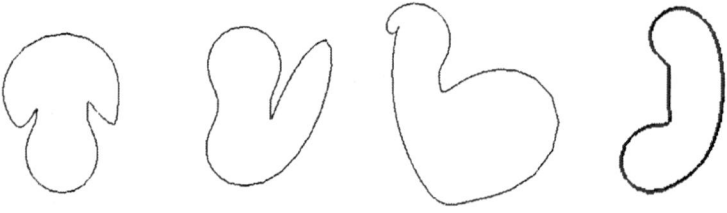

Fig. 4. Examples of "snake pedals" using an ellipse generator

The pedal curve definition can be modified slightly by subtracting the second term from the first in (1). *This allows for larger local deformations including shrinkage and expansion.* A pedal surface is the surface analog of the pedal curve. It is the locus of the points on the foot of the perpendicular from a fixed pedal point to a variable tangent plane of the surface. As in the 2D case, we can let the pedal point vary for each point on the generator surface. Thus we have the snake pedal surfaces in 3D whose shape can be controlled by snakes which are either curves or surfaces in 3D [14].

Fitting the "snake pedal" to data is posed as a nonlinear minimization and we use the Levenberg-Marquardt nonlinear optimization algorithm [11] in conjunction with an efficient version of the alternating direction implicit (ADI) technique [14] to achieve the fitting. Fig. 2.1 presents a model fitting example to sparse 3D data points placed by an expert neunro-scientist along the boundaries of a gyrus in selected slices of an MR brain scan. Such a scenario arises in the semi-automatic construction of anatomical models for possible use as a prior model in shape recovery from unknown data. In this example, from left to right, the images depict a slice of an MR brain scan in which the shape of interest – a gyrus – has been identified by a neuro-scientist via sparsely placed points on the shape boundary. The next image shows the collection of these 3D points in red and the initialized snake pedal model followed by an image depicting the intermediate stage of fitting and the final fitted model respectively. As evident, the model achieves a visually accurate fit to the data. In addition, the model fit has been validated against manual segmentation from an expert neuro-scientist.

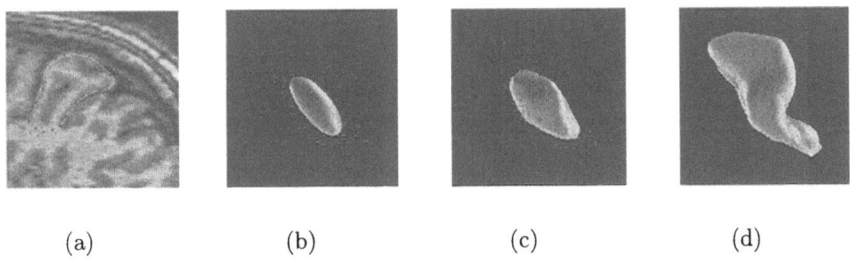

(a)   (b)   (c)   (d)

Fig. 5. Left to right: MR brain scan depicting a region of interest (a gyrus), initialized model, intermediate fitting stage and final model fit

2.2 Evolving Snake Pedals

As described in the earlier sections, the traditional PDE-based geometric curve evolution algorithms do not provide a mechanism to characterize the global shape of an object. In this section, we describe how the level set formulation of the geometric curve evolution can be applied to our snake pedal model to realize topological changes (when necessary) as well as capture the global shape representation of an object.

In our approach, to incorporate a smoothing constraint on the snake pedal, we impose regularization via Euclidean arc-length minimization of the snake pedal. This leads to the standard geodesic/geometric active contour. Let us consider a snake pedal denoted by $\mathcal{P}_e(t)$, with its position denoted by $\mathbf{p}_e = \{p_{e1}, p_{e2}\}$, then the standard geometric curve evolution formula for the snake pedal can be written as

$$\frac{\partial \mathbf{p}_e}{\partial t} = F(k_e)\mathbf{N}_e, \tag{3}$$

where k_e and $\mathbf{N}_e$ are the curvature and normal of the snake pedal respectively. We now examine how the "snake" would evolve if the snake pedal were evolving as a function of its local curvature. Indeed, we will not evolve the snake pedal curve directly, instead, we will first solve for the snake position under the constraint that the arc-length of the snake pedal is minimized, and the pedal curve can then be determined by the pedaling operation defined in Section 2.1, given the position of the generator. The problem therefore can be solved by the following procedure:

1. Derive the curve evolution equation for the snake $\mathcal{P}(t)$ by minimizing the arc-length of the snake pedal $\mathcal{P}_e(t)$;
2. Embed the evolving curve $\mathcal{P}(t)$ in a higher dimensional surface ϕ_1 and formulate the equation of motion for ϕ_1;
3. Solve the equation of motion for ϕ_1 using proper numerical techniques;
4. Determine the snake pedal curve from the evolving snake via the pedaling operation, given the generator.

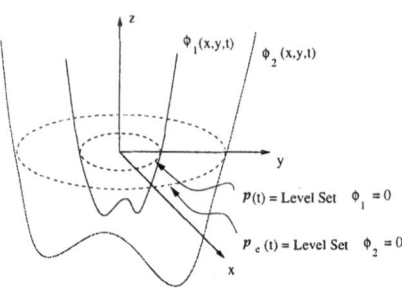

Fig. 6. Relation between $\mathcal{P}(t)$, $\mathcal{P}_e(t)$, ϕ_1, and ϕ_2, the level-sets of the higher dimensional surfaces ϕ_1 and ϕ_2 respectively. They are related by the pedaling operation

We remind the reader that in the above procedure, the snake pedal curve also evolves, but it evolves as a standard geometric active contour embedded in another higher dimensional surface ϕ_2. We do not need to solve the equation of motion for ϕ_2 directly instead, ϕ_2 can be regarded as being *implicit* in the procedure. Thus, we do not determine the level-set curve $\mathcal{P}_e(t)$ of the surface ϕ_2 instead, we first evaluate ϕ_1 and determine its zero set, then we apply the pedaling operation to obtain the snake pedal $\mathcal{P}_e(t)$. In addition, even though ϕ_2 is not involved in the final algorithm, it is very useful in the derivation of the governing PDE for the function ϕ_1. Note that the snake model discussed here is no longer the classical energy-minimizing model, since its deformation is not obtained by minimizing some internal deformation energy, but we will still use the name "snake" to represent the controlling active contours in the snake pedal model. Fig. 6 depicts this important relationship between $\mathcal{P}(t), \mathcal{P}_e(t), \phi_1$, and ϕ_2.

Note that *an important feature of this modeling technique is the incorporation of a global parameterized shape, namely, the generator, into the curve evolution framework.* As already mentioned earlier, this global parameterized shape can be very useful in applications involving objects recognition as well as in shape learning (by collecting statistics on the global shape parameters of the model). Since a geometric active contour is used to represent the controlling "snake" in the model, and also the model can capture the "global orientation" of an object or a group of objects, this snake pedal model is referred to as a *hybrid geometric active contour* model. Detailed discussion of the related concepts will be given in the following sections, starting with the derivation of the relationship between the snake and the snake pedal evolution.

Relation Between the Snake and Snake Pedal Curve Evolution Consider a snake $\mathbf{p} = (p_1, p_2)^T$ and a generator $\boldsymbol{\alpha} = (\alpha_1, \alpha_2)^T$ with normal $\mathbf{J}'_{\alpha} = (n_1, n_2)^T$, where $\mathbf{p}$ and $\boldsymbol{\alpha}$ are related by an association scheme – a radial association produced by using the same parameterization for both the curves [4]. We obtain the corresponding snake pedal $\mathbf{p}_e = (p_{e1}, p_{e2})^T$ via the following pedaling operation:

$$\mathbf{p}_e = \mathbf{p} - \frac{(\boldsymbol{\alpha} - \mathbf{p}) \cdot \mathbf{J}'_{\alpha}}{\|\mathbf{J}'_{\alpha}\|^2} \cdot \mathbf{J}'_{\alpha}, \tag{4}$$

or simply,

$$\mathbf{p}_e = \mathbf{J}_A \, \mathbf{p} - \mathbf{b}, \tag{5}$$

where

$$\mathbf{J}_A = \begin{bmatrix} 1 + \dfrac{n_1^2}{n_1^2 + n_2^2} & \dfrac{n_1 \cdot n_2}{n_1^2 + n_2^2} \\ \dfrac{n_1 \cdot n_2}{n_1^2 + n_2^2} & 1 + \dfrac{n_2^2}{n_1^2 + n_2^2} \end{bmatrix}, \tag{6}$$

and

$$\mathbf{b} = \frac{\alpha_1 \cdot n_1 + \alpha_2 \cdot n_2}{n_1^2 + n_2^2} \begin{bmatrix} n_1 \\ n_2 \end{bmatrix}. \tag{7}$$

Let the inverse of $\mathbf{J}_A$ be denoted by $\mathbf{J}_B$, which is also a function of n_1 and n_2. We remind the reader that because the generator does not evolve over time, the forms of $\mathbf{J}_B$ and $\mathbf{b}$ do not change over time, but their contents change only during the iterative estimation process. Thus, we can treat $\mathbf{J}_B$ as a constant matrix and $\mathbf{b}$ as a constant vector with respect to time when evolving $\mathbf{p}(t)$ or $\mathbf{p}_e(t)$. Therefore, (5) can be explicitly written as a function of time:

$$\mathbf{p}_e(t) = \mathbf{J}_A\,\mathbf{p}(t) - \mathbf{b}. \tag{8}$$

Taking partial derivative on both sides of (8) with respect to time t yields

$$\frac{\partial \mathbf{p}_e(t)}{\partial t} = \mathbf{J}_A \frac{\partial \mathbf{p}(t)}{\partial t}, \quad \text{or} \quad \frac{\partial \mathbf{p}(t)}{\partial t} = \mathbf{J}_B \frac{\partial \mathbf{p}_e(t)}{\partial t}. \tag{9}$$

Equation (9) reveals a very crucial relationship between the snake and snake pedal evolution: the evolution of two curves are linearly related by a Jacobian matrix. We remind the reader that the relationship between the snake and snake pedal is not linear, but their evolutions over time are related by a linear transformation.

PDE for the Snake and Snake Pedal Evolution When embedding the snake $\mathcal{P}(t)$ as the zero set of a higher dimensional surface ϕ_1, we have:

$$\{\mathcal{P}(t) \in \mathfrak{R}^2 : \phi(\mathbf{p}, t) = 0\}, \tag{10}$$

Differentiating (10) with respect to t yields: $\frac{\partial \phi_1}{\partial t} + \nabla \phi_1 \cdot \frac{\partial \mathbf{p}}{\partial t} = 0$. Similarly, for the higher dimensional function ϕ_2, we have the following formula: $\frac{\partial \phi_2}{\partial t} + \nabla \phi_2 \cdot \frac{\partial \mathbf{p}_e}{\partial t} = 0$. From the discussion in the previous section, we have

$$\begin{cases} \frac{\partial \mathbf{p}_e}{\partial t} = \mathbf{J}_A \cdot \frac{\partial \mathbf{p}}{\partial t}, \\ \quad \text{or} \\ \frac{\partial \mathbf{p}}{\partial t} = \mathbf{J}_B \cdot \frac{\partial \mathbf{p}_e}{\partial t}. \end{cases} \tag{11}$$

As described earlier, we want to minimize the arc-length of the snake pedal, which amounts to imposing a smoothness constraint on the snake pedal curve, hence we require that: $\frac{\partial \mathbf{p}_e}{\partial t} = F(k_e)\mathbf{N}_e$, where $F(k_e)$ is the speed function, which depends on the curvature of the snake pedal k_e. $\mathbf{N}_e$ is the unit normal of the snake pedal. Similar to the relation between the normal of the snake and its higher dimensional function $\phi_1 : \mathbf{N} = -\frac{\nabla \phi_1}{\|\nabla \phi_1\|}$. For the zero level set of ϕ_2, the following relation holds: $\mathbf{N}_e = -\frac{\nabla \phi_2}{\|\nabla \phi_2\|}$ Combining the above three equations we obtain,

$$\frac{\partial \phi_2}{\partial t} = F(k_e)\|\nabla \phi_2\|. \tag{12}$$

Equation (12) is the standard level-set evolution. Similarly, for the governing equation of the snake curve, we have:

$$\frac{\partial \phi_1}{\partial t} = F(k_e)\nabla \phi_1 \cdot \mathbf{J}_B \frac{\nabla \phi_2}{\|\nabla \phi_2\|}. \tag{13}$$

The above two equations are the equations of motion for ϕ_1 and ϕ_2, respectively. We rewrite them together as follows:

$$\begin{cases} \frac{\partial \phi_2}{\partial t} = F(k_e)\|\nabla\phi_2\| \\ \frac{\partial \phi_1}{\partial t} = F(k_e)\nabla\phi_1 \cdot \mathbf{J}_B \frac{\nabla\phi_2}{\|\nabla\phi_2\|} \end{cases}. \tag{14}$$

Eq. (14) represents the PDEs for the evolution of ϕ_1 and ϕ_2 (note that they are not coupled). One approach to solve these PDEs is to use a combination of central and upwind finite differences [10] to solve the first equation in every iteration, and then solve the second equation using a similar method subsequently. We will discuss the up-wind finite difference method in Section 2.3. This approach is straightforward, but needs large amounts of storage for both ϕ_1 and ϕ_2. Note that in (14), only the gradients of ϕ_1 and ϕ_2 are involved on the right hand sides of both equations, we propose a more elegant approach to solve the PDEs in (14) with much less storage, by employing the intrinsic relation between $\nabla\phi_1$ and $\nabla\phi_2$ as discussed in [4]. In [4], a surprisingly simple relation between ϕ_1 and ϕ_2 is obtained after a tedious derivation. This relationship is given by,

$$\nabla\phi_1 = \mathbf{J}_A \cdot \nabla\phi_2, \quad \text{or} \quad \nabla\phi_2 = \mathbf{J}_B \cdot \nabla\phi_1. \tag{15}$$

Where the Jacobian between the evolution of the snake and snake pedal curve $\mathbf{J}_A$ and $\mathbf{J}_B = \mathbf{J}_A^{-1}$ are defined as before. At first glance, this relation is seemingly contradictory to our intuition. One would think that since $\frac{\partial \mathbf{p}_e(t)}{\partial t} = \mathbf{J}_A \frac{\partial \mathbf{p}(t)}{\partial t}$, if there is any Jacobian between the gradients of ϕ_1 and ϕ_2, the relation should be $\nabla\phi_2 = \mathbf{J}_A\nabla\phi_1$, rather than $\nabla\phi_1 = \mathbf{J}_A\nabla\phi_2$.

Since our objective is to obtain the equation of motion for the higher dimensional surface ϕ_1, we substitute ϕ_2 with $\mathbf{J}_B\ \phi_1$ in (13) to get

$$\frac{\partial \phi_1}{\partial t} = F(k_e)\ \|\mathbf{J}_B\nabla\phi_1\|. \tag{16}$$

The representation of k_e in terms of ϕ_1 is quite complicated, we refer the reader to [4] for these details. Equation (16) is the equation of motion for ϕ_1 and constitutes the primary equation in our application. When using the snake pedal model for recovery of the shape of interest from image data, we need to solve the more general equation of motion for the higher dimensional function ϕ_1: $\frac{\partial \phi_1}{\partial t} = g(x, y)\ F(k_e)\ \|\mathbf{J}_B\nabla\phi_1\| + \nabla\phi_1 \cdot \nabla g$, where $g(x, y)$ is an image feature based function and is used to stop the curve evolution when the contour is close to the desired edges. $\nabla\phi_1$ and ∇g must be evaluated at locations on the snake and the snake pedal, respectively.

2.3   Numerical Solution

In this section, we discuss application of the snake pedal to recover the boundaries of the shape of interest from an image using a novel global plus local shape estimation procedure. For the global shape estimation, we employ the well known

Levenberg-Marquardt (LM) method; while for the local shape estimation, we present a *modified* level-set method.

In Section 2.2, we illustrated that the solution for the snake pedal evolution can be achieved by first solving the snake evolution, which is embedded in a higher dimensional surface ϕ_1, then applying the pedaling operation on the snake. Therefore, developing a reliable and efficient numerical algorithm for solving the governing equation of ϕ_1, i.e., (16) is the primary task in applying the snake pedal model for extracting shapes of interest from image data. The governing equation of motion for ϕ_1, in the simplest form is given in (16).

As discussed in [10], the speed function $F(.)$ in (16) consists two terms, namely, the advection term F_A and the diffusion term F_G. The diffusion term smooths the curve while the advection term may result in sigularities during the curve evolution even with smooth initial data. A variety of entropy-satisfying algorithms have been proposed to evolve the curve beyond the formation of sigularities.

In our numerical approach, to solve the equation of motion (16), for the diffusion term, we use the standard central difference approximation. Whereas, for the advection term, we need to solve the following hyperbolic initial-value problem:

$$\phi_{1t} = \sqrt{a(x,y)\phi_{1x}^2 + b(x,y)\phi_{1y}^2 + c(x,y)\phi_{1x}\phi_{1y}}, \tag{17}$$

where $a(x,y), b(x,y)$ and $c(x,y)$ are determined by the entries of $\mathbf{J}_B$ and do not change over time. ϕ_{1x}^2 and ϕ_{1y}^2 can be approximated by the upwind finite difference scheme discussed in [10]. But for the $\phi_{1x}\phi_{1y}$ term, we use the *minmod finite difference* approximation discussed in Kimmel *et al.* [7]. The minmod finite derivative is defined as:

$$minmod\{a,b\} = \begin{cases} sign(a)min(|a|,|b|) & \text{if } ab > 0 \\ 0 & \text{otherwise.} \end{cases} \tag{18}$$

Using this definition to approximate $\phi_{1x}\phi_{1y}$ leads to

$$\phi_{1x}\phi_{1y}|_{\substack{x=i\Delta x \\ y=j\Delta y}} = minmod(D_x^+\phi_{1,(i,j)}, D_x^-\phi_{1,(i,j)}) \; minmod(D_y^+\phi_{1,(i,j)}, D_y^-\phi_{1,(i,j)}), \tag{19}$$

where D_x^+, D_x^- are as defined are

$$D_x^-\phi_{1i} = \frac{\phi_{1i}^n - \phi_{1(i-1)}^n}{\Delta x}, \qquad D_x^+\phi_{1i} = \frac{\phi_{1(i+1)}^n - \phi_{1i}^n}{\Delta x}, \tag{20}$$

and similar definitions apply to D_y^+ and D_y^-.

Combining these finite differences yields a first order numerical scheme for solving (17), the advection term in (16):

$$\begin{aligned} \phi_{1,(i,j)}^{n+1} = \phi_{1,(i,j)}^n + \Delta t \\ [a_{i,j}((max(D_x^-\phi_{1,(i,j)},0))^2 + (min(D_x^+\phi_{1,(i,j)},0))^2) \\ + b_{i,j}((max(D_y^-\phi_{1,(i,j)},0))^2 + (min(D_y^+\phi_{1,(i,j)},0))^2) \\ - c_{i,j}minmod(D_x^+\phi_{1,(i,j)}, D_x^-\phi_{1,(i,j)})minmode(D_y^+\phi_{1,(i,j)}, D_y^-\phi_{1,(i,j)})]^{1/2} \end{aligned} \tag{21}$$

This numerical scheme is stable and provides a natural way to handle the topological changes in the snake evolution.

3   Implementation Results

In this section, we present the level-set implementation of the hybrid geometric active model with ellipse and super-ellipse generators described in Section 2.2 respectively. The examples contain 2D slices from an MR scan of the human heart. In each row of Fig. 7, from left to right, images show the model initializations, intermediate stages of fitting and the final model fits. The model is initialized to capture the endocardium structure. In the top row, we used an ellipse generator and in the bottom row, a superellipse was used. AS evident from the results, the super-ellipse captures the global shape better for this example. The snake pedal is shown in green (light gray) and the global shape in red (dark gray). We use image-based speed function to deter the model evolution in both examples.

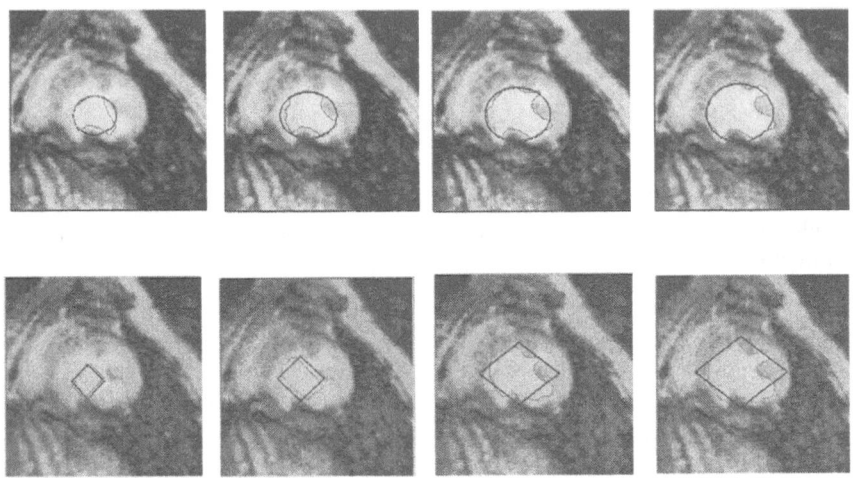

Fig. 7. Hybrid geometric active contour fitting examples: Left to right, model initialization (snake pedal in green (light gray) and generator in red (dark gray)), intermediate stages of evolution and final fit. The first row uses an ellipse generator while the second row uses a super-ellpise generator

Fig. 8 depicts a topological change example for synthetic data. From left to right, images depict model initialization, intermediate stage of evolution and final fit respectively. In this example, the snake pedal is initialized as a single small ellipse, as the fitting proceeds, the model expands and splits, and finally fits to all the object contours in the whole image. The global shapes of the generator is not shown here since the meaning of the "global" shape in these examples is not very useful.

By replacing the ellipse generator with a super-ellipse, we can obtain a more general/powerful representation of the global shape in the snake pedal model.

In all these examples, we implemented the level-set form of the equation:

$$\frac{\partial \phi_1}{\partial t} = g(x, y) \, F(k_e) \, \|\mathbf{J}_B \nabla \phi_1\| + \nabla \phi_1 \cdot \nabla g,$$

where, $g(\nabla I) = 1/(1 + \|\nabla(G * I)\|^2/K)$ with $G * I$ being a Gaussian convolved with the image and K being a scaling constant. More sophisticated stopping criteria may be synthesized to yield better accuracy in shape recovery. We use the upwind difference and minmod difference method described in Section 2.3 to implement this Hamilton-Jacobi equation of motion.

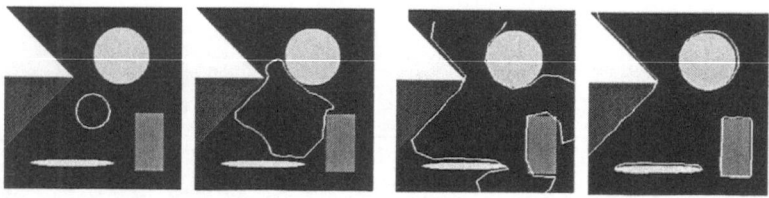

Fig. 8. Topological change examples with hybrid geometric active contour models: Left to right, initialization (snake pedal in yellow (white)), intermediate stages of evolution and final fit

4   Conclusions

In this paper, we proposed novel extensions to a powerful geometric shape modeling scheme called the snake pedals, introduced in [14]. The extension involved methods for automatically coping with topological changes and for the first time, the introduction of the concept of a global shape into geometric/geodesic snake models. The ability to characterize global shape of an object using very few parameters facilitates shape learning and recognition. Unlike the deformable superquadrics, the geometric snake pedals have the ability to cope with large bending and twists in a shape without explicitly introducing parameters to characterize the same. This leads to reduced numerical complexity and increased numerical stability in the resulting shape recovery algorithms used. The modeling scheme was applied to recover shapes of interest from a variety of medical image data using numerically stable algorithms.

Acknowledgments

We thank Dr. C. M. Leonard for the MR brain scans and acknowledge the data source http://ipagwww.med.yale.edu/chakrab/pap1/pap1figs.html for the endocardium in Fig. 7.

References

1. Caselles, V., Catte, F., Coll, T., and Dibos, F.: A geometric model for active contours in image processing. Numerische Mathematik **66** (1993) 1–31
2. Caselles, V., Kimmel, R., and Sapiro, G.: Geodesic active contours. In Fifth International Conference on Computer Vision (1995) 694–699
3. Gray, A.: Modern differential geometry of curves and surfaces. CRC Press, Boca Raton (1993)
4. Guo, Y.: Snake Pedals: Active Geometric Models for Shape Modeling and Recovery. PhD thesis, University of Florida (1998)
5. Kass, M., Witkin, A., Terzopoulos, D.: An active contour models. Int. Journal of Computer Vision **1** (1987) 321–331
6. Kichenassamy, S., Kumar, A., Olver, P., Tannenbaum, A., Yezzi, A.: Gradient flows and geometric active contour models. In Fifth International Conference on Computer Vision (1995) 810–815
7. Kimmel, R., Amir, A., Bruckstein, A.M.: Finding shortest paths on surfaces using level sets propogation. IEEE Trans. on Pattern Analysis and Machine Intelligence **17** (1995) 635–640
8. Malladi, R., Sethian, J.A., Vemuri, B.C.: A topology independent shape modeling scheme. In SPIE Proc. on Geometric Methods in Computer Vision II, SPIE **2031** (1993) 246–256
9. Malladi, R., Sethian, J.A., Vemuri, B.C.: Shape modeling with front propagation : A level set approach. IEEE Trans. Pattern Analysis and Machine Intelligence **17** (1995) 158–175
10. Osher S., Sethian, J.A.: Fronts propagating with curvature dependent speed: Algorithms based on halmiton-jacobi formulation. Journal of Computational Physics **79** (1988) 12–49
11. Press, W.H., Teukolsky, S.S., Vetterling, W.T., Flannery, B.P. Nemurical Recipes in C. Cambridge University Press (1992)
12. Tek H., Kimia, B.B.: Image segmentation by reaction-diffusion bubbles. In Fifth International Conference on Computer Vision, Boston, MA, (1995)
13. ter Haar Romeny, B.M. (ed.): Geometry Driven Diffusion in Computer Vision. Kluwer (1994)
14. Vemuri, B.C., Guo, Y.: Snake pedals: Geometric models with physics–based control. In International Conference on Computer Vision, Bombay, India (1998) 427–432
15. Wickert, J.: A review of nonlinear diffusion filtering. In: Koenderink, J., ter Haar Romeny, B.M., Florack, L., Viergever, M. (eds.): Scale–space Theory in Computer Vision, Lecture Notes in Computer Science, Vol. 1252, Springer (1997) 3–28

Co–dimension 2 Geodesic Active Contours for MRA Segmentation

Liana M. Lorigo[1], Olivier Faugeras[1,2], W. E. L. Grimson[1], Renaud Keriven[3], Ron Kikinis[4], and Carl-Fredrik Westin[4]

[1] MIT Artificial Intelligence Laboratory, Cambridge MA, USA
`liana@ai.mit.edu`
[2] INRIA, Sophia Antipolis, France
[3] Cermics, ENPC, France
[4] Harvard Medical School, Brigham & Women's Hospital, Boston MA, USA

Abstract. Automatic and semi-automatic magnetic resonance angiography (MRA) segmentation techniques can potentially save radiologists large amounts of time required for manual segmentation and can facilitate further data analysis. The proposed MRA segmentation method uses a mathematical modeling technique which is well-suited to the complicated curve-like structure of blood vessels. We define the segmentation task as an energy minimization over all 3D curves and use a level set method to search for a solution. Our approach is an extension of previous level set segmentation techniques to higher co-dimension.

1 Introduction

The high-level goal of this research is to develop computer vision techniques for the segmentation of medical images. Automatic and semi-automatic vision techniques can potentially assist clinicians in this task, saving them much of the time required to manually segment large data sets. Specifically, we consider the segmentation of volumetric vasculature images, such as the magnetic resonance angiography (MRA) image pictured in Fig. 1.

As shown here, blood vessels appear in MRA images as bright curve-like patterns which may be noisy and have gaps. What is shown is a "maximum intensity projection". The data is a stack of slices where most areas are dark, but vessels tend to be bright. This stack is collapsed into a single image for viewing by performing a projection through the stack that assigns to each pixel in the projection the brightest voxel over all slices. This image shows projections along three orthogonal axes.

Thresholding is one possible approach to this segmentation problem and works adequately on the larger vessels. The problem arises in detecting the small vessels, and that is the objective of our work. Thresholding cannot be used for the small vessels for several reasons. The voxels may have an intensity that is a combination of the intensities of vessels and background if the vessel is only partially inside the voxel. This sampling artifact is called *partial voluming*. Other imaging conditions can cause some background areas to be as bright as other

A. Kuba et al. (Eds.): IPMI'99, LNCS 1613, pp. 126–139, 1999.
© Springer-Verlag Berlin Heidelberg 1999

vessel areas, complicating threshold selection. Finally, the images are often noisy, and methods using local contextual information can be more robust.

Our method uses the fact that the underlying structures in the image are indeed 3D curves and evolves an initial curve into the curves in the data (the vessels). In particular, we explore techniques based on the concept of *mean curvature flow*, or *curve-shortening flow*, from the field of differential geometry.

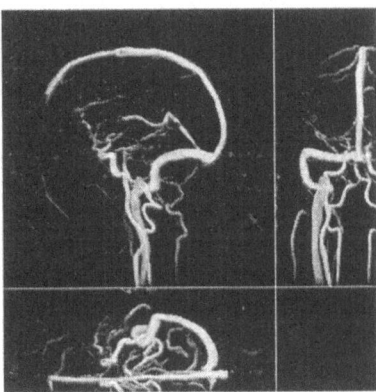

Fig. 1. Maximum intensity projection of a phase-contrast MRA image of blood vessels in the brain

2   Curvature Evolution Methods

Mean curvature evolution schemes for segmentation, implemented with level set methods, have become an important approach in computer vision [5,10,11]. This approach uses partial differential equations to control the evolution. An overview to the superset of techniques using related partial differential equations can be found in [4]. The fundamental concepts from mathematics from which mean curvature schemes derive were explored several years earlier when smooth closed curves in 2D were proven to shrink to a point under mean curvature motion [8,9]. Evans and Spruck and Chen, Giga, and Goto independently framed mean curvature flow of any hypersurface as a level set problem and proved existence, uniqueness, and stability of viscosity solutions [7,6]. For application to image segmentation, a vector field was induced on the embedding space, so that the evolution could be controlled by an image gradient field or other image data. The same results of existence, uniqueness, and stability of viscosity solutions were obtained for the modified evolution equations for the case of planar curves, and experiments on real-world images demonstrated the effectiveness of the approach [3,5].

Curves evolving in the plane became surfaces evolving in space, called *minimal surfaces* [5]. Although the theorem on planar curves shrinking to a point could not be extended to the case of surfaces evolving in 3D, the existence, uniqueness, and stability results of the level set formalism held analogously to the 2D case. Thus the method was feasible for evolving both curves in 2D and surfaces in 3D. Beyond elegant mathematics, spectacular results on real-world data sets established the method as an important segmentation tool in both domains. One fundamental limitation to these schemes has been that they describe only the flow of hypersurfaces, i.e., surfaces of co-dimension 1.

Altschuler and Grayson studied the problem of curve-shortening flow for 3D curves [1], and Ambrosio and Soner generalized the level set technique to arbitrary manifolds in arbitrary dimension. They provided the analogous results and extended their level set evolution equation to account for an additional vector field induced on the space [2].

We herein present the first implementation of geodesic active contours in 3D, based on Ambrosio and Soner's work. Specifically, our system uses these techniques for automatic segmentation of blood vessels in MRA images. The dimension of the manifold is 1, and its co-dimension is 2.

3   Mean Curvature Flow

Intuitively, *mean curvature flow* refers to some curve evolving in time so that at each point, the velocity vector normal to the curve is equal to the mean curvature vector. This concept is normally defined for arbitrary generic surfaces, but only curves are necessary for this paper, so we have restricted the definition. More formally, let $C(t)$, $t \geq 0$ be a family of curves in $\Re^2$ or $\Re^3$, N the normal for a given orientation. That is, C is a curve, and t represents the "time" parameter or the index into the family of curves, not position. The mean curvature flow equation is then given by the vector equation

$$C_t = \kappa N \tag{1}$$

with given initial curve $C(0) = C_0$, κ the curvature of the curve, and C_t the time derivative of the curve. Note that since we consider only 1D curves here, as opposed to evolving surfaces, the mean curvature is just the usual curvature of the curve. This motion is also called "curve-shortening flow" since it is the solution, obtained by Euler-Lagrange equations, to the problem of minimizing curve length:

$$\min_C \int |C'(p)| dp$$

where p is the spatial parameter of the curve.

4   Level Set Method for Planar Curves

We give the basic idea of the level set method [12] to evolve a *planar* curve C. Define a function $u : \Re^2 \to \Re$ so that C is a level-set of u. We follow the convention that C is, in particular, the zero level set of u, although this choice is not necessary for the method. The function u is now an implicit representation of the curve C. The advantages of this representation are that it is intrinsic (independent of parameterization) and that it is topologically flexible since different topologies of C are represented by the constant topology of u. Let C_0 be the initial curve.

It is shown in [7] and [6] that evolving C according to

$$C_t = \beta N \tag{2}$$

with initial condition $C(\cdot, 0) = C_0(\cdot)$ for any function β, is equivalent to evolving u according to

$$u_t = \beta |\nabla u| \tag{3}$$

with initial condition $u(\cdot, 0) = u_0(\cdot)$ and $u_0(C_0) = 0$.

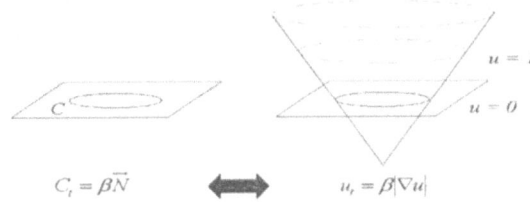

Fig. 2. Level sets of an embedding function u, for a closed curve in $\Re^2$

This result is independent of the choice of function u [7,6]. As customary in the literature, we choose u_0 to be the signed distance function to the curve C (Fig. 2).

5   Level Set Method for Curves in Higher Codimension

The level set evolution equations that follow were proven in [2]. They enable us to evolve space curves, with evolution driven by both mean curvature and image information. In the following discussion, C is a curve in 3D.

5.1   Mean Curvature Flow

Let $v : \Re^3 \to [0, \infty)$ be an auxiliary function whose zero level set is identically C, that is smooth near C, and such that ∇v is non-zero outside C. For a nonzero vector $\mathbf{q} \in \Re^n$, define

$$P_\mathbf{q} = I - \frac{\mathbf{q}\mathbf{q}^T}{|\mathbf{q}|^2}$$

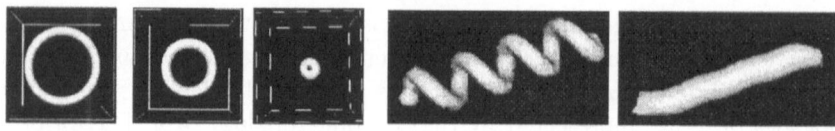

Fig. 3. Evolving curves under mean curvature flow. The first three images show a circle shrinking to a point, and the last two images show a helix shrinking to its axis

as the projector onto the plane normal to **q**. Further define $\lambda(\nabla v(x,t), \nabla^2 v(x,t))$ as the smaller nonzero eigenvalue of $P_{\nabla v}\nabla^2 v P_{\nabla v}$. The level set evolution equation is then

$$v_t = \lambda(\nabla v(x,t), \nabla^2 v(x,t)).$$

That is, this evolution is equivalent to evolving C according to $\boldsymbol{C}_t = \kappa\boldsymbol{N}$ in the sense that C is the zero level set of v throughout the evolution.

Figure 3 demonstrates this evolution. As discussed above, a circle shrinks to a point under mean curvature motion. Under this motion, a helix evolves into its axis.

5.2   Incorporation of Vector Field

This section discusses the situation where there is an underlying vector field driving the evolution, in combination with the curvature term. Assume the desired evolution equation is of the form

$$\boldsymbol{C}_t = \kappa\boldsymbol{N} - \Pi\boldsymbol{d},$$

where Π is the projection operator onto the normal space of C (which is a vector space of dimension 2) and $\boldsymbol{d}$ is a given vector field in $\Re^3$. The evolution equation for the embedding space then becomes

$$v_t = \lambda(\nabla v, \nabla^2 v) + \nabla v \cdot \boldsymbol{d}.$$

5.3   3D Image Segmentation

For the case of 1D structures in 3D images, we wish to minimize

$$\int_0^1 g(|\nabla I(C(p))|)|C'(p)|dp$$

where $C(p) : [0,1] \rightarrow \Re^3$ is the 1D curve, $I : [0,a] \times [0,b] \times [0,c] \rightarrow [0,\infty)$ is the image, and $g : [0,\infty) \rightarrow \Re^+$ is a strictly decreasing function such that $g(r) \rightarrow 0$ as $r \rightarrow \infty$ (analogous to [5]). For our current implementation, we use $g(r) = exp(-r)$ because it works well in practice. Another common choice is

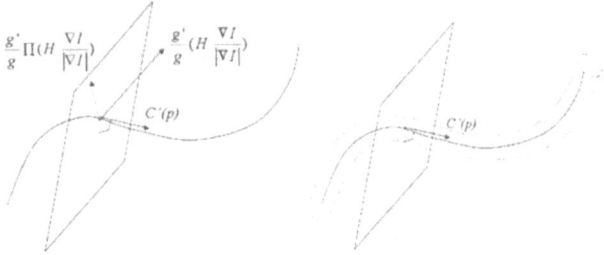

Fig. 4. (a) The tangent to C at p, the normal plane, the image-based vector, and its projection onto the normal plane. (b) ε-level set method

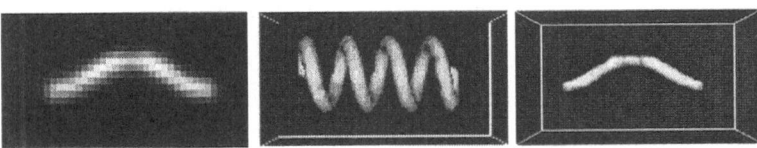

Fig. 5. Evolving helix under mean curvature flow with additional vector field: target curve, initial level set, level set after evolution with endpoints constrained

$g(|\nabla I|) = \frac{1}{1+|\nabla I|^2}$. By computing the Euler-Lagrange equations, we find that the curve evolution equation is

$$C_t = \kappa N - \frac{g'}{g}\Pi(\mathbf{H}\frac{\nabla I}{|\nabla I|}), \qquad (4)$$

where $\mathbf{H}$ is the Hessian of the intensity function. The second term in the above equation is illustrated in Fig. 4(a). That is,

$$d = \frac{g'}{g}\mathbf{H}\frac{\nabla I}{|\nabla I|},$$

so the equation for the embedding space is

$$v_t = \lambda(\nabla v(x,t), \nabla^2 v(x,t)) + \frac{g'}{g}\nabla v(x,t)\cdot\mathbf{H}\frac{\nabla I}{|\nabla I|}. \qquad (5)$$

Thus, Ambrosio and Soner's work has provided the basis for the use of mean curvature flow and level set methods to segment 1D structures in 3D. Figure 5 illustrates how underlying image information can attract the evolving tube. The underlying volumetric image data is shown, as a maximum intensity projection, in the first image. This volume was generated by drawing a cosine curve in the volume, then smoothing with a Gaussian filter. The second image shows the initial curve, a helix. The result of the evolution is shown in the rightmost image.

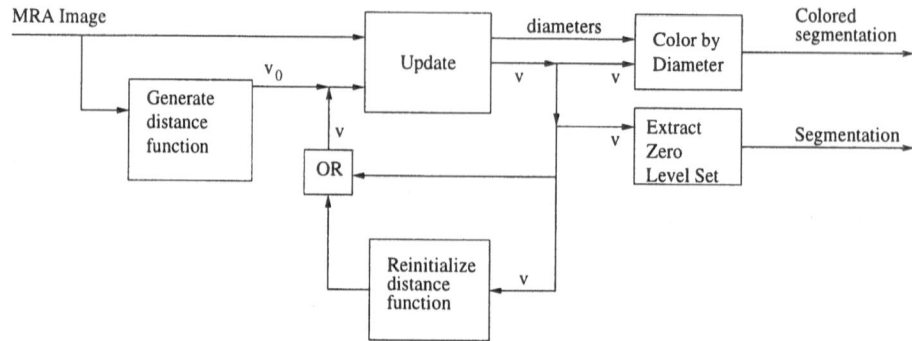

Fig. 6. Overview of segmentation algorithm

6   MRA Segmentation System

This section describes our system for segmentation of vessels from MRA using the described level set method. A flowchart is shown in Fig. 6. We discuss issues that have arisen in converting the theory above to practice for this application.

ε-**Level Set Method:** Since the projection operator $P_{\mathbf{q}}$ is defined only for non-zero vectors q, the method is undefined at $\nabla v = \mathbf{0}$, which is the curve itself, and is numerically unstable near the curve. For this reason, we regard v as a distance function to a "tube" of small radius ε around the curve, instead of extracting the true 1D curve. That is, we evolve the ε-level set instead of evolving the true curve (Fig. 4(b)). Note that ε does not denote a fixed value here: we mean simply that the evolving shape is a "tubular" surface of some (unspecified and variable) nonzero width. In addition to being more robust, this method better captures the geometry of blood vessels, which have nonzero diameter.

Banding: Instead of evolving the entire volume, we evolve only the portion of the volume within a narrow band of the zero level set (the current surface). This technique is commonly used in level set methods. Normally, we set the band to include voxels that are up to 6 voxels away from the surface. We have increased this distance up to 12 for some experiments. The advantage of this technique is efficiency, and the disadvantage is that we may miss structures that are outside the band if the potential function g does not have a large enough capture range to attract the segmentation to these structures. This issue can be addressed by ensuring that g is compatible with the band size.

Curvature Instead of Eigenvalues: For computational efficiency and because of numerical instability of the gradient computations and thus the evolution equation near $\nabla v = \mathbf{0}$, we remark that the level sets of the function v flow in the direction of the normal with velocity equal to the sum of their smaller principal curvature and the dot product of ∇v with the image-based vector field d. Therefore, we compute the smaller curvature directly from v instead of as an eigenvalue of $P_{\nabla v} \nabla^2 v P_{\nabla v}$.

Image Scaling: To control the trade-off between fitting the surface to the image data and enforcing the smoothness constraint on the surface, we add an *image scaling* term *imscale* to Equation 5 to obtain

$$v_t = \lambda(\nabla v(x,t), \nabla^2 v(x,t)) + imscale * \frac{g'}{g} \nabla v(x,t) \cdot \mathbf{H} \frac{\nabla I}{|\nabla I|} \qquad (6)$$

imscale is set by the user or can be pre-set to a default value.

Gradient Directionality: Because vessels appear brighter than the background, we weight the image term by the cosine of the angle between the normal to the surface and the gradient in the image. This cosine is given by the dot product of the respective gradients of v and I, so the update equation becomes

$$v_t = \lambda(\nabla v(x,t), \nabla^2 v(x,t)) + imscale * (\nabla v \cdot \nabla I) * \frac{g'}{g} \nabla v(x,t) \cdot \mathbf{H} \frac{\nabla I}{|\nabla I|}. \qquad (7)$$

For example, if the two vectors point in the same direction, then the brighter region is inside the surface and the darker region is outside; the angle between the vectors is 0, whose cosine is 1, so the image term is fully counted. However, if they point in opposite directions, the negative weighting prevents the evolving vessel walls from being attracted to image gradients that point in the opposite direction.

Reinitializing Volume: As customary in level set segmentation methods, the volume v is periodically reinitialized to be a distance function: the zero level set S is extracted, then each point in the volume is set to be its distance to S. For our implementation, this reinitialization is itself a level set method. To obtain the positive distances, the surface is propagated outward at constant speed of 1, and the distance at each point is determined to be the time at which the surface crossed that point. A second step propagates the surface inward to obtain the negative distances analogously. For some experiments, we have used the Fast Marching Method [12] to implement these steps.

Initial Surface: Figure 7 shows additional detail on the generation of the initial surface. This initial surface (and thus the initial volume) is normally

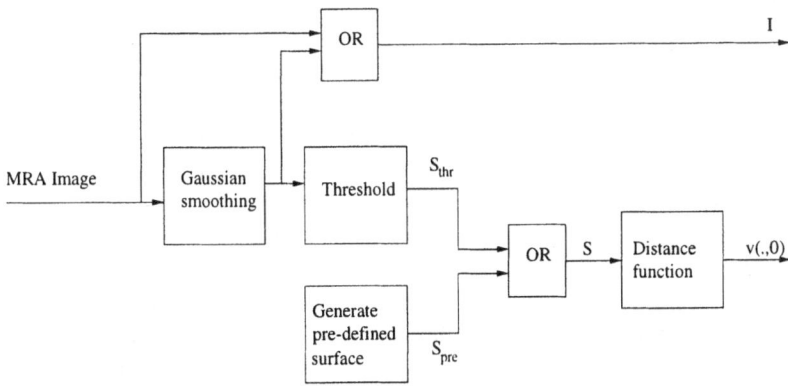

Fig. 7. More detailed illustration of initialization part of algorithm

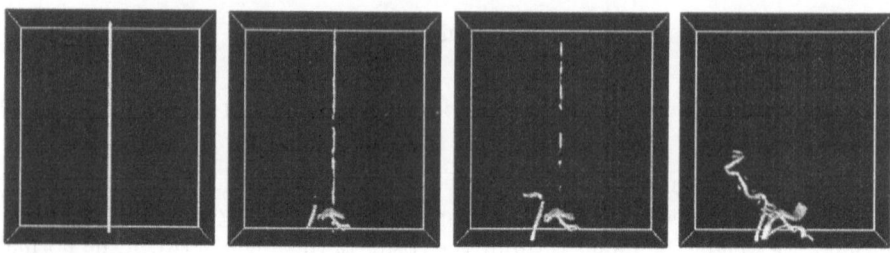

Fig. 8. Illustration of a vertical bar evolving in a segmentation of the first dataset in Fig. 10

generated by thresholding the MRA dataset. However, the method does not require that the initial surface be near the target surface but may use any initial surface. Figure 8 illustrates a vertical bar evolving into the segmentation of the first dataset in Fig. 10.

Smoothing: As shown in Fig. 7, the datasets may be pre-processed to reduce noise. For the results presented here, the raw datasets were convolved with an isotropic Gaussian of $\sigma = 0.5$.

Cleaning: We post-process the segmentations to remove any surface patches whose surface area is less than some threshold (a parameter of the method) to eliminate patches corresponding to noise in the original data.

Vessel Radii Estimation: The larger principal curvature can be useful in measuring the radii of the vessels for a particular application, since radius is the inverse of curvature. This curvature can be easily computed when the smaller principal curvature is computed for the segmentation. We have added the option to color-code our segmentations based on vessel radii, as estimated from the local larger principal curvature of the tubular surface.

7   Results

We demonstrate segmentation results on four datasets, courtesy of the Surgical Planning Laboratory, Brigham and Womens Hospital and Harvard Medical School (Figs. 9, 10, and 11). All datasets had an initial resolution of .9375x.9375x 1.5mm^3 (256x256x60 voxels). The final example only was resampled to .9375x .9375x.9375mm^3 (256x256x96 voxels) before segmentation; the other segmentations were performed directly on the raw data. The images are not square (256x256) because uninteresting portions were cropped for efficiency. In Fig. 10, the initial surface for the segmentation was a surface obtained by thresholding the raw dataset whereas in Fig. 9 it was a tube as in Fig. 8; *imscale* also varied as discussed below. For comparison, Fig. 10 first shows results obtained by thresholding alone. Figure 11 shows an enlargement of a portion of the segmentations and corresponding maximum intensity projection considered in Fig. 10.

The following parameters were used in these experiments; all settings were chosen empirically. For our method, *imscale* varied across the datasets depending

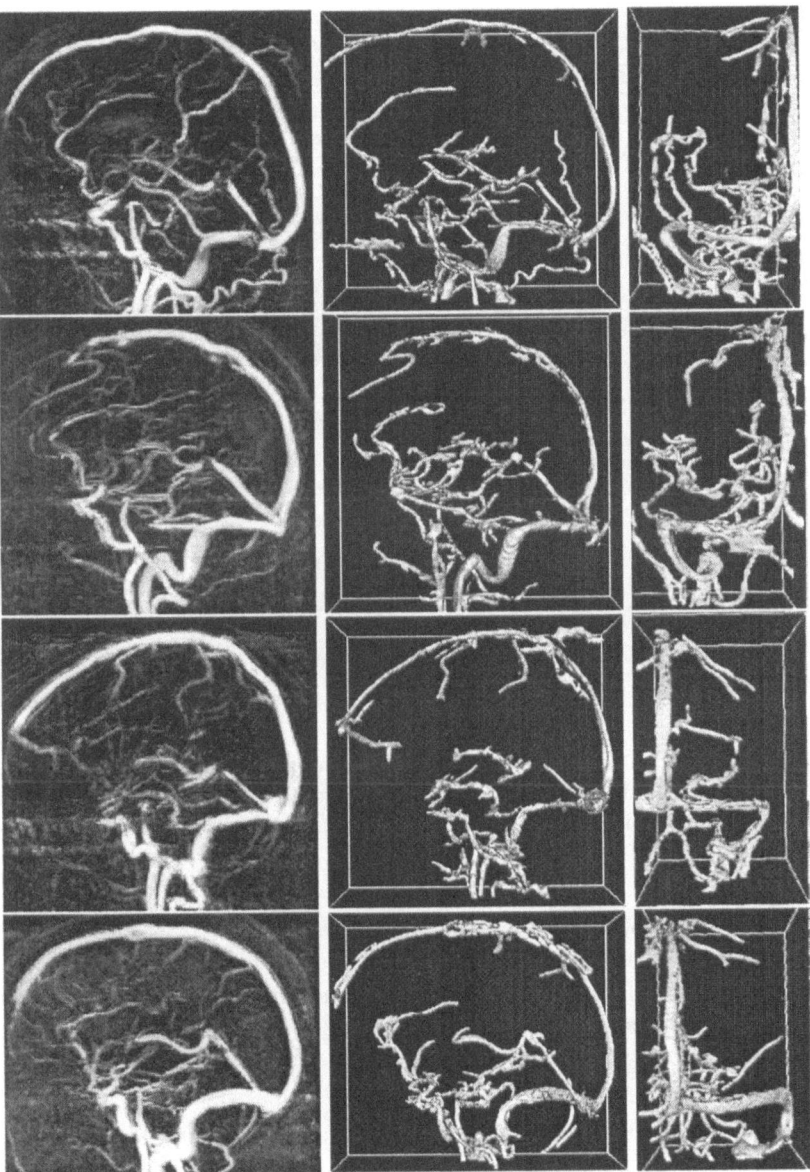

Fig. 9. The first image in each row is the maximum intensity projection of the raw data, and the second and third are the segmentation result from two orthogonal viewpoints. These results are obtained by our method where the initial surface was a vertical bar as showed in Fig. 8

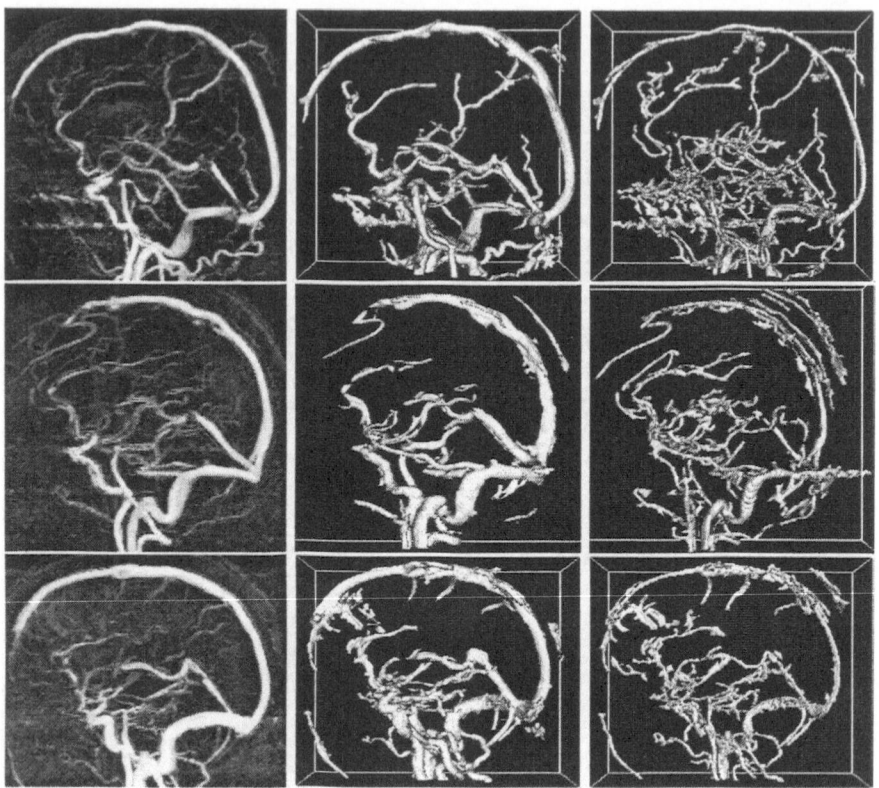

Fig. 10. Results on three datasets are shown. For each image pair, the first image is the maximum intensity projection of the raw data, the second is the segmentation result from thresholding only and the third is the segmentation result using our method

on the noise present. A threshold t_{init} was used in Fig. 10 to obtain the initial surface from the dataset; such a threshold was obviously not needed in Fig. 9. A cleaning threshold c indicated the minimum surface area of connected components of the surface to be retained in the post-processing "cleaning" step.

For thresholding only, the threshold t_{thresh} was chosen and also the cleaning threshold c. For all datasets, t_{init} was slightly higher than t_{thresh} for the same dataset: although using a lower t_{thresh} alone looks better after the cleaning step, the noise before cleaning worsened our results and led us to use a slightly higher value for initialization.

Recall that obtaining the very small vessels is the goal of this work since the large vessels are easily segmented by thresholding. For this reason, *imscale* was set fairly high in the experiments in Fig. 10 to obtain the small vessels, at the expense of also obtaining many imaging artifacts. A coarser segmentation is obtained in Fig. 9 by choosing lower values for *imscale*. Although the results in this figure are only similar to those obtained by simple thresholding, the objective of the demonstration is academic: it shows that we capture the vasculature shape even when the initial guess is meaningless. In practice, better results are obtained using thresholding for initialization.

When considering that the *imscale* parameter controls the trade-off between noise and small vessels in our method, and when comparing our method to thresholding alone, it is important to note that it would not be possible to similarly lower t_{thresh} to obtain the small vessels (and noise) by thresholding alone. Lowering the threshold obtains large blobs in the volume which do not correspond to vessels. Our method is thus more powerful than thresholding alone.

Finally, we demonstrate the capability to color-code the vasculature surface based on local curvature. Notice (Fig. 12) that for a ribbon-like vessel, the flatter sides shows a large radius, and the sharply curved edges show a small radius. In this example, the colorscale is continuous from darkest to lightest intensities, with darkest indicating a radius of curvature $\leq$ 1mm and lightest indicating a radius of curvature $\geq$ 2mm. The curvatures output by our evolution have been smoothed by a 3x3x3 filter prior to coloring the surface.

8   Future Work

Vessels tend to appear thinner in our segmentations than in those obtained by thresholding. One possible reason is that our method uses gradients instead of intensities, so the vessel wall is found attracted to the strongest gradients, which may be fully inside the bright region indicated by thresholding. A second option is that the underlying mathematics of our algorithm assume that the vessels are 1D curves, not tubular surfaces. We believe that our ε-level set method allows the method to successfully handle tubular surfaces, but have not yet verified this analytically. A final potential reason for the discrepancy is that the segmentations obtained by thresholding may be thicker than the true blood vessels due to noise around the vessels. Future work will involve comparisons to manual segmentations which will provide ground truth to evaluate both methods.

We also observe a lot of noise in our segmentations of the first and second datasets. As mentioned above, we could obtain much less noise at the expense of the thinnest vessels by lowering *imscale*. For the large amounts of noise in these datasets, noise is often indistinguishable from small vessels when only a small local neighborhood is considered, as in our algorithm. To address this problem, one could reduce noise prior to segmentation by filtering or incorporate a more sophisticated image measure into Equation 5.

On the positive side, the segmentation of small vessels that were not obtainable by thresholding encourages us to continue in the development of this algorithm. Although still in preliminary stages, we believe that it has the potential to yield effective segmentations of very thin vessels.

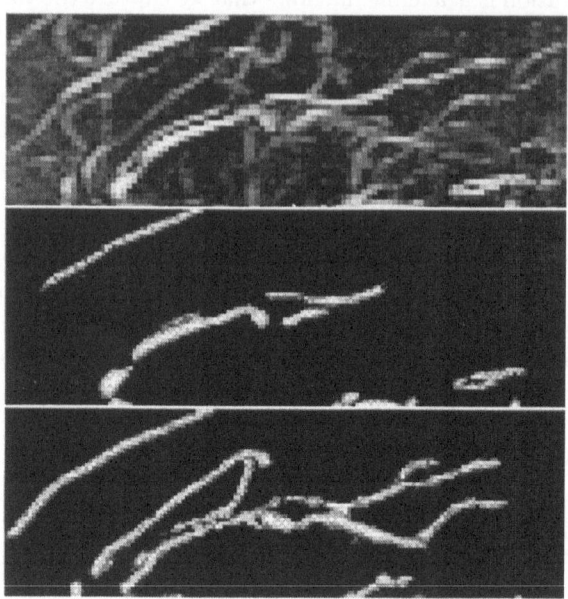

Fig. 11. Enlargement of a portion of the second example from Fig. 10. As above, the second image is the segmentation obtained by thresholding alone, and the third image is the result of our method

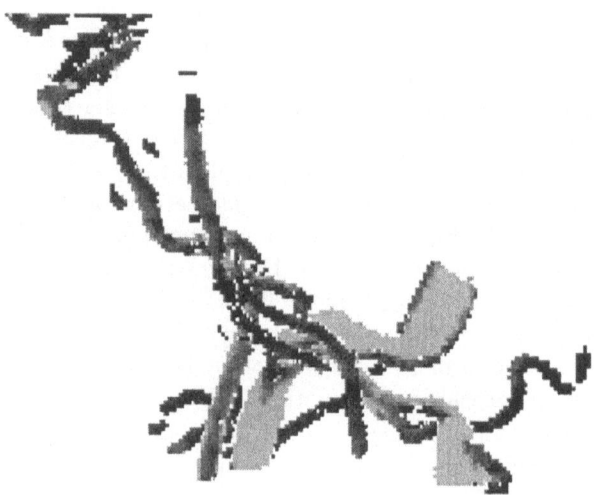

Fig. 12. Our method naturally allows estimation of local radii of curvature of the segmented vessels. In this image of a partial segmentation of the first dataset in Fig. 10, the colorscale is continuous from darkest to lightest intensities, with darkest indicating a radius of curvature $\leq$ 1mm and lightest indicating a radius of curvature $\geq$ 2mm

Acknowledgments

This work was supported in part by NSF Contract IIS-9610249, in part by NSF ERC (Johns Hopkins University agreement) 8810-274, and in part by MERL, A Mitsubishi Electric Research Laboratory.

References

1. Altschuler, S. and Grayson, M.: Shortening space curves and flow through singularities. Journal of Differential Geometry **35** (1992) 283–298
2. Ambrosio, L. and Soner, H.M.: Level set approach to mean curvature flow in arbitrary codimension. Journal of Differential Geometry **43** (1996) 693–737
3. Caselles, V., Catte, F., Coll, T. and Dibos, F.: A geometric model for active contours. Numerische Mathematik **66** (1993) 1–31
4. Caselles, V., Morel, J.M., Sapiro, G. and Tannenbaum, A.: Introduction to the special issue on partial differential equations and geometry-driven diffusion in image processing and analysis. IEEE Trans. Image Processing **7(3)** (1998) 269–273
5. Caselles, V., Kimmel, R. and Sapiro, G.: Geodesic active contours. Int'l Journal of Computer Vision **22(1)** (1997) 61–79
6. Chen, Y.G., Giga, Y. and Goto, S.: Uniqueness and existence of viscosity solutions of generalized mean curvature flow equations. J. Differential Geometry **33** (1991) 749–786
7. Evans, L.C. and Spruck, J.: Motion of level sets by mean curvature: I. Journal of Differential Geometry **33** (1991) 635–681
8. Gage, M. and Hamilton, R.S.: The heat equation shrinking convex plane curves. Journal of Differential Geometry **23** (1986) 69–96
9. Grayson, M.: The heat equation shrinks embedded plane curves to round points. Journal of Differential Geometry **26** (1987) 285–314
10. Kichenassamy, A., Kumar, A., Olver, P., Tannenbaum, A. and Yezzi, A.: Gradient flows and geometric active contour models. In Proc. IEEE Int'l Conf. Computer Vision (1995) 810–815
11. Sapiro, G.: Vector-valued active contours. In Proc. IEEE Conf. Computer Vision and Pattern Recognition (1996) 680–685
12. Sethian, J.A.: Level Set Methods. Cambridge University Press (1996)

An Adaptive Fuzzy Segmentation Algorithm for Three-Dimensional Magnetic Resonance Images

Dzung L. Pham[1][2] and Jerry L. Prince[1]

[1] Center of Imaging Science,
Department of Electrical and Computer Engineering,
The Johns Hopkins University, Baltimore MD 21218
{pham, prince}@jhu.edu
[2] Laboratory of Personality and Cognition,
Gerontology Research Center,
National Institute on Aging, Baltimore, MD 21224

Abstract. An algorithm is proposed for the fuzzy segmentation of two and three-dimensional multispectral magnetic resonance (MR) images that have been corrupted by intensity inhomogeneities, also known as shading artifacts. The algorithm is an extension of the two-dimensional adaptive fuzzy C-means algorithm (2-D AFCM) presented in previous work by the authors. This algorithm models the intensity inhomogeneities as a gain field that causes image intensities to smoothly and slowly vary through the image space. It iteratively adapts to the intensity inhomogeneities and is completely automated. In this paper, we fully generalize 2-D AFCM to three-dimensional (3-D) multispectral images. Because of the potential size of 3-D image data, we also describe a new, faster multigrid-based algorithm for its implementation. We show using simulated MR data that 3-D AFCM yields significantly lower error rates than both the standard fuzzy $C-$means algorithm and several other competing methods when segmenting corrupted images. Its efficacy is further demonstrated using real 3-D scalar and multispectral MR brain images.

1 Introduction

Tissue classification is a necessary step in many medical imaging applications including the quantification of tissue volumes, study of anatomical structure, and computer integrated surgery. Classification of voxels exclusively into distinct classes, however, is problematic due to artifacts such as noise and the partial volume effect, which occurs when multiple tissues are present in a single voxel. To compensate for these artifacts, there has recently been growing interest in fuzzy segmentation methods. In fuzzy segmentations, voxels may be classified into multiple classes with a varying degree of membership. The membership thus gives an indication of where noise and partial volume averaging have occurred in the image. Standard fuzzy segmentation algorithms, however, do not effectively compensate for intensity inhomogeneities, a common artifact in magnetic resonance (MR) images.

A. Kuba et al. (Eds.): IPMI'99, LNCS 1613, pp. 140–153, 1999.

In MR images, intensity inhomogeneities are typically caused by non-uniformities in the RF field during acquisition, although other factors also play a role [15]. The result is a shading effect where the pixel or voxel intensities of the same tissue class vary over the image domain. It has been shown that the shading in MR images is well modeled by the product of the original image and a smooth, slowly varying gain field [7,18]. Corrupted images may be segmented by first applying a correction algorithm (cf. [7,16]) to remove intensity inhomogeneities, and then applying a standard segmentation algorithm that assumes no inhomogeneities are present.

Several methods have also been proposed that simultaneously compensate for the shading effect while segmenting the image. These methods have the advantage of being able to use intermediate information from the segmentation while performing the correction. Most of these methods, however, have focussed on classifying each voxel into distinct tissue classes [19,13,17]. An expectation-maximization algorithm has also been proposed [18,8] that models the inhomogeneities as a bias field of the image logarithm. This method is capable of obtaining fuzzy segmentations based on posterior probabilities, but for most data sets some manual interaction is required to provide training data.

Recently, we presented some initial results on an unsupervised segmentation algorithm called the adaptive fuzzy C-means algorithm (AFCM), designed for segmenting two-dimensional (2-D) scalar images corrupted by intensity inhomogeneities [10,11]. Based on the fuzzy C-means algorithm (FCM) [1], the advantages of 2-D AFCM are that it automatically produces fuzzy segmentations, it is robust to inhomogeneities, and it computes a smooth gain field based on all pixels in the image. Although this algorithm is suitable for the segmentation of MR images obtained using single or multi-slice acquisitions, it cannot be used in volumetric acquisitions where the inhomogeneities are three-dimensional (3-D) in nature, nor can it be used on multispectral data.

In this paper, we generalize AFCM to 3-D multispectral images. Our generalization also allows for the adjustment of the "crispness" or "fuzziness" of the resulting segmentation and for the segmentation of data with ellipsoidal shaped clusters. A novel algorithm is presented for computing the gain field that typically yields a threefold improvement in speed over a standard multigrid approach without reducing accuracy. This speed improvement is especially significant when working with large 3-D data sets. We also provide in this paper several new results using simulated data that show that the segmentations obtained using FCM on uncorrupted images and AFCM on corrupted images are accurate both in terms of classification and modeling of partial volume effects. Moreover, we show that under default initializations, AFCM's performance on corrupted 3-D images is superior to the performance of methods presented in [16] and [19].

2   Background

In this section, we give a brief overview of FCM and 2-D AFCM. FCM has previously been used with some success in the fuzzy segmentation of magnetic resonance (MR) images (cf. [12,1]) as well as for the estimation of partial volumes [3]. It clusters data by computing a measure of membership, called the *fuzzy membership*, at each voxel for a specified number of classes. The fuzzy membership function, constrained to be between zero and one, reflects the degree of similarity between the data value at that location and the prototypical data value or *centroid*, of its class. Thus, a high membership value near unity signifies that the data value at that location is "close" to the centroid for that particular class.

FCM is formulated as the minimization of the following objective function with respect to the fuzzy membership functions u_j and the centroids $\mathbf{v}_k$ [1]:

$$J_{\mathrm{FCM}} = \sum_{j\in\Omega}\sum_{k=1}^{C} u_{jk}^{q} \|\mathbf{y}_j - \mathbf{v}_k\|^2 \tag{1}$$

Here, Ω is the set of voxel locations in the image domain, q is a parameter that is constrained to be greater than one, u_{jk} is the membership value at voxel location j for class k such that $\sum_{k=1}^{C} u_{jk} = 1$, $\mathbf{y}_j$ is the observed (vector) image intensity at location j, and $\mathbf{v}_k$ is the centroid of class k. The total number of classes C is assumed to be known. The parameter q is a weighting exponent on each fuzzy membership and determines the amount of "fuzziness" of the resulting classification. For $q = 1$, J_{FCM} reduces to the classical within-group sum of squared errors objective function and FCM becomes equivalent to the K-means or ISODATA clustering algorithms [1]. A commonly used value is $q = 2$ (cf. [12]). The operator $\|\cdot\|$ is any inner product norm on $\mathbf{R}^P$, where P is the number of channels in the image, and $\|\cdot\| = \sqrt{<\cdot,\cdot>}$. By specifying the appropriate norm, FCM can be applied to data that possess ellipsoidal shaped clusters, although typically the Euclidean norm is used.

The FCM objective function (1) is minimized when high membership values are assigned to voxels whose intensities are close to the centroid for its particular class and low membership values are assigned when the voxel intensity is far from the centroid. The resulting fuzzy segmentation can be converted to a hard or crisp segmentation by assigning each voxel solely to the class that has the highest membership value for that voxel. This is known as a *maximum membership segmentation*. The advantages of FCM are that it is unsupervised (i.e. it does not require training data), and it is robust to initial conditions [6]. However, FCM assumes that the centroids of the image are spatially invariant, which is not true of images that have been corrupted by intensity inhomogeneities.

In order to preserve the advantages of FCM, we proposed the following objective function [11,10] for segmenting 2-D scalar images possessing intensity inhomogeneities:

$$J_{\text{AFCM2D}} = \sum_{j \in \Omega} \sum_{k=1}^{C} u_{jk}^2 (y_j - g_j v_k)^2$$

$$+ \lambda_1 \sum_{j \in \Omega} \sum_{r=1}^{2} (D_r * g)_j^2 + \lambda_2 \sum_{j \in \Omega} \sum_{r=1}^{2} \sum_{s=1}^{2} (D_r * D_s * g)_j^2 \qquad (2)$$

where y_j is the pixel intensity, v_k is the centroid, g_j is an unknown gain field to be estimated, and D_r is a (known) finite difference operator along the rth dimension of the image. The notation $(D * g)_j$ refers to the operation of convolving g with the difference kernel D and taking the resulting value at the jth pixel. Note that J_{AFCM2D} assumes $q = 2$. Equation (2) models the brightness variation of the inhomogeneity by allowing the centroids to spatially vary according to the gain field g_j. The last two terms are first and second order regularization terms used to ensure g_j is spatially smooth and slowly varying. The finite difference operators act like derivatives, except they are performed on a discrete domain. AFCM, like FCM, does not place any assumption of spatial smoothness on the membership functions u_j.

In [11], (2) was minimized by taking its first partial derivatives with respect to u, v, and g, and performing iterating through these three necessary conditions. The necessary condition on g leads to a difference equation with spatially varying coefficients that was solved using a standard multigrid approach (see Sect. 3.3).

3   Adaptive Fuzzy C-Means

In this section, we generalize the AFCM objective function to 3-D, multispectral images and describe an algorithm for minimizing the objective function. We also describe an implementation that yields much faster results than the standard multigrid approach.

3.1   Objective Function

When working with multispectral MR data corrupted by intensity inhomogeneities, there are two possible assumptions one can make about the gain field: 1) the gain field is a scalar field; 2) the gain field is a vector field. The first assumption implies that the brightness variation in each component or spectra of the acquired image is identical, while the second assumes that they can be different. In practice, we have found in double-echo MR data that the scalar gain field assumption provides nearly identical segmentation results to the vector gain field assumption and is also faster, requiring fewer computations. Furthermore, the algorithm derived from the scalar case is notationally cleaner and therefore more easily explained. For these reasons, we focus mainly on the scalar assumption for the remainder of this paper.

Using the scalar gain field assumption, we define AFCM to be an algorithm that seeks to minimize the following objective function with respect to membership functions u_j, the centroids $\mathbf{v}_k$, and the gain field g:

$$J_{\text{AFCM}} = \sum_{j \in \Omega} \sum_{k=1}^{C} u_{jk}^q \|\mathbf{y}_j - g_j \mathbf{v}_k\|^2$$

$$+ \lambda_1 \sum_{j \in \Omega} \sum_{r=1}^{R} (D_r * g)_j^2 + \lambda_2 \sum_{j \in \Omega} \sum_{r=1}^{R} \sum_{s=1}^{R} (D_r * D_s * g)_j^2. \qquad (3)$$

This equation is applicable to 2-D images when $R = 2$ and to 3-D images when $R = 3$. For $R = 2$, $q = 2$, and scalar image data, Eq. (3) reduces to the 2-D AFCM objective function given in (2).

If we assume that the membership values u_{jk} and the centroids $\mathbf{v}_k$ are known in (3), then the gain field that minimizes J_{AFCM} is the field that makes the centroids close to the data, but is also slowly varying and smooth. Without the regularization terms, a gain field could always be found that would set the objective function to zero. If λ_1 and λ_2 are set sufficiently large, then the gain field is forced to be constant and the AFCM objective function essentially reduces to the standard FCM objective function.

The scalar gain field objective function J_{AFCM} in Eq. (3) can be minimized by taking the first derivatives of J_{AFCM} with respect to u_{jk}, $\mathbf{v}_k$, and g_j, setting them equal to zero, and iterating through these three necessary conditions for J_{AFCM} to be at a minimum. This yields the following algorithm:

Algorithm 1: AFCM

1. Provide initial values for the centroids, $\mathbf{v}_k, k = 1, \dots, C$, and set the gain field g_j equal to one for all $j \in \Omega$.
2. Compute membership functions as follows:

$$u_{jk} = \frac{\|\mathbf{y}_j - g_j \mathbf{v}_k\|^{-2/(q-1)}}{\displaystyle\sum_{l=1}^{C} \|\mathbf{y}_j - g_j \mathbf{v}_l\|^{-2/(q-1)}} \qquad (4)$$

for all $j \in \Omega$ and $k = 1, \dots, C$.

3. Compute new centroids as follows:

$$\mathbf{v}_k = \frac{\displaystyle\sum_{j \in \Omega} u_{jk}^q g_j \mathbf{y}_j}{\displaystyle\sum_{j \in \Omega} u_{jk}^q g_j^2}, \quad k = 1, \dots, C. \qquad (5)$$

4. Compute a new gain field by solving the following space-varying difference equation for g_j:

$$\sum_{k=1}^{C} u_{jk}^q \langle \mathbf{y}_j, \mathbf{v}_k \rangle = g_j \sum_{k=1}^{C} u_{jk}^q \langle \mathbf{v}_k, \mathbf{v}_k \rangle + \lambda_1 (H_1 * g)_j + \lambda_2 (H_2 * g)_j$$

where the convolution kernels H_1 and H_2 are given by

$$H_1 = \sum_{r=1}^{R}(D_r + \check{D}_r)_j \tag{6}$$

$$H_2 = \sum_{r=1}^{R}\sum_{s=1}^{R}\left((D_r * D_s) + (\check{D}_r * \check{D}_s)\right)_j \tag{7}$$

where $\check{D}$ is the mirror reflection of the finite difference operator D. Standard forward differences were used in this work.

5. If the algorithm has converged, then quit. Otherwise, go to Step 2.

We define convergence to be when the maximum change in the membership functions over all pixels between iterations is less than a given threshold value. In practice, we used a threshold value of 0.01. Methods for determining initial centroids in Step 1 are described in Sect. 3.2. Solution to the difference equation in Step 4 is described in Sect. 3.3.

3.2   Initial Centroids

AFCM requires an initial estimate of centroid values. Like FCM, AFCM is fairly robust to the selection of these initial estimates; however, proper selection will generally improve accuracy and convergence of the algorithm. We propose two methods for automatically selecting initial centroids: the first method may be applied generally to all scalar data, while the second method is specific to multispectral MR images.

If the given data is scalar-valued, then one can apply the approach described in [11,10], where the modes of a critically smoothed kernel estimator of the image histogram are used to determine the initial centroids. The approach is essentially the same as the "bump-hunting" algorithm described by Silverman in [14]. Briefly, a kernel estimator of the histogram is smoothed in an iterative fashion until it possesses a number of modes equal to the desired number of classes, C. These modes are then numerically computed using first and second derivatives of the kernel estimator and used as initial centroids.

For multispectral data, manipulation of a multidimensional kernel estimator can be computationally prohibitive. In this case, one can obtain initial centroids by applying the approach described in [12]. This approach requires *a priori* knowledge of the approximate T_1, T_2, and proton spin density of the tissue classes being segmented. Most of these values for different tissue classes have been documented in the literature (cf. [2]). These values can then be used in an imaging equation derived for the corresponding pulse sequence (e.g. spin echo) to obtain expected intensity values. This rough initialization is normally sufficient for AFCM to yield good convergence properties.

3.3   Solution to Gain Field

In Step 4 of AFCM, a new gain field is computed given the current values of the centroids and membership functions. This is the most computationally intensive

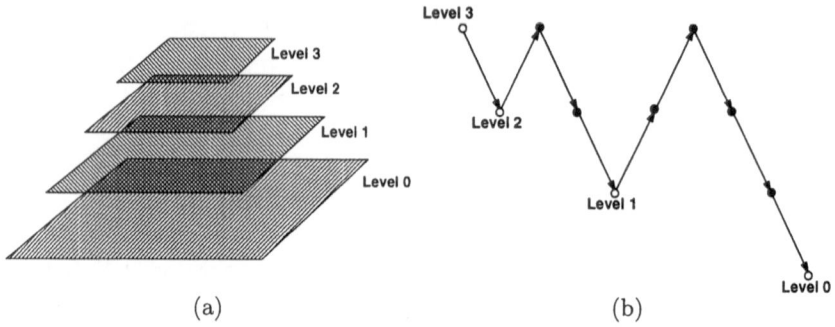

Fig. 1. Multigrid: (a) a four-level multigrid pyramid, (b) a full multigrid V-cycle

step in AFCM and deserves special attention in its numerical implementation. Because the difference equation (4) is space-varying, the gain field cannot be found using standard frequency domain filters. The equation could be solved iteratively using the Jacobi or Gauss-Seidel schemes [4], but these methods take a large number of iterations to converge. In [11,10], this equation was solved using a standard multigrid algorithm at each iteration of AFCM (for a general overview of multigrid algorithms, see [17] or [4]). For 2-D images, this approach is sufficiently fast, but for large 3-D images, execution times can grow to several hours. We now describe a modified multigrid algorithm that yields significantly faster overall execution time without loss of accuracy. Its premise is that during early iterations of AFCM, only an approximate solution to the gain field is required. Thus, a subsampled solution is used and later refined as the number of iterations increases.

Figure 1a illustrates the structure of a multigrid pyramid. Level 0 represents the original resolution of the data, while the higher levels represent increasingly coarser representations of the data. The basis of a multigrid algorithm is the substitution of fine grid iterations for solving Eq. (4), with iterations on a coarse grid, thereby reducing the number of computations required. In addition, the multiresolution update scheme used in a multigrid algorithm yields much faster convergence. In [11,10], the gain field was computed by applying one full multigrid V-cycle [4] at each iteration of 2-D AFCM. A four level full multigrid V-cycle is illustrated in Fig. 1b.

For 3-D images, we propose a new, faster method that takes advantage of the fact that during early iterations of AFCM, the estimates of the centroid and membership functions are poor and an exact solution to the gain field is not necessary. We define a *truncated multigrid cycle* at level L to be a full multigrid V-cycle that terminates the first time the Lth pyramid level is reached. In Fig. 1b, the termination points of a truncated multigrid cycle are shown as open circles. For a truncated multigrid cycle at level $L > 0$, the estimated gain field is an approximation of the final solution on a coarse grid but it can be computed quickly. The implementation of AFCM using a truncated full multigrid cycle proceeds as follows:

Algorithm 2: AFCM using truncated multigrid cycle

1. Set the size of the multigrid pyramid to some value K. Set $L = K - 2$.
2. Run entire AFCM algorithm until convergence using a truncated multigrid cycle at level L to solve for the gain field at each iteration.
3. If $L > 0$, decrease L by 1. Using the most recent values of $u, \mathbf{v}$, and g as initial values, go to Step 2. Else if $L = 0$, terminate.

This modified multigrid algorithm greatly increases the speed of AFCM during its early iterations. As the number of iterations increase, the truncation level reduces towards the original resolution and the iterations become slower. If a result is required quickly, one can terminate Algorithm 2 at some value of $L > 0$. This provides an approximation of the final solution. We have found that since the gain field is smooth, the approximation error decreases rapidly as the resolution increases.

4   Results

AFCM was implemented in C on a Silicon Graphics O2 system with an R10000 processor running IRIX 6.3. It has been tested on both real MR data as well as simulated MR brain images obtained from the Brainweb simulated brain database at the McConnell Brain Imaging Centre of the Montreal Neurological Institute, McGill University [5]. (Simulated brain data sets of varying noise, inhomogeneity, and contrast are available on the World Wide Web at the website listed under References.) In this section, we present the application of AFCM only to 3-D images. For 2-D results, readers are referred to [11]. In all results that follow, the value of q was set to 2, and the standard Euclidean distance norm was used. We denote the AFCM results computed with the full multigrid V-cycle as FM-AFCM and the results computed with the truncated multigrid V-cycle as TM-AFCM. Using FM-AFCM, execution times for a 3-D, T1-weighted, MR data set with 1mm cubic voxels are typically between 45 minutes and 3 hours. Using TM-AFCM, execution times are between 10 minutes and 1 hour. We show in this section that this speed increase does not result in reduced accuracy.

4.1   Visual Evaluation of Performance on Simulated Data

Figure 2 shows the results of applying FCM and AFCM on a Brainweb simulated MR brain image. This brain image was simulated with T1-weighted contrast, 1mm cubic voxels, 3% noise and 40% image intensity inhomogeneity. All extracranial tissue was removed prior to applying the segmentation algorithms. The number of tissue classes was assumed to be three, corresponding to gray matter (GM), white matter (WM), and cerebrospinal fluid (CSF) tissue classes. Background pixels were ignored. Figure 2a shows a slice from the simulated data set and Fig. 2b shows the true partial volume model of the gray matter (GM) tissue class that was used to generate the simulated image. Figures 2c and 2d show the GM membership function obtained by applying FCM and TM-AFCM,

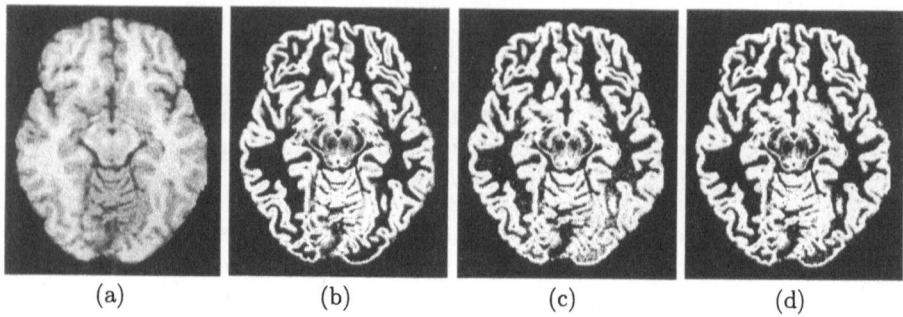

Fig. 2. FCM and AFCM membership functions: (a) Simulated MR phantom, (b) GM partial volume truth model, (c) FCM GM membership function, (d) TM-AFCM GM membership function.

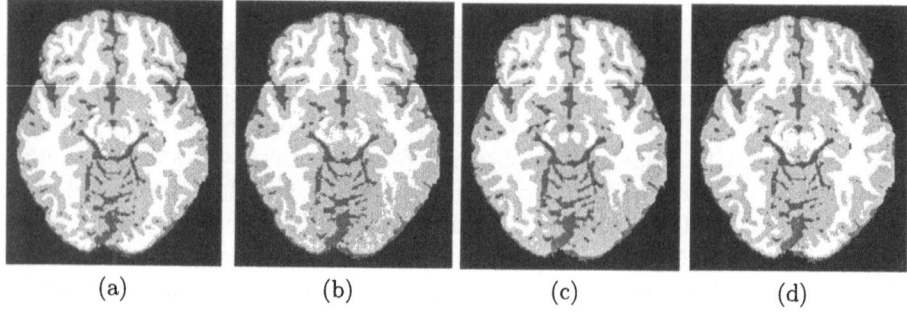

Fig. 3. Comparison of hard segmentations: (a) truth model, (b) FCM max membership segmentation, (c) AMRF segmentation, (d) TM-AFCM max membership segmentation.

respectively, to the 3-D data set. Bright areas represent where the membership function is close to one. Because of the shading effect present in the data, the FCM membership function deteriorates near the bottom of the image. The AFCM result, however, shows less speckling at the bottom of the image and is very similar to the true partial volume image. Both results do, however, show some overall grain because of the effects of noise.

Figure 3 shows the results of three different segmentation algorithms applied to the same data set described in the previous example. Figure 3a shows the true hard segmentation of the simulated data. CSF is labeled as dark gray, GM as light gray, and WM as white. Figures 3b-d show the maximum membership segmentation produced by FCM, the segmentation produced by the adaptive Markov random field (AMRF[1]) method used in [19], and the maximum membership segmentation produced by TM-AFCM, respectively. Clearly, the AFCM segmentation is most similar to the truth model. Both the FCM and AMRF

---

[1] This method is also very similar to the one described in [13].

Table 1. Error measures from simulated data results

Method	Error measure					
	0% MSE	20% MSE	40% MSE	0% MCR	20% MCR	40% MCR
FCM	0.0194	0.0272	0.0517	3.988%	5.450%	9.046%
FM-AFCM	0.0210	0.0242	0.0251	4.171%	4.322%	5.065%
TM-AFCM	0.0210	0.0214	0.0244	4.168%	4.322%	4.938%
EM	0.0437	0.0491	0.0770	6.344%	7.591%	13.768%
AMRF	–	–	–	3.876%	4.795%	6.874%
MNI-FCM	–	–	–	4.979%	4.970%	5.625%

results segment much of the WM as GM near the bottom of the image. The AMRF segmentation is also spatially smoother than the other methods. This is because it takes into account pixel dependency while both FCM and AFCM classify pixels independently.

4.2   Quantitative Evaluation of Performance on Simulated Data

Table 1 summarizes error measures resulting from applying the FCM, FM-AFCM, TM-AFCM and the AMRF algorithms to Brainweb simulated T1-weighted data sets (1mm cubic voxels, 3% noise) with varying levels of inhomogeneity. Also shown are the errors using an expectation-maximization (EM) algorithm for finite Gaussian mixture models [9]. In addition, error measures were also computed for a segmentation obtained by first applying the N3 inhomogeneity correction software [16] obtained from the Montreal Neurological Institute, then applying FCM. The results of this method are given in the row labeled MNI-FCM. Two error measures were used. The first measure was the mean squared error (MSE) between the true GM partial volume and the GM fuzzy membership function. For the EM algorithm, the posterior probability of each tissue class given the data was compared with the GM partial volume. The second error measure used was the misclassification rate (MCR), defined as the number of pixels misclassified by the algorithm divided by the total number of pixels in the image. For FM-AFCM and TM-AFCM, the parameters λ_1 and λ_2 were fixed to a default value of 2×10^4 and 2×10^5 respectively. Default parameters were also used for all other segmentation methods.

Columns 1-3 show the MSE resulting from segmenting data sets with 0%, 20%, and 40% inhomogeneity, respectively. Similarly, columns 4-6 show the MCR for the same respective data sets. The MSE columns show that AFCM is capable of estimating partial volume coefficients with a reasonable accuracy even in the presence of inhomogeneities. The MCR columns show that as the inhomogeneity is increased, the errors for all methods also increase. However, the AFCM methods are much more robust to increased inhomogeneity than the other methods, with TM-AFCM achieving slightly lower errors than FM-AFCM. The EM algorithm performs poorly with respect to both error criteria, possibly because the Gaussian mixture model assumption is incorrect. In the case of 40% inhomogeneity, AFCM provides an improvement of nearly 50% over FCM, nearly 30% over the MRF methods, and over 10% over the MNI-FCM method. At zero inhomogeneity, both the FCM and AMRF methods perform slightly better than AFCM, while AMRF yields the lowest error. This is expected since the AMRF method provides some smoothing of noise, while FCM and AFCM do not. The increase in error of AFCM over FCM in the zero inhomogeneity case is due to the additional freedom of the gain field. This effect is also seen in the errors resulting from the MNI-FCM method. One could easily reduce the error by increasing the regularization terms, if the amount of inhomogeneity was known to be low. The difference in error is small, however, and overall, AFCM performs well on images of varying inhomogeneity without the need for modifying the regularization parameters. Note that one can potentially achieve much lower errors in each of the AFCM, AMRF, and MNI-FCM methods if more information about the inhomogeneity is known *a priori*, thereby allowing some tailoring of their parameters.

4.3   Correction of Inhomogeneities

Figure 4 shows the results of using AFCM to correct the inhomogeneity in an actual 3-D T1-weighted MR image data set. Figure 4a shows a slice from the original data set. Figure 4b shows the same slice after correction by AFCM. The correction was obtained by multiplying the original image by the reciprocal of the estimated gain field. The corrected image does not exhibit the left to right shading present in the original image. Figure 4c shows the computed gain field for that slice. The gain field is actually computed everywhere in the image domain but for visual purposes, it has been masked by the brain area. Note the bright area on the upper left quadrant of the image has been captured by the gain field.

Figures 4d and 4e show histograms of the slice before and after the correction has been performed. On a typical histogram of an uncorrupted MR image, three modes are present corresponding to (from left to right) CSF, GM, and WM. The original histogram in Fig. 4d, however, exhibits an additional mode around an intensity of 80 that corresponds to the bright WM on the upper left of the image slice. The corrected histogram does not possess this additional mode and also shows a significant improvement in contrast between the modes corresponding to GM and WM.

4.4   Multispectral Data

Figure 5 shows the results of FCM and TM-AFCM when applied to a 3-D spin echo (T_2-weighted and proton spin density (PD) weighted) multispectral MR data set that has been preprocessed to removed extracranial tissues. Figures 5a and 5b show a PD–weighted and the corresponding T2–weighted slice, respectively, from the data set. Figures 5c and 5d show the GM membership functions

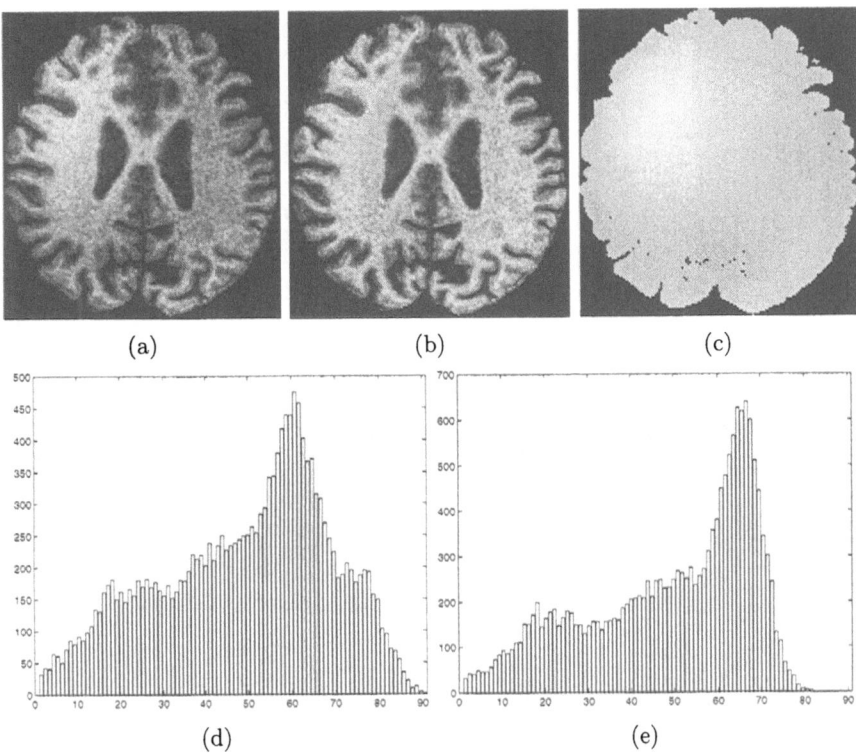

Fig. 4. Correction of inhomogeneity using TM-AFCM: (a) slice from original MR image, (b) MR slice after AFCM correction, (c) gain field computed using AFCM, (d) histogram of slice before correction, (e) histogram after correction.

computed by FCM and AFCM, respectively. One can see that the FCM membership function has a noticeable fading on the left side. There is also an increased speckling in the FCM membership function on the right side of the image. The AFCM membership function, however, is markedly cleaner and does not exhibit the same fading. Figures 5e and 5f show the contour of where the GM membership function is equal to the white matter membership function, overlayed on the PD-weighted slice. The inhomogeneity can have the effect of shifting the apparent boundaries between tissue classes. On the upper right hand side of Fig. 5e, the FCM contour has shifted inward towards the center of the image while on the left of the image, the contour has shifted outward. The AFCM contour however, conforms to the GM-WM boundary as seen on the original images much more accurately.

Acknowledgments

The authors would like to thank Chenyang Xu, Maryam Etemad, Daphne Yu and Dr. Carey Priebe for their support in this work. The authors would also

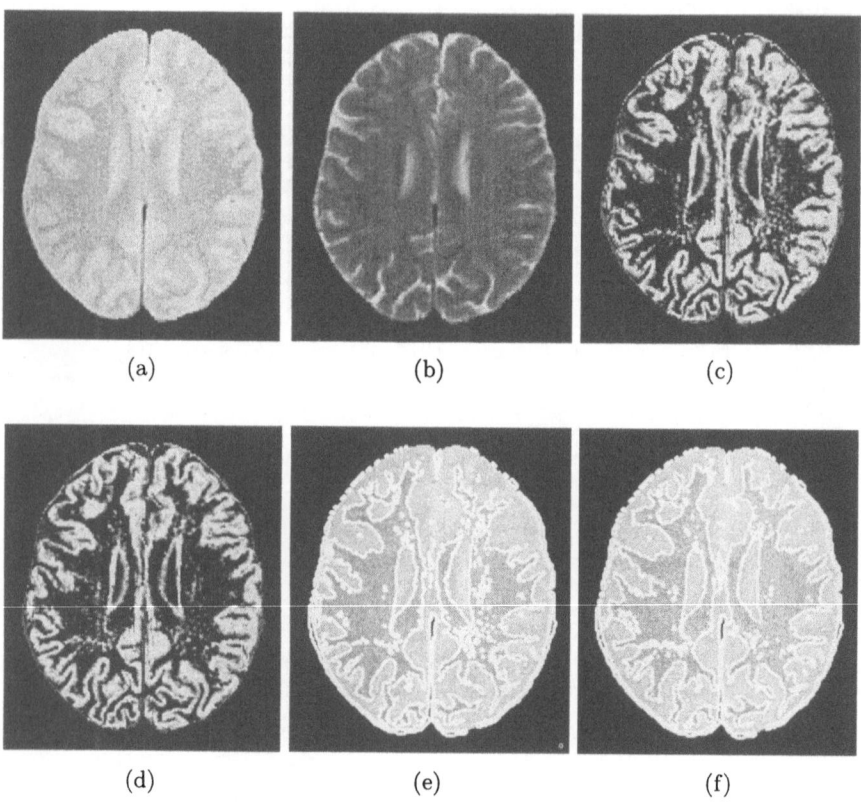

Fig. 5. FCM vs. AFCM for double-echo MR data: (a) slice from PD-weighted MR image, (b) slice from T2-weighted MR image, (c) FCM GM membership function, (d), TM-AFCM GM membership function, (e) FCM isocontour superimposed on PD-weighted image, (f) TM-AFCM isocontour superimposed on PD-weighted image.

like to thank Michelle Yan for use of the AMRF segmentation software and the McConnell Brain Imaging Centre of the Montreal Neuroimaging Institute for the use of their simulated brain database and N3 inhomogeneity correction software. This work was supported in part by an NSF Presidential Faculty Grant (MIP-9350336) and by NIH Grant 1RO1NS37747-01.

References

1. Bezdek, J., Hall, L., and Clarke, L.: Review of MR image segmentation techniques using pattern recognition. Medical Physics **20** (1993) 1033–1048
2. Bottomley, P., Foster, T., Argersinger, R., and Pfeifer, L. M.: A review of normal tissue hydrogen NMR relaxation times and relaxation mechanisms from 1-100 MHz: Dependence on tissue type, NMR frequency, temperature, species, excision, and age. Medical Physics **11** (1984) 425–448

3. Brandt, M., Bohan, T., Kramer, L., and Fletcher, J.: Estimation of CSF, white and gray matter volumes in hydrocephalic children using fuzzy clustering of MR images. Computerized Medical Imaging and Graphics **18** (1994) 25–34

4. Briggs, W.: A Multigrid Tutorial. Society for Industrial and Applied Mathematics (1987)

5. Collins, D., Zijdenbos, A., Kollokian, V., Sled, J., Kabani, N., Holmes, C., and Evans, A.: Design and construction of a realistic digital brain phantom. IEEE Trans. on Medical Imaging **17** (1998), 463–468, See `http://www.bic.mni.mcgill.ca/brainweb`

6. Davenport, J., Bezdek, J., and Hathaway, R.: Parameter estimation for finite mixture distributions. Comput. Math. Applic. **15** (1988) 810–828

7. Dawant, B., Zijdenbos, A., and Margolin, R.: Correction of intensity variations in MR images for computer-aided tissue classification. IEEE Trans. on Medical Imaging **12** (1993) 770–781

8. Kapur, T., Grimson, W., Kikinis, R., and Wells, W.: Enhanced spatial priors for segmentation of magnetic resonance imagery. In Proc. of the First Int. Conf. on Medical Image Computing and Computer Assisted Interventions (MICCAI98) (1998) 457–468

9. Liang, Z.: Tissue classification and segmentation of MR images. IEEE Eng. in Med. and Bio. (1993) 81–85

10. Pham, D., and Prince, J.: An adaptive fuzzy c-means algorithm for image segmentation in the presence of intensity inhomogeneities. In Proc. of SPIE Medical Imaging 1998: Image Processing vol. 3338 (1998) 555–563

11. Pham, D., and Prince, J.: An adaptive fuzzy c-means algorithm for image segmentation in the presence of intensity inhomogeneities. Pattern Recognition Letters **20** (1999) 57–68

12. Pham, D., Prince, J., Dagher, A., and Xu, C.: An automated technique for statistical characterization of brain tissues in magnetic resonance imaging. International Journal on Pattern Recognition and Artificial Intelligence **11** (1997) 1189–1211

13. Rajapakse, J., Giedd, J., and Rapoport, J.: Statistical approach to segmentation of single-channel cerebral MR images. IEEE Trans. on Medical Imaging **16** (1997) 176–186

14. Silverman, B.: Density estimation for statistics and data analysis. Chapman and Hall (1993)

15. Simmons, A., Tofts, P., Barker, G., and Arridge, S.: Sources of intensity nonuniformity in spin echo images at 1.5T. Magnetic Resonance in Medicine **32** (1994) 121–128

16. Sled, J., Zijdenbos, A., and Evans, A.: A nonparametric method for automatic correction of intensity nonuniformity in MRI data. IEEE Trans. on Medical Imaging **17** (1998) 87–97

17. Unser, M.: Multigrid adaptive image processing. In Proc. of the IEEE Conference on Image Processing (ICIP95) (1995) 49–52

18. Wells, W., Grimson, W., Kikins, R., and Jolesz, F.: Adaptive segmentation of MRI data. IEEE Trans. on Medical Imaging **15** (1996) 429–442

19. Yan, M., and Karp, J.: An adaptive Bayesian approach to three-dimensional MR brain segmentation. In Proc. of XIVth Int. Conf. on Information Processing in Medical Imaging (1995) 201–213

Automatic Detection and Segmentation of Evolving Processes in 3D Medical Images: Application to Multiple Sclerosis

David Rey, Gérard Subsol, Hervé Delingette, and Nicholas Ayache

INRIA Sophia Antipolis, EPIDAURE project, France
David.Rey@sophia.inria.fr

Abstract. Physicians often perform diagnoses based on the evolution of lesions, tumors or anatomical structures through time. The objective of this paper is to automatically detect regions with apparent local volume variation with a vector field operator applied to the local displacement field obtained after a non-rigid registration between successive temporal images. In studying the information of apparent shrinking areas in the direct and reverse displacement fields between images, we are able to segment evolving lesions. Then we propose a method to segment lesions in a whole temporal series of images. In this paper we apply this approach to the automatic detection and segmentation of multiple sclerosis lesions in time series of MRI images of the brain.

1 Introduction

1.1 Multiple Sclerosis Data

Multiple sclerosis is a progressive disease that requires an evolution study through time. The evolution of the disease can be followed on a patient with a temporal series of examinations. A time series of 3D images of a patient is acquired from the same modality and with a definite protocol to have similar properties: similar histogram, field of view, voxel size, image size, etc. In this paper we use two sets of multiple sclerosis time series composed of T2 weighted MRI images. These two time series come from the Brigham and Women's Hospital [1] and from the BIOMORPH [2] European project. The data from the Brigham and Women's Hospital consist in $256 \times 256 \times 54$ images, with a voxel size of $0.9 \times 0.9 \times 3.0$ mm. The temporal interval between two images of the series is about one week. The data from the BIOMORPH project consist in $256 \times 256 \times 24$ images with a voxel size of $0.9 \times 0.9 \times 5.0$ mm. The temporal interval between two images of the series is about four weeks.

---

[1] Dr Guttman and Dr Kikinis

[2] http://www.cs.unc.edu/~styner/biomorph/biomorph.html

A. Kuba et al. (Eds.): IPMI'99, LNCS 1613, pp. 154–167, 1999.

1.2   Quantitative Measurements

A quantitative analysis is required to give accurate and reproducible results, and because the data are large. Between two examinations, a patient does not have the same position in the acquisition device. Therefore images at different times are not directly comparable. We have to apply a transformation to each image to compensate for the difference in position (translation) and orientation (rotation). Then we can compare the two images, and apply automatic computerized tools to detect and quantify evolving processes There are several existing automatic methods to study the lesions of multiple sclerosis in time series:

- With a single image, it is possible to threshold or to study the image intensity to segment lesions [1]. Unfortunately, thresholding does not always make it possible to distinguish the lesions from the white matter.
- It is possible to subtract two successive images to find areas where the lesions have changed. But this method has two major problems. First, the subtraction is extremely dependent on the rigid registration [2], [3]. For instance, we show in Fig. 13 an evolving lesion that appears in the image of the subtraction as a dark hole. But when the registration is inaccurate, it is hard to distinguish evolving lesions: the edges of the anatomical structures appear (cortex, ventricles, etc.) and give the same apparent information as the lesions. Secondly, the subtraction only characterizes the difference of intensity between two images. The image of the subtraction does not give a contrasted image with respect to the evolution ratio, but only with respect to the difference between the intensity of the lesion and the intensity of the background. For example we show in Fig. 1 that if we threshold the image of the subtraction, only some parts of the evolving structures are detected. Moreover the threshold value is not related to the amplitude of the evolutions as can be seen in Fig. 1 where a series of threshold values is applied to a synthesis example.

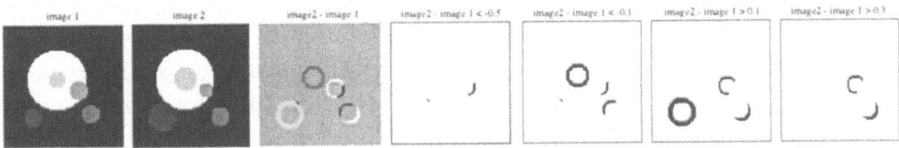

Fig. 1. Different threshold values applied to an image of subtraction. For each value, only some parts of the evolving structures are detected. Moreover, the threshold value is not related to the amplitude of the evolutions

- With n images, it is possible to follow the intensity of each voxel in time [4]. Although very nice results are obtained with perfectly rigidly aligned, the approach remains sensitive to the rigid registration, and there is no direct relation between the amplitude of evolution and the variation of voxels

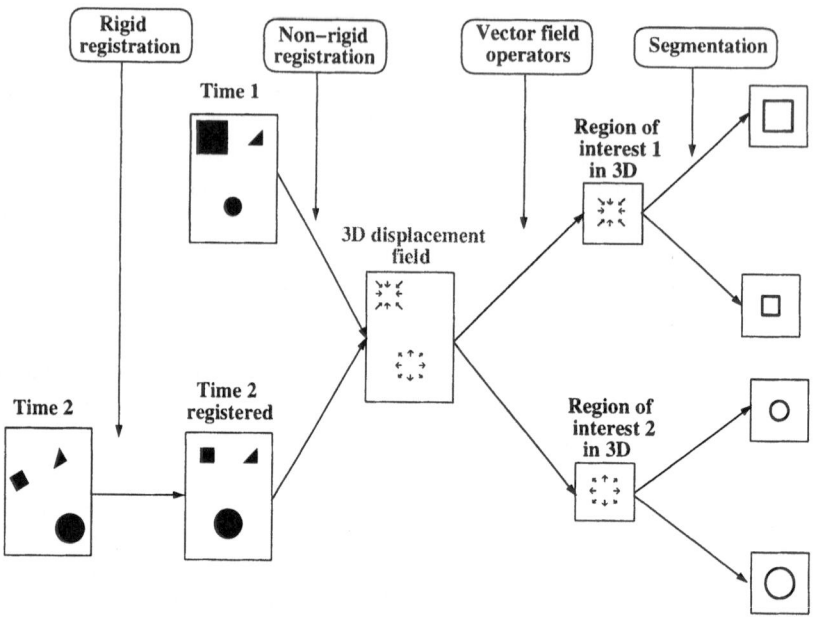

Fig. 2. Method of detection and segmentation of evolving processes using the displacement field

intensity. Moreover, this method does not take into account the spatial correlation between neighboring voxels.

1.3 A New Method Based on the Displacement Field

Our idea is thus to avoid a voxel by voxel comparison and to use the "apparent" motion between two images. Figure 2 shows the different stages of the automatic processing and gives an overview of this paper. First, images are aligned by a rigid registration. Then we compute the displacement field to recover the "apparent" motion between images with a non-rigid registration algorithm. We focus on the detection of the regions of interest of the field thanks to vector field operators, and use them to segment evolving lesions. This work is a natural continuation of the previous research work of Thirion and Calmon [5].

2 Computation of the Displacement Field

2.1 Rigid Registration

First we compute a rigid registration with an algorithm which matches "extremal" points defined as the maxima of the crest lines of the images [6]. Feature points called "extremal" points are automatically extracted from the 3D image. They are defined as the loci of curvature extrema along the "crest lines"

image 1   image 2   displacement field (zoom)

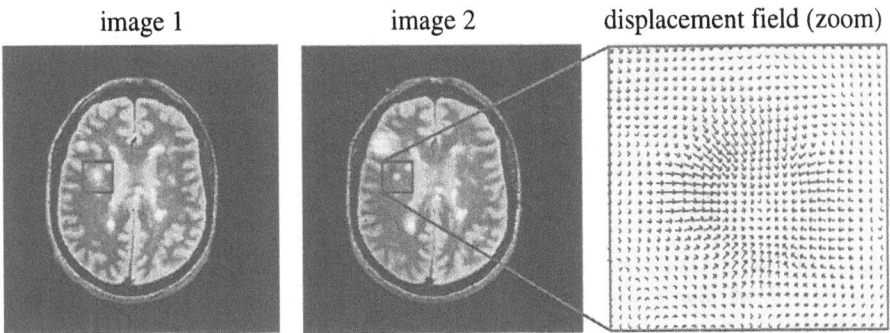

Fig. 3. An example of the computation of the "apparent" displacement field thanks to a non-rigid registration algorithm. Notice how it emphasizes the shrinking lesion

of the isosurface corresponding to the zero-crossing of the Laplacian of the image. Based on those stable points, a two-step registration algorithm computes a rigid transformation. The first step called "prediction" looks for triplets of points from the two sets which can be put into correspondence with respect to their invariant attributes. The second step called "verification" checks whether the 3D rigid transformation computed from the two corresponding triplets is valid for all the other points. A study of the accuracy of this algorithm, especially for aligning MS data, can be found in [7].

2.2   Non-rigid Registration

We compute the 3D displacement field with a non-rigid algorithm based on local diffusion [8]. This algorithm diffuses the first image into the second one. Each point of the second image "attracts" or "repels" the point that has the same coordinates as the first image according to their difference of intensity. All these forces are regularized and deform the second image. The process is iterated based on a multi-scale scheme. At the end, each point $P(x, y, z)^T$ of the reference image has a vector $\mathbf{u}(u_1(P), u_2(P), u_3(P))$ that gives its apparent **displacement** (cf Fig. 3). We can also define the **deformation** which is a function $\Phi(\Phi_1(P), \Phi_2(P), \Phi_3(P))$ that transforms the point $P(x, y, z)^T$ into the point $P'(x', y', z')^T$. We have thus:

$$\begin{cases} x' = x + u_1(x, y, z) = \Phi_1(x, y, z) \\ y' = y + u_2(x, y, z) = \Phi_2(x, y, z) \\ z' = z + u_3(x, y, z) = \Phi_3(x, y, z) \end{cases}$$

This apparent displacement field $\mathbf{u}$ gives an idea of the time evolution between two images. We can compute the two fields: from image 1 to image 2, and from image 2 to image 1, which contain complementary information as we will see in section 4.1. Figure 3 shows the vector field from 1 to 2 around a lesion, emphasizing a radial shrinking. The vector field operators should transform a 3D vector

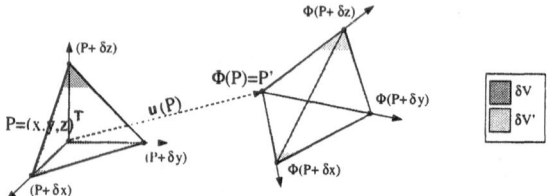

Fig. 4. $\mathbf{u}(P)$ is the apparent displacement of P at time 1. $P' = P + \mathbf{u}(P)$ is the apparent location of P at time 2. The Jacobian of the apparent deformation measures the local volume variation $\frac{\delta V'}{\delta V}$ (see text)

field in a simpler representation that is a 3D scalar image. This scalar image should be contrasted with respect to the time evolutions. Moreover we need to introduce operators that have a physical meaning for a better interpretation.

3   The Jacobian Operator

3.1   Mathematical Expression and Physical Meaning

We introduce as an operator the Jacobian of the deformation function at point P, as suggested from [9]: $\Phi(\Phi_1(P), \Phi_2(P), \Phi_3(P))$. This operator is widely used in continuum mechanics [10] [11]. The Jacobian of Φ at point P is defined as:

$$Jacobian = det(\nabla_p\Phi) = \begin{vmatrix} \frac{\partial \Phi_1}{\partial x} & \frac{\partial \Phi_1}{\partial y} & \frac{\partial \Phi_1}{\partial z} \\ \frac{\partial \Phi_2}{\partial x} & \frac{\partial \Phi_2}{\partial y} & \frac{\partial \Phi_2}{\partial z} \\ \frac{\partial \Phi_3}{\partial x} & \frac{\partial \Phi_3}{\partial y} & \frac{\partial \Phi_3}{\partial z} \end{vmatrix}.$$

It can also be written with the vector displacement field $\mathbf{u}(u_1, u_2, u_3)$ at P:

$$det(\nabla_p\Phi) = det(Id + \nabla_p\mathbf{u}) = \begin{vmatrix} \frac{\partial u_1}{\partial x} + 1 & \frac{\partial u_1}{\partial y} & \frac{\partial u_1}{\partial z} \\ \frac{\partial u_2}{\partial x} & \frac{\partial u_2}{\partial y} + 1 & \frac{\partial u_2}{\partial z} \\ \frac{\partial u_3}{\partial x} & \frac{\partial u_3}{\partial y} & \frac{\partial u_3}{\partial z} + 1 \end{vmatrix}.$$

It is useful to recall a physical interpretation of the Jacobian operator in terms of local variation of volume. With the notations of the Fig. 4, $\mathbf{u}(P)$ is the apparent displacement of P at time 1. $P' = P + \mathbf{u}(P)$ is the apparent location of P at time 2. The volume δV of the elementary tetrahedron defined by $(P, P + \delta x, P + \delta y, P + \delta z)$ is given by:

$$\delta V = \frac{1}{6} \begin{vmatrix} 1 & 1 & 1 & 1 \\ x & x + \delta x & x & x \\ y & y & y + \delta y & y \\ z & z & z & z + \delta z \end{vmatrix} = \frac{1}{6} \begin{vmatrix} 1 & 1 & 1 & 1 \\ 0 & \delta x & 0 & 0 \\ 0 & 0 & \delta y & 0 \\ 0 & 0 & 0 & \delta z \end{vmatrix} = \frac{1}{6}\delta x \delta y \delta z.$$

As we assume that δx is small, a first order approximation of the deformation Φ in P is given by $\Phi(P + \delta x) = \Phi(P) + \frac{\partial \Phi}{\partial x}\delta x + o(\delta x^2)$. We have the same approximation in y and z directions. Thus the volume $\delta V'$ of the deformed elementary tetrahedron is:

$$\delta V' \simeq \frac{1}{6} \begin{vmatrix} 1 & 1 & 1 & 1 \\ 0 & \frac{\partial \Phi_1}{\partial x}\delta x & \frac{\partial \Phi_1}{\partial y}\delta y & \frac{\partial \Phi_1}{\partial z}\delta z \\ 0 & \frac{\partial \Phi_2}{\partial x}\delta x & \frac{\partial \Phi_2}{\partial y}\delta y & \frac{\partial \Phi_2}{\partial z}\delta z \\ 0 & \frac{\partial \Phi_3}{\partial x}\delta x & \frac{\partial \Phi_3}{\partial y}\delta y & \frac{\partial \Phi_3}{\partial z}\delta z \end{vmatrix} = \frac{1}{6} Jac_p(\Phi)\delta x \delta y \delta z.$$

Therefore:

$$\delta V' \simeq Jac_p(\Phi) \cdot \delta V.$$

Thus, the local variation $\frac{\delta V'}{\delta V}$ of an elementary volume is given (as a first order approximation) by the Jacobian of the deformation function Φ. When $Jac_p(\Phi) > 1$ there is a local expansion at point P, and when $Jac_p(\Phi) < 1$ there is a local shrinking at point P. The transformation is locally preserving the volume when $Jac_p(\Phi) = 1$.

3.2 Robustness of the Jacobian with Respect to Misalignment

Figure 5 shows what happens when two images are not perfectly aligned: the deformation function Ψ, which is measured, is different from the ideal one Φ. The misregistration is given by a residual rotation R and translation t. We have $\Psi = R \circ \Phi + t$.

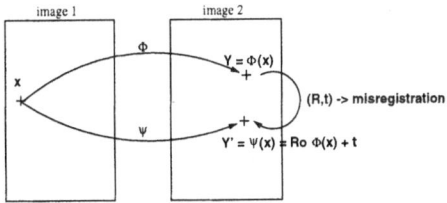

Fig. 5. Φ is the deformation function for a perfect rigid registration, and Ψ is the deformation function when there is a misregistration (R,t). We have $\Psi = R \circ \Phi + t$

Then we have:

$$Jac(\Psi) = det(\nabla \Psi) = det(\nabla(R \circ \Phi + t)) = det(R \cdot \nabla \Phi) = Jac(\Phi).$$

Therefore the Jacobian of the theoretical deformation function (for a perfect rigid registration) is equal to the Jacobian of a measured deformation function (whatever the misregistration). Of course this requires that, even in the case of an approximate alignment of images, the non-rigid registration still computes a correct displacement field. In our case the rigid registration is performed because our non-rigid registration algorithm requires a proper initial alignment to give a good result. Nevertheless, the rigid registration does not have to be as accurate as for the subtraction method where a precision better than or equal to one voxel is required.

3.3   Computation and Application of the Jacobian

We have seen that the computation of the Jacobian of the deformation Φ can be performed directly with the displacement field $\mathbf{u}$. We need to compute the first 9 derivatives of the displacement field $\mathbf{u}$: $\frac{\partial u_x}{\partial x}, \frac{\partial u_x}{\partial y}, \frac{\partial u_x}{\partial z}, \ldots, \frac{\partial u_z}{\partial z}$. For a faster computation we use recursive filtering that gives an image for each derivative. Then, we need to store in memory the 9 derivatives to compute the Jacobian and for an image of $256 \times 256 \times 180$ this requires about 425M-bytes of memory. So to avoid overfilling the memory space we compute the Jacobian on sub-images and then we fuse the different sub-results which include an overlapping border to avoid side effects.

The Jacobian gives a contrasted image with respect to the evolution amplitude. The most contrasted areas tend to correspond to shrinking or growing lesions. In Fig. 6 we see that an important shrinking of a lesion between two images gives a dark region in the Jacobian image. On other areas, the value is almost constant and very close to 1, which indicates no apparent variation of volume. A zoom around a lesion shows that darker areas correspond to shrinking lesions.

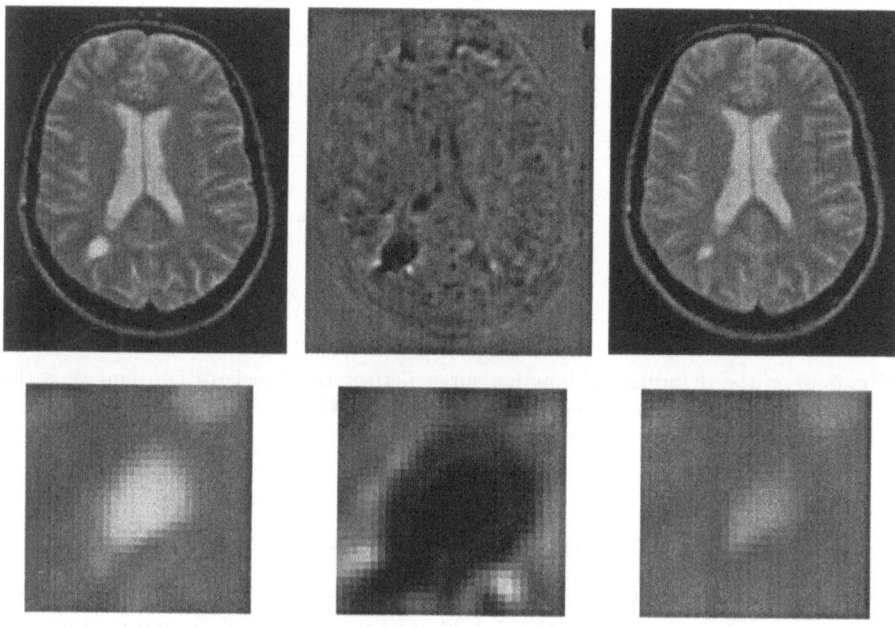

Fig. 6. Application of the Jacobian: we can see a lesion that shrinks

3.4   Other Operators

Calmon and Thirion have developed another vector field operator based on the divergence and the norm of the displacement field **u** [12] [13]:

$$norm \cdot div(P) = \|\mathbf{u}(P)\| div\ \mathbf{u}(P) = \|\mathbf{u}(P)\|(\frac{\partial u_1}{\partial x} + \frac{\partial u_2}{\partial y} + \frac{\partial u_3}{\partial z}).$$

This operator has no simple physical meaning even if the sign of the operator gives information about shrinking (negative values) or expansion (positive values). As we have no physical interpretation of the value, it is difficult to threshold the image automatically in order to extract the regions of interest.

Prima et al. proposed another operator which gives the local variation of volume [14]. A cell of voxels of volume is V_1 is deformed to a complex polyhedron which volume V_2 is computed. Then $\frac{V2-V1}{V1}$ is calculated. Note that another algorithm to compute V_2 is given in [15]. This operator is directly related to the Jacobian:

$$\frac{V_2 - V_1}{V_1} = \frac{V_2}{V_1} - 1 \simeq Jac - 1.$$

Figure 7 shows the application of these three operators on the same displacement field. In particular we can notice how the Jacobian and the discrete computation of the relative variation of volume are similar. The advantage of our approach is that it provides a continuous framework for a computation of the Jacobian at any scale.

(a)   (b)   (c)

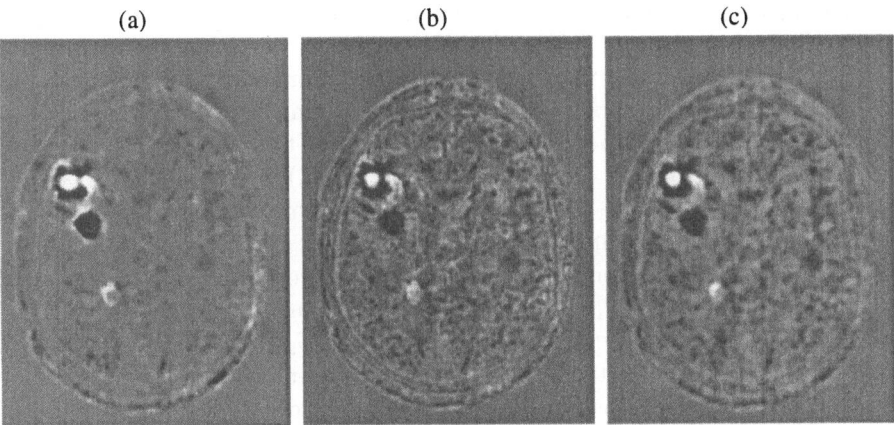

Fig. 7. Comparison between different existing operators. (a): $\|\mathbf{u}\| div\ \mathbf{u}$. (b): discrete computation of $\frac{V_2-V_1}{V_1} \sim (Jac\ (\varPhi) - 1)$. (c): Jacobian

4   Results

4.1   Thresholding and Segmentation

We can extract the areas that correspond to a significant time evolution. It is possible to find a uniform threshold over the whole Jacobian image relying on its physical interpretation in terms of local variation of volume. We chose an empiric threshold of 0.3 for significant shrinking. An example in Fig. 8 shows that it gives a good segmentation of a shrinking lesion. correspond to shrinking lesions. In

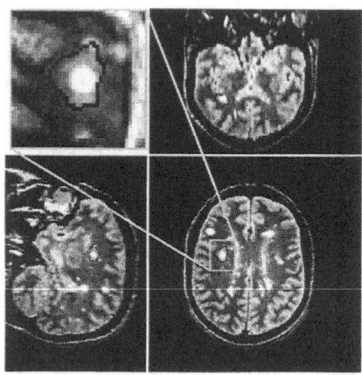

Fig. 8. The threshold $det(\nabla\Phi) < 0.3$ makes it possible to segment shrinking lesions

fact, we are going to focus only on the shrinking areas. We can see in Fig. 9 that a better description is provided with the shrinking field. If there is an important expansion locally between images 1 and 2, we would need a one to many mapping due to limited resolution of the image. To avoid this, we consider only shrinking regions from 1 to 2, and then shrinking regions from 2 to 1. By thresholding shrinking areas we obtain the segmentations $s_{1\rightarrow2}$ in the first image, and $s_{2\rightarrow1}$ in the second image. Then we have to combine those two information: the whole segmentations in image 1 and 2 are given by $S_{12}(t1) = [s_{1\rightarrow2}] \cup [\mathbf{u}_{2\rightarrow1}(s_{2\rightarrow1})]$, and $S_{12}(t2) = [s_{2\rightarrow1}] \cup [\mathbf{u}_{1\rightarrow2}(s_{1\rightarrow2})]$. Figures 10 show automatic segmentation results obtained at two times.

With the fields between images 1 and 2 and between images 2 and 3, we can compute segmentations S_{12} in the images 1 and 2 and S_{23} in the images 2 and 3. Then we propagate the segmentations S_{12} and S_{23} respectively to times $t3$ and $t1$, thanks to the vector fields $\mathbf{u}_{21}$ and $\mathbf{u}_{23}$. Then by addition, we obtain a segmentation of the lesions in all the images of a series ([16]). In Fig. 11, we can see the result of this method on three successive instances.

4.2   Study on a Synthetic Example

We have created two images I_1 and I_2, by including two artificial evolving 3-D lesions into the same 3-D T2 weighted image of a brain without lesions. The

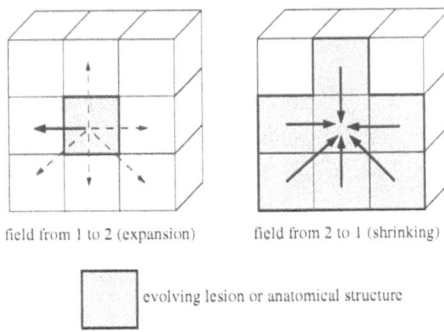

field from 1 to 2 (expansion)   field from 2 to 1 (shrinking)

evolving lesion or anatomical structure

Fig. 9. The information is richer when we look at the shrinking field. Left: If there is a large expansion, the direct displacement field cannot express that one voxel should deform to several voxels. We would need a one to many mapping due to limited resolution of the image. Right: Thanks to the reverse field, a better description of the phenomenon is possible

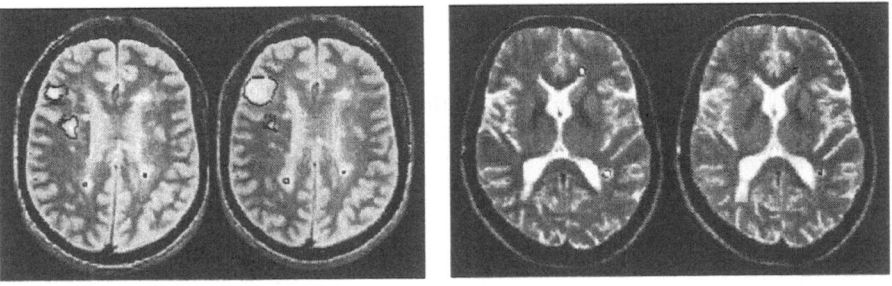

Fig. 10. Segmentation of evolving lesions. Left: Brigham & Women's Hospital data. Right: BIOMORPH data

artificial lesions are represented by spheres of radius respectively 10mm and 4mm in I_1, and 6mm and 8mm in I_2 (Fig. 12a). Because the global rigid registration of I_1 and I_2 is the identity in this case, we have only applied the non-rigid registration algorithm to compute the direct and reverse local displacement field everywhere. We have then applied our method to extract the boundary of evolving regions, with $Jac(\Phi) < 0.3$. Results on Fig. 12c show that the evolving regions are correctly detected. The accuracy of the delimitation of the boundary is qualitatively correct, but we observed a difference between 5 and 20 percent between the correct diameter of lesions and the measured one.

4.3   Robustness with Respect to Imperfect Rigid Registration

From the previous example, we also created an image I_2' by translating I_2 by 3 voxels in one direction. As expected, our method provides similar results when

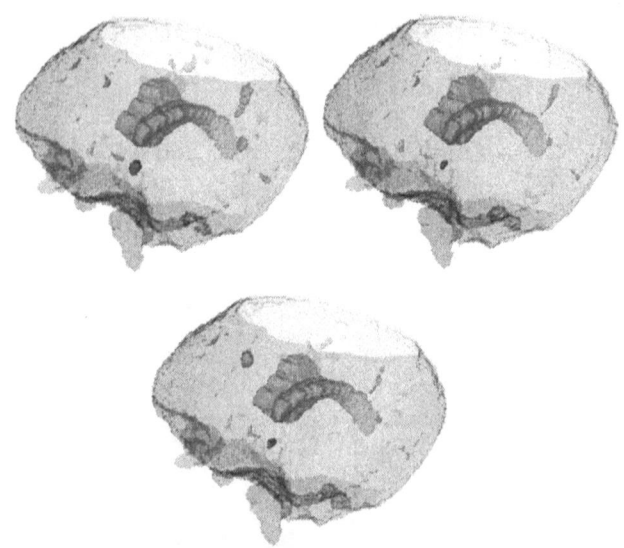

Fig. 11. Thanks to the segmentation of the evolutions between times 1 and 2, and between times 2 and 3, it is possible to visualize the lesions evolution between the 3 successive acquisitions

applied to I_1 and I_2' (Fig. 12e) , while a simple difference yields very noisy results (Fig. 12d).

We also considered the application of our method between two real T2 weighted MR image, Im_1 and Im_2 (same 3D images as the ones presented in Fig. 3). When Im_1 and Im_2 are perfectly rigidly registered, our method produces the segmentation of an evolving lesion in the cross-section shown in Fig. 13b, which can be compared to a simple difference analysis between the registered images (Fig. 13a). We also created an image Im_2' by adding a misalignment to I_2 corresponding to a rotation of 1 degree around an axis orthogonal to this cross-section and passing through its center, plus a translation of 1 voxel in the two directions of the plane of this cross-section. We observe that the results provided by our method (Fig. 13c) remain similar to the results of Fig. 13b, whereas a simple difference now produces very noisy results (Fig. 13d).

5   Conclusion

In this article we proposed a new method to study multiple sclerosis lesions evolution through time based on the apparent displacement field between images. We believe that our approach will be useful to detect evolving regions corresponding to local apparent expansion or shrinking. As this method is robust with respect to imperfect rigid alignment, we plan to use it in combination with

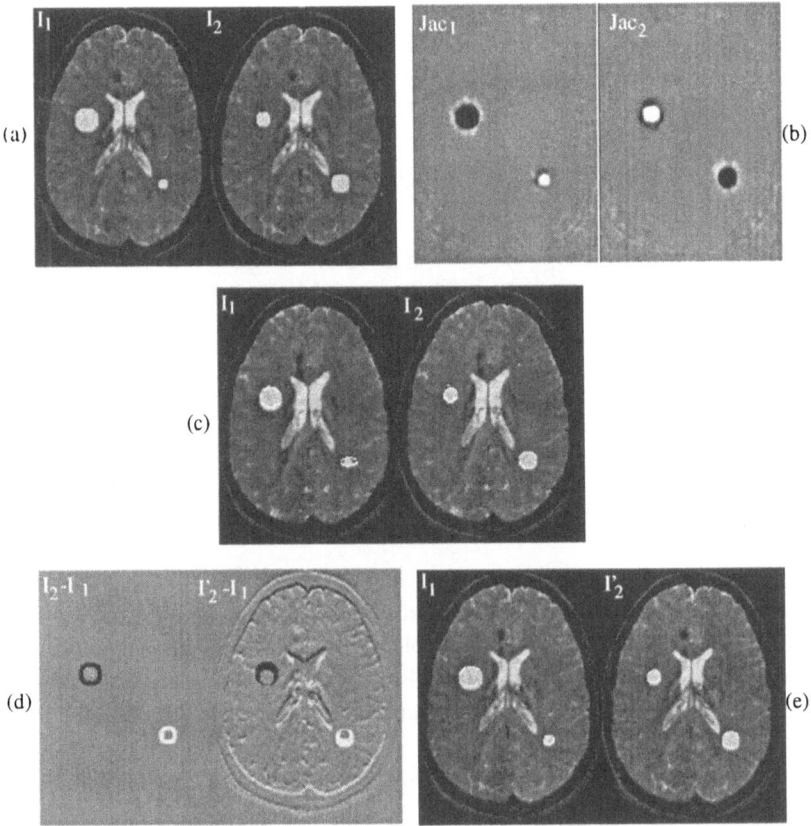

Fig. 12. (a): two synthetic temporal images I_1 and I_2. (b): the Jacobian image of the field from I_1 to I_2 and I_2 to I_1. (c): automatic segmentation of evolving lesions in I_1 and I_2 using $Jac(\Phi) < 0.3$. (d): $I_2 - I_1$ on the left. On the right $I_2' - I_1$ where I_2' is a translated version of I_2. (e): automatic segmentation of evolving lesions in I_1 and I_2', which shows robustness to imperfect rigid registration of images

other segmentation algorithms in order to delineate more precisely the boundary of the lesions in temporal sequences. Then we will compare our results with manual and other automatic segmentation results [17]. This will be done within the BIOMORPH project. Finally we plan to apply our approach to study the "mass effect" by quantifying the evolution of anatomical structures such as the cerebral ventricles or the interface between grey matter and white matter.

Acknowledgments

This work was supported by the EC-funded BIOMORPH project 95-0845, a collaboration between the Universities of Kent and Oxford (UK), ETH Zürich (Switzerland), INRIA Sophia Antipolis (France) and KU Leven (Belgium). Many

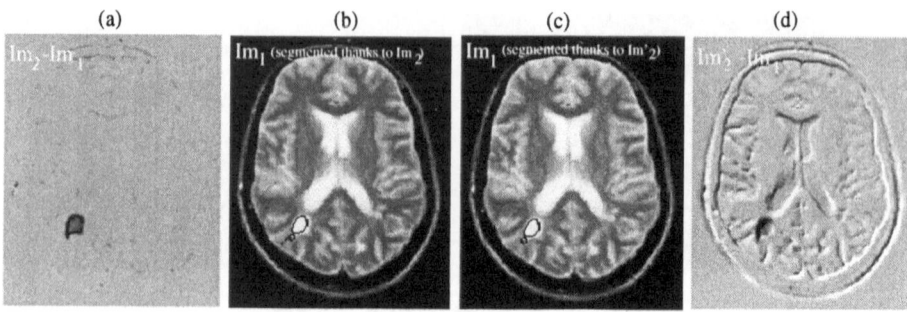

Fig. 13. Segmentation of evolving lesions in Im_1 thanks to the study between Im_1 and Im_2 (perfectly rigidly registered) and between Im_1 and Im'_2 where Im'_2 is a misregistered version of Im_2. This study shows the robustness with respect to imperfect rigid registration. (a): $Im_2 - Im_1$. (b): automatic segmentation in Im_1 thanks to the study between Im_1 and Im_2. (c): automatic segmentation in Im_1 thanks to the study between Im_1 and Im'_2. (d): $Im'2 - Im_1$

thanks to Alan Colchester and Fernando Bello (University of Kent at Canterbury) for long discussions about multiple sclerosis and lesions segmentation.

We would like to thank to Charles Guttmann and Ron Kikinis, Brigham and Women's Hospital, and Harvard Medical School, who provided us with multiple sclerosis images time series.

We warmly thank Héléne Rastouil for proofreading this paper.

References

1. Zijdenbos, A. and Forghani, R. and Evans, A.: Automatic Quantification of MS Lesions in 3D MRI Brain Data Sets: Validation of INSECT. In: Wells, W.M. and Colchester, A. and Delp, S. editors, the First International Conference on Medical Image Computing and Computer-Assisted Intervention MICCAI'98, volume 1496 of Lecture Notes in Computer Science, 439-448, Boston (1998).
2. Hajnal, J.V. and Saeed, N. and Oatridge, A. and Williams, E.J. and Young, I.R. and Bydder, G.: Detection of Subtle Brain Changes Using Subvoxel Registration and Substraction of Serial MR Images. Journal of Computer Assisted Tomography, **5** (1995) 677-691
3. Lemieux, L.: The Segmentation and Estimation of Noise in Difference Images of Co-registered MRI Scan Pairs. In: Medical Image Understanding and Analysis (MIUA'97), Oxford (1997). Electronic version : http://www.robots.ox.ac.uk/mvl/frame_proceedings.html#Registration
4. Gerig, G. and Welti, D. and Guttman, C. and Colchester, A. and Székely, G.: Exploring the Discrimination Power of the Time Domain for Segmentation and Characterization of Lesions in Serial MR Data. In: Wells, W.M and Colchester, A. and Delp, S. editors, the First International Conference on Medical Image Computing and Computer-Assisted Intervention, MICCAI'98, volume 1496 of Lecture Notes in Computer Science, 469-480, Boston (1998)

5. Thirion, J.P. and Calmon, G.: Measuring Lesion Growth from 3D Medical Images. In: IEEE Nonrigid and Articulated Motion Workshop (NAN'97), Puerto Rico (1997). Electronic version: http://www.inria.fr/RRRT/RR-3101.html

6. Thirion, J.P.: New Feature Points Based on Geometric Invariants for 3D Image Registration. International Journal of Computer Vision, **2** (1996) 121-137. Electronic version: http://www.inria.fr/RRRT/RR-1901.html

7. Pennec, X. and Thirion, J.P.: A Framework for Uncertainty and Validation of 3D Registration Methods based on Points and Frames. IJCV, **3** (1997) 203-229. Electronic version: http://www.inria.fr/epidaure/personnel/pennec/Publications.html

8. Thirion, J.P.: Image matching as a diffusion process: an analogy with Maxwell's demons. Medical Image Analysis, **2** (1998) 243-260. Electronic version: http://www.inria.fr/RRRT/RR-2547.html

9. Davatzikos, C. and Vaillant, M. and Resnick, S. and Prince, J.L. and Letovsky, S. and Bryan, R.N.: Morphological Analysis of Brain Structures Using Spatial Normalization. In: Höhne, K.H. and Kikinis, R. editors, Visualization in Biomedical Computing, volume 1131 in Lecture Notes in Computer Science, 355-360, Hamburg (1996). Electronic version : http://iacl.ece.jhu.edu/prince/jlp_pubs.html.

10. Bro-Nielsen, M.: Medical Image Registration and Surgery Simulation. PhD thesis, IMM, (1997)
Electronic version: http://www.imm.dtu.dk/documents/users/bro/phd.html.

11. Weiss, J.A. and Maker, B.N. and Govindjee, S.: Finite Element Implementation of Incompressible, Transversely Isotropic Hyperelasticity. Computer Methods in Applied Mechanics and Engineering, number 135 (1997) 107-128

12. Thirion J.P. and Calmon, G.: Deformation Analysis to Detect and Quantify Active Lesions in 3D Medical Image Sequences. Research Report 3101, INRIA (1997). Electronic version: http://www.inria.fr/RRRT/RR-3101.html

13. Thirion, J.P. and Prima, S. and Subsol, G.: Statistical Analysis of Dissymmetry in Volumetric Medical Images. Research Report 3178, INRIA (1997). Electronic version: http://www.inria.fr/RRRT/RR-3178.html

14. Prima, S. and Thirion, J.P. and Subsol, G. and Roberts, N.: Automatic Analysis of Normal Brain Dissymmetry of Males and Females in MR Images. In: Wells, W.M. and Colchester, A. and Delp, S. editors, the First International Conference on Medical Image Computing and Computer-Assisted Intervention, MICCAI'98, volume 1496 of Lecture Notes in Computer Science, 770-779, Boston (1998)

15. Calmon, G. and Roberts, N. and Eldridge, P. and Thirion, J.P.: Automatic Quantification of Changes in the Volume of Brain Structures. In: Wells, W.M. and Colchester, A. and Delp, S. editors, the First International Conference on Medical Image Computing and Computer-Assisted Intervention, MICCAI'98, volume 1496 of Lecture Notes in Computer Science, 964-973, Boston (1998)

16. Rey, D and Subsol, G. and Delingette, H. and Ayache, N.: Automatic detection and segmentation of evolving processes in 3D medical images: application to multiple sclerosis. Research Report 3559, INRIA (1998). Electronic version: http://www.inria.fr/RRRT/RR-3559.html

17. Bello, F. and Colchester, A.: Measuring Global and Local Spatial Correspondence Using Information Theory. In: Wells, W.M. and Colchester, A. and Delp, S. editors, the First International Conference on Medical Image Computing and Computer-Assisted Intervention, MICCAI'98, volume 1496 of Lecture Notes in Computer Science, 964-973, Boston (1998)

Registration of Cortical Anatomical Structures via Robust 3D Point Matching

Haili Chui, James Rambo, James Duncan, Robert Schultz,
and Anand Rangarajan

Departments of Diagnostic Radiology, Electrical Engineering
and Yale Child Study Center
Yale University, New Haven, CT 06520, USA
haili.chui@yale.edu

Abstract. Inter-subject non-rigid registration of cortical anatomical structures as seen in MR is a challenging problem. The variability of the sulcal and gyral patterns across patients makes the task of registration especially difficult regardless of whether voxel- or feature-based techniques are used. In this paper, we present an approach to matching sulcal point features interactively extracted by neuroanatomical experts. The robust point matching (RPM) algorithm is used to find the optimal affine transformations for matching sulcal points. A 3D linearly interpolated non-rigid warping is then generated for the original image volume. We present quantitative and visual comparisons between Talairach, mutual information-based volumetric matching and RPM on five subjects' MR images.

1 Introduction

The recent development of brain imaging technologies (PET, MRI, fMRI) has provided rich information on the human brain. A potentially fruitful emerging area of research is human brain mapping [25] which requires a comprehensive statistical analysis of brain structure and function across diverse populations and different imaging modalities. A major requirement in brain mapping is that the imaging data from different subjects and modalities have to be placed in a common reference frame. Recent efforts have focused on using anatomical MR as the basis for such registration.

Inter-subject anatomical registration is a difficult task due to the complexity and variability of brain structures. This is most obvious in the cortical regions. The folding of the cortical surfaces – the sulci and gyri – vary dramatically from person to person and, in some cases [25] are not even always present in each subject. However, the folding pattern is not completely arbitrary. In fact, the sulci often serve as important cortical landmarks. Furthermore, many cortical areas have been associated with critical brain functionalities (vision, language, motor control etc.) with the sulci often representing important functional boundaries. Cortical registration, despite its enormous difficulty, is hence highly desirable as a basis for further statistical quantitative analysis.

A. Kuba et al. (Eds.): IPMI'99, LNCS 1613, pp. 168–181, 1999.

Our approach is based on matching feature points representing the sulcal structures. The points were obtained using a tool [17] which allows a neuroanatomy expert to interactively trace sulci on a 3D skull-stripped MRI brain volume. In contrast to just choosing a few landmarks, the tool allows us to represent sulci using hundreds of 3D points. Also, major sulci can be identified and easily labeled.

We then match two sets of labeled sulci (extracted from two subjects' MRI) using a *robust point matching* (RPM) algorithm [20]. The method first determines the best global 3D affine transformation that brings the two sets of sulci into register. Then piecewise affine transformations are solved for each sulcus to further refine the registration. Afterward, a linearly weighted 3D volumetric warping is generated from the piecewise affine mapping.

RPM has been previously developed and used for 2D rigid alignment [20] and 2D affine warping [11]. For the first time, we have developed the technique for 3D affine and piecewise affine warping and applied it to real 3D sulcal features. Embedded within a *deterministic annealing* scheme, RPM allows us to jointly estimate the spatial mapping (affine, piecewise affine) and the point-to-point sulcal correspondences. Moreover, some sulcal structures in one subject may not have corresponding homologies in the other. RPM is able to reject a fraction of such non-homologies as *outliers*. Unlike other methods of point feature registration, RPM returns a one-to-one correspondence between sulcal points. Except for the extraction of the sulci, the whole process is done automatically and the registration and warping of one pair of brains only takes a few minutes.

2   Review

There are two principal approaches to non-rigid brain registration: voxel-based methods and feature-based methods.

Voxel-based approaches try to find the optimal transformation such that a local image intensity similarity measure is maximized. Most methods in this class allow highly complex transformations which are normally proportional to the size of the volume. Elastic media models, viscous fluid models [4] or local smoothness models [6] are introduced as constraints to guide the non-rigid spatial mapping. From these efforts, the need for non-rigid transformations is by now quite clear. Note, however that these algorithms are driven by local voxel intensities. Each voxel is treated equally without taking advantage of higher level geometric information (such as the sulcal and gyral patterns used here). In these methods, further anatomic validation is necessary to ensure that homologous sulci are indeed matched. Aware of this lack, landmarks were used as an initial step in [4]. As [5] also pointed out in their recent work, the voxel intensity approach worked well for deep subcortical structures, but sometimes had difficulty aligning sulci and gyri. To correct this, in their recent work, [5] used a chamfer distance measure [3] on sulcal points and combined it with their former voxel-based matching (ANIMAL) framework. All of these efforts are attempting to incorporate neuroanatomic geometric feature expertise into their registration engines.

Feature-based methods, as the name implies, capitalize on the information from different identifiable brain structures. Features which represent important brain structures are extracted. The features run the gamut of landmark points [2], curves [22] or surfaces [24,8]. Subsequently, these methods attempt to solve for the correspondence and transformation between the features. The spatial transformations resulting from feature matching are then propagated to the whole volume. Underlying the philosophy of feature matching is that homologous features always provide an effective anchor for registration. However, enthusiasm for these methods is usually tempered not only by the difficulty of feature extraction but also by the difficulty of simultaneously determining the correspondences or homologies and the spatial mapping. The first problem – feature extraction – usually calls for some residual manual intervention while the second problem – automated matching – involves the computationally demanding task of determining the correspondences and the spatial mapping. As our method basically belongs to this category, we discuss previous methods in some detail and compare them to ours.

Bookstein [2] pioneered the usage of landmark points for registration and shape analysis. The thin-plate-spline is used as the spatial mapping between the two landmark point sets to generate a elastic transformation in which the bending energy is minimized. Since this method basically relies on a few landmark points, the accuracy of their locations is essential. The homologies between all landmark points is deemed known (in advance). In contrast, in our approach, the correspondences and the spatial mapping are co-determined from hundreds of sulcal feature points. In addition, the anatomical variability between subjects can create many outliers, i.e., sulcal points which do not match. Since we are using hundreds of points to represent the structural information, it is statistically much more robust and the noise or point "jitter" which may be caused by various sources such as the tracing process or sampling error, should not significantly affect the final result.

In [24], 3D active surfaces are used to extract the surfaces of lateral ventricle and outer cortex which are developmentally fundamental for the brain. An initial surface is first constructed from some fiducial points and is then relaxed towards the edges until a final balance is reached between the edge attraction force and the surface smoothness measure. To better represent the deep cortical structures (sulci), parametric mesh surfaces are also interactively extracted. A point-to-point mapping between the two *surfaces* is then calculated and a linearly weighted 3D volumetric warping is generated. [8] has a similar framework where surface curvature maps at different scales are used for different brain structures. More consideration is given to the inhomogeneity within the brain. A more sophisticated elasticity model makes the algorithm more flexible at the ventricles and more powerful to account for some abnormal cases where, for example, tumors are involved. Both methods emphasize the importance of sulcal alignment and not surprisingly, the validation in [24] has shown that anatomically homogeneous points can be accurately aligned. As our method is based on matching cortical structures, it is quite similar to both of these approaches. However, we use point-sets as a representation for the sulci rather than surfaces. The major sulci are labeled which imposes strong constraints on the matching. Moreover, the non-rigid matching of 3D surfaces (parameterized by surface normals for example) is a difficult problem. The parameterization of cortical structures as point-sets allows us to easily utilize Procrustes methods of shape analysis [12,18] (by equating the atlas with the Procrustes mean). Eigenanalysis of the error covariance matrix (around the Procrustes mean atlas) also yields valuable information regarding the dominant modes of deformation present in a population [7].

We have presented a detailed review of competing approaches to solving point correspondence problems elsewhere [20]. Here we briefly discuss chamfer distances [3,5] and the iterated closest point (ICP) matching algorithm [1]. The chamfer distance has been used in cortical registration by [22] and [5]. The main problem with the chamfer distance is that it uses a brittle nearest neighbor measure to assign correspondence. Nearest neighbor methods used in chamfer matching and ICP are problematic in the vicinity of outliers since they generate local minima [19]. Unlike the chamfer matching in [5] where a distance image is calculated from the Euclidean distance from each voxel to its nearest sulcal point feature, we directly use the sulcal point feature locations for the matching. Finally, we should mention the work presented in [13] where a maximum clique approach is taken to matching relational sulcal representations. Maximum cliques is a very difficult NP-complete problem [10] which in this case increases the likelihood of getting stuck in local minima. Also, it is difficult to explicitly model non-rigid spatial mappings in the maximum clique approach [13]. Consequently, the "engine" that does the work has to be pure sulcal correspondences making the problem more difficult.

3   Robust Sulcal Matching

3.1   Softassign and Deterministic Annealing

There are two important factors that make RPM different from other point matching methods. These two factors mostly account for RPM's robustness, which proved to be well suited for matching of the complex sulcal patterns.

The first is the *softassign* technique. Let's suppose we have two point sets $\{X_i, i = 1, 2, \ldots, N_1\}$ and $\{Y_j, j = 1, 2, \ldots, N_2\}$, where N_1 and N_2 are the numbers of points in each set. ($X_i = (1, X_i^1, X_i^2, X_i^3)^T$: we are using homogeneous coordinates with a 4x4 affine spatial mapping so that the whole transformation could be simply written as AX_i.) The point matching problem is then equivalent to solving the following optimization problem:

$$\min_{M,A} E(M, A) = \min_{M,A} \sum_{i=1}^{N_1} \sum_{j=1}^{N_2} M_{ij} ||X_i - AY_j||^2 - \alpha \sum_{i=1}^{N_1} \sum_{j=1}^{N_2} M_{ij} \tag{1}$$

subject to: $\sum_{i=1}^{N_1+1} M_{ij} = 1, \forall j \in \{1, \dots, N_2\}$, $\sum_{j=1}^{N_2+1} M_{ij} = 1, \forall i \in \{1, \dots, N_1\}$, where $M_{ij} \in \{0, 1\}$. Matrix A represents the set of transformation parameters we are trying to solve. M is the *binary* correspondence matrix [20,11] with an extra row and an extra column introduced to account for outliers. The second term in (1) controls the degree of robustness. Greater the value of α, less points are rejected as outliers and vice-versa.

Obviously, the transformation parameters, represented by A, belong to the set of continuous variables; on the other hand, the correspondence matrix M is binary. The softassign technique provides a way to solve the optimizaton problem with two such variables of different natures. Instead of forcing M_{ij} to be binary, we relax it to be continuous in the interval $[0, 1]$, but with the row and column sum constraints still intact. In addition to being just a numerical technique, it also gives us a new way of treating correspondence. Now, one point does not necessarily just correspond to only one other point; it could have multiple memberships with all others with one membership being much larger than the rest. This property is clearly desirable if you have one point in one set lying in between two points in the other set. It does not have to choose immediately which one it belongs to but instead keeps a degree of "fuzziness" while preferring the closest one a little bit more. This also suggests that during the registration process when the transformation is optimized gradually, the correspondence memberships would change continuously and gradually as well without jumping around in the space of permutation matrices (and outliers). In more formal terms, making the correspondences fuzzy smoothes the energy function ridding it of poor local minima [19]. The fuzzy correspondence matrix still has to satisfy the row and column constraints. It turns out that the Sinkhorn balancing procedure of alternating row and column normalizations is an ideal vehicle to satisfy the row and column constraints [20]. The softassign essentially keeps all correspondences positive and then uses Sinkhorn's theorem to ensure that all rows and columns sum to one (except for the outlier row and column).

Another classic point matching method is the ICP algorithm [1,9]. ICP uses a nearest neighbor heuristic to set binary correspondences. The algorithm iterates between the spatial mapping and the nearest neighbor correspondences until convergence. As in the chamfer distance [3], the brittleness of the nearest neighbor measure can in many cases create local minima [19]. Some efforts have been made to improve ICP's robustness by including an adaptive thresholding [9]. Also, there is no guarantee that ICP will return one-to-one correspondences. While correspondence does not have to be a pre-requisite for registration, it does play a more significant role in the creation of probabilistic atlases [15]; the atlas formation step requires averages and covariance matrices to be computed over all the corresponding points in a training set. We expect the one-to-one correspondence returned by RPM to play a significant role in the formation of probabilistic atlases.

Deterministic Annealing [27] is the other important technique used in RPM, which is a good companion to softassign. It is closely related to simulated annealing except that all operations are deterministic. The temperature parameter T

in deterministic annealing specifies the degree of fuzziness of the correspondence matrix – the higher the temperature, the greater the fuzziness. At each temperature, the initial condition from the previous temperature is used and a straightforward deterministic descent is performed on the energy function. The process is repeated at lower and lower temperatures until M becomes almost binary. The method is more robust than classical gradient methods in that more configurations are allowed at higher temperature, and this makes the energy function smoother and less vulnerable to local minima. At very low temperatures, RPM is very similar to ICP with the added benefit of one-to-one correspondence.

3.2   The Spatial Mapping – 3D Affine Transformations

With the above background regarding softassign and deterministic annealing in place, it is reasonably straightforward to develop the method for a 3D affine spatial mapping. The complete form of the energy function is:

$$\min_{M,A} \max_{\mu\nu} E(A, M)$$

$$= \min_{M,A} \max_{\mu\nu} \{ \sum_{i,j}^{N_1,N_2} M_{ij}||X_i - (A+I)Y_j||^2 + \lambda \operatorname{trace}(A^T A) - \alpha \sum_{i,j}^{N_1,N_2} M_{ij}$$

$$+ \sum_i^{N_1} \mu_i (\sum_j^{N_2+1} M_{ij} - 1) + \sum_j^{N_2} \nu_j (\sum_i^{N_1+1} M_{ij} - 1)$$

$$+ T \sum_{i,j}^{N_1,N_2} M_{ij}(\log M_{ij} - 1) \}. \tag{2}$$

Even though there are six terms, only the first two will be directly involved when we are going to solve for the transformation A (actually $A+I$ where I is the identity transformation). The transformation A is now in 3D. The first term is the error measure. Assume for the moment that the correspondence M is known. The second term is the regularization on A. Basically we are assuming that the affine transformation should be close to identity. The degree of deviation from identity depends on λ. Typically, we begin with a high value of λ and quickly decrease it, with the consideration being that at first the correspondences are still far from the right answer and the transformation should not be too committed. Though this may add some complexity to the algorithm, we have found it worthwhile for two reasons. The first is that the algorithm does not seem to be very sensitive for slightly different choices of λ annealing schedules, i.e. as long as the starting value is high enough so that the transformations are not too large in the beginning and the final value small enough so that the transformations won't always forced too close to identity. The second reason stems from an observation that because of the extra constraint we put on the transformation, we could then choose not to use that robustness term $-\alpha \sum_{i,j}^{N_1,N_2} M_{ij}$ at all. Actually, in all our experiments α was set to 0.

With M held fixed, the energy function w.r.t. A is:

$$E_{\text{affine}}(A)|_M = \sum_{i,j}^{N_1,N_2} M_{ij}||X_i - (A+I)Y_j||^2 + \lambda \, \text{trace}(A^T A) \qquad (3)$$

which is a standard least squares problem for the matrix A . By taking the derivative $\frac{\partial E_{\text{affine}}}{\partial A} = 0$, we can get the closed-form solution for A.

$$A = [\sum_{i,j}^{N_1,N_2} M_{ij}(X_iY_j^T - Y_jY_j^T)] \cdot [\sum_{i,j}^{N_1,N_2} M_{ij}Y_jY_j^T + \lambda I]^{-1} = P \cdot Q. \qquad (4)$$

We will briefly describe the solution for the correspondence mainly for the sake of completion. The fourth and fifth terms are the row and column constraints expressed via Lagrange parameters. The Sinkhorn algorithm within the softassign process will automatically satisfy these constraints so we do not need to explicitly solve for the Lagrange parameters μ_i and ν_j [20]. The sixth term is an entropy term which can also be regarded as a barrier function [14]. Solving for M_{ij} (keeping the Lagrange parameters μ_i and ν_j fixed), we get:

$$M_{ij} = e^{-\frac{||X_i-(A+I)Y_j||^2-\alpha-\mu_i-\nu_j}{T}}. \qquad (5)$$

Having specified both the spatial mapping in (4) and the correspondences in (5), we summarize the algorithm in the following pseudo-code.

The Robust Point Matching (RPM) Algorithm

Initialize M, T, A, λ
Begin A: Deterministic Annealing. Do A until $T < T_{\text{final}}$
  Begin B: Softassign and Relaxation. Do B until M converges or # of iterations $> I_0$
    $Q_{ij} \leftarrow ||X_i - (A+I)Y_j||^2 - \alpha$
    $M_{ij} \leftarrow \exp(-\frac{Q_{ij}}{T})$
    Begin C: Sinkhorn. Do C until M converges or # of iterations $> I_1$
      $M_{ij} \leftarrow \frac{M_{ij}}{\sum_{j=1}^{N_2+1} M_{ij}}$ (row normalization)
      $M_{ij} \leftarrow \frac{M_{ij}}{\sum_{i=1}^{N_1+1} M_{ij}}$ (column normalization)
    End C
    $A \leftarrow [\sum_{i,j}^{N_1,N_2} M_{ij}(X_iY_j^T - Y_jY_j^T)] \cdot [\sum_{i,j}^{N_1,N_2} M_{ij}Y_jY_j^T + \lambda I]^{-1}$
  End B
  $T \leftarrow T * T_{\text{anneal-rate}}$
  $\lambda \leftarrow \lambda * \lambda_{\text{anneal-rate}}$
End A

3.3   Global/Piecewise Affine Registration and Warping

Given two brains' sulcal point-sets, the registration is done in two steps. The first step finds the global affine transformation to account for the overall translation, orientation, scale and skew. After that, we further allow each sulcus to move locally to refine the alignment by solving for a piecewise affine transformation for each of them. To make sure that the sulcus only does *local* adjustment, the regularization is increased compared to the first step so that only small transformations are allowed.

We then tried to propagate the transformations found for the sulcal points to the whole 3D volume to generate a 3D warping. A weighted linear combination of all the sulci's piecewise affine transformations is calculated based on the shortest distance between a voxel and each sulcus. More specifically, we have a total number of N sulci with each of them (nth) denoted by a set of points, $\{X_l^{(n)}, l = 1, 2, \dots \}$ and a set of affine transformations $A^{(n)}, n = 1, 2, \dots, N$. For the current voxel Y_{ijk} (other than the sulcal points locations, where the transformation is unknown and need to be calculated), the shortest distance to the nth sulcus is found, $d_{ijk}^{(n)} = \min_l ||Y_{ijk} - X_l^{(n)}||$, $n = 1, 2, \dots, N$. A set of weights is then defined as:

$$w_{ijk}^{(n)} = \frac{\frac{1}{d_{ijk}^{(n)}}}{\sum_{n=1}^{N} \frac{1}{d_{ijk}^{(n)}}} \tag{6}$$

and the final voxel transformation is the weighted summation of all $A^{(n)}$. This is done for each voxel to warp the entire volume.

$$A_{ijk} = \sum_{n=1}^{N} w_{ijk}^{(n)} \cdot A^{(n)}. \tag{7}$$

4   Experiments and Results:

The sulcus tracing was done on an SGI graphics platform [17] with a ray-casting technique that allows drawing in 3D space by projecting 2D coordinates of the tracing onto the exposed cortical surface. A screenshot of the tool is shown on the left in Fig. 1. The inter-hemispheric fissure and 10 other major sulci (superior frontal, central, post-central, Sylvian and superior temporal on both hemispheres) were extracted as point features. A sulcal point-set extracted from one subject is shown on the right in Fig. 1.

4.1   RPM Applied to Sulcal Point Sets

The original sulcal point-sets normally contain around 3,000 points each. The point-set is first sub-sampled to have around 300 points by taking every tenth point. The original MRI volume's size is 106(X) x 75(Y) x 85(Z, slices). With

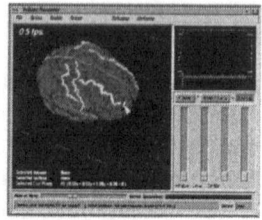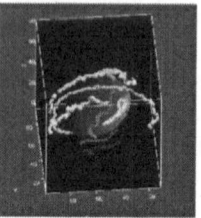

Fig. 1. Left: A screenshot of the sulcus tracing tool with some traced sulci on the 3D MR brain volume. Right: Sulci extracted and displayed as point-sets

that in mind, it is reasonable to assume that the average distances between points before registration should be in the range of 10 - 100. We set our starting temperature to be roughly in the same scale. After registration, we would expect the average distance between corresponding points to be within a few voxels (say, 1 - 10). Our final temperature should be slightly smaller. From these considerations, we set the RPM annealing parameters to be the following: $T_{\text{init}} = 50$, $T_{\text{final}} = 1$, $T_{\text{anneal-rate}} = 0.95$. The regularization parameter λ is set to force A to be small at first. We use the value of $\lambda_{init} = \max_{ij}[P_{ij}]$ (P, as defined in (4)) and decrease it by $\lambda_{\text{anneal-rate}} = 0.8$ at the end of every temperature iteration. As mentioned above, the idea is that the regularization should prevent the affine to be over determined by the initial fuzzy correspondence at first; once the algorithm starts moving towards the right correspondence, which usually happens within the first few iterations, the regularization should be relaxed by decreasing λ faster than the temperature. Actually, we observed that normally any annealing rate between 0.7 and 0.9 works quite well.

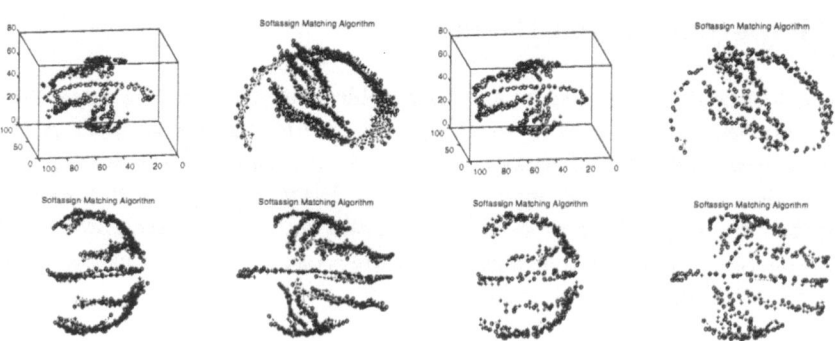

Fig. 2. Demonstration of the robust point matching process. Left four: 3D point sets and their three 2D projections in the middle of the matching. 3D point sets are shown as circles and crosses. Their most significant correspondences are shown as dotted lines. Right four: Towards the end of the matching

Figure 2 shows one example of RPM in action. The circles and crosses stand for two sets of sulcal points and the gray links indicate the most significant correspondences (($M_{ij} > \frac{1}{N_1}$ or $\frac{1}{N_2}$)) between the two point-sets at that moment. The first is taken in the middle of the registration procedure in which clearly one can see that correspondence is still "fuzzy". The second is taken towards the end of the process and the correspondence is close to binary so fewer links are seen.

4.2   A Comparison between Talairach, Voxel-based matching and RPM.

We applied RPM to five sulcal point-sets and compared it with two other methods which also use affine (and piecewise-affine) transformations for brain registration.

As mentioned in the review section, we suspected that the voxel-based methods' performance would not be as satisfying as feature-based methods for sulcal alignment. To test this, we compare RPM with a voxel-based affine matching method [23] which maximizes the mutual information between the two volumes.

By defining a common coordinate system, the Talairach method is a standard technique for brain alignment. A piecewise affine transformation is applied to 12 rectangular regions of brains defined by landmark points of anterior and posterior commissures and extrema of the cortex. We used the Talairach program available as part of the MEDx package (from Sensor Systems Inc.) to align 5 brains. Sulcal points were traced on the resulting brain volumes.

The volumes were then matched by the voxel-based method described in [23] and the resulting spatial mapping was applied to the sulcal points. RPM was separately run on the sulcal point-sets, and both the result from a simple global affine transformation and piecewise affine transformations are shown in Fig. 3. Since we register every brain to the first one, after registration, the minimum distance from each sulcal point in the current brain to the first is calculated. The mean and variance of such minimum distances for each sulcus is calculated for quantitative comparison. The results are shown in Fig. 4. The above comparison of Talairach with RPM and voxel-based approaches shows that RPM can significantly improve upon Talairach in most cases even though it may have less degrees of freedom. The voxel-based method's performance is mixed; it gives bigger errors for 5 of the 11 sulci. The significant improvement from the global affine transformations by allowing piecewise transformations confirmed the belief of the importance of non-rigid transformations.

4.3   3D Warping and Comparison.

The three dimensional warping of the brain volumes is calculated from the transformations found for the sulci as described above. The insufficiency of the Talairach alignment for the sulcal structure is clearly seen. Even though our warping strategy based on piecewise affine transformations is quite simple, the results show further improvement upon the global affine transformation.

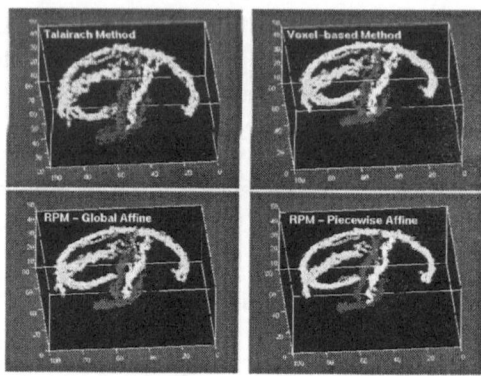

Fig. 3. Sulcal points alignment. The alignment results of five brains' sulcal point-sets on the left side of the brain are shown together. Denser, closely packed distributions of sulcal points suggest that they are better aligned. We clearly see the improvement of RPM over both Talairach and the voxel-based approach, especially for RPM with the piecewise affine mapping

Two subjects' brains as well as some of their major sulci are shown in Fig. 5. The variability of the sulci can be appreciated from this figure.

By displaying the reference brain's sulci on the other brain volumes warped using the Talairach technique, global affine transformation from RPM and piecewise affine transformations from RPM, we can see the improvement of sulcal structure alignment by our method. We should also note that the better alignment is accompanied by increased degree of brain deformation. These are shown in Figs. 6, 7, and 8.

5   Discussion and Conclusion

Our simulation and experiments with real data indicate that sulcal point matching is a fast, robust and accurate tool for the registration of cortical anatomical structures. We now mention several enhancements that could further improve our point feature-based non-rigid registration. First, statistical shape models can be computed using the correspondence information returned by RPM. From these models, more meaningful deformation modes based on principal components can be constructed. Also, an arc length-based ordering of the points (akin to curves) can be imposed. This would have the effect of radically reducing the correspondence search. Finally, using a mixture model [21], we can extend the matching algorithm to the problem of matching a labeled sulcal atlas to an unlabled or partially labeled sulcal point-set. This would allow us to automatically label the sulci extracted from a new brain image. We have reported preliminary work on matching labeled point-sets to unlabeled features (though not sulcal point features) elsewhere [16].

Since we are using point-sets, which are quite flexible – i.e. it does not matter if those points all lie on a curve, a surface or a more complicated geometrical

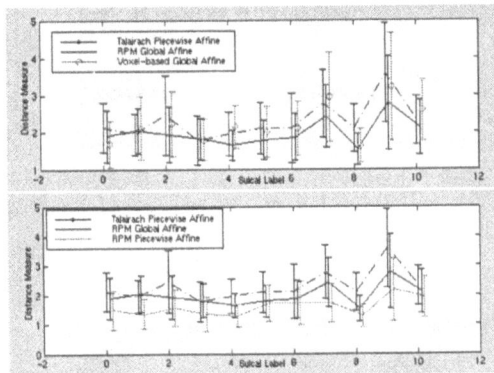

Fig. 4. The minimum distance measure (as described in text) for each sulcus (sulcal label: 0 - interhemispheric fissure; 1,2 - central sulcus; 3,4 - Sylvian fissure; 5,6 - superior temporal sulcus; 7,8 - post-central sulcus; 9,10 - superior frontal sulcus.) Top figure shows the comparison between Talairach (dashed line), voxel-based method (light dotted line) and RPM with a global affine transformation (solid line). Bottom figure shows the first two again with results of RPM with piecewise affine transformation (light line)

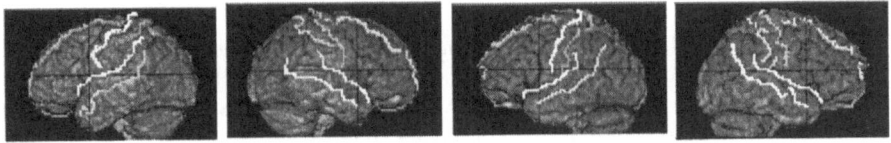

Fig. 5. Two brain volumes after Talairach alignment with their sulci are shown here. Left to right: Both sides of one brain A, both sides of another brain B

object – deep cortical structures (for example representations like *sulcal ribbons* [26]) can be easily incorporated into our framework. Future work will focus on hierarchical (labeled and unlabeled) point-set representations of the cortical structures.

6   Acknowledgments

We thank Larry Staib, Colin Studholme and Larry Win for their generous help. A.R and H. C are partially supported by a grant from the Whitaker Foundation.

References

1. Besl, P.J. and McKay, N.D.: A method for registration of 3-D shapes. IEEE Trans. Patt. Anal. Mach. Intell. **14(2)** (1992) 239–256
2. Bookstein, F.L.: Principal warps: Thin-plate splines and the decomposition of deformations. IEEE Trans. Patt. Anal. Mach. Intell. **11(6)** (1989) 567–585

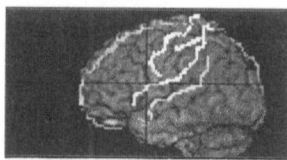 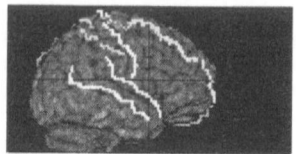

Fig. 6. One brain's (A) sulci overlay on the other's (B) volume after Talairach alignment for both side.Clear mismatch can been seen at the temporal lobe area near the Sylvian fissure and the superior temporal sulcus

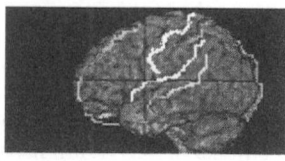 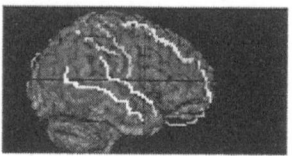

Fig. 7. Same except that the volume shown here is deformed by the global affine transformation found by RPM. An improvement over the previous Talairach result can be seen. Locally around the Sylvian fissure area, a small misalignment is seen in the left figure

3. Borgefors, G.: Hierarchical chamfer matching: a parametric edge matching algorithm. IEEE Trans. Patt. Anal. Mach. Intell. **10(6)** (1988) 849–865
4. Christensen, G., Joshi, S., Miller, M.: Volumetric transformation of brain anatomy. IEEE Trans. Med. Imag. **16(6)** (1997) 864–877
5. Collins, D., Goualher, G., Evans, A.: Non-linear cerebral registration with sulcal constraints. Medical Image Computing and Computer-Assisted Intervention *Lecture Notes in Computer Science* **volume 1496** (1988) 974–984
6. Collins, D., Holmes, C., Peters, T., Evans, A.: Automatic 3D model-based neuroanatomical segmentation. Human Brain Mapping **3(3)** (1995) 190–208
7. Cootes, T., Taylor, C., Cooper, D., and Graham, J.: Active shape models: Their training and application. Computer Vision and Image Understanding **61(1)** (1995) 38–59
8. Davatzikos, C.: Spatial transformation and registration of brain images using elastically deformable models. Computer Vision and Image Understanding: Special Issue on Medical Imaging **6(2)** (1997) 207–222
9. Feldmar, J., Ayache, N.: Rigid, affine and locally affine registration of free-form surfaces. Intl. J. Computer Vision **18(2)** (1996) 99–119
10. Garey, M.R., Johnson, D.S.: Computers and intractability: a guide to the theory of NP–completeness. Freeman, W.H., San Francisco, CA (1979)
11. Gold S., Rangarajan A., Lu, C.P., Pappu, S., Mjolsness, E.: New algorithms for 2-D and 3-D point matching: pose estimation and correspondence. Pattern Recognition **31(8)** (1998) 1019–1031
12. Goodall, C.: Procrustes methods in the statistical analysis of shape. J. R. Statist. Soc. B **53(2)** (1991) 285–339
13. Lohmann, G., von Cramon D.: Sulcal basin and sulcal strings as new concepts for describing the human cortical topography. Workshop on Biomedical Image Analysis, IEEE Press (1998) 41–54

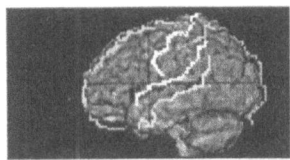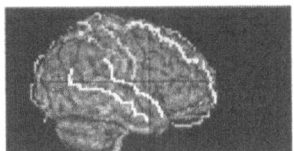

Fig. 8. Same as above except that the volume shown is deformed by the 3D warping based on piecewise affine transformations from RPM. The better global alignment seen from the figure above is maintained and some further local refinement could also be seen (again, notice the area around Sylvian fissure in the left figure). We could also see that the brain's shape has been noticeably deformed

14. Luenberger, D.: Linear and Nonlinear Programming. Addison–Wesley, Reading, MA (1984)

15. Mazziotta, J., Toga, A., Evans, A., Fox, P., Lancaster, J.: A probabilistic atlas of the human brain: theory and rationale for its development. NeuroImage **2(2)** (1995) 89–101

16. Pappu, S., Gold, S., Rangarajan, A.: A framework for non-rigid matching and correspondence. Advances in Neural Information Processing Systems, MIT Press, Cambridge, MA **8** (1996) 795–801

17. Rambo, J., Zeng, X., Schultz, R., Win, L.,Staib, L., Duncan, J.: Platform for visualization and measurement of gray matter volume and surface area within discrete cortical regions from MR images. NeuroImage **7(4)** (1998) 795

18. Rangarajan, A., Chui, H., Bookstein, F.: The softassign Procrustes matching algorithm. Information Processing in Medical Imaging (IPMI '97), Springer (1997) 29–42

19. Rangarajan, A., Chui, H., Duncan, J.: Rigid point feature registration using mutual information. Medical Image Analysis (1999) (accepted).

20. Rangarajan, A., Chui, H., Mjolsness, E., Pappu, S., Davachi, L., Goldman-Rakic, P., Duncan, J.: A robust point matching algorithm for autoradiograph alignment. Medical Image Analysis **4(1)** (1997) 379–398

21. Redner, R.A., Walker, H.F.: Mixture densities, maximum likelihood and the EM algorithm. SIAM Review **26(2)** (1984) 195–239

22. Sandor, S., Leahy, R.: Surface based labeling of cortical anatomy using a deformable atlas. IEEE Trans. Med. Imag. **16(1)** (1997) 41–54

23. Studholme, C., Hill, D., Hawkes, D.: An overlap invariant entropy measure of 3d medical image alignment. Pattern Recognition **32** (1999) 71–86

24. Thompson, P., Toga, A.W.: A surface-based technique for warping three-dimensional images of the brain. IEEE Trans. Med. Imag. **5(4)** (1996) 402–417

25. Toga, A., Mazziotta, J.: Brain Mapping: The Methods. Academic Press (1996)

26. Vaillant, M., Davatzikos, C., Bryan, R.: Finding 3D parametric representations of the deep cortical folds. Proc. of the Workshop on Mathematical Methods in Biomedical Image Analysis, IEEE Computer Society Press (1996) 151–159

27. Yuille, A.L.: Generalized deformable models, statistical physics, and matching problems. Neural Computation **2(1)** (1990) 1–24

Hierarchical Matching of Cortical Features for Deformable Brain Image Registration

Marc Vaillant[1,2] and Christos Davatzikos[2]

[1] Department of Biomedical Engineering, Johns Hopkins University School of
Medicine, Baltimore MD 21287, USA
marc@jhu.edu
[2] Neuroimaging Laboratory, Department of Radiology, Johns Hopkins University
School of Medicine, Baltimore MD 21287, USA
hristos@parthenon.rad.jhu.edu

Abstract. This paper builds upon our previous work on elastic registration, using surface-to-surface mapping. In particular, a methodology for finding a smooth map from one cortical surface to another is presented, using constraints imposed by a number of sulcal and gyral curves. The outer cortical surface is represented by a map from the unit sphere to the surface which is obtained by a deformable surface algorithm. The sulcal and gyral constraints are defined as landmark curves on the outer cortical surface representation. The unit sphere is then elastically warped to itself in 3D using the predefined sulcal and gyral constraints, yielding a reparameterization of the original surface. This method is tested on MR images from 8 subjects, showing improved registration in the vicinity of the sulci used as constraints. We also describe a hierarchical framework for automating this procedure, by using conditional spatial probability distributions of cortical features on the spherical parametric domain, in order to automatically identify cortical features. This approach is demonstrated on the central and precentral sulci.

1   Introduction

Deformable registration has received a great deal of attention by the brain imaging community in the past decade [1,2,3,4,5,6,7,8,9,10]. Finding a spatial transformation that morphs one brain to another is important in several applications, including computational anatomy [2,11,12], functional image analysis [13], and image guided neurosurgery.

The several methods that have been proposed in the literature can be broadly classified into image-matching and feature-matching methods. The former are based on the assumption that two images to be matched have similar signal characteristics. Accordingly, these methods look for transformations that maximize some measure of overlap or similarity between the transformed and the target images [2,5]. Feature-based approaches utilize distinct anatomical features that are first extracted from images, in order to find the morphing transformation [1,3,7,8,9,10]. We have previously reported a method that uses open or

A. Kuba et al. (Eds.): IPMI'99, LNCS 1613, pp. 182–195, 1999.

closed surfaces as features that drive a 3D elastic transformation [7]; similar approaches have been pursued by other investigators [3,6,10]. Features can be the boundaries of brain structures, or the cortical sulci, which can be modeled as thin convoluted ribbons embedded in 3D [14].

One of the important issues that needs to be considered in a surface matching paradigm is that there is an infinite number of possible ways in which one surface can be mapped to another. In the context of deformable registration, however, only the map that preserves anatomical homologies is meaningful. In this paper we present an approach for defining such a map, using distinct features of the cortex (Sect. 2). Moreover, in Sect. 3 we describe a framework for automating this procedure, by using spatial probability distributions of cortical features on a spherical reference domain, in conjunction with geometric properties of an individual's cortical surface, in order to automatically identify these features. In this paper we restrict our attention to the outer cortical surface. Our methods, however, are applicable to any anatomical surface that is parameterized on the unit sphere. Of particular interest is the application of our methods to the problem of spatial normalization of the whole cortical surface, the accurate extraction of which is still an open research problem [10,15,16,17], in order to normalize structural and functional data to a common reference system.

Using prior spatial distributions for identifying cortical sulci has been recently shown to be a promising approach [18]. The method presented in [18] was based on 3D spatial distributions of the sulci, after an overall shape normalization of the corresponding brain images via a 3D linear transformation. The work we present herein is similar in nature, but it differs in three respects. First, our spatial priors pertain to curves that belong to surfaces parameterized on the unit sphere, and are therefore applicable to any surface matching paradigm using the unit sphere as parametric domain. In addition to reducing the dimensionality of the problem by one dimension, we believe that our approach might turn out to produce tighter spatial priors, since the fact that we work in the parametric domain implies that variability in the overall shape of the brain is factored out. Moreover, in Sect. 3 we propose a hierarchical approach, which starts with the identification of the major and less variable cortical features, and then proceeds with more variable ones. Effectively, our method removes a certain degree of variability at each stage of the hierarchical matching. Our assumption, which is tested on variability measurements gathered from the precentral and central sulci of 20 subjects, is that having identified the location of, e.g. the central sulcus, gives us a better idea of where to look for the precentral sulcus, as opposed to looking for the precentral sulcus directly.

2   Elastic Registration

2.1   Overall Framework

In [7] we treated the problem of finding a map from one surface to another as a problem of finding an elastic reparameterization of one of the two surfaces, so that the geometric structures (quantified by the principal curvatures) of the two surfaces are similar on surface points with the same parametric coordinates. That approach has been tested on a large sample of 250 images [19], and it has demonstrated an overall good registration. However, accurate registration of individual sulci or gyri could not be achieved. This is due primarily to the complexity of the cortical structure. In particular, because of the convoluted nature of the cortex, we only used global geometric properties of the brain, in order to find a map from one surface to another. Typically, these global shape measures highlight structures such as the inter-hemispheric and Sylvian fissures, or at the tips of the temporal and occipital lobes. Figure 1a shows the gray matter and white matter distributions of 100 subjects after elastic warping to the Talairach space [20]. Achieving a better registration in the cortical region is the main goal of the work reported in this paper.

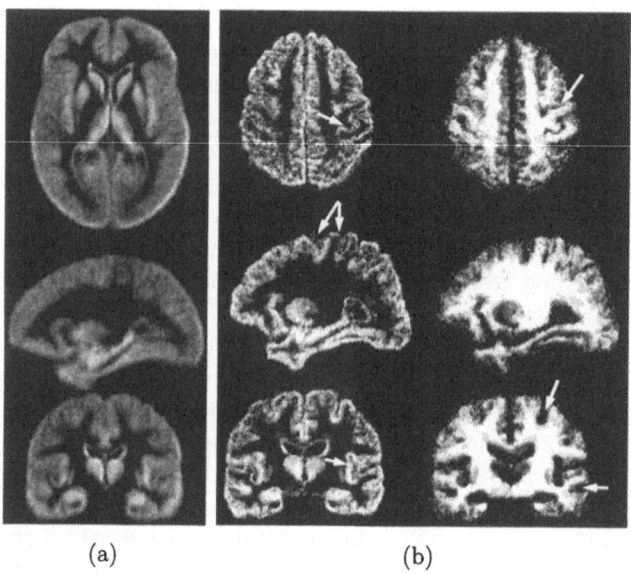

(a)   (b)

Fig. 1. (a) Triplanar display of the average distribution of gray matter from 100 normal subjects, after segmented images of these subjects were mapped to Talairach space. Individual cortical folds were not brought into perfect registration as reflected by the fuzziness in the average image. (b) The average distributions of gray and white matter for 8 subjects, after elastic warping using 9 landmark curves primarily in the left hemisphere (right in the images). Arrows indicate regions of good registration (low fuzziness) around landmark curves. Note the good registration around the central sulcus (top left, arrow)

In particular, we first present a method for morphing one cortical surface to another, using a map between corresponding sulci and gyri; these are curves defined on a parameterized surface. Some investigators have previously used flattened representations of surfaces in order to find a morphing transformation from one surface to another [7]. An issue that arises in the reparameterization of flat maps is singularities at corner points of the parametric grids or boundary constraints. In the approach we describe in this paper, we get around this problem by using an iterative procedure which consists of 3D surface warping steps followed by projections onto the parametric domain. Upon convergence, this procedure results in a reparameterization of a surface under constraints imposed by sulcal or gyral curves. We now describe each step of our algorithm in further detail.

2.2   Surface Construction

We represent each surface by a map from the unit sphere to the surface. In this paper we focus on the outer cortical surface. A spherical map is obtained by shrink wrapping a deformable surface [21], which is initialized at a spherical configuration. After convergence of the deformable surface to a configuration conforming to the outer cortex, we readily obtain a map from the sphere to the surface by simply following the trajectory of each point on the initial sphere.

For the numerical implementation of the algorithm, the sphere is represented as a tessellated icosahedron. We typically start with 2,500 vertices in order to speed up the deformation of the deformable surface, and as the surface conforms to the outer cortical boundary, we increase the number of vertices by subdividing the triangles. The final resolution surface is sampled with with 40,000 vertices, and at convergence, each point on the tessellated sphere is mapped to a point on the outer cortical surface. This map will be denoted by $\mathbf{x}(u,v)$, where (u,v) is a pair of parametric coordinates on the sphere, such as longitude and latitude.

2.3   Curvature Estimation

The geometric structure around each point of the triangular grid of a surface is determined via a least-squares estimation procedure, which finds the bi-quadratic patch that best fits the shape of the surface in the neighborhood of a point [21]. The major difficulty in the least-squares estimation procedure is that the optimal size of the neighborhood used to estimate the parameters of the bi-quadratic patch are not known in advance. In order to optimally capture the local variations of the sulcal shape, while maximally smoothing out the noise, the optimal size of the neighborhood is found adaptively, as described in [21]. Although we do not impose any continuity constraints on the curvature estimates of neighboring vertices, the fact that the surface patches used to estimate the curvature on neighboring vertices overlap, for the most part, results in smoothly varying curvature estimates. Figure 2a,b show three-dimensional renderings of two outer cortical surfaces. Overlaid on the surfaces is shown one of the two principal curvatures as blue.

2.4   Defining Constraints on the Surface

The initial parameterization, $\mathbf{x}(u,v)$, of the surface depends on how the deformable surface shrink-wraps around a particular brain boundary, and therefore it depends on initialization as well as on the shape of the individual brain. Therefore, there is no reason to expect that the parametric coordinates (u, v) on the unit sphere, $\mathcal{S}$, correspond to the same anatomically region in two different brains. Consider two different brain images, $\mathcal{I}_1$ and $\mathcal{I}_2$, and the corresponding outer cortical surfaces, $\mathbf{x}_1(u, v)$ and $\mathbf{x}_2(u, v)$, with

$$\mathbf{x}_1 : \mathcal{S} \longrightarrow \mathcal{I}_1 , \tag{1}$$

and similarly for $\mathbf{x}_2(\cdot)$. A map from $\mathcal{I}_1$ to $\mathcal{I}_2$ can be implicitly defined as a reparameterization, $\mathbf{r}(u, v)$, of $\mathbf{x}_1(u, v)$. In particular if

$$\mathbf{r} : \mathcal{S} \ni (u, v) \longrightarrow \mathbf{r}(u, v) \in \mathcal{S} , \tag{2}$$

then

$$\chi : \mathcal{I}_1 \ni \mathbf{x}_1(\mathbf{r}(u, v)) \longrightarrow \mathbf{x}_2(u, v) \in \mathcal{I}_2 \tag{3}$$

defines a map from one cortical surface to the other. Our goal here is to find the reparameterization, $\mathbf{r}(\cdot)$, which brings the two cortical anatomies into good correspondence. That is, $\mathbf{x}_1(\mathbf{r}(u, v))$ and $\mathbf{x}_2(u, v)$ should be anatomically corresponding regions.

We define this parameterization based on a number of landmark-curves on the sphere. In particular, let $\mathbf{c}_1^j(l)$, and $\mathbf{c}_2^j(l)$, $j = 1, \ldots, K$, $l \in [0, 1]$, be two sets of curves parameterized on the unit interval and positioned on $\mathcal{S}$. These curves are parameterized by piece-wise constant speed parameterizations, i.e. their points are evenly spaced in-between break points along the curves. Typical curves we use are the inter-hemispheric fissure, the central, precentral, postcentral, superior frontal, lateral, superior temporal sulci, or the ridge curves of the adjacent gyri. Examples of break points are the precentral knob, intersection points of sulci (e.g. precentral with superior frontal, central sulcus with inter-hemispheric fissure), or distinct points such as the tips of the temporal or occipital lobes. For the experiments of this section, the K pairs of curves are defined manually on three-dimensional renderings of the surfaces, using an OpenGl-based interface (see Fig. 2). These curves are then mapped onto the sphere via the inverse of the maps $\mathbf{x}_1(\cdot)$ and $\mathbf{x}_2(\cdot)$. In the following section we describe a framework for automatically defining these curves using prior probability spatial distributions in conjunction with geometric properties of the surface, such as its curvature.

2.5   Surface Reparameterization

By construction, the K pairs of curves provide point correspondences on the surface. In particular,

$$\forall l \in [0, 1], \mathbf{c}_1^j(l) \longrightarrow \mathbf{c}_2^j(l) .$$

We use these point correspondences to elastically warp the sphere to itself, and therefore find the reparameterization function, $\mathbf{r}(u, v)$. In principle, this can be formulated as a 2D transformation problem. However, in order to avoid difficulties introduced by discontinuities on singular points (e.g. on the two poles of a polar coordinate system) or along boundaries of flat maps, we have formulated this problem as a 3D problem, i.e. as a problem of warping S onto itself via an iterative procedure. Successive projections back on S warranties that the result is the desired two dimensional transformation, $\mathbf{r}(\cdot)$ from S to S. This iterative algorithm is described in detail below.

Let $\mathbf{p}(u, v)$ be the position of a vertex of S at some time point during the iterative procedure. As we will discuss below, $\mathbf{p}(u, v)$ does not necessarily remain on S during our iterative algorithm, but is continuously projected onto S. Let, also, $\mathbf{s}(u, v)$ be the 3D unit vector of the point on the unit sphere that has parametric coordinates (u, v). Finally, let $\mathbf{f}(\mathbf{p}(u, v))$ be a force field defined for each vertex point (u, v) as follows:

$$
\mathbf{f}(\mathbf{p}(u,v)) = \begin{cases} \mathbf{s}(\mathbf{c}_2^j(l)) - \mathbf{p}(u,v) \text{ , if } (u,v) = \mathbf{c}_1^j(l), \text{ for some } l \in [0,1], \\ \qquad\qquad\qquad j \in \{1, \dots, K\} \text{ ,} \\ 0 \qquad\qquad\qquad\qquad \text{, otherwise .} \end{cases}
$$

That is, $\mathbf{f}(\cdot)$ is nonzero only on the K landmark curves. Let, also, $\mathbf{e}(u, v)$ be the sum of elastic forces applied from the neighbors of $\mathbf{p}(u, v)$. [Since the vertices of the grid on the sphere result from successive tessellations of an icosahedron, all but 12 points of this grid have 6 neighbors; the rest have 5 neighbors]. Then, we find the function $\mathbf{r}(u, v)$ with the following iterative algorithm:

$$
\begin{aligned}
\mathbf{p}^0(u, v) &= \mathbf{s}(u, v) \\
\mathbf{p}^{t+1}(u, v) &= \mathcal{P}\left\{\mathbf{p}^t(u, v) + \delta^t\left[\mathbf{f}(\mathbf{p}^t(u, v)) + L\mathbf{e}(\mathbf{p}^t(u, v))\right]\right\} \qquad (4) \\
\mathbf{r}(u, v) &= \mathbf{s}^{-1}(\mathbf{p}^T(u, v))
\end{aligned}
$$

where T is the maximum number of iterations, and $\mathcal{P}\{\}$ denotes the operator that projects a point radially onto the unit sphere.

According to this iterative algorithm, the vertices of the unit sphere move in the three-dimensional space under the influence of attractive forces between corresponding curves, which are interpolated by elastic forces. As soon as a vertex moves away from the unit sphere, however, it is projected back on the unit sphere, and the algorithm continues until convergence. Convergence is achieved when the K curves in S that correspond to landmark curves in $\mathcal{I}_1$ are very close to (in the absence of elastic forces, they coincide with) their counterparts corresponding to $\mathcal{I}_2$. Convergence is generally achieved after 200 iterations.

2.6   3D Elastic Warping

After the surface correspondences are defined via the map χ (see (3)), $\mathcal{I}_1$ is elastically transformed to $\mathcal{I}_2$. This transformation (STAR) has been described in detail elsewhere [7]. Since most of our research subjects are elderly individuals, we have adopted a framework of prestrained elasticity in order to account for ventricular expansion that is typical in these individuals.

2.7   Experiments

In our first experiment we considered two MR images, and we outlined several
sulci, as shown in Fig. 2. The maximum curvature is shown in gray, in the 3D
renderings of the outer cortical surface. The positions of the outlined curves on
the unit sphere are shown in the Fig. 2c, with white corresponding to Fig. 2b and
black to Fig. 2a. We then elastically reparameterized the surface of Fig. 2b. The
new positions of the white curves, together with the target (black) curves are
shown in Fig. 2d. The grid is overlaid on the two renderings of the unit sphere
in order to appreciate how the curve deformation is interpolated in the rest of
the vertices.

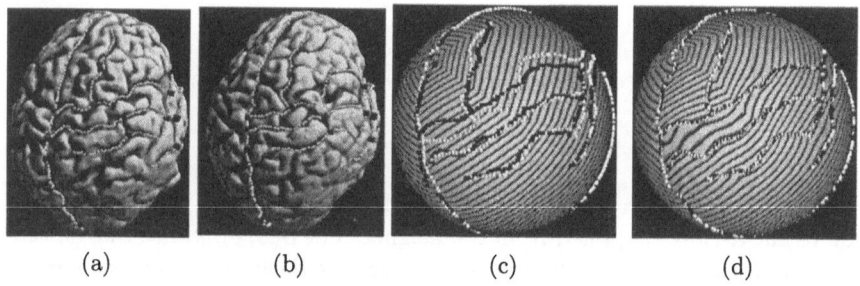

(a)   (b)   (c)   (d)

Fig. 2. (a),(b) 3D renderings of two outer cortical surfaces, with landmark curves
overlaid on them (white). (c) The position of the landmark curves in the parametric
domain (the unit sphere). The curves corresponding to (a) are shown in black and the
curves corresponding to (b) are shown in white. (d) An elastic reparameterization of
the sphere, so that the two sets of curves have similar parametric coordinates

We then applied this method to 3D MR images from 8 individuals. These
images were first segmented into gray matter, white matter, and CSF, using a
Markov Random Field method described in [22]. A deformable surface was then
fitted to the gray matter/CSF boundary of each image. Based on the resulting
surfaces, we then defined the following curves: inter-hemispheric and Sylvian
fissures, central, precentral, postcentral, superior frontal, and superior temporal
sulci, and the medial axis of the inferior aspect of the temporal lobe, for the left
hemisphere only (right in the images, according to the radiology convention). We
used the first of the 8 images as the target image, and we applied our algorithm
to reparameterize the remaining 7 images. Finally, we used the STAR algorithm
to warp the 7 images into conformation to the target.

In order to visualize the degree to which the warped images were in registration, we calculated the average distributions of the gray and white matter,
which are displayed in Fig. 1b. In Fig. 1b, relatively fuzzier regions imply a relatively poorer registration, whereas crisp regions imply a good registration, since
in these regions cortical gyri are aligned and therefore averaged together. Notable is the very good registration in the vicinity of regions in which constraining
sulcal curves were used. Those regions are marked with arrows in the triplanar

display; notable is the almost perfect registration in the precentral knob (upper left), which is thought to be the region controlling hand movement. Note that even though we only used sulcal constraints on one of the two hemispheres, a relatively good registration is also apparent in the contralateral sites. This is primarily due to the symmetry of the brain, and to the elastic forces. For example, if we correctly map the intersection of the left central sulcus with the inter-hemispheric fissure across individuals, then we are very likely to also map the intersection of the right central sulcus with he inter-hemispheric fissure, since these two points are identical under perfect symmetry.

3   Hierarchical Labeling of the Sulci

3.1   Overall Framework

Our experiments in the previous section demonstrated that cortical constraints are important in bringing the highly variable cortical regions into registration. However, the manual definition of the sulcal curves is a laborious procedure (in the experiments of the previous section, defining the set of curves for each brain required approximately 25 minutes of a trained person's time). Therefore, we have investigated an approach for automatically labeling major cortical features.

Our approach is based on a hierarchical labeling of a number of landmark curves in the parametric domain, i.e. in the unit sphere S; the labels propagate to the sulcal curves that are embedded in 3D via the surface parameterization $\mathbf{x}(u, v)$. Labeling of the landmark curves is achieved by elastically matching a "template unit sphere", which contains statistics of each landmark curve that are collected from a training set, to the unit sphere holding the parameterization of a particular brain's surface. The statistics currently provide prior knowledge of the expected location of each landmark curve and its variability. This matching is done hierarchically. In the simplest case, at each stage of this hierarchical procedure, one landmark curve is considered only.

One could, in principle, use the spatial distributions on S to label all cortical features simultaneously. However, the high variability of many cortical features, such as the folds of the prefrontal cortex, might be an impediment. Our reason for using a hierarchical scheme is that the variability of certain cortical features can be reduced if measured relative to other, less variable features. For example, the precentral sulcus is a relatively more variable feature than the central sulcus. However, if we know the location of the central sulcus, we can make a better guess as of where the precentral sulcus might be; this is shown quantitatively using data from a sample of 20 of our subjects in Sect. 3.2. Accordingly, in our hierarchical matching scheme, we use *conditional spatial probability distributions* of sulci on S, which we will refer to as *CSPD's*. For example, assume that, in a particular subject, the central sulcus has been somehow labeled. Then, the outer cortical surface of that subject can be reparameterized as described in the previous section, so that its central sulcus has the same position on the unit sphere as the average central sulcus of the training set. The CSPD of the precentral sulcus, conditioned on the fact that the central sulcus is coincident with its average in the training set, is presumably tighter, i.e. it has lower variance, and it can subsequently used for labeling the precentral sulcus. We now describe the details of this algorithm. We have focused on the central and precentral sulci, in order to better understand how our methods behave.

3.2   The Spatial Probability Distributions

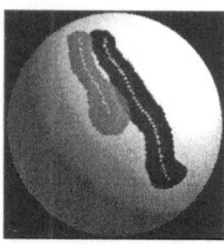

Fig. 3. The CSPD's(90% regions) derived from 20 normal subjects, of the central sulcus (black), and the lateral portion of the precentral sulcus (gray) conditioned on the alignment of the central sulcus with its average

A training set of 20 normal subjects was randomly selected from our database. Parameterizations of the outer cortical surface were then found for these subjects, as described in Sect. 2.2. The central and precentral sulcal curves were then outlined for all subjects. This resulted in 20 pairs of curves, each parameterized in the unit interval by a piece-wise constant speed parameterization, as described in Sect. 2.4. For each $l \in [0, 1]$, the corresponding sulcal curve point was assumed to follow a Gaussian distribution, which was estimated via the mean and the covariance matrix.

The spatial distribution of the precentral sulcus was calculated conditioned on the fact that the location of the central sulcus was known. More specifically, we reparameterized all 20 surfaces so that the central sulci were all aligned to their average position on the unit sphere. The precentral sulci were transformed accordingly. Subsequently, the CSPD of the (transformed) precentral sulci was calculated. Figure 3 shows the 90%-thresholded regions of the central sulcus, and of the precentral sulcus after alignment of the central sulcus.

In order to test the hypothesis behind the hierarchical formulation of the sulcal matching, we calculated the variance along each point of the precentral sulcus with and without aligning the central sulcus first. The resulting variances are shown in Fig. 4a. The reduction in the variance is clear, and it is due to the fact that the locations of the central and precentral sulci are correlated with each other. In Fig. 4b we show the variance along the superior frontal sulcus, before and after alignment of the central sulcus. As expected, the variance doesn't change much, since the positions of these two sulci are not highly correlated.

3.3   Hierarchical Labeling

Consider, for example, the average shape of the curves on $\mathcal{S}$ that correspond to the central sulcus in the training set. We will loosely refer to this curve as the average central sulcus, having in mind that the true shape of the average central sulcus is actually found via the map from its average position on $\mathcal{S}$ to 3D. We achieve the labeling of an individual's central sulcus by mapping $\mathcal{S}$ onto itself, so that the average central sulcus is mapped to the individual's central sulcus,

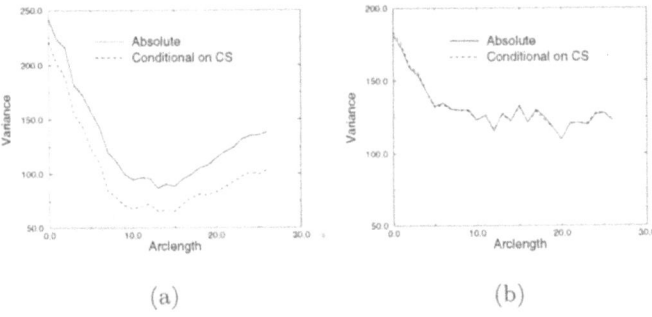

Fig. 4. Plots of the variance along the precentral sulcus (a), and the superior frontal sulcus (b) before (solid line) and after (dotted line) alignment of the central sulcus with a fixed curve (namely, the average of its spatial distribution)

thereby transferring its label. This is accomplished via the procedure described in (4), with the force field $\mathbf{f}(u, v)$ being nonzero only on the central sulcus. More generally, a different curve (or set of curves) is considered at different hierarchical levels of our algorithm. Therefore, in general, the force field $\mathbf{f}(u, v)$ is nonzero on the curve(s) considered at a particular stage of the hierarchical matching procedure.

In (4), the target curves, $\mathbf{c}_2^j(l)$, which determined the force field $\mathbf{f}(u, v)$, were predefined on $\mathcal{S}$ since they were manually drawn in advance. However, here, the target curve is not known in advance, but is calculated at each iteration. In particular, consider the hierarchical level in which the central sulcus is to be labeled in an individual's surface. At each iteration in this stage, a search in the neighborhood of each point on the average central sulcus is performed, looking for points for which the subject's surface has high curvature; for sulcal curves we use the minimum principal curvature, whose absolute value is high on the sulci, while for gyral curves we use the maximum curvature. The center of mass of the high curvature points is then calculated. The collection of the center of mass points forms the target curve, $\mathbf{c}_2(l)$, at each iteration in (4). Clearly, as an average sulcus deforms towards its shape in an individual's brain, the target curve, formed by the collection of the center of mass points, is reevaluated continuously. This mechanism is shown schematically in Fig. 5.

In equilibrium, the average central sulcus is mapped to the central axis of the subject's sulcus, and the rest of the points on the unit sphere are mapped accordingly to some other location on the unit sphere. The inverse of this transformation is a reparameterization of the subject's surface, for which the subject's central sulcus has exactly the coordinates of the average central sulcus of the training set. In the subsequent stage of the hierarchical matching procedure, the precentral sulcus, which has been mapped to a new location during the previous stage, is used as the driving-force curve. The central sulcus is fixed to its average configuration.

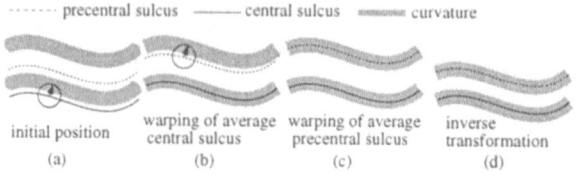

Fig. 5. A schematic representation of the hierarchical labeling of the sulci. (a) The average central and precentral sulci overlaid on the curvature map of an individual surface. (b) Stage during which the average central sulcus is mapped to the individual's central sulcus, via the center of mass forces originating from high curvature regions, as shown schematically by the arrow. (c) Stage during which the precentral sulcus is labeled, after alignment of the central sulcus. (d) The inverse transformation, which effectively reparameterizes the individual's surface so that its central and precentral sulci have the parametric coordinates of the sample average

We have used two different mechanisms for calculating the center of mass forces. First, we have weighted the center of mass force by the probability of the corresponding location, using the corresponding CSPD. Second, we use the CSPD only to define the maximum search window, but we don't weight the forces by the value of the probability. The former mechanism is, in some cases, slightly more robust. However, the latter allows more flexibility in the transformation, and hence we have adopted it in our experiments.

3.4   Experiments

Figure 6a shows the average central sulcus (bottom curve in white) overlaid on a subject's surface; this curve was obtained by following the map $\mathbf{x}(\cdot)$ of that subject, starting from the average parametric coordinates of the central sulcus on $\mathcal{S}$. The lateral part of the precentral sulcus is also shown (top curve in white). Figure 6b shows the same curves after reparameterization of the subject's surface in the first level of the hierarchical procedure, in which the central sulcus was used as the driving curve. The result of the subsequent stage is shown in Fig. 6c, in which the precentral sulcus was used as driving curve. The corresponding transformations of the unit sphere, demonstrating the elastic reparameterization of the subject's surface, are shown in Figs. 6d-f.

One could, in principle, apply this mechanism without computing the inverse transformation, as follows. First, transform the unit sphere so that the average central sulcus is mapped to the central sulcus of the individual's surface, as described above. Then do the same with the precentral sulcus, and so on. The difficulty in this approach would be in estimating how the probability distribution of the precentral sulcus (and all the other sulci) is warped from its initially Gaussian form, as the surface itself is warped. In contrast, when mapping the individual's curvature pattern to match the average sulci through the inverse transformation described above, the CSPD's of all sulci remain Gaussian and easily computable.

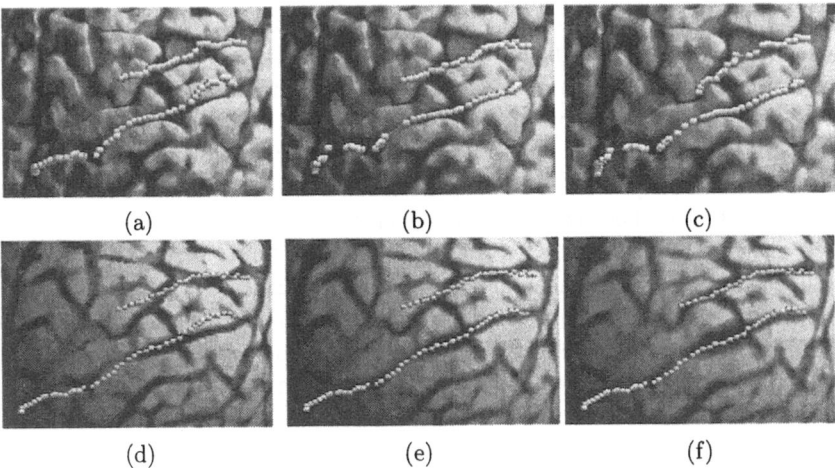

Fig. 6. An example of the automated labeling of the central sulcus and the lateral portion of the precentral sulcus. (a) The curves having the parametric coordinates of the average central sulcus (bottom curve in each figure) and average precentral sulcus (top curve in each figure) on the unit sphere, which is shown in (d). (b) The same curves, after elastic reparameterization of the unit sphere, as shown in (e), using the central sulcus as driving curve. (c) The same curves, after the reparameterization of the unit sphere at the second hierarchical level (f), in which the precentral sulcus was used as driving curve

4   Summary and Discussion

We presented a methodology for deformable brain registration, which aims at improving registration accuracy in the cortical region, by using landmark curves such as the outer edge of a sulcus or a gyrus. In this work we have focused on the outer cortical surface. The landmark curves are used to find a map between two surfaces to be registered.

We presented a framework for obtaining the surface reparameterization, which avoids problems introduced by singularities of the parametric domain, such as poles. In particular, we determine the reparameterization of a surface parameterized on the unit sphere by a sequence of three-dimensional elastic transformations followed by projections onto the unit sphere.

We also presented a framework for automatically determining this surface-to-surface map via a hierarchical procedure using conditional spatial probability distributions. This procedure is based on the premise that the variability of a highly variable curve is a composite of its own intrinsic variability and of the variability of certain less variable curves. For example, the variability of the precentral sulcus is a composite of its own intrinsic variability and of the variability of the adjacent central sulcus. Therefore, if the central sulcus is identified, then it is reasonable for one to look for the precentral sulcus in the vicinity of the central sulcus and at a certain distance from it. We use use conditional spatial distributions of the sulci in order to define the region in which to look for a particular sulcus, given that all the sulci in the previous stages of this hierarchical procedure have been identified.

Our work on the automated identification of cortical curves is still at a preliminary stage. Several issues need to be addressed. First, we need to precisely determine strong correlations between sulci and gyri, which will define which landmark curves depend highly on others, and therefore it will determine the sequence in which these curves must be visited by our hierarchical procedure. Purely based on the development of the brain, one would expect that the most stable features are the inter-hemispheric and Sylvian fissures, which are formed in relatively early embryonic life. The central sulcus is one of the features appearing next. Although the adjacent precentral and postcentral sulci do not necessarily follow, it is reasonable to consider them after the central sulcus in our hierarchical scheme, since their position naturally depends on the position of the central sulcus.

The second issue to be investigated is a model for representing variability on the structure of landmark curves, in addition to our current model of variability in their position. For example, certain sulci are often interrupted. Moreover, parts of certain sulci tend to be interrupted more often than others. This information can be readily incorporated into our CSPD's. For example, labels attached to each point on a sulcal curve, in addition to its average position on the unit sphere and its covariance matrix, can be the probability of being interrupted, its average depth [21,14], curvature and torsion [23]. This information can help resolve ambiguities introduced by the high variability of the cortical morphology.

5   Acknowledgments

This work was supported in part by the NIH grant 1R29AG/NS14971-01, by a Whitaker grant, and by NIH contract NIH-AG-93-07. The MR images we acquired as part of the Baltimore Longitudinal Study of Aging.

References

1. Bookstein, F.L.: Principal warps: Thin-plate splines and the decomposition of deformations. IEEE Trans. on Pattern Analysis and Machine Intelligence **11(6)** (1989) 567–585
2. Miller, M.I., Christensen, G.E., Amit, Y., Grenander, U.: Mathematical textbook of deformable neuroanatomies. Proc. of the National Academy of Sciences **90** (1993) 11944–11948
3. Joshi, S.C., Miller, M.I., Christensen, G.E., Banerjee, A., Coogan, T., Grenander, U.: Hierarchical brain mapping via a generalized Dirichlet solution for mapping brain manifolds. Proc. of the SPIE Conf. on Geom. Methods in Applied Imaging **2573** (1995) 278–289
4. Friston, K.J., Ashburner, J., Frith, C.D., Poline, J.B., Heather, J.D., Frackowiak, R.S.J.: Spatial registration and normalization of images. Human Brain Mapping **2** (1995) 165–189

5. Christensen, G.E., Rabbitt, R.D., Miller, M.I.: Deformable templates using large deformation kinematics. IEEE Trans. on Image Processing **5(9)** (Sept. 1996)
6. Thompson, P., and Toga, A.W.: Thompson, P., Toga, A.W.: A surface-based technique for warping three-dimensional images of the brain. IEEE Trans. on Med. Imaging **15** (1996) 402–417
7. Davatzikos., C.: Spatial transformation and registration of brain images using elastically deformable models. Comp. Vision and Image Understanding **66(2)** (1997) May 207–222
8. Chen, M., Kanade, T., Rowley, H.A., Pomerleau, D.: Quantitative study of brain analtomy. Proc. of Biomed. Image Anal. Workshop (1998) 84–92
9. Rangarajan, A., Duncan, J.S.: Matching point features using mutual information. Proc. of Biomed. Image Anal. Workshop (1998) 172–181
10. McInerney, T., Kikinis, R.: An object-based volumetric deformable atlas for the improved localization of neuroanatomy in MR images. Lecture Notes in Comp. Sci., MICCAI'98 **1496** (1998) 861–869
11. Subsol, G., Roberts, N., Doran, M., Thirion, J.P., Whitehouse, G.H.: Automatic analysis of cerebral atrophy. Magnetic Resonance Imaging **15** (1997) 917–927
12. Davatzikos, C., Resnick, S.M.: Sex differences in anatomic measures of interhemispheric connectivity: correlations with cognition in men but not in women. Cerebral Cortex **8** (Oct./Nov. 1998) 635–640
13. Friston, K.J., Holmes, A.P., Worsley, K.J., Poline, J.P., Frith, C.D., Frackowiak, R.S.J.: Statistical parametric maps in functional imaging: a general linear approach. Human Brain Mapping (1995) 189–210
14. Vaillant M., Davatzikos, C.: Finding parametric representations of the cortical sulci using an active contour model. Medical Image Analysis **1(4)** (1997) 295–315
15. Xu, C., Pham, D.L., Prince, J.L., Etemad, M.E., Yu, D.N.: Reconstruction of the central layer of the human cerebral cortex from MR images. Lecture Notes in Comp. Sci., MICCAI'98 **1496** (1998) 481–488
16. Zeng, X., Staib, L.H., Schultz, R.T., Duncan, J.S.: Segmentation and measurement of the cortex from 3D MR images. Lecture Notes in Comp. Sci. MICCAI'98 **1496** (1998) 519–530
17. MacDonald, D., Avis, D., Evans, A.C.: Proximity constraints in deformable models for cortical surface identification. Lecture Notes in Comp. Sci. MICCAI'98 **1496** (1998) 650–659
18. Le Goualher, G., Collines, D.L., Barillot, C., Evans, A.C.: Automatic identification of cortical sulci using a 3D probabilistic atlas. Lecture Notes in Comp. Sci. MICCAI'98 **1496** (1998) 509–518
19. Resnick SM., Goldszal A., Davatzikos C., Golski S., Kraut M.A., Metter E.J., Bryan R.N., Zonderman A.B., Age differences and one-year age changes in MRI volumes: Findings from the Baltimore Longitudinal Study of Aging. (Submitted January 1999)
20. Talairach, J., Tournoux, P.: Co-planar Stereotaxic Atlas of the Human Brain. Thieme, Stuttgart, (1988)
21. Davatzikos, C., Bryan, R.N.: Using a deformable surface model to obtain a shape representation of the cortex. IEEE Trans. on Med. Imaging **15** (Dec. 1996) 785–795
22. Goldszal, A.F., Davatzikos, C., Pham, D., Yan, M., Bryan, R.N., Resnick, S.M.: An image processing protocol for the analysis of MR images from an elderly population. J. Comp. Assist. Tomogr. **22(5)** (1998) 827–837
23. Bakircioglu, M., Grenander, U., Khaneja, N., Miller, M.I.: Curve matching on brain surfaces using Frenet distances. Human Brain Mapping **6** (1998) 329–333

Using Local Geometry to Build 3D Sulcal Models

A. Caunce[1] and C. J. Taylor[2]

Wolfson Image Analysis Unit, Department of Medical Biophysics, University of Manchester, Manchester M13 9PT, UK
ac@sv1.smb.man.ac.uk, ctaylor@man.ac.uk

Abstract. This paper presents a series of 3D statistical models of the cortical sulci. They are built from points located automatically over the sulcal fissures, and corresponded automatically using variants on the Iterative Closest Point algorithm. The models are progressively improved by adding in more and more structural and configural information, and the final results are consistent with findings from other anatomical studies. The models can be used to locate and label anatomical features automatically in 3D head images for analysis, visualisation, classification, and normalisation.

1 Introduction

The aim of this work is to build statistical models of the cortical sulci from a set of example (training) images. These models can provide an insight into the biological variability present in cortical configurations and can be used in Active Shape Model (ASM) [10] searches to locate and label the sulci in unseen images. Since many of the sulci demarcate functional areas [29], this provides a basis for labelling the cortical surface providing a standard frame within which to analyse functional and structural change in disease. The form of the statistical models and their incorporation into ASM search are described briefly in Sect. 3. The method requires that 'landmark' points are found for each member of a set of training images and that a one-to-one correspondence be established between these sets of landmark points for each pair of training images. Because the structures are so complex, it was desirable to develop automated methods for finding the landmark points and establishing the correspondences. We have developed a simple data-driven method, described in Sect. 4, was developed for generating the landmark points over the mouths of the sulcal fissures. Automatic correspondence is based on the iterative closest point (ICP) algorithm [4,41]. Naive ICP gives poor results, but incorporating structural and configural information (Sect. 6) results in significantly better models that capture forms of variability already known to be present in the configuration of the cortical surface [3]. Quantitative and visualisation results are given in Sect. 8 and examples of sulcal and cortical labelling using ASM search are shown in Sect. 9.

A. Kuba et al. (Eds.): IPMI'99, LNCS 1613, pp. 196–209, 1999.

2   Background

We are interested in methods for locating brain structures automatically. Many attempts to segment the cortex have relied on clustering (which tends to be more effective with multi-sequence data) [5] or image morphology [6,26], but these techniques only provide gross structure for visualisation and not information about the location of particular areas. Generally anatomical labelling has required an expert user to label structures of interest manually [19,34]. Computerised anatomical atlases have been developed [31], but these tend to be derived from as little as one subject brain. Such atlases usually deform to the new example using intensity information [9,38] or a combination of prescribed transformations [2,11], sometimes user driven [12]. These take little or no account of the variation of the object class; the resulting labelling may therefore be unreliable. In order to extract and label structures automatically the information must be incorporated into the model used [1,22], as in [13,21,37] where 3D models of structures in the head were developed from a training set of examples. In these cases the structures chosen were considerably simpler than the cortical surface, which meant that manual delineation and point correspondence was possible. Subsol et al. [35,36] developed more complex 3D models of skull and cortical ridges from sets of examples. The ridges were detected and matched automatically to produce an atlas but the authors chose to use mathematical modal analysis based on physical structure [23] rather than statistical observation. Sandor & Leahy [33] developed a model which could locate and label a small number of sulci, but had no built in knowledge of their structural variations and configurations. Other authors have analyzed the sulcal variability with a view to labelling automatically [17,32,39] or interactively [24] detected structures, but generally this has been restricted to a small number of major fissures or only a small number of manually labelled and corresponded examples are used[20]. The work presented here is fully 3D, uses automatically marked and corresponded data, and considers the whole of the exposed surface, building on earlier less complex experiments which used poorer data [8].

3   Active Shape Models

Active Shape Models (ASM) have as their basis the Point Distribution Model (PDM). PDMs have been used to model many classes of variable objects ranging from faces [16] to electrical components [10]. Full details of the PDM can be found in [10] but the following gives a brief description. Given a set of example pattern vectors $\{x_i \epsilon R^n\}$, where correspondence is established between the values at each index of x_i, then each vector can be rewritten:

$$x_i = \bar{x} + E p_i \qquad (1)$$

where $\bar{x}$ is the mean pattern vector, E is the matrix whose columns are the eigenvectors of the co-variance matrix of the set, and p_i is an n-dim vector of parameters describing the degree to which x_i varies from $\bar{x}$ in a way described by the corresponding eigenvectors. Each eigenvector describes the way in which linearly correlated x_{ij} move together over the set, referred to as a 'mode of variation'. New examples, not included in the training set, can be generated by manipulating the elements of p. To model objects in three-dimensions the $\{x_i\}$ are constructed using the co-ordinates of descriptive features of each example. The features must correspond to the same 'points' on each object. Given co-ordinates (x_{ij}, y_{ij}, z_{ij}) at each feature j of object i, the shape vector is:

$$x_i = (x_{i1}, y_{i1}, z_{i1}, x_{i2}, y_{i2}, z_{i2}, \ldots , x_{in}, y_{in}, z_{in})^T. \tag{2}$$

Appropriate features may be corners, edges, borders, surface patterns, etc. These can often be identified and corresponded by hand, but for extremely complex subjects, like the cortical surface, an automated approach preferable. A PDM can be adapted for search by recording grey-level intensity data in a neighbourhood around each point and progressively adapting the model shape through an unseen image until the neighbourhood matches are optimal (within model constraints). The final positions of the model enable those specific features to be labelled (see Sect. 9).

4   Automatically Placing Landmarks

In order to generate PDMs, landmark points must be placed on significant features over a set of training examples. The sulcal fissures were chosen because they provide anatomical landmarks [28,40] and can be used as a diagnostic aid [34]. Since the cortical surface is extremely convoluted with complex sulcal configurations [25], it was necessary to develop some automated process to do this. Inspired by volume visualisation techniques [18], a projection method was developed which locates points above the mouths of the sulcal fissures on the cortical envelope or hull. The images used were 22 full 3D acquisitions obtained on a 1.5T machine with a 3D Fourier-transform spoiled-gradient-recalled sequence. Each has 124 slices, 1.5mm thick, at 256x256 resolution, optimised for good T1 contrast. Firstly the brain is segmented from the skull semi-automatically using region growing in ANALYZE [30]. Using a closing operation the cortical hull is produced and the grey levels of the brain image are averaged along the surface normals up to a specified depth. The averaged intensity is then projected onto the hull. The intensity values can then be thresholded to leave a representation of the sulcal fissures on the hull which is finally thinned [27] to produce the landmark points. Fig. 1 illustrates the projection approach and Fig. 2 shows the whole process.

Once the points are obtained they can be allocated to curve segments. This is done automatically and curves are delimited by joins (more than 2 neighbours) and endpoints (1 neighbour). Fig. 3 shows a point set labelled in this way. The grey-level intensities were projected onto the hull to a depth of 5 units and the grey-level threshold was set at 0.8 standard deviations below the mean of the distribution.

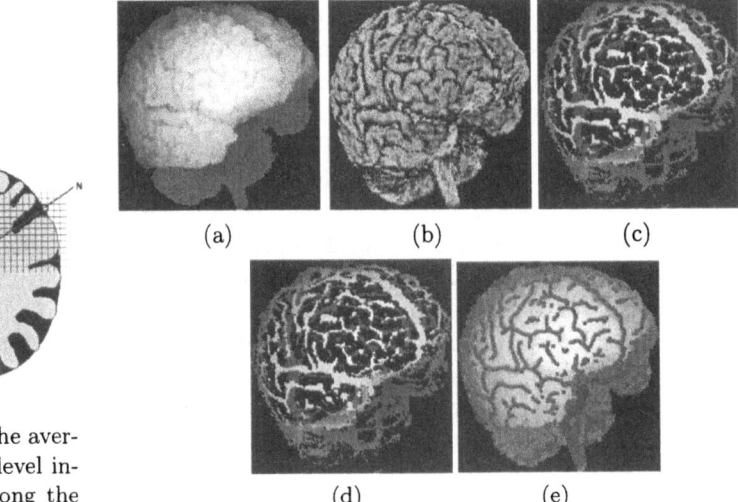

(a)   (b)   (c)

(d)   (e)

Fig. 1. The average grey-level intensity along the surface normal is projected on to the cortical envelope

Fig. 2. The projection process: Segmented brain (a), cortical envelope (b), projection image (c), thresholded projection (d), thinned point set (e)

5   Iterative Closest Point Matching

The problem of establishing matches between the point sets falls into two parts: finding the global alignment of the points and then the specific point correspondences. The ICP algorithm [4,41] tackles both of these problems simultaneously, although the first rather better than the second. The algorithm is run through a series of iterations; at each step the closest points (Euclidean distance) between sets are found and then, based on these matches, one (or both) of the sets is brought more closely into alignment with the other by adjusting global pose parameters. Specifically, for this application, each training example is matched to a master example chosen arbitrarily. This is not an ideal method and future

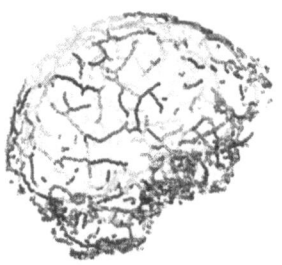

Fig. 3. Point set labelled with short curve segments

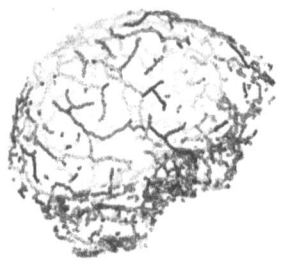

Fig. 4. Point set labelled with long curve segments (Sect. 6.4.1)

work will attempt to use pairwise-tree matching [14] to eliminate the dominance of one set. The point correspondences are established in both directions and any matches outside a particular distance limit (2 standard deviations above the mean) are disallowed. The pose of the matched set only is modified to bring it into alignment with the master [15]. This is continued until either the pose adjustment is sufficiently small or a specific number of iterations have been performed. In order to build the model, all allowed matches (in either direction) to each point on the master are averaged to produce matches for that set. Due to the distance limit imposed, not all points in each set will be included in the model. This basic algorithm produced a model with good shape descriptive properties but with poor configurational representation. I.e. simply matching the closest point has taken no account of the actual variability of structures (and their mutual configuration) between examples, therefore the model can readily represent shape variations but cannot accurately reproduce the variability of cortical patterns (see Sect. 6). To rectify this, certain modifications were made to the basic algorithm by incorporating local shape and pattern information into the matching metric, and by taking into consideration the branching and breaking of structures. This improved the way the algorithm tackled part two of the matching problem: the specific point correspondences.

6   Incorporating Structural and Configural Information

6.1   Local Attributes

There are several local attributes that are suitable for inclusion in some kind of similarity measure in order to find the 'closest' point for the ICP. Over the course of the experiments presented here, items used were as follows.

6.1.1 3D co–ordinates. Compared using Euclidean distance:

$$d_{ij}^e = \sqrt{(x_i - x_j)^2 + (y_i - y_j)^2 + (z_i - z_j)^2} \tag{3}$$

where d_{ij}^e is the distance between two points i on one set and j on the other.

6.1.2 Surface normal. Considering angles between 0 and 180 degrees:

$$d_{ij}^n = \frac{2 + \delta}{\overrightarrow{n}_i \cdot \overrightarrow{n}_j + 1 + \delta} \tag{4}$$

where $\overrightarrow{n}_i$ is the unit surface normal at point i and δ is a small value designed to prevent division by 0, say 1e-5.

6.1.3 Curve segment direction. The principal directions of the curve segments containing the points i and j are compared considering angles between 0 and 90 degrees:

$$d_{ij}^a = \frac{1 + \delta}{\overrightarrow{a}_i \cdot \overrightarrow{a}_j + \delta} \tag{5}$$

where $\overrightarrow{a}_i$ is the unit vector principal direction.

6.1.4 Neighbourhood histogram. This is a 2D low-resolution representation of the local configuration of sulcal fissures about a point, see Fig. 5. The histogram is centred on each point and aligned with the direction of its associated curve. The bins represent the number of points in a particular area of the local neighbourhood as projected from 3D into 2D. Since a curve effectively has 2 directions and a point can belong (join) to several curves, each point can have many histograms associated with it.

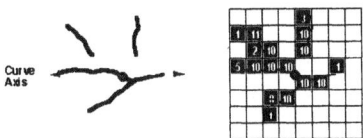

Fig. 5. The neighbourhood histogram about a point. The grid is centred over the point and aligned with the principal direction of its curve segment. The bins represent the number of points in that area of the neighbourhood

They are compared by concatenating the rows into a 1D normalised vector and using a dot product:

$$d_{ij}^{h} = \frac{1 + \delta}{max_{kl}\{\overrightarrow{h}_{i_k} \cdot \overrightarrow{h}_{j_l} + \delta\}} \tag{6}$$

where $\overrightarrow{h}_{i_k}$ is the normalised vector representing the kth histogram of point i. This assumes that corresponding points will have similar sulcal configurations around them.

6.2   Curve Segments

Although the basic ICP algorithm attempts to match corresponding points, there is no provision for ensuring that points from the same structures did correspond. To do this, the curve segment information was introduced, and curve matching was decided on a voting basis; i.e. after point correspondences were established (by whatever means) each curve is considered matched to the curve with the most point matches. After that, corresponding points between curves were established using simple Euclidean distance.

6.3   Size Variation

Not only is the variation in sulcal configuration extreme but each structure can vary in size. In order to ensure that points are correctly matched between such structures, they are aligned at their centres of gravity (COG), and then one is scaled to match the extent of the other. Fig. 6 illustrates the process and it can be seen that this correspondence is superior to taking the closest point on the original structures.

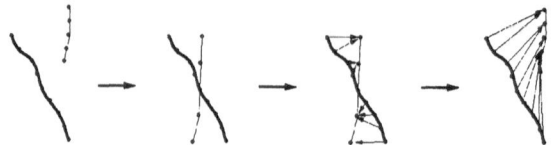

Fig. 6. Matched structures are aligned and scaled before points are corresponded

6.4   Combining Curves

Due to the effects of breaking and branching in particular, a large structure can consist of several small curve segments as described in Sect. 4. The basic ICP algorithm is not affected by this but, once the concept of curve segments is introduced, it becomes an issue. One-to-one matching of curves using a voting scheme will in many cases fail to match some parts correctly, if at all, and two methods were introduced to combat this as follows.

6.4.1 Joining curve segments. By examining the principal directions and proximity of curve segments, suitable candidates could be joined to form longer curves. The three angles between the axes and the line joining the COGs must all be close to 0, and the curves must be sufficiently close to allow joining, see Fig. 7. The same point set of Fig. 3 is shown in Fig. 4 with long curve segments.

6.4.2 Matched linked sets. This method relies on linking curves after matching. For this scheme a chain of matches is established and all the included points on each set are considered as one structure for the purposes of establishing closest points. Figure 8 shows this process which should allow varying numbers of segments on the same structure to match successfully.

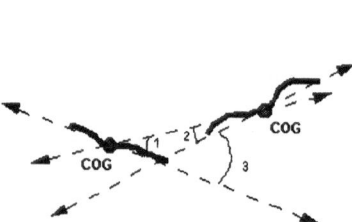

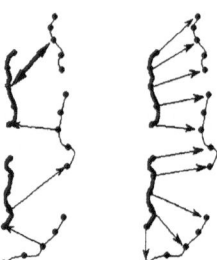

Fig. 7. Testing for a valid join. The angles and distance are considered. (It is unlikely these two curves would be joined)

Fig. 8. Matched linked sets. A chain of curve matches is established (left) and all the points in each set are allowed to match as one structure to give uniform closest points (right)

7   Experiments

Various combinations of the modifications described in the previous section were used to generate models. However, for the purposes of this paper we present the most significant.

Method 1. Basic ICP (Euclidean distance - eqn (3)).

Method 2. Adding normals and axes (6.1.2 & 6.1.3) and then matching curve segments (6.2). The distance between points i and j becomes:

$$d_{ij} = d_{ij}^e * d_{ij}^n * d_{ij}^a. \tag{7}$$

Method 3. As Method 2 but allowing matched linked sets (6.4.2) and scaling and aligning (6.3.1).

Method 4. As Method 3 but using long curve segments (6.4.1) and incorporating neighbourhood histograms of size 40 with a resolution of 8 pixels (6.1.4).

$$d_{ij} = d_{ij}^e * d_{ij}^n * d_{ij}^a * d_{ij}^h. \tag{8}$$

8   Assessing the Models

Since ground truth is not known, a self-contained method had to be developed to assess the models. A PDM represents an object class by combining the mean shape with a linear combination of the principal components of the variation over the set. Each principal component is one way in which all the points move together and is referred to as a 'mode of variation'. Since these models represent the configurations of structures rather than isolated features, it is reasonable to assume that most neighbouring points should be connected. This means that they should move in a similar fashion within each mode. A measure was devised, therefore, which assesses the degree to which neighbours move together. A coherence value is calculated for each mode:

$$c_k = \frac{1}{N} \sum_{i=1}^{N} \frac{1}{n_i} \| \sum_{j=1}^{n_i} \overrightarrow{m}_j \| \tag{9}$$

where N is the total number of points in the model, is the number of points in the neighbourhood of point i, and the unit vectors are the displacement directions of the points. Fig. 9 shows the principle. In theory this can take values between 0 and 1 but in practice will never reach the extremes. Fig. 10 shows the coherence values for the 4 methods described in Sect. 5 when a neighbourhood size of 0.05 was used (the model is scaled to unit size). The Wilcoxon paired signed ranks test statistics give $p<0.005$ for all hypotheses that the coherence values from one method to the next are not improved.

Coherence for NBH = 0.05

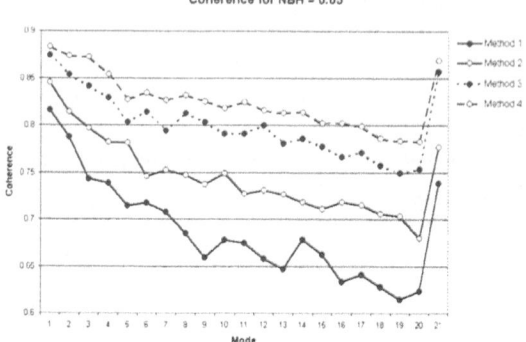

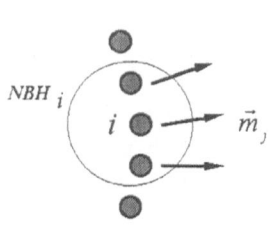

Fig. 9. Calculating Coherence. The direction vectors of neighbours are examined for each point

Fig. 10. Coherence values for Methods 1–4

It is clear from these results that adding in local geometric and topographical information has improved the matching metric and that the countermeasures to branching and breaking have been successful. It is also reasonable to assume that, as point correspondence becomes more precise, the number of points in the model may fall as structures become excluded on some examples. Table 1 shows the number of points for each method and this supports that assumption.

Table 1. The numbers of points in each model

Method	1	2	3	4
No. Points	7234	6719	6715	6613

Visual inspection of the models was particularly important and a method was devised of displaying the shape changes (movement normal to the surface - Fig. 12) present in the model, and the pattern changes (tangential movement -

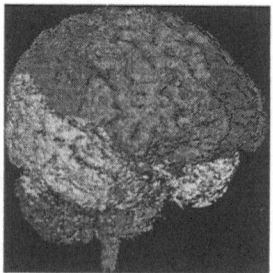
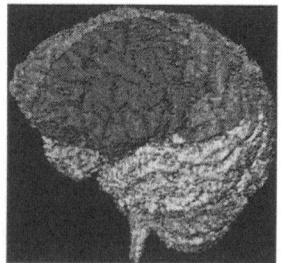

Fig. 11. The labelled cortex of the unseen image of Fig. 14 (right & left views)

Fig. 13). In all cases the mean shape is shown. The size of the point indicates the amount it moves and the colour indicates direction, for positive model parameters, as shown in the key. These directions are reversed for negative parameters. It is important to note that point sizes are relative within mode only. Table 2 gives the percentage of variance explained by each mode of Method 4, these were similar for all the models.

Table 2. The percentage variation represented by each mode from Method 4

Mode	% Variance	Mode	% Variance	Mode	% Variance
1	8.14738	8	5.01766	15	4.02958
2	7.85342	9	4.84648	16	3.94542
3	6.56275	10	4.64844	17	3.84594
4	6.41422	11	4.43208	18	3.54666
5	5.58816	12	4.36429	19	3.49159
6	5.33754	13	4.2875	20	3.18029
7	5.11439	14	4.2394	21	1.1068

From Figs. 12 and 13 it can be seen that, as the matching method is improved, the emphasis moves from shape to pattern change and the model becomes visibly more coherent (neighbouring points show similar size and colour). In fact the asymmetrical pattern changes of modes 1 & 4 for Method 4, localised around the temporal lobe and sylvian fissure, agree with observations in other anatomical studies [3]. Also the shape change of Mode 2 in Method 1, and Mode 3 in Method 4, shows a diagonal squashing which can be interpreted as the relationship of the two hemispheres to each other, or torque, which is an acknowledged source of variation.

9   Active Shape Model Search

Taking the labelling scheme of Fig. 4, the model from Method 4 was used to search an unseen original (unsegmented) image. The grey-level templates at each model point were derived from the unprocessed images of the training set. All the modes of the model were used since the sulcal configurations are extremely complex, and it can be seen from Table 2 that even the minor modes account for a substantial amount of variation. Figure 14 shows the final position superimposed on the cortex. Ultimately anatomical labels will be attached to the model points. Similarly, since the fissures are used to demarcate cortical areas [29,40] the model can be used to locate these also. For example, the model was fitted to one of the original training examples using an ICP-like fitting process. At each iteration, the model points were modified (within the scope of the PDM) towards their closest neighbour on the target set. Using the point locations as a guide, the hull for that example was labelled for lobar regions. Using the model

Mode 1   Mode 2   Mode 3   Mode 4

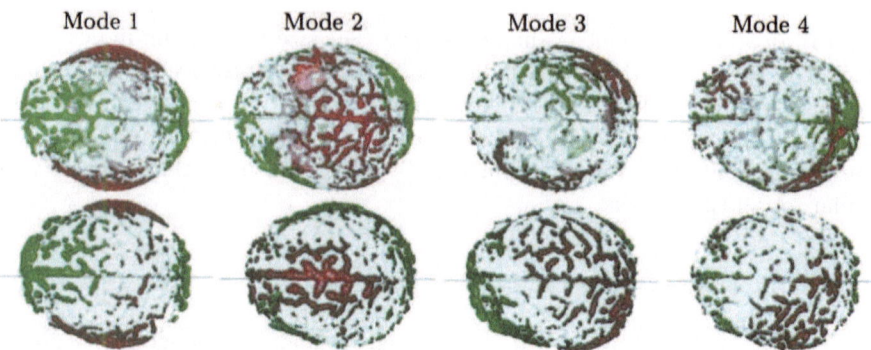

Fig. 12. Modes 1-4 of Methods 1 (top) & 4. Showing shape change, i.e. movement normal to the surface. Top views are shown

Key: Red & Green indicate opposite directions

Mode 1   Mode 2   Mode 3   Mode 4

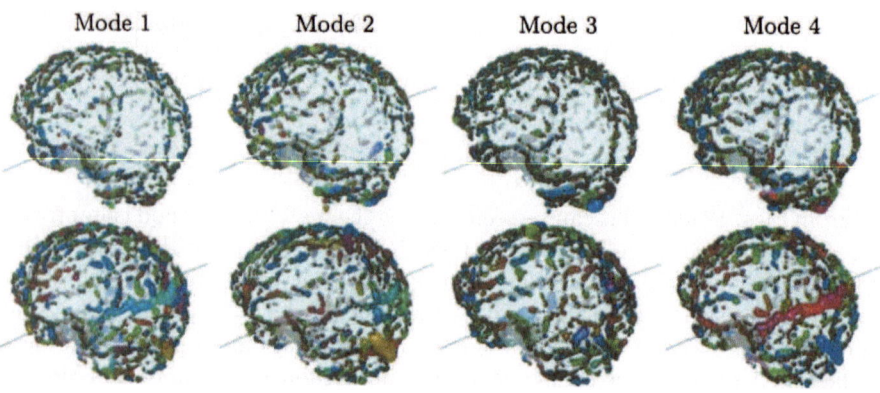

Fig. 13. Modes 1-4 of Methods 1 (top) & 4. Showing pattern change, i.e. movement tangential to the surface. 3/4 views are shown

Key: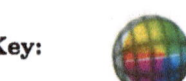

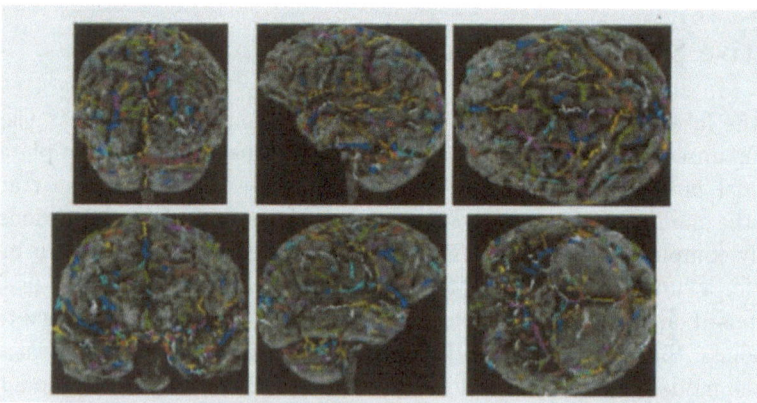

Fig. 14. The final model position after searching an unseen original (unsegmented) image. The labels are those from Fig. 4

points on the unseen example of Fig. 14 to calculate a 3D mapping (3D Thin Plate Spline, TPS [7]), the labelled hull was warped to the new example. From that position, labels were transferred to the pre-segmented cortex on a closest point basis. Fig. 11 shows the results. It can be seen that some labels have 'bled' into adjoining regions. These are due to innaccuracies in the model search. This should be alleviated by adding more examples to the model, improving its ability to represent such complex structures.

10 Summary

We have shown that adding in local structural and configural information to the point matching metric has improved PDMs generated automatically from unlabelled feature data. In addition special measures to account for the variable fragmentation of structures have also made improvements. These models can then be used to search for, and label, specific features in unseen 3D images, and can provide a 3D mapping for an atlas to an unlabelled image. The potential applications include visualisation, measurement, diagnosis and normalisation.

Acknowledgements

We would like to thank to Dr. Tonmoy Sharma of The Institute of Psychiatry, London (UK), for the images used in these experiments.

References

1. Ayache, N., Cinquin, P., Cohen, I., Cohen, L., Leitner, F., and Monga, O.: Segmentation of Complex Three-Dimensional Medical Objects: A Challenge and a Requirement for Computer-Assisted Surgery Planning and Performance. Computer-Integrated Surgery, MIT Press (1996) 59–74
2. Bajcsy, R., Kovacic, S.: Multiresolution Elastic Matching. Computer Vision, Graphics, and Image Processing **46** (1989) 1–21
3. Barta, P.E., Petty, R.G., McGilchrist, I., Lewis, R.W., Jerram, M., Casanova, M.F., Powers, R.E., Brill II, L.B., Pearlson, G.D.: Asymmetry of the planum temprale: methodological considerations and clinical associations. Psychiatry Research: Neuroimaging **61** (1995) 137–150
4. Besl, P.J., McKay, N.D.: A Method for Registration of 3-D Shapes. IEEE Trans. PAMI **14**(2) (1992) 239–256
5. Bezdek, J.C., Hall, L.O., Clarke, L.P.: Review of MR Image Segmentation Techniques Using Pattern Recognition. Medical Physics **20**(4) (1993) 1033–1048
6. Bomans, M., Hohne, K-H., Tiede, U., Riemer, M.: 3-D Segmentation of MR Images of the Head for 3-D Display. IEEE Trans. on Medical Imaging **9**(2) (1990) 177–183
7. Bookstein, F.L.: Principle Warps: Thin-Plate Splines and the Decomposition of Deformations. Trans. Pattern Analysis and Machine Intelligence **11**(6) (1989) 567–585
8. Caunce, A., Taylor, C.J.: 3D Point Distribution Models of the Cortical Sulci. Proc. ICCV (1998) 402–407

9. Collins, D.L., Holmes, C.J., Petetrs, T.M., Evans, A.C.: Automated 3-D Model-Based Neuroanatomical Segmentation. Human Brain Mapping **3** (1995) 190–208

10. Cootes, T.F., Taylor, C.J., Cooper, D.H., Graham, J.: Active Shape Models - Their Training and Application. Computer Vision and Image Understanding **61**(1) (1995) 31–59

11. Gee, J.C., Revich, M., Bajcsy, R.: Elastically Deformaing 3D Atlas to Match Anatomical Barian Images. J. Comp Assist. Tomog. **17**(2) (1993) 2250–236

12. Grietz, T., Bohn, C., Holte, S., Eriksson, L.: A Computerised Brain Atlas: Construction, Anatomical Content, and Some Applications. J. ComAssist. Tomog. **15**(1) (1991) 26–38

13. Hill, A., Thornham, A., Taylor, C.J.: Model-Based Interpretation of 3D Medical Images. Proc. BMVC (1993)

14. Hill, A. and Taylor, C.J., Automatic Landmark Generation for Point Distribution Models. Proc. BMVC **2** (1994) 429–438

15. Horn, B.K.P.: Closed-form solution of absolute orientation using unit quaternions. J. Opt. Soc. Am. A **4**(4) (1987) 629–642

16. Lanitis, A., Taylor, C.J., Cootes, T.F.: An Automatic Face Identification System Using Flexible Appearance Models. Proc. BMVC, York, UK. **1** (1994) 65–74

17. Le Goualher, G.: Automatic Identification of Cortical Sulci Using a 3D Probabilistic Atlas. Proc. MICCAI (1998) 509–518

18. Levoy, M.: Display of Surfaces from Volume Data. IEEE Computer Graphics and Applications **May** (1998) 29–37

19. Loftus, W.C., Tramo, M.J., Gazzaniga, M.S.: Coritcal Surface Modeling Reveals Gross Morphometric Correlates of Individual Differences. Human Brain Mapping **3** (1995) 257–270

20. Lohmann, G., von Cramon, Y.: Automatic detection and Labelling of the Human Cortical Folds in Magnetic Resonance Data Sets. Proc. ECCV (1998) 369–381

21. Martin, J., Pentland, A., Kikinis, R.: Shape Analysis of Brain Structures Using Physical and Experimental Modes. CVPR, Seattle, Washington **June** (1994) 752–755

22. McInery, T., Terzopoulos, D. Deformable models in medical image analysis: a survey. Medical Image Analysis **1**(2) (1996) 91–108

23. Nastar, C., Ayache, N.: Frequency-Based Nonrigid Motion Analysis: Application to Four Dimensional Medical Images. IEEE Trans. Pattern Analysis and Machine Intelligence **18**(11) (1996) 1067–1079

24. Nieman, K., Keyserlingk, D.G.v., Wasel, J.: Superimposition of an Averaged Three-Dimensional Pattern of Brain Structures on CT Scans. Acta. Neurochirurgica **93** (1998) 61–67

25. Ono, M., Kubik, S., Abernathy, C.D.: Atlas of the Cerebral Sulci. New York: Georg Thieme Verlag (1990)

26. Orphanoudakis, S., Tzirita, G., Haris, K.: A Hybrid Algorithm for the Segmentation of 2D/3D Images. Information Processing in Medical Imaging, ed. Y.B.e. al., Netherlands: Kluwer Academic Publishers (1995) 385–386

27. Palagyi, K., Kuba, A.: A Thinning Algorithm to Extract Medial Lines from 3D Medical Images. Proc. IPMI (1997) 411–416.

28. Rademacher, J., Galaburda, A.M., Kennedy, D.N., Filipek, P.A., Caviness, Jr., V.S.: Human Cerebral Cortex: Localization, Parcellation, and Morphometry with Magnetic Resonance Imaging. J. of Cognitive Neuroscience, **4**(4) 354–374

29. Rademacher, J., Caviness, V.S., Steinmetz, H., Gallaburda, A.M.: Topographical Variation of the Human Primary Cortices: Implications for Neuroimaging, Brain Mapping, and Neurobiology. Cerebral Cortex **3** (1993) 313–329

30. Robb, R.A., Barillot, C.: Interactive Display and Analysis of 3D Medical Images. IEEE Trans. Medical Imaging **8**(3) (1989) 217–226

31. Roland, P.E., Zilles, K.: Brain Atlases - A New Research Tool. Trends in Neurosciences **17**(11) (1994) 458–467

32. Royakkers, N., Fawal, H., Desvignes, M., Revenu, M., Travere, J-M.: Morphometry and Identification of Brain Sulci on Three–Dimensional MR Images. Information Processing in Medical Imaging, ed. Y.e.a. Bizais. Netherlands: Kluwer Academic Publishers (1995)

33. Sandor, S. Leahy, R.M.: Towards Automated Labelling of the Cerebral Cortex Using a Deformable Atlas. Information Processing in Medical Imaging, ed. Y.e.a. Bizais. Netherlands: Kluwer Academic Publishers (1995) 127–138

34. Sasodya, S., Stevens, J.M., Fish, D.R., Free, S.L., Shorvon, S.D.: The Demonstration of Gyral Abnormalities in Patients with Cryptogenic Partial Epilepsy Using Three-Dimensional MRI. Arch. Neurology **53** (1996) 28–34

35. Subsol, G., Thirion, J-P., Ayache, N.: A General Scheme for Automatically Building 3D Morphometric Anatomical Atlases: Application to a Skull Atlas. INRIA: Tech. Rep. 2586 (1995)

36. Subsol, G., Thirion, J-P., Ayache, N.: Application of an Automatically Built 3D Morphometric Brain Atlas: Study of Cerebral Ventricle Shape. Visualisation in Biomedical Computing, eds: Hohne, K.H., and Kikinis, R., LEC **1131** (1996) 373–382

37. Szekely, G., Kelemen, A., Brechbuhler, C., Gerig, G.: Segmentation of 2-D and 3-D objects from MRI volume data using constrained elastic deformations of flexible Fourier contour and surface models. Medical Image Analysis **1**(1) (1996) 19–34

38. Thirion, J-P.: Fast Non-Rigid Matching of 3D Medical Images. INRIA technical Report 2547, May (1995)

39. Thompson, P.M., Schwartz, C., Lin, R.T., Khan, A.A., Toga, A.W.: Three-dimensional Statistical Analysis of Sulcal Variability in the Human Brain. The Journal of Neuroscience **16**(13) (1997) 4261–4274

40. Tramo, M.J. Loftus, W.C., Thomas, C.E., Green, R.L., Mott, L.A., Gazzaniga, M.S.: Surface Area of Human Cerebral Cortex and Its Gross Morphological Subdivisions: In Vivo measurements in Monozygotic Twins Suggest Differential Hemisphere effects on Genetic Factors. Journal of Cognitive Neuroscience **7**(2) (1995) 292–301

41. Zhang, Z.: On Local Matching of Free-Form Curves. Proc. BMVC (1992) 347–356

ANIMAL+INSECT: Improved Cortical Structure Segmentation

D. Louis Collins[1], Alex P. Zijdenbos[1], Wim F. C. Baaré[2], and Alan C. Evans[1]

[1] McConnell Brain Imaging Centre, Montréal Neurological Institute,
McGill University, 3801 University St., Montréal, Canada H3A 2B4
{louis, alex, alan}@bic.mni.mcgill.ca
[2] Dept. Psychiatry, University Hospital Utrecht, Utrecht,the Netherlands
wim@ni.azu.nl

Abstract. An algorithm for improved automatic segmentation of gross anatomical structures of the human brain is presented that merges the output of a tissue classification process with gross anatomical region masks, automatically defined by non-linear registration of a given data set with a probabilistic anatomical atlas. Experiments with 20 real MRI volumes demonstrate that the method is reliable, robust and accurate. Manually and automatically defined labels of specific gyri of the frontal lobe are similar, with a Kappa index of 0.657.

1 Introduction

Quantitative analysis of neuro-anatomical or neuro-functional data often requires explicit regional identification of gross anatomical structures. Unfortunately, manual segmentation is time-consuming, subjective and error prone. Furthermore, inter- and intra-observer variability may reduce detectability of subtle differences when making comparisons. Automatic structure identification from medical images is a difficult task, due to the anatomical variability between subjects, differences in subject positioning (between patients and with respect to standard anatomical texts), the distinct physical properties measured by the imaging modalities, and variability of acquisition parameters such as slice thickness and pixel size.

It is important to note that we differentiate between *classification* and *segmentation*. We define segmentation to be the top-down regional parceling of an image into anatomically meaningful continuous groups of voxels; classification is defined to be the bottom-up (or data driven) labelling of individual voxels with a tissue class label without demanding spatial contiguity for a class of voxels. The image data represent only one measure (or a few measures in the case of multi-spectral data) concerning the underlying anatomy, and by itself is sufficient only for classification. Anatomically distinct regions of the brain are differentiated on the basis of histology, cyto-architecture, connectivity, cyto-chemistry or function. As such, data from external sources are required to constrain and guide the segmentation process.

A. Kuba et al. (Eds.): IPMI'99, LNCS 1613, pp. 210–223, 1999.

These external data can be represented in at least two basic forms, and this distinction is used here as a basis to identify two main classes of methods that have been proposed to solve the segmentation problem for different applications. In the first, a symbolic mapping is created between features extracted from the image volume (usually small homogeneous regions) and a symbolic model of the anatomical structures to be segmented.

Expert rule-based systems are often used to achieve this mapping where anatomical knowledge is stored explicitly along with segmentation heuristics in semantic form such as an 'if-then' rule. Example of these procedures can be found in the work of Raya *et. al.* [1], Chen *et. al.* [2], Dellepiane *et. al.* [3], Arata and Dhawan [4,5] and Davis *et. al.* [6]. Other algorithms do not explicitly employ if-then rules to drive the segmentation. Instead, anatomical constraints are implicitly incorporated into the procedure. Kaneda *et. al.* [7] use model-guided contour extraction and 3-D reconstruction to identify dilated ventricles in CT images. Anatomical constraints have also been used by Brummer [8,9] to extract brain contours from MRI. Pathology (i.e. MS lesions) can be identified using similar techniques [10].

Registration-based segmentation procedures differ from those previously described since they estimate a spatial transformation function that best maps features of one data set onto another pre-labelled volume that serves as an iconic model. These procedures are all based on the assumption that there exists a one-to-one mapping between the brain to be segmented and the one used as a model. In one of the first 2D examples, Broit *et. al.* [11] used elastically-constrained non-linear registration between a computed tomography (CT) image and a corresponding atlas slice. This work has been continued by Bajcsy *et. al.* , extended to 3D and reposed in a probabilistic formulation [12,13,14]. Miller *et. al.* also use a probabilistic formulation with physically based models [15,16,17] in order to segment individual brains by registering them to a target. We too have developed a registration-based segmentation procedure named ANIMAL (Automatic Nonlinear Image Matching and Anatomical Labeling) to automatically identify structures in the brain (described in more detail in Sect. 2.4). It has been shown to successfully segment basal ganglia structures [18] but it has not been able to segment cortical structures satisfactorily (voxel-based overlap indices with manual segmentations have been typically around 40-50%). There are two reasons for this: i) there exists important variability in the topology of sulcal and gyral patterns cortex. For example, how should one account for the existence of a double Heschl's Gyrus in a subject when the pre-labeled target has only one? This is an example of where the one-to-one relationship that ANIMAL depends on does not hold at the cortex[1]. ii) the deformation field estimated by ANIMAL does not have the power to unfold the cortex of one brain and then refold it back onto a target brain. The deformation field is bandlimited and therefore does not have high enough frequencies to introduce (or remove) cortical folds

---

[1] Note that this problem affects not only ANIMAL, but all registration-based segmentation procedures. Even though fluid-based methods may recover a continuous mapping, point correspondence between model and model is ill-defined.

where needed. Still, the ANIMAL procedure is able to correctly identify structure location, position and smooth structure boundaries.

The procedure presented here addresses these problems. By merging the complementary information from ANIMAL's non-linear deformation (i.e. low resolution region identification) with the output of a classification technique (i.e. voxel class labels), it is possible to accurately identify specific cortical structures from a subject's MRI. The work presented here is most similar to that of Zachmann et. al. [19], where an iconic model (represented by a voxelated volume, where the value in each voxel represents the probability of existence of a structure) is used for identification of the different fluid spaces of the brain. The work here is different in that it is fully 3D, uses non-linear registration (instead of linear), and is applied to the entire cerebral volume including not only the cerebrospinal fluid (CSF) filled spaces, but deep brain structures and cortical gyri and sulci as well.

2   Methods

2.1   Stereotaxy

The methodology presented here is highly dependent on the notion of stereotaxic space, i.e. a standardized brain-based coordinate system that yields a method of identification of structure location and position so that regions of interest can be compared between brains using standard coordinates. Like many groups in brain mapping research, we have selected to use a coordinate system similar to that defined by Talairach [20] with the origin placed at the anterior commissure, the x-axis running from left to right, the y-axis running from posterior to anterior and the z-axis running from inferior to superior.

When image volumes are transformed into this space and resampled on the same voxel grid such that all brains have the same orientation and size, voxel-by-voxel comparisons across data volumes from different populations are possible, since each voxel (i, j, k) corresponds to the same (x, y, z) point in the brain-based coordinate system. The transformation to this coordinate system also provides a means for enhancement of functional signals by averaging images in this space [21]. This paradigm allows information (anatomical, metabolic, electrophysiological, chemical, architectonic) from different brains to be spatially organized and catalogued by mapping all brains into the same coordinate system [22]. Finally, in the original Talairach spirit, the coordinate corresponding to a particular structure, as defined by an atlas in this coordinate system, can be used to predict its location in a subject's brain volume when mapped into the same space. However, normal anatomical morphometric variability limits this predictive value since there remains variability in structure position even after linear transformation.

We represent this variability by a statistical probability anatomy maps (SPAM) [23]. By definition, the SPAM for any given structure is a volumetric data set sampled in stereotaxic space, where the value at each voxel position represents the probability of existence of that structure at that location within the brain-based coordinate system. At each voxel, the probability is proportional to the number of volumes containing the structure label, divided by the total number of volumes. For example, SPAMs can be created with voxel-by-voxel averaging of label volumes from tissue classified data from many subjects to yield spatial priors that can be used in classification procedures. Here the SPAMs are created from the segmented structure labels from many subjects (see Sect. 2.5) and used as prior anatomical model information to drive the segmentation.

2.2   MRI Preprocessing

A number of processing steps are required to achieve segmentation. We have combined preprocessing steps (image intensity non-uniformity correction [24]), linear registration (ANIMAL in linear mode [25]) and resampling into stereotaxic space, cortical surface extraction (Multiple surface deformation or MSD [26,27]), tissue classification (INSECT [28]), and non-linear registration (ANIMAL in non-linear mode [18]) into a processing pipeline. These are represented schematically in Fig. 1. Since the ANIMAL and INSECT procedure are merged to improve segmentation, the new procedure is termed ANIMAL+INSECT. After running this pipeline, a subject's MRI volume can be visualized in stereotaxic space with its corresponding tissue labels, anatomical structure labels and cortical surface — all in 3D. The following sections describe the classification (INSECT) and nonlinear registration (ANIMAL) procedures in more detail.

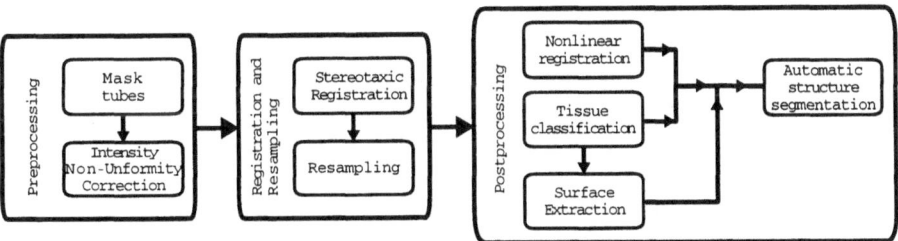

Fig. 1. Processing pipeline. All MRI data are processed through the pipeline shown above. After preprocessing to correct for intensity non-uniformity, the data are linearly registered into stereotaxic space and resampled onto a 1mm isotropic grid. The resulting volume is automatically classified into GM, WM, and CSF components and the cortical surface is automatically extracted. The non-linear transformation to stereotaxic space is used to warp the standard probabilistic atlas onto the classified data, defining structures by masking tissue classes. The cortical surface is used to mask non-brain from cerebral structures

2.3   INSECT

After image intensity non-uniformity correction, stereotaxic registration and resampling, the classification strategy used by INSECT relies on a standard feedforward error-backpropagation artificial neural network (ANN). Since after re-sampling an (x,y,z) location in the image lattice corresponds to the same physical (brain) location in all MRI modalities, the intensity values of all MRI modalities at that location are used as the ANN inputs. As such, the number of ANN input nodes is equal to the number of MRI modalities, whereas the number of out-put nodes is equal to the number of tissue classes (typically white matter, gray matter, CSF, and background). The ANN is fully connected between layers, and contains one hidden layer with 10 nodes. Training of the network is accomplished using a collection of fixed stereotaxic coordinates, derived from the SPAMs (or probability maps, see Sect. 2.1) of WM, GM, and CSF. Based on these SPAMs, any spatial location included in the training set belongs to one of the three tissue classes with a minimum likelihood of 90%. The MRI intensity values of the sub-ject's MRI acquisition at these locations are used as training input to the ANN, with the corresponding tissue class label as the target output. After training, the ANN is used to classify each voxel of the subject data set into WM, GM, or CSF.

2.4   ANIMAL

Identification of individual brain regions, such as the caudate nucleus, planum temporale or superior frontal gyrus, faces two major problems. First, while anatomists may generally agree where a structure is located, there is often no consensus on exactly which part of the structure should be included or excluded. Secondly, the manual labelling process is both time-consuming and the position identified of chosen boundary is subjective, and dependent on the level and con-trast of the image displayed. To address these difficulties we have developed ANIMAL, an algorithm to perform this labelling automatically in 3D [18].

The ANIMAL algorithm deforms one MRI volume to match another, previ-ously labelled, target MRI volume. It builds up a 3D non-linear deformation field in a piecewise linear fashion, recursively fitting local spherical neighbourhoods. Each local neighbourhood from one volume is translated to achieve an optimal match within the other volume. The local neighbourhoods are arranged on a 3-D grid to fill the volume and each grid node moves within a range defined by the grid spacing. The algorithm is applied iteratively in a multi-scale hierarchy. At each step image volumes are convolved with a 3D Gaussian blurring kernel where blurring and neighbourhood size (sphere diameter) are reduced after each stage. Local neighbourhood fit is measured by correlation of the blurred image intensities. Initial fits are obtained rapidly since at lower scales, only gross dis-tortions are considered, but later iterations at finer scales accommodate local differences at the price of increasing computational cost. Anatomical segmenta-tion is achieved by transforming labels from the second (target) volume onto the first volume, via the inverse of spatial mapping of the 3D deformation field (see Fig. 4-c for an example of an ANIMAL segmentation).

This method has the important advantage that it is atlas independent, since the labels do not take part in the fitting process. In fact, multiple atlases defined for different applications or by different anatomists can co-exist on the target volume, and each one can be mapped through the non-linear transformation without recomputation of the latter.

2.5   ANIMAL+INSECT

In the standard application of ANIMAL, the target is an MRI volume from a single subject where all of the voxels within the volume have been anatomically labelled by a neuroanatomist to form an atlas [29]. In the ANIMAL+INSECT paradigm described here, the target is an voxel-by-voxel intensity average of 305 MRI volumes, where each volume was automatically registered and resampled in stereotaxic space [30]. The atlas used for segmentation was created by averaging anatomical labels from 152 subjects young normal subjects, collected as part of the ICBM project [31].

Probabilistic Atlas There are a number of problems associated with an anatomical atlas that is based on a single subject. For example, even though the subject may be normal, certain brain regions may represent an extreme of the normal distribution. Also, the use of a single brain atlas does not contain any notions of anatomical variability, so it is impossible to evaluate the normality of shape, size or position of specific structures from other subjects by comparing them with the atlas. Finally, only one cortical topology (sulcal/gyral pattern) is represented even though large variability is known to exist [32]. Since all registration-based segmentations strategies (ANIMAL included) are based on the assumption that there exists a 1-to-1 homology for all structures between source and target brains, these strategies are undefined and may fail when this correspondence does not exist, especially at the cortex.

Many of the problems listed above are addressed by using a probabilistic atlas, or SPAM, created from the labellings of a large ensemble of normal subjects [23]. The SPAM atlas used here models the anatomical variability of shape, size and topology of 91 gross anatomical structures, where each structure is represented by a SPAM volume in stereotaxic space (see Sect. 2.1). The ANIMAL+INSECT segmentation paradigm requires that the atlas labels be transformed from the target space and resampled onto the subject's MRI volume. Resampling a large number of SPAM volumes is inefficient, since only the label of the most likely structure at each voxel position need be transferred to the subject's volume for masking. Therefore, a max-probability atlas (MPA) was created in the target space, where only the label of the most probable structure is stored at each voxel. This volume is created once by traversing the stereotaxic volume, voxel-by-voxel, and storing only the label of the SPAM with the highest probability at that voxel.

In practice, labelled data from large number of subjects is needed to create the atlas. Ideally, manual segmentations of all atlas structures on all subjects should be used. Unfortunately manual identification is very time consuming (e.g., 1 man-month required to segment the thalamus on 200 subjects [33]), making the ideal situation unrealistic. Here, as proof of principal, the standard ANIMAL

[18] procedure was used with a gross anatomical atlas containing 91 structures [29] to segment 150 data sets of young normal adults [34]. Validations of the ANIMAL procedure have demonstrated that on average, automatic segmentations are comparable to manual labellings for basal ganglia [18] and cortical gyri[2] [35], making this solution only slightly less than ideal. These 150 segmentations were used to create 91 SPAM volumes that were in turn used to produce the MPA shown in Fig 2. In addition, three other MPA models were created from 1) the set of 71 grey matter SPAMs to create a gMPA, 2) the set of 16 white matter SPAMs to create a wMPA and 3) the set of 4 CSF SPAMs to create a vMPA (v for ventricular).

Merge Method Application of ANIMAL, using the MNI305 intensity average target and the corresponding MPA results in a *customized maximum probabilistic atlas* (c-MPA) for the given subject (see Fig. 3). This paradigm is similar to the typical use of the Talairach atlas in brain mapping for structure interpretation and localization. The major advantage is that the customized atlas indicates the most likely structure label for each voxel for a particular subject given anatomical variability of a normal population, instead of only a structure label of the single target brain. The ANIMAL+INSECT methodology makes a further improvement by incorporating tissue class information derived from the subject in question in the following manner.

After the three c-MPA models corresponding to GM, WM and CSF are warped and resampled, they are used as masks to assign labels to regions of the corresponding tissue types classified by INSECT. The c-gMPA is applied to the GM tissue class to identify the gyri of the different cerebral lobes, basal ganglia structures and the thalamus. The c-wMPA is applied to the WM tissue class to label the corpus collosum, the anterior and posterior limbs of the internal capsule and the WM voxels belonging to the lobes. In the same fashion, the c-vMPA is applied to the CSF tissue class to segment the lateral, third and forth ventricles. Note that while the c-MPAs actually overlap and thus may yield several different labels for a given voxel, only the c-MPA label corresponding to the voxel's tissue is applied. In the same manner, partial volume effects may be accounted for if the classification procedure outputs continuous (instead of discrete) data. For example, sulcal CSF can be labelled as such with the c-vMPA, even though the classifier outputs CSF voxels with a magnitude less than 1.0.

Some cortical SPAMs extend past the inner table of the skull and may extend into the scalp with a very low (but non-null) probability, since there are no other cerebral structure SPAMs that will compete for the maximum probability label. When the original MPA is created, these extra voxel labels remain and will erroneously apply a cortical label to voxels located in the skull or scalp that were classified as GM or WM. In order to remove these incorrect labels, the

---

[2] It is interesting to note that while individual cortical structure labellings may be in error, SPAMs generated by averaging either manual or automatic labellings are very similar.

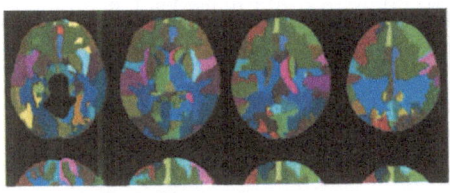
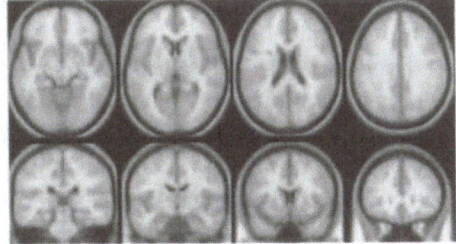

Fig. 2. Max-probability atlas. These images show slices through the maximum probability atlas (left) and the corresponding slices through the ICBM150 T1-weighted average brain (right)

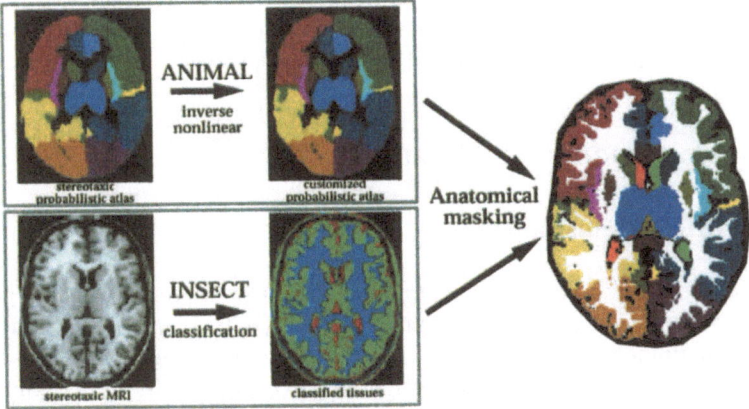

Fig. 3. Schematic of ANIMAL+INSECT merge. The non-linear transformation required to customized the stereotaxic MPA for the subject is estimated by ANIMAL. The subject's MRI is classified in to WM, GM and CSF classes by INSECT. The classified data are masked by the regions in the c-MPA to segment regions on the subjects MRI volume

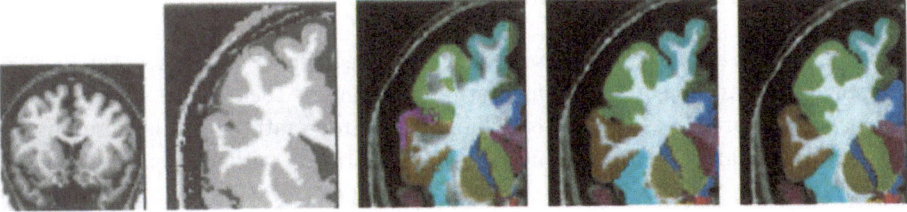

Fig. 4. ANIMAL-only vs ANIMAL+INSECT. (Left to right) Coronal slice through original MRI volume; typical zoomed result (upper left quadrant) result of INSECT classification; of ANIMAL-only segmentation; of ANIMAL+INSECT segmentation; or manual segmentation. Note how the ANIMAL+INSECT result improves segmentation at the cortex and the ventricles and agrees with the expert labelling.

cortical surface extracted by MSD is used to create a brain mask that is applied against the label volume.

Some structures cannot be segmented using only the method described above. For example, in the T1-weighted volumes from the ICBM data base, the medial half of the thalamus is usually classified as GM, while the lateral half is classified as WM and cannot be distinguished from the adjacent white matter of the posterior limb of the internal capsule. In this case, it is impossible to apply a regional mask to a single tissue class to extract and label the structure. Therefore, some structure-specific segmentation rules are required. For the thalamus, the medial border is easily defined by masking the GM tissue class with the c-gMPA. The definition of the lateral border is completely model-based using the standard ANIMAL(-only) segmentation technique and is equal to the lateral border of the thalamus in the cMPA. Similar rules are used for the head of the caudate nucleus, putamen and globus pallidus. Once these structures are segmented, their labels are overlaid on top of the previous segmentation result, overwriting any labels already specified by the initial cMPA masking process.

3   Experiments and Results

3.1   MRI Acquisition

The data used for the experiments described below were acquired as part of the International Consortium for Brain Mapping (ICBM) project, a Human Brain Mapping funded research project with the goal of building a probabilistic atlas of human neuro-anatomy [31]. T1-weighted MRI volumes from 152 young normal volunteers (86 male, 66 female, age 24.6 ± 4.8) were acquired using a 3-D spoiled gradient-echo acquisition with sagittal volume excitation (TR=18, TE=10, flip angle=30°, 140-180 sagittal slices). As described below in Sect. 3, frontal lobe gyri were manually identified on twenty of these volumes.

3.2   Comparison of Segmentations

Figure 4 shows a comparison of an ANIMAL-only segmentation, an ANIMAL+INSECT segmentation and a manual segmentation. Not only is the ANIMAL+INSECT segmentation improved at the cortex, where some grey-matter regions were missed with the standard ANIMAL technique, the segmentation of the lateral ventricles is much better as well. Where the ANIMAL technique overestimated the size of the ventricle, the ANIMAL+INSECT is in complete agreement with the MRI anatomy and with the expert's labelling. Note that there remain some discrepancies between the ANIMAL+INSECT and the manual segmentations - especially at the boundaries between gyri.

In order to determine how well the segmentation procedure works in general, we used manually segmented labels of gyri of the frontal lobes and compared these to automatic labellings.

3.3   Manual Labelling

In each hemisphere, the gray matter of five pre-frontal regions (superior, medial and inferior frontal gyrus, the anterior cingulate gyrus and the orbito-frontal gyri) were labelled by hand. The voxels for each structure were manually identified by voxel painting using *Display*, a computer program developed in our lab [36] that shows four 2D orthogonal slices (transverse, coronal, sagittal and user-defined oblique) through the volume with arbitrary pan, zoom and intensity mapping on each slice. Display also includes a 3D graphics window that is capable of displaying 3D geometric objects such as the cortical surface. The cursor can be placed in any of the 2D or 3D windows, and its position is simultaneously updated in the other views. Voxel labels are painted on any of three orthogonal views with simultaneous update in the other two. Cortical landmarks such as the precentral, superior and inferior frontal, cingulate, fronto-orbital, fronto-marginal and superior rostral sulci are identified in the 3D window and are used to guide the manual segmentation. Manual segmentation of the ten gyri listed above required approximately 10-15 hours per subject.

3.4   Automatic Labelling

Qualitatively, the images in Fig 5 demonstrate that the automatic labellings of the left superior frontal gyrus are very similar to the manual segmentations. In fact, the grey-white border and grey-CSF borders are very similar. In some cases however, the ANIMAL+INSECT method includes the opposite sulcal bank in the gyral labels.

In order to compare the two methods quantitatively, we have used a similarity measure first proposed by Dice [37]. As shown by Zijdenbos [38], this measure is a variant of the standard chance-corrected Kappa (κ) coefficient first developed by Cohen [39]. This measure is the same as κ when the background is infinitely large.

When averaged over the 20 segmentations, the mean and standard deviation of the κ variant is 0.657 ± 0.037. In order to interpret this value and put it into context, the right-most image on the third row of Fig 5 has a value of 0.728 (best κ value in this experiment), while the third image in the top row has a value of 0.573 (worst κ value). Finally, the labelling of the superior frontal gyrus from a single subject was deliberately dilated by one voxel, and the κ variant was evaluated between on the original and dilated labelling, yielding 0.725. Dilating by 2 voxels yields 0.593.

4   Discussion

We have presented an improved method for automatic segmentation of brain structures by merging the complementary information from ANIMAL's non-linear deformation regional identification with the output of INSECT's classification technique. The procedure presented here is completely automatic and therefore

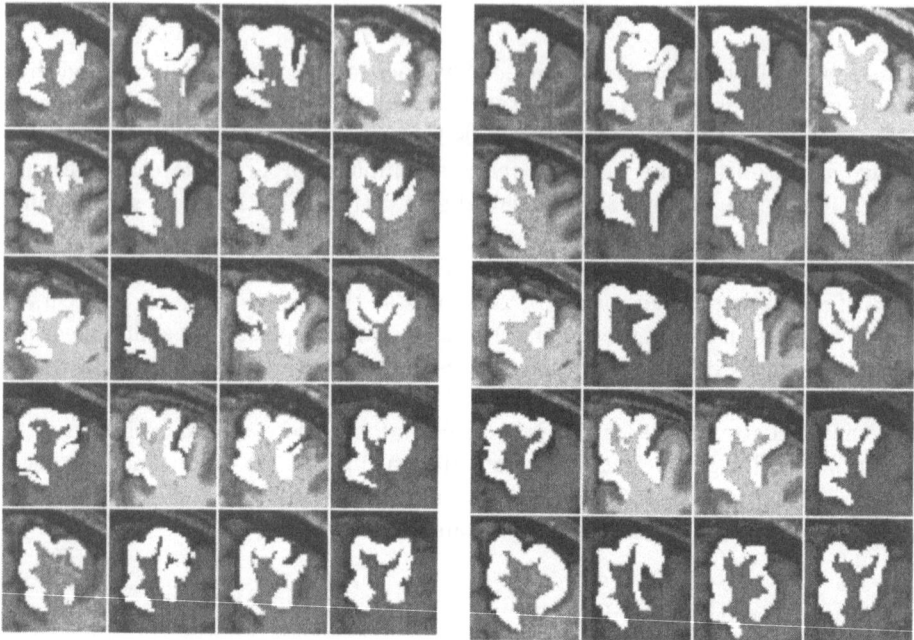

Fig. 5. Segmentation of the Superior Frontal Gyrus. These images compare the manual (left) and automatic (right) segmentations of the left superior frontal gyrus on coronal slices from 20 subjects

fully objective and applicable to large ensembles of brain volumes. While the new procedure uses two algorithms that were developed at the Montreal Neurological Institute, the new improved segmentation method is not dependent on these particular methods. In fact, any classification method that differentiates tissue types and any non-linear registration method may be merged to maximize the complementary information of both techniques. Since INSECT yields high resolution structure information, it is no longer necessary to run ANIMAL to fine resolutions, thus providing a considerable improvement in speed. In fact, running times are reduced from approximately 10 hours for estimation of the high resolution non-linear fit to less than 2 hours, including both classification and low-resolution warping.

The qualitative results shown in Fig 5 demonstrate that the ANIMAL+INSECT methodology can segment individual gyri from MRI data. While the quantitative measures presented here are not as high as we would like, we are currently working on estimating intra- and inter-observer variability estimates to put these values into context.

At least three methodological problems remain for future work: 1) In their current form, the cortical SPAMs do not explicitly represent multiple topological patterns that exist for cortical gyri. We plan to use an atlas that contains multiple SPAM representations for specific cortical regions, where each SPAM corresponds to a given cortical pattern for that region. 2) Structures that have a high anatomical variability are represented by SPAMs whose size is smaller than their true average size. These structures must be segmented using a model-only method, similar to those described above for the segmentation of the thalamus, caudate, putamen and globus pallidus. 3) Surface data, extracted by MSD, will be used to refine over-defined cortical regions (e.g., where the opposite sulcal bank is included in the segmentation of a gyrus). By using the surface information, it will be possible to separate small disconnected regions on the cortical surface, and then correct the gyral labelling in 3D.

Acknowledgments

The authors would like to express their appreciation for support from the Human Frontier Science Project Organization, the Canadian Medical Research Council (SP-30), the McDonnell-Pew Cognitive Neuroscience Center Program, the U.S. Human Brain Map Project (HBMP), NIMH and NIDA. W.F.C.Baaré was supported by the Netherlands Organization for Scientific Research and the Foundation "De Drie Lichten" in the Netherlands. This work forms part of a continuing project of the HBMP-funded International Consortium for Brain Mapping (ICBM) to develop a probabilistic atlas of human neuroanatomy.

References

1. S. P. Raya, "Low-level segmentation of 3D magnetic resonance brain images - a rule based system," *IEEE Transactions on Medical Imaging*, vol. 9, pp. 327–337, Sept. 1990.
2. L.-S. Chen and M. R. Sontag, "Representation, display and manipulation of 3D digital scenes and their medical applications," *Computer Vision, Graphics, and Image Processing*, vol. 48, pp. 190–216, 1989.
3. S. Dellepiane, S. Serpico, and G. Vernazza, "Approximate reasoning and knowledge in NMR image understanding," in *8th International Conference on Pattern Recognition*, (Paris, France), pp. 943–946, IEEE, Oct. 1986.
4. L. Arata, A. P. Dhawan, J. Broderick, and M. Gaskil, "Model-based analysis of MR images of the brain," *IEEE Engineering in Medicine and Biology*, vol. 13, no. 3, pp. 1331–1332, 1991.
5. A. P. Dhawan and L. Arata, "Knowledge-based multi-modality three-dimensional image analysis of the brain," *American Journal of Physiologic Imaging*, vol. 7, pp. 210–9, Jul-Dec 1992.
6. D. N. Davis and C. J. Taylor, "A blackboard architecture for automating cephalometric analysis," *Med Inf (Lond)*, vol. 16, pp. 137–49, Apr-Jun 1991.
7. Y. Kaneda, S. Fujii, Y. Kobashiri, M. Yoshirda, and M. Matsuo, "Pattern recognition and three dimensional construction from CT images," in *Proceedings of the International Conference on Cybernetics and Society*, (Tokyo and Kyoto, Japan), pp. 281–284, IEEE, Nov 3-7 1978.
8. M. E. Brummer, "Hough transform detection of the longitudinal fissure in tomographic head images," *IEEE Transactions on Medical Imaging*, vol. 10, Mar. 1991.

9. M. E. Brummer, R. M. Mersereau, R. L. Eisner, and R. R. J. Lewine, "Automatic detection of brain contours in MRI data sets," in *Information Processing in Medical Imaging* (A. C. F. Colchester and D. J. Hawkes, eds.), (Wye, UK), p. 188, IPMI, July 1991.

10. I. Kapouleas, "Automatic detection of white matter lesions in magnetic eesonance brain images," *Comput Methods Programs Biomed*, vol. 32, pp. 17–35, May 1990.

11. C. Broit, *Optimal registration of deformed images*. PhD thesis, University of Pennsylvania, Philadelphia, 1981.

12. R. Bajcsy and C. Broit, "Matching of deformed images," in *Proceedings of the 6th International Conference on Pattern Recognition*, (Munich, Germany), pp. 351–353, IEEE, Oct 19-22 1982.

13. R. Dann, J. Hoford, S. Kovacic, M. Reivich, and R. Bajcsy, "Three-dimensional computerized brain atlas for elastic matching: Creation and initial evaluation," in *Medical Imaging II*, (Newport Beach, Calif.), pp. 600–608, SPIE, Feb. 1988.

14. J. Gee, L. LeBriquer, and C. Barillot, "Probabilistic matching of brain images," in *Information Processing in Medical Imaging* (Y. Bizais and C. Barillot, eds.), (Ile Berder, France), IPMI, Kluwer, July 1995.

15. M. Miller, Y. A. G.E. Christensen, and U. Grenander, "Mathematical textbook of deformable neuroanatomies," *Proceedings of the National Academy of Sciences*, vol. 90, no. 24, pp. 11944–11948, 1990.

16. G. Christensen, R. Rabbitt, and M. Miller, "3D brain mapping using a deformable neuroanatomy," *Physics in Med and Biol*, vol. 39, pp. 609–618, 1994.

17. G. Christensen, R. Rabbitt, and M. Miller, "Deformable templates using large deformation kinematics," *IEEE Transactions on Image Processing*, vol. 5, no. 10, pp. 1435–1447, 1996.

18. D. L. Collins, C. J. Holmes, T. M. Peters, and A. C. Evans, "Automatic 3D model-based neuroanatomical segmentation," *Human Brain Mapping*, vol. 3, no. 3, pp. 190–208, 1995.

19. H. Zachmann, "Interpretation of cranial MR-images using a digital atlas of the human head," *IEEE Transactions on Medical Imaging*, pp. 99–110, 1991.

20. J. Talairach and P. Tournoux, *Co-planar stereotactic atlas of the human brain: 3-Dimensional proportional system: an approach to cerebral imaging*. Stuttgart, New York: Georg Thieme Verlag, 1988.

21. P. T. Fox, M. A. Mintun, E. M. Reiman, and M. E. Raichle, "Enhanced detection of focal brain responses using intersubject averaging and change-distribution analysis of subtracted PET images," *Journal of Cerebral Blood Flow and Metabolism*, vol. 8, pp. 642–653, 1988.

22. P. T. Fox, S. Mikiten, G. Davis, and J. L. Lancaster, "BrainMap: A database of functional brain mapping," in *Functional Neuroimaging, technical foundations* (R. W. Thatcher, M. Hallett, T. Zeffiro, E. R. John, and M. Heurta, eds.), pp. 95–105, San Diego, Ca.: Academic Press, 1994.

23. A. Evans, D. Collins, and C. Holmes, "Automatic 3D regional MRI segmentation and statistical probability anatomy maps," in *Quantification of Brain Function: Tracer kinetics and image analysis in brain PET* (T. Jones, ed.), pp. 123–130, 1995.

24. J. G. Sled, A. P. Zijdenbos, and A. C. Evans, "A non-parametric method for automatic correction of intensity non-uniformity in MRI data," *IEEE Transactions on Medical Imaging*, vol. 17, Feb. 1998.

25. D. L. Collins, P. Neelin, T. M. Peters, and A. C. Evans, "Automatic 3D intersubject registration of MR volumetric data in standardized talairach space," *Journal of Computer Assisted Tomography*, vol. 18, pp. 192–205, March/April 1994.

26. D. MacDonald, D. Avis, and A. C. Evans, "Multiple surface identification and matching in magnetic resonance images," in *Proceedings of Conference on Visualization in Biomedical Computing*, SPIE, 1994.

27. D. MacDonald, *Identifying geometrically simple surfaces from three dimensional data*. PhD thesis, McGill University, Montreal, Canada, December 1994.

28. A. P. Zijdenbos, A. C. Evans, F. Riahi, J. Sled, J. Chui, and V. Kollokian, "Automatic quantification of multiple sclerosis lesion volume using stereotaxic space," in *Proceedings of the 4th International Conference on Visualization in Biomedical Computing, VBC '96:*, (Hamburg), pp. 439–448, September 1996.

29. N. Kabani, D. Collins, and A. Evans, "A 3d neuroanatomical atlas," in *4th International Conference on Functional Mapping of the Human Brain* (A. Evans, ed.), (Montreal), Organization for Human Brain Mapping, June 1998. submitted.

30. A. C. Evans, D. L. Collins, and B. Milner, "An MRI-based stereotactic atlas from 250 young normal subjects," *Soc.Neurosci.Abstr.*, vol. 18, p. 408, 1992.

31. J. Mazziotta, A. Toga, A. Evans, P. Fox, and J. Lancaster, "A probabilistic atlas of the human brain: theory and rationale for its development. the international consortium for brain mapping," *NeuroImage*, vol. 2, no. 2, pp. 89–101, 1995.

32. M. Ono, S. Kubik, and C. Abernathey, *Atlas of Cerebral Sulci*. Stuttgart: Georg Thieme Verlag, 1990.

33. J. Absher, "A probabilistic atlas of the thalamus," tech. rep., McConnell Brain Imaging Centre, Montreal Neurological Institute, McGill University, Montreal, Sept 1993.

34. D. L. Collins, N. J. Kabani, and A. C. Evans, "Automatic volume estimation of gross cerebral structures," in *4th International Conference on Functional Mapping of the Human Brain* (A. Evans, ed.), (Montreal), Organization for Human Brain Mapping, June 1998. abstract no. 702.

35. W. Baaré, D. Collins, N. Kabani, D. MacDonald, C. Liu, M. Petrides, R. Kwan, and A. Evans, "Automated and manual identification of frontal lobe gyri," in *Third International Conference on Functional Mapping of the Human Brain*, vol. 5, (Copenhagen), p. S348, Human Brain Map, May 1997.

36. D. MacDonald, "Display: a user's manual," tech. rep., McConnell Brain Imaging Centre, Montreal Neurological Institute, McGill University, Montreal, Sept 1996.

37. L. R. Dice, "Measures of the amount of ecologic association between species," *Ecology*, vol. 26, no. 3, pp. 297–302, 1945.

38. A. P. Zijdenbos, B. M. Dawant, R. A. Margolin, and A. C. Palmer, "Morphometric analysis of white matter lesions in MR images: Method and validation," *IEEE Transactions on Medical Imaging*, vol. 13, pp. 716–724, Dec. 1994.

39. C. J, "A coefficient of agreement for nominal scales," *Educational and Psychological Measurements*, vol. 20, pp. 37–46, 1960.

Consistent Linear-Elastic Transformations for Image Matching

Gary E. Christensen

Department of Electrical and Computer Engineering
The University of Iowa, Iowa City, Iowa 52242, USA
gary-christensen@uiowa.edu

Abstract. A fundamental problem with a large class of image registration techniques is that the estimated transformation from image A to B does not equal the inverse of the estimated transform from B to A. This inconsistency is a result of the matching criteria's inability to uniquely describe the correspondences between two images. This paper seeks to overcome this limitation by jointly estimating the transformation from A to B and from B to A while enforcing the consistency constraint that these transforms are inverses of one another. The transformations are further restricted to preserve topology by constraining them to obey the laws of continuum mechanics. A new parameterization of the transformation based on a Fourier series in the context of linear elasticity is presented. Results are presented using both Magnetic Resonance and X-ray Computed Tomography Imagery. It is shown that joint estimation of a consistent set of forward and reverse transformations constrained by linear-elasticity gives better registration results than using either constraint alone or none at all.

1 Introduction

A reasonable but perhaps not always desirable assumption is that the mapping of one anatomical image (source) to another (target) is diffeomorphic, i.e., continuous, one-to-one, onto, and differentiable. By definition, a diffeomorphic mapping has an unique inverse that maps the target image back onto the source image. Thus, it is reasonable goal to estimate a transformation from image A to B that should equal the inverse of the transformation estimated from B to A assuming a diffeomorphic mapping exists between the images. However, this consistency between the forward and reverse transformations is not guaranteed with many image registration techniques.

Depending on the application, the diffeomorphic assumption may or may not be valid. This assumption is valid for registering images collected from the same individual imaged by two different modalities such as MRI and CT, but it is not necessarily valid when registering images before and after surgery. Likewise, a diffeomorphic mapping assumption may be valid for registering MRI data from two different normal individuals if the goal is to match the deep nuclei of the

A. Kuba et al. (Eds.): IPMI'99, LNCS 1613, pp. 224–237, 1999.

brain, but it may not be valid for the same data sets if the goal is to match the sulcal patterns.

Alternatively, diffeomorphic transformations may be used to identify areas where two image volumes differ topologically by analyzing the properties of the resulting transformation. For example, consider the problem of matching an MRI image with a tumor to one without a tumor. A possibly valid diffeomorphic transformation would be one that registers all of the corresponding brain structures by shrinking the tumor to a small point. Such a transformation would have an unusually small Jacobian which could be used to detect or identify the location of the tumor. Conversely, consider the inverse problem of matching the image without the tumor to the one with the tumor. A valid registration in this case may be to register all of the corresponding brain structures by allowing the transformation to "tear" (i.e., not be diffeomorphic) at the site of the tumor. Just as valid could be a diffeomorphic transformation that registers all of the corresponding brain structures by allowing the transformation to stretch at the site of the tumor.

As in the previous examples, we will assume that a valid transformation is diffeomorphic everywhere except possibly in regions where the source and target images differ topologically, e.g., in the neighborhood of the tumor. For the remainder of the this paper, we will consider registration problems that the diffeomorphic transformation assumption is valid. These ideas can be extended to certain non-diffeomorphic mapping problems by including boundary conditions to model, isolate or remove regions that differ topologically.

Transformations that are diffeomorphic maintain topology guaranteeing that connected subregions remain connected, neighborhood relationships between structures are preserved, and surfaces are mapped to surfaces. Preserving topology is important for synthesizing individualized electronic atlases; the knowledge base of the atlas maybe transferred to the target anatomy through the topology preserving transformation providing automatic labeling and segmentation. If total volume of a nucleus, ventricle, or cortical sub region are an important statistic it can be generated automatically. Topology preserving transformations that map the template to the target also can be used to study the physical properties of the target anatomy such as mean shape and variation. Likewise, preserving topology allows data from multiple individuals to be mapped to a standard atlas coordinate space [1]. Registration to an atlas removes individual anatomical variation and allows information from many experiments to be combined and associated with a single conical anatomy.

The forward transformation h from image T to S and the reverse transformation g from S to T are pictured in Fig. 1. Ideally, the transformations h and g should be uniquely determined and should be inverses of one another. Estimating h and g independently very rarely results in a consistent set of transformations due to a large number of local minima. As a result, we propose to jointly estimate h and g while constraining these transforms to be inverses of one another. The joint estimation makes intuitive sense in that the invertibility constraint will reduce the number of local minima because the problem is being solved from two different directions. Although uniqueness is very difficult to achieve in medical image registration, the joint estimation should lead to more consistent and biologically meaningful results.

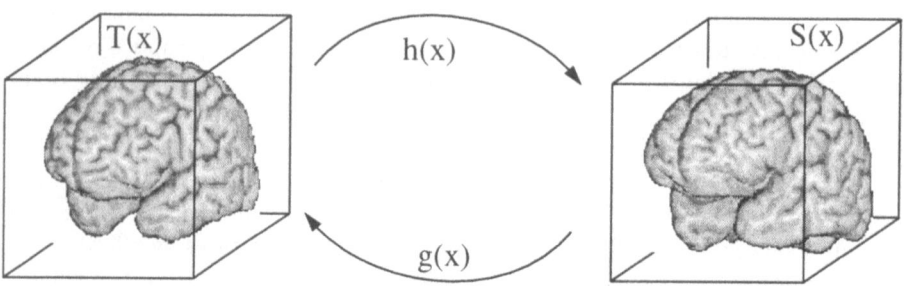

Fig. 1. The transformation h maps the image volume T to S and the transformation g maps S to T. In order for the mappings to be biologically meaningful, h and g should be inverses of one another

The need to impose the invertibility consistency constraint depends on the particular application and on the correspondence model used for registration. In general, registration techniques that do not uniquely determine the correspondence between image volumes should benefit from the consistency constraint. This is because such techniques often rely on minimizing/maximizing a similarity measure which has a large number of local minima/maxima due to correspondence ambiguity. Examples include similarity measures based on features in the source and target images such as image intensities, object boundaries/surfaces, etc. In theory, similarity measures have more local minima as the dimension of the transformation increases. A registration method that determines the correspondence between images by minimizing an image intensity similarity measure is considered in this paper.

Methods that use specified correspondences for registration will benefit less or not at all from the invertibility consistency constraint. For example, landmark based registration methods implicitly impose an invertibility constraint because the correspondence defined between landmarks is the same for estimating the forward and inverse transformations. However, the drawbacks of specifying correspondences include requiring user interaction to specify landmarks, unique correspondences can not always be specified, and such methods usually only provide coarse registration due to the small number of correspondences specified.

2   Registration Algorithm

2.1   Problem Statement

The image registration problem is usually stated as: Find the transformation h that maps the template image volume T into correspondence with the target image volume S. Alternatively, the problem can be stated as: Find the transformation g that transforms S into correspondence with T. For this paper, the previous two statements are combined into a single problem and restated as:

> **Problem Statement:** Jointly estimate the transformations h and g such that h maps T to S and g maps S to T subject to the constraint that $h = g^{-1}$.

It is assumed that the 3D image volumes T and S are medical imaging modalities such as MRI, fMRI, CT, cryosection imagery, etc. collected from similar anatomical populations. Each image is defined as a function of $x \in \Omega = [0,1]^3$ where Ω is called the image coordinate system. The transformations are vector-valued functions that map the image coordinate system Ω to itself, i.e., $h : \Omega \mapsto \Omega$ and $g : \Omega \mapsto \Omega$. Diffeomorphic constraints are placed on h and g so that they preserve topology. Throughout it is assumed that $h(x) = x + u(x)$, $h^{-1}(x) = x + \tilde{u}(x)$, $g(x) = x + w(x)$ and $g^{-1}(x) = x + \tilde{w}(x)$ where $h(h^{-1}(x)) = x$ and $g(g^{-1}(x)) = x$. All of the fields h, g, u, $\tilde{u}$, w, and $\tilde{w}$ are (3×1) vector-valued functions of $x \in \Omega$.

Registration is defined using a symmetric cost function $C(h, g)$ that describes the distance between the transformed template $T(h)$ and target S, and the distance between the transformed target $S(g)$ and template T. To ensure the desired properties, the transformations h and g are jointly estimated by minimizing the cost function $C(h, g)$ while satisfying diffeomorphic constraints and inverse transformation consistency constraints. The diffeomorphic constraints are enforced by constraining the transformations to satisfy laws of continuum mechanics [2].

2.2 Symmetric Cost Function

The main problem with image similarity registration techniques is that minimizing the similarity function does not uniquely determine the correspondence between two image volumes. In addition, similarity cost functions generally have many local minima due to the complexity of the images being matched and the dimensionality of the transformation. It is these local minima (ambiguities) that cause the estimated transformation from image T to S to be different from the inverse of the estimated transformation from S to T. In general, this becomes more of a problem as the dimensionality of the transformation increases. To overcome this problem for 3×3 linear transformations, Woods et al. [3] averages the forward and inverse linear transformations to reconcile differences between pairwise registrations.

To overcome correspondence ambiguities, we jointly estimate the transformations from image T to S and from S to T. This is accomplished by defining a cost function to measure the shape differences between the deformed image $T(h(x))$ and image $S(x)$ and the differences between the deformed image $S(g(x))$ and image $T(x)$. Ideally, the transformations h and g should be inverses of one another, i.e., $h(x) = g^{-1}(x)$. The transformations h and g are estimated by minimizing a cost function that is a function of $(T(h(x)) - S(x))$ and $(S(g(x)) - T(x))$. The cost function used in this work is given by

$$C_1(T(h), S) + C_1(S(g), T) = \int_\Omega |T(h(x)) - S(x)|^2 dx + \int_\Omega |S(g(x)) - T(x)|^2 dx.$$
(1)

Alternatively, the mutual information cost function given in [4,5] could be used. Notice that this joint estimation approach applies to both linear and non-linear transformations.

2.3   Transformation Parameterization

A 3D Fourier series representation is used to parameterize the forward and inverse transformations. This parameterization is simpler than the parameterizations used in our previous work [6,7,8] and each basis coefficient can be interpreted as the weight of a harmonic component in a single coordinate direction. The displacement fields are constrained to have the form

$$u(x) = \sum_{k=0}^{N-1} \sum_{j=0}^{N-1} \sum_{i=0}^{N-1} \mu_{ijk} e^{\hat{j}<x,\omega_{ijk}>} \quad \text{and} \quad w(x) = \sum_{k=0}^{N-1} \sum_{j=0}^{N-1} \sum_{i=0}^{N-1} \eta_{ijk} e^{\hat{j}<x,\omega_{ijk}>}$$
(2)

where μ_{ijk} and η_{ijk} are (3×1), complex-valued vectors and $\omega_{ijk} = [\frac{2\pi i}{N}, \frac{2\pi j}{N}, \frac{2\pi k}{N}]$. Notice that this parameterization is periodic in x and therefore has cyclic boundary conditions for x on the boundary of Ω . The coefficients μ_{ijk} and η_{ijk} are constrained to have complex conjugate symmetry during the estimation procedure.

Proposition 1. *Each displacement field in (2) is real and can be written as*

$$u(x) = 2 \sum_{k=0}^{N-1} \sum_{j=0}^{N-1} \sum_{i=0}^{N/2-1} \left(a_{ijk} Re\{e^{\hat{j}<x,\omega_{ijk}>}\} - b_{ijk} Im\{e^{\hat{j}<x,\omega_{ijk}>}\} \right)$$
(3)

if the (3×1) vector $\mu_{ijk} = a_{ijk} + \hat{j}b_{ijk}$ has complex conjugate symmetry.

Proof. Notice that (2) can be written as

$$u(x) = \sum_{k=0}^{N-1} \sum_{j=0}^{N-1} \sum_{i=0}^{N/2-1} (a_{ijk} + \hat{j}b_{ijk}) e^{\hat{j}<x,\omega_{ijk}>} + (a_{ijk} - \hat{j}b_{ijk}) e^{-\hat{j}<x,\omega_{ijk}>}$$

because the μ_{ijk} are complex conjugate symmetric. Simplifying the summand gives the result.   □

2.4   Inverse Transformation Consistency Constraint

Minimizing the cost function in (1) is not sufficient to guarantee that the transformations h and g are inverses of each other. The inverse transformation consistency constraint is enforced by minimizing the squared difference between the transformation h and and the inverse transformation of g, and vice versa. To state this mathematically we define the following relationships: $h(x) = x + u(x)$, $h^{-1}(x) = x + \tilde{u}(x)$, $g(x) = x + w(x)$ and $g^{-1}(x) = x + \tilde{w}(x)$. The consistency constraint is enforced by minimizing

$$C_2(u, \tilde{w}) + C_2(w, \tilde{u}) = \int_\Omega ||u(x) - \tilde{w}(x)||^2 dx + \int_\Omega ||w(x) - \tilde{u}(x)||^2 dx. \quad (4)$$

The inverse transformation h^{-1} is estimated from h by solving the minimization problem $h^{-1}(y) = \arg\min_x ||y - h(x)||^2$ for each y on a discrete lattice in Ω. The inverse h^{-1} exists and is unique if h is a diffeomorphic transformation, i.e., continuous, one-to-one, and onto.

2.5   Diffeomorphic Constraint

Minimizing the cost function in (4) does not ensure that the transformations h and g are diffeomorphic transformations except for when $C_2(u, \tilde{w}) + C_2(w, \tilde{u}) = 0$. To enforce the transformations to be diffeomorphic, we use continuum mechanical models such as linear elasticity [7,9] and viscous fluid [9,10]. For this paper, a linear-elastic constraint of the form

$$C_3(u) + C_3(w) = \int_\Omega ||Lu(x)||^2 dx + \int_\Omega ||Lw(x)||^2 dx \quad (5)$$

was used to enforce the diffeomorphic property where $h(x) = x + u(x)$ and $g(x) = x + w(x)$. The operator L has the form $Lu(x) = -\alpha\nabla^2 u(x) - \beta\nabla(\nabla \cdot u(x)) + \gamma$ for linear elasticity, but in general can be any nonsingular linear differential operator [8].

Following the approach in [8], the operator L can be considered a (3×3) matrix operator. Discretizing the continuous partial derivatives of L, it can be shown that (5) has the form

$$C_3(u) + C_3(w) = N^3 \sum_{k=0}^{N-1} \sum_{j=0}^{N-1} \sum_{i=0}^{N-1} \mu_{ijk}^\dagger D_{ijk}^2 \mu_{ijk} + \eta_{ijk}^\dagger D_{ijk}^2 \eta_{ijk} \quad (6)$$

where † is the complex conjugate transpose. D_{ijk} is a real-valued, (3×3) matrix with elements

$$d_{11} = 2\alpha\left[\beta\left(1 - \cos\left(\tfrac{2\pi i}{N}\right)\right) + \left(1 - \cos\left(\tfrac{2\pi j}{N}\right)\right) + \left(1 - \cos\left(\tfrac{2\pi k}{N}\right)\right)\right] + \gamma$$

$$d_{22} = 2\alpha\left[\left(1 - \cos\left(\tfrac{2\pi i}{N}\right)\right) + \beta\left(1 - \cos\left(\tfrac{2\pi j}{N}\right)\right) + \left(1 - \cos\left(\tfrac{2\pi k}{N}\right)\right)\right] + \gamma$$

$$d_{33} = 2\alpha\left[\left(1 - \cos\left(\tfrac{2\pi i}{N}\right)\right) + \left(1 - \cos\left(\tfrac{2\pi j}{N}\right)\right) + \beta\left(1 - \cos\left(\tfrac{2\pi k}{N}\right)\right)\right] + \gamma$$

$$d_{12} = d_{21} = \beta\left[\cos\left(\tfrac{2\pi}{N}(i-j)\right) - \cos\left(\tfrac{2\pi}{N}(i+j)\right)\right]$$

$$d_{13} = d_{31} = \beta\left[\cos\left(\tfrac{2\pi}{N}(i-k)\right) - \cos\left(\tfrac{2\pi}{N}(i+k)\right)\right]$$

$$d_{23} = d_{32} = \beta\left[\cos\left(\tfrac{2\pi}{N}(j-k)\right) - \cos\left(\tfrac{2\pi}{N}(j+k)\right)\right].$$

2.6   Minimization Problem

By combining (1), (4), and (5), the image registration problem becomes

$$\hat{h}(x), \hat{g}(x) = \underset{h(x),g(x)}{\arg\min} \int_\Omega |T(h(x)) - S(x)|^2 + |S(g(x)) - T(x)|^2 dx$$
$$+ \lambda \int_\Omega ||u(x) - \tilde{w}(x)||^2 + ||w(x) - \tilde{u}(x)||^2 dx \qquad (7)$$
$$+ \rho \int_\Omega ||Lu(x)||^2 + ||Lw(x)||^2 dx$$

where the constants λ and ρ are Lagrange multipliers used to enforce/balance the constraints.

2.7   Estimation Procedure

The transformations $\hat{h}$ and $\hat{g}$ that satisfy (7) were estimated using a gradient descent algorithm to determine the basis coefficients $\{\mu_{ijk}, \eta_{ijk}\}$. The estimation was accomplished by solving a sequence of optimization problems from coarse to fine scale via increasing the number of the basis coefficient vectors $\{\mu_{ijk}, \eta_{ijk}\}$ during the estimation. This is analogous to multi-grid methods but here the notion of refinement from coarse to fine is accomplished by increasing the number of basis components. As the number of basis functions is increased, smaller and smaller variabilities between the template and target images are accommodated.

3   Results

Two MRI and two CT image volumes were used to evaluate the registration algorithm. The data sets were collected from different individuals using the same MR and CT machines and the same scan parameters. The MRI data sets correspond to two normal adults and the CT data sets correspond to two 3-month-old infants, one normal and one abnormal (bilateral coronal synostosis). The MRI and CT data sets were chosen to test registration algorithm when matching anatomies with similar and dissimilar shapes, respectively.

The MRI data were preprocessed by normalizing the image intensities, correcting for translation and rotation, and segmenting the brain from the head using Analyze^{TM}. The translation aligned the anterior commissure points, and the rotation aligned the corresponding axial and sagittal planes containing the anterior and posterior commissure points, respectively. The data sets were then down-sampled and zero padded to form a $64 \times 64 \times 64$ voxel lattice. The CT data sets were corrected for translation and rotation and down-sampled to form a $64 \times 64 \times 50$ voxel lattice. The translation aligned the basion skull landmarks, and the rotation aligned the corresponding Frankfort Horizontal and midsagittal planes, respectively.

The data sets were registered initially with zero and first order harmonics. After every 40th iteration, the maximum harmonic was increased by one. The MRI-to-MRI registration was terminated after 300 iterations and the CT-to-CT registration was terminated after 200 iterations. Tables 1, 2, and 3 show the results of four MRI experiments and four CT experiments. In order to isolate the contribution of each term of (7), one experiment was done with no priors, one with the linear-elastic model, one with the inverse consistency constraint, and one with both priors. The four MRI experiments used the parameters 1. $\lambda = \rho = 0$, 2. $\lambda = 0$ and $\rho = 50$, 3. $\lambda = 0.07$ and $\rho = 0$, and 4. $\lambda = 0.07$ and $\rho = 50$; and four CT experiments used the parameters: 1. $\lambda = \rho = 0$, 2. $\lambda = 0$ and $\rho = 25$, 3. $\lambda = 0.02$ and $\rho = 0$, and 4. $\lambda = 0.02$ and $\rho = 25$. The labels MRI1 and CT1 are used to refer to results from the Case 1 experiments, and likewise for 2 to 4.

Table 1. Cost Terms Associated with Transforming Image Volume T to S

Experiment	$C_1(T(h), S)$ orig.	final	$\lambda C_2(u, \tilde{w})$ final	$\rho C_3(u)$ final	Total
MRI1	1980	438	0	0	438
MRI2	1980	606	0	85.7	692
MRI3	1980	482	33.4	0	516
MRI4	1980	639	13.0	74.6	727
CT1	454	27.0	0	0	27.0
CT2	454	38.8	0	28.1	66.9
CT3	454	28.5	3.15	0	31.6
CT4	454	40.8	3.34	28.3	72.4

Case 1. corresponds to unconstrained estimation in which h and g are estimated independently. The numbers in the tables are consistent with this observation. First, $C_2(u, \tilde{w})$ and $C_2(w, \tilde{u})$ show the largest error between the forward and inverse mapping for each group of experiments. Secondly, the Jacobian for these cases are the lowest in their respective groups. This is expected because the unconstrained experiments find the best match between the images without any constraint preventing the Jacobian from going negative (singular). This is further supported by the fact that the final values of $C_1(T(h), S)$ and $C_1(S(g), T)$ are the lowest in there groups.

Table 2. Cost Terms Associated with Transforming Image Volume S to T

Experiment	$C_1(S(g), T)$		$\lambda C_2(w, \tilde{u})$	$\rho C_3(w)$	Total
	orig.	final	final	final	
MRI1	1980	512	0	0	512
MRI2	1980	660	0	78.3	738
MRI3	1980	539	33.6	0	573
MRI4	1980	676	13.0	73.7	727
CT1	454	30.6	0	0	30.6
CT2	454	47.7	0	32.4	80.1
CT3	454	34.6	3.43	0	38.0
CT4	454	50.8	3.78	31.9	86.5

Case 2. corresponds to independently estimating h and g while requiring each transformation to satisfy the diffeomorphic constraint enforced by linear elasticity. Just as in Case 1, the large difference between the forward and reverse displacement fields as reported by $C_2(u, \tilde{w})$ and $C_2(w, \tilde{u})$ confirms that linear elasticity alone is not sufficient to guarantee that h and g are inverses of one another. We do however, see that the linear elasticity constraint did improve the transformation over the unconstrained case because the minimum Jacobian and the inverse of the maximum Jacobian is far from being singular.

Case 3. corresponds to the estimation problem that is constrained only by the inverse transformation consistency constraint. The $C_2(u, \tilde{w})$ and $C_2(w, \tilde{u})$ values for these experiments are much lower than those in Cases 1. and 2. because they are being minimized. The transformations h and g are inverses of each other when $C_2(u, \tilde{w}) + C_2(w, \tilde{u}) = 0$ so that the smaller the costs $C_2(u, \tilde{w})$ and $C_2(w, \tilde{u})$ are, the closer h and g are to being inverses of each other.

Table 3. Transformation Measurements

Experiment	Jacobian(h)		Jacobian(g)		$C_2(u, \tilde{w})$	$C_2(w, \tilde{u})$
	min	1/max	min	1/max		
MRI1	0.257	0.275	0.100	0.261	28,300	29,500
MRI2	0.521	0.459	0.371	0.653	10,505	10,460
MRI3	0.315	0.290	0.226	0.464	478	479
MRI4	0.607	0.490	0.410	0.640	186	186
CT1	0.340	0.325	0.200	0.49	73,100	76,400
CT2	0.552	0.490	0.421	0.678	28,700	28,300
CT3	0.581	0.361	0.356	0.612	158	171
CT4	0.720	0.501	0.488	0.725	167	189

Case 4. is the joint estimation of h and g with both the inverse consistency constraint and the linear-elastic constraint. We can see that this produced the

best results because the differences between the inverse transformations were so small, i.e., $C_2(u, \tilde{w})$ and $C_2(w, \tilde{u})$. Also, the minimum Jacobian of h is nearly the inverse of the maximum Jacobian of g, and vice versa. In addition, the minimum and one over the maximum Jacobian of h and g have their largest values for this experiment (excluding one entry from MRI2). The MRI4 experiment shows a better than twofold improvement over MRI3 with respect to the difference in the inverse transformations, while the the inverse transformations difference for the CT4 and CT3 experiments are nearly equal. This may suggest that the inverse consistency constraint may be used without the linear-elasticity constraint. However, the minimum and one over the maximum Jacobian values are larger for CT4 than CT3 and similarly for MRI4 and MRI3 suggesting less distortion. The closer the minimum Jacobian is to one, the smaller the distortion of the images.

Figure 2 shows three slices from the 3D result of Case 4 for both the MRI and CT experiments. The first two columns show the template T and target S images before transformation. The third and forth columns show the transformed template $T(h)$ and target $S(g)$. Columns 5,6, and 7 show the x-,y-, and z-components of the displacement field u used to deform the template and columns 8,9, and 10 show the same for the displacement field w. The near invertibility in gray-scale between the displacement fields u and w gives a visual impression that h and g are nearly inverses of each other.

The time series statistics for MRI4 and CT4 experiments are shown in Figs. 3 and 4. These graphs show that the gradient descent algorithm converged for each set of transformation harmonics. In both cases, the cost functions $C_1(T(h), S)$ and $C_1(S(g), T)$ decreased at each iteration while the prior terms increased before decreasing. Notice that the inverse consistency constraint increased as the images deformed for each particular harmonic resolution. Then when the number of harmonics were increased, the inverse constraint decreased before increasing again. This is due to the fact that a low-dimensional Fourier series does not have enough degrees of freedom to faithfully represent the inverse of a low-dimensional Fourier series. This is easily seen by looking at the high dimensionality of a Taylor series representation of the inverse transformation. Finally, notice that the inverse consistency constraint caused the extremal Jacobian values of the forward and reverse transformations to track together. This is easiest to see in the CT4 experiment. Note that these extremal Jacobian values correspond to the worst case distortions produced by the transformations.

4   Discussion

The experiments presented in this paper were designed to test the validity of the new inverse transformation consistency constraint as applied to a linear-elastic transformation algorithm. As such, there was no effort made to optimize the rate of convergence of the algorithm. The convergence rate of the algorithm can be greatly improved by using a more efficient optimization technique than gradient descent such as conjugate gradient at each parameterization resolution. In

T	S	T(h)	S(g)	u1	u2	u3	w1	w2	w3

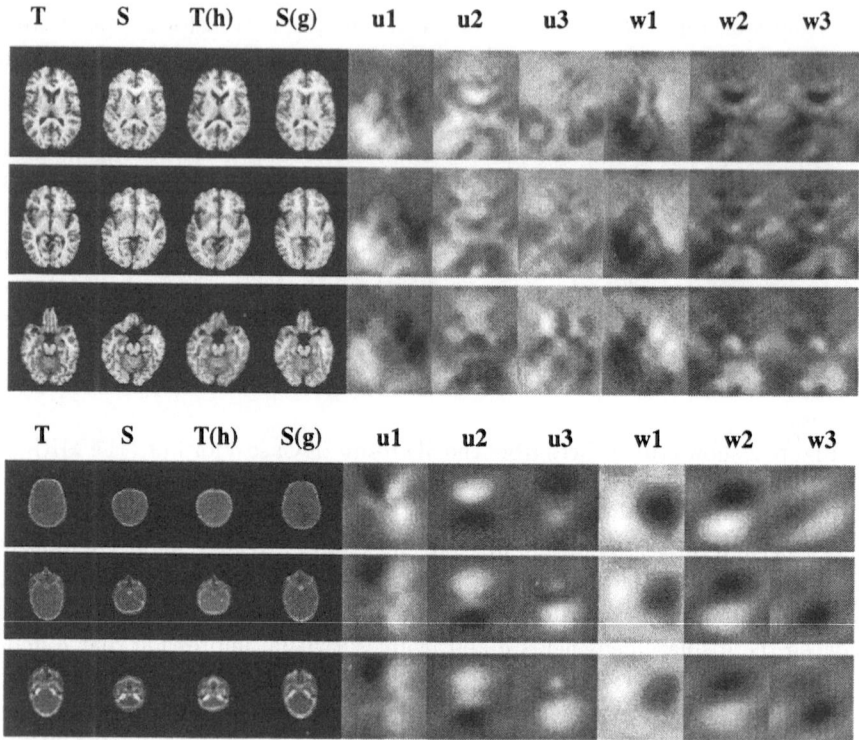

T	S	T(h)	S(g)	u1	u2	u3	w1	w2	w3

Fig. 2. Images associated with the MRI4 and CT4 experiments

addition, a convergence criteria can be used to determine when to increment the number of parameters in the model. The CT data used in the experiments was selected to stress the registration algorithm. The convergence of the algorithm would have been much faster if the data sets were adjusted for global scale initially.

It is important to track both the minimum and maximum values of the Jacobian during the estimation procedure. The Jacobian measures the differential volume change of a point being mapped through the transformation. At the start of the estimation, the transformation is the identity mapping and therefore has a Jacobian of one. If the minimum Jacobian goes negative, the transformation is no longer a one-to-one mapping and as a result folds the domain inside out [11]. Conversely, the reciprocal of the maximum value of the Jacobian corresponds to the minimum value of the Jacobian of the inverse mapping. Thus, as the maximum value of the Jacobian goes to infinity, the minimum value of the Jacobian of the inverse mapping goes to zero. In the present approach, the inverse transformation consistency constraint was used to penalize transformations that deviated from their inverse transformation. A limitation of this approach is that cost function in (4) is an average metric and can not enforce the pointwise constraints that $\min_x\{J(h)\} = 1/\max_x\{J(g)\}$ and $\min_x\{J(g)\} = 1/\max_x\{J(h)\}$. This

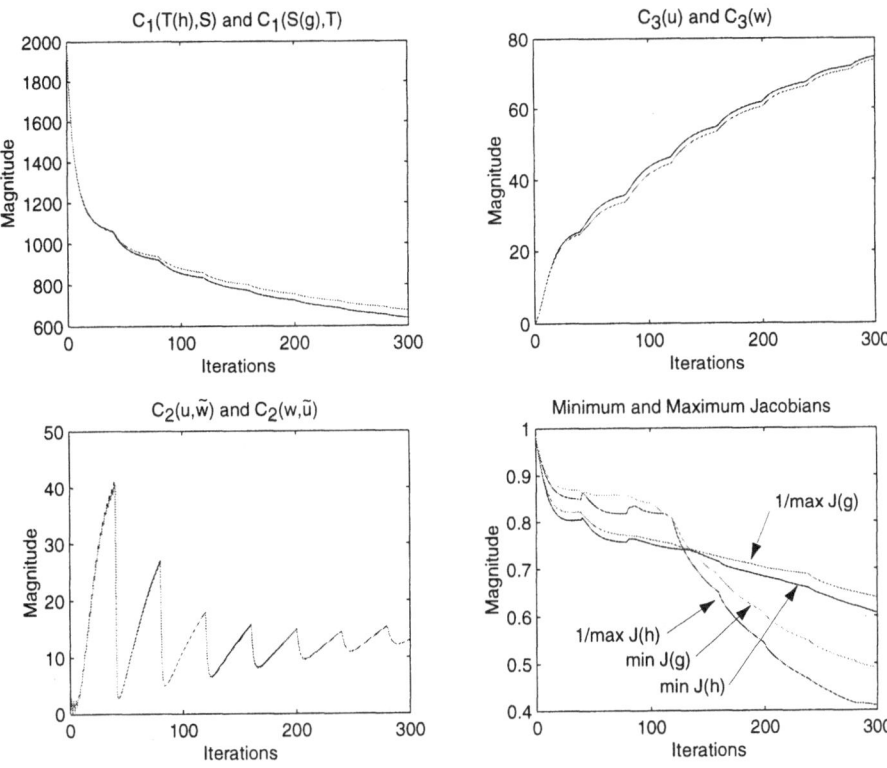

Fig. 3. Statistics associated with the MRI4 experiment

point is illustrated by Table 3 by the fact that the minimum values of $J(h)$ and $J(g)$ differ from the reciprocal of the maximum values of $J(g)$ and $J(h)$, respectively, However, these extremal Jacobian values do give an upper-bound on the worst case distortions produced by the transformations demonstrating the consistency between the forward and reverse transformations.

5   Summary and Conclusions

This paper presented a new algorithm for jointly estimating a consistent set of transformations that map one image to another and vice versa. A new parameterization based on the Fourier series was presented and was used to simplify the discretized linear-elasticity constraint. The Fourier series parameterization is simpler than our previous parameterizations and each basis coefficient can be interpreted as the weight of a harmonic component in a single coordinate direction. The algorithm was tested on both MRI and CT data. It was found that the unconstrained estimation leads to singular or near transformations. It was also shown that the linear-elastic constraint alone is not sufficient to guarantee that the forward and reverse transformations are inverses of one another. Results

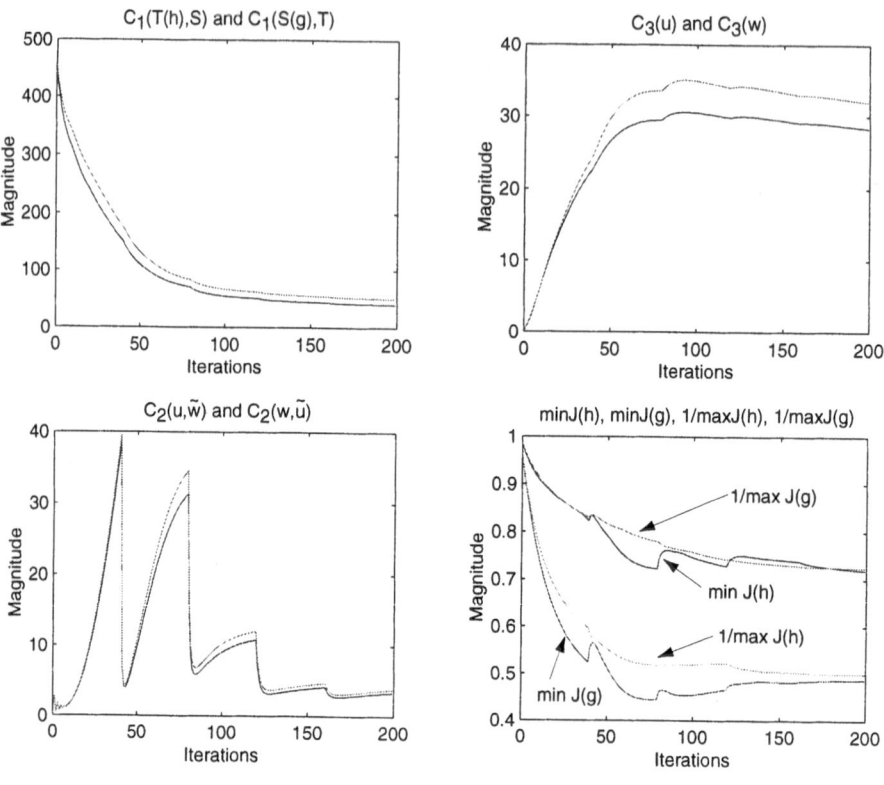

Fig. 4. Statistics associated with the CT4 experiment

were presented that suggest that even thought the inverse consistency constraint is not guaranteed to generate nonsingular transformations, in practice it may be possible to use the inverse consistency as the only constraint. Finally, it was shown that the most consistent transformations were generated using both the inverse consistency and the linear-elastic constraints.

Acknowledgments

I would like to thank my graduate students Hans Johnson and Peng Yin for their help in preparing this manuscript. I would like to thank John Haller and Michael W. Vannier of the Department of Radiology, The University of Iowa for providing the MRI data. I would like to thank Jeffrey L. Marsh of the Department of Surgery, Washington University School of Medicine for providing the CT data. I would like to thank Michael I. Miller and Sarang C. Joshi for their helpful insights over the last eight plus years. This work was supported in part by the NIH grant NS35368 and a grant from the Whitaker Foundation.

References

1. Talairach, J., Tournoux, P.: Co-Planar Stereotactic Atlas of the Human Brain. Beorg Thieme Verlag, Stuttgart, 1988
2. Segel, L.A.: Mathematics Applied to Continuum Mechanics. Dover Publications, New York, 1987
3. Woods, R.P., Grafton, S.T., Watson, J.D., Sicotte, N.L., Mazziotta, J.C.: Automated Image Registration: II. Intersubject Validation of Linear and Nonlinear Models. Journal of Computer Assisted Tomography **22** (1998) 153–165
4. Maes, F., Collignon, A., Vandermeulen, D., Marchal, G., Suetens, P.: Multimodality image registration by maximization of mutual information. IEEE Transactions on Medical Imaging **16** (1997) 187–198
5. Wells III, W.M., P.Viola, P., Atsumi, H., Nakajima, S., Kikinis R.: Multi-modal volume registration by maximization of mutual information. Medical Image Analysis **1** (1996) 35–51
6. Miller, M.I., Christensen, G.E., Amit, Y., Grenander, U.: Mathematical textbook of deformable neuroanatomies. Proceedings of the National Academy of Sciences **90** (1993) 11944-48
7. Christensen, G.E., Rabbitt, R.D., Miller, M.I.: 3D brain mapping using a deformable neuroanatomy. Physics in Medicine and Biology **39** (1994) 609–618
8. Miller, M.I., Banerjee, A., Christensen, G.E., Joshi, S.C., Khaneja, N., Grenander, U., Matejic, L.: Statistical methods in computational anatomy. Statistical Methods in Medical Research **6** (1997) 267–299
9. Christensen, G.E., Joshi, S.C., Miller, M.I.: Volume geometric transformations for mapping anatomy. IEEE Trans. on Med. Imaging **16** (1997) 864–877
10. Christensen, G.E., Rabbitt, R.D., Miller, M.I.: Deformable templates using large deformation kinematics. IEEE Transactions on Image Processing **5** (1996) 1435–1447
11. Christensen, G.E., Rabbitt, R.D., Miller, M.I., Joshi, S.C.,, Grenander, U., Coogan, T.A., Van Essen, D.C.: Topological properties of smooth anatomic maps. In Bizais, Y., Braillot, C., Di Paola, R.. editors, Information Processing in Medical Imaging, Kluwer Academic Publishers, Boston (1995) 101–112

Non-linear Registration with the Variable Viscosity Fluid Algorithm

Hava Lester[1], Simon R Arridge[1], Kalvis M Jansons[2], Louis Lemieux[3], Joseph V Hajnal[4], and Anjela Oatridge[4]

[1] Dept Computer Science, University College London, London WC1E 6BT, UK
hava@bic.mni.mcgill.ca, s.arridge@cs.ucl.ac.uk
[2] Dept Mathematics, University College London, London WC1E 6BT, UK
[3] Institute of Neurology, Queen Square, London WC1N 3BG, UK
[4] The MRC Cyclotron Unit, Hammersmith Hospital, London W12 OHS, UK

Abstract. In this paper we classify inhomogeneous non-linear registration algorithms into those of variable data influence, of variable deformability and of variable model type. As examples we introduce three modifications of the viscous fluid registration algorithm: passing a filter over the computed force field, adding boundary conditions onto the velocity field, and re-writing the viscous fluid PDE to accommodate a spatially-varying viscosity field. We demonstrate their application on artificial test data, on pre-/post-operative MR head slices and on MR neck volumes.

1 Introduction

Image registration requires finding an optimal transformation between an image pair, the *source* $S(\boldsymbol{x})$ and *target* $T(\boldsymbol{x})$. Single-level registration algorithms are divided between those which apply linear transformations and those which allow higher order deformations. Generally higher order deformations are performed after an initial registration by a linear method, so linear and non-linear are combined sequentially. In [1] we examined the application of hierarchies of data, warp and model, where complexity increases *temporally* with the progress of registration. It is rare that an algorithm allows simultaneous or parallel application of both linear and non-linear models within one image, so that only selected areas of the image deform. Many medical images contain regions representing both soft and hard tissue, and whereas the former often require high order deformations to achieve a good registration, in an intra-subject study the hard tissue regions should remain rigid. Registration of such image pairs requires algorithms where the model varies *spatially* within the image domain, using prior information on the variation of tissue types within the deforming image. These are instances of *inhomogeneous* non-linear registration algorithms. This paper classifies types of inhomogeneity and reviews those available in the literature. We then present three modifications to the fluid algorithm which introduce inhomogeneities into its application. Section 4 describes inhomogeneities in applying the force field and in computing the velocity field, and presents the varying-viscosity fluid registration algorithm. Finally, Sect. 5 shows results of application of these algorithms to 2- and 3-dimensional data.

A. Kuba et al. (Eds.): IPMI'99, LNCS 1613, pp. 238–251, 1999.
© Springer-Verlag Berlin Heidelberg 1999

2   Spatial Inhomogoneneities in Registration Algorithms

We [1] classify temporal hierarchies of registration into those of *data*, those of descriptors of deformation or *warp*, and those of complexity of *model*. In a similar vein, we classify spatial inhomogeneities as those in the *data influence*, in the strength of *deformation constraints*, and in the application of *model type*.

2.1   Variable Data Influence

The first type of inhomogeneity varies the importance attached to information content in the domain of the image pair when computing the transformation required at each point in the source. In terms of a Bayesian approach [2], where the deformation is determined by the solution of a weighted sum of likelihoods and priors, the weight assigned to the likelihood is varied according to assumptions about the relevance of the data in different regions of the image. In terms of regularisation, where the equation solved is a weighted sum of driving forces and constraints on the deformation, the influence of the driving force is weakened or strengthened relative to the deformation constraints.

By ignoring the contribution of the driving force, we can force a region to be *passive*, whose deformation is due solely to its proximity to *active* regions.

Let $\Omega = \{x\}$ be the domain of the image. We make the following definitions:

Definition 1 (Active and passive regions). *Let* $\Theta \subset \Omega$ *be a region whose deformation is given by* $u(x)$ *satisfying a regularisation equation*

$$g(u(x)) + \tau f\left(S(u(x)), T(x)\right) = 0 \qquad (1)$$

where f *is the likelihood and* g *is the prior constraint dependent on the deformation. We define* Θ *to be passive if for all pixels* $x \in \Theta$, *the regularisation parameter* τ *weighting the likelihood is equal to zero, and active otherwise.*

A medical application would be an intra-modality pair of which the source contains known segmented structures whose homologues are absent in the target but which may be confused, due to similarities of intensity, with regions nearby.

2.2   Variable Deformability

The second inhomogeneity paradigm varies the strength of deformation constraint. Regions of the image are then classified as *strongly* or *weakly deformable*. In the case of registration modelled on the behaviour of a physical material, the deformability is described by one or more parameters of the material properties - the elasticity of an elastic medium (Sect. 3.3) or the viscosity of a fluid (Sect. 4.3). Allowing these parameters to vary spatially requires the derivation of modified Partial Differential Equations (PDEs) to account for the parameter gradients.

Definition 2 (Strongly and weakly deformable). *Let $\Theta \subset \Omega$ be a region whose deformation is given by $u(x)$ satisfying a regularisation equation*

$$g(u(x); \mu(x)) + \tau f\left(S(u(x)), T(x)\right) = 0 \tag{2}$$

where f is the likelihood and g is a prior constraint dependent on the deformation and on an independent parameter $\mu \in [0, 1]$ varying spatially within the image, such that $g(\mu) \to 0$ as $\mu \to 0$. We define Θ to be strongly *or* weakly deformable *according to the range of μ from 0 (strongest) to 1 (weakest).*

The strength of the deformation parameter is supplied at every position in the source image, using prior information obtained from one of two sources: physical or statistical. In the first case, prior information is available on the deformability of the physical tissues which the images represent. For example, [3] demonstrate the estimation of tissue elasticity using certain scanning protocols, and we assume the rigidity of hard tissue. Basing the variability of the deformation constraint on such physical information is valid only in intra-subject studies, where the registration of the source to the target attempts to reproduce actual physical movements of tissue. A second type of prior information is applicable to and derived from cross-population studies, where the variation in the deformation constraint is a function of the statistical cross-population variability in the shape of each structure in the images. Structures which have been found to display little variance in size and shape across a population of normals will be labelled with a high value of μ, while other areas exhibiting greater variability will be labelled with a low value of μ and allowed greater deformations in registering to their homologues in the target image. For instance, [4] allows high variability in ventricular and cortical fold regions, and low variability in subcortical structures, in a variable-elasticity algorithm (Sect. 3.3).

2.3   Variable Model Type

Finally it is possible to vary spatially the models or equations causing deformation. This type of inhomogeneity can achieve completely affine transformations within selected regions while deforming intervening or surrounding areas. Boundary conditions are set between model type regions such that a continuity of mapping is ensured across the image. Examples of such algorithms are the Combination MultiQuadric (C-MTQ), Sect. 3.2, the three component Finite Element (3C-FEM), Sect. 3.1, and a version of the modified fluid 2 (MF2), Sect. 4.2. In the case of 3C-FEM and MF2, the updating of nodal displacements or of pixel velocities is prohibited within selected areas. This is an easy and effective method of ensuring that these regions remain rigid; additionally they remain *motionless*.

We define here the concept of a rigid body within the deforming source, together with two paradigms of a rigid region.

Definition 3. *A region $\Theta \subset \Omega$ is said to be* rigid *within a non-linear deformation of source $S(\Omega)$ to target $T(\Omega)$ if the transformation $u(\Theta)$ is linear.*

Definition 4. *A region $\Theta \subset \Omega$ is said to be* motionless *if $\forall x \in \Theta$, the transformation $u(x) = 0$. Where the registration $S(u(\Omega, t)) \rightarrow T(\Omega)$ is a function of time, Θ is motionless if $\frac{\partial}{\partial t} u(\Theta, t) = 0 \ \forall x \in \Theta, \forall t$ and if $u(\Theta, 0) = 0$.*

It may be desirable to have rigid but *independently-moving* regions:

Definition 5. *A region $\Theta \subset \Omega$ is said to be* independently-moving *if $\forall x \in \Theta$, the transformation $u(x, t) = c(x, t)$ is a non-zero linear function of x where $c(x_i) = c(x_j) \ \forall x_i, x_j \in \Theta$ at any time t and where $\exists x \in \Omega, x \notin \Theta$ such that $u(x, t) \neq c(x, t)$ satisfies the regularisation of a likelihood and prior.*

The main application of such algorithms will be in the modelling of movement of hard and soft tissue during surgery.

3 Review of Inhomogeneous Registration Methods

3.1 Three-component Finite Element Model (3C-FEM)

[5] gives a finite-element model based on three tissue types, labelled rigid, deformable and 'fluid'. The deformations are driven by user-supplied landmark displacements and deformations of the deformable regions are constrained by three energy terms:

$$E_{\text{tension}}(N_i, N_j) = \left| N_j - N_i - N_{ij}^0 \right|^2$$

$$E_{\text{stiffness}}(N_i, N_j, N_k) = \left| N_j + N_k - 2N_i \right|^2$$

$$E_{\text{fold}}(N_k, N_l, N_m) = \begin{cases} \frac{A^2}{\gamma^2 A_0^2} + \frac{\gamma^2 A_0^2}{A^2} & \text{if } \frac{A}{A_0} \leq \gamma \\ 2 & \text{otherwise} \end{cases}$$

where N_{ij}^0 is the original distance between the nodes N_i and N_j and the nodes N_i, N_j and N_k are collinear before deformation; nodes N_k, N_l and N_m form a triangle with initial area A_0 and deformed area A and γ is a threshold of triangular area reduction. The 'fluid' deformations are constrained only by E_{fold} which prevents folding of the image. Rigid regions are obtained by prohibiting the updating of their nodal displacements.

3.2 Combination Multiquadric Spline (C-MTQ)

Little *et. al.* [6] have constructed a variant of the landmark spline, incorporating regions which undergo independent linear transformations only. The method is applied to pre-segmented images, with regions classified as hard or soft tissue. The hard tissue regions form a set $\mathcal{O}$ of n rigid bodies $\{O_i\}$ such that $\mathcal{O} = \bigcup_{i=1}^{n} O_i$, where one body O_i, can consist of separate parts (all undergoing the same linear transformation) but no two bodies may overlap. The method uses a distance transform to weight differently the linear and non-linear components of the overall image mapping, such that the non-linear terms are smoothly reduced to zero as the rigid bodies are approached, and each rigid body is constrained to its own linear mapping while contributing to the underlying linear drift of the non-rigid areas.

3.3   Elastic Registration with Variable Elasticity

Davatzikos [4] presents an elastic registration model applied to images of the head where the elasticity parameters vary spatially within the image. The deformation is driven by distances between parametrically-defined pre-segmented cortical and ventricular surfaces in the source and target, and also incorporates a pre-strained elasticity term. The latter allows for voluntary growth in specified image areas, for example to model the growth of a tumour.

First the brain tissue is segmented from the images and a deformable surface is applied to the source and target brain volumes, giving for each a parametric description of the shape of the outer cortical surface. At each point on the ventricular surface in the deforming source, a force is computed from the distance to the nearest point on the boundary of the target ventricular surface, weighted by the scalar product of outward normals at these points. These ventricular forces together with cortical forces derived from matching cortical surfaces by curvature measures provide a total external driving force field f which is supplied to the *variable-elasticity* equation:

$$\{f + \lambda \nabla^2 u + (\lambda + \mu)\nabla(\nabla \cdot u)\}+$$
$$\{(\nabla u + (\nabla u)^T - 2\bar{\bar{I}})\nabla\lambda + (\nabla \cdot u - 3)\nabla\mu\}+$$
$$\{\epsilon(2\nabla\lambda + 3\nabla\mu) + (2\lambda + 3\mu)\nabla\epsilon\} = 0. \qquad (3)$$

The first bracketed term is the regularisation between driving forces f and the elasticity constraints on the displacements vector $u(x)$. The second contains gradients in the elasticity parameters λ and μ, allowing variation in the elasticity field. ventricular and cortical surface regions are set lower elasticity values, allowing for greater ease of deformation. The third term contains gradients in a parameter ϵ determining an additional strain tensor $\bar{\bar{E}}_0 = \epsilon(x)\bar{\bar{I}}$ which forces extra expansion or contraction in pre-selected regions. Hence the algorithm also contains inhomogeneities in activity, or data influence.

4   Modifications to the Viscous Fluid Registration Model

The fluid PDE is summarised by

$$\nabla \cdot \bar{\bar{\sigma}} + f = 0 \qquad (4)$$

where f is the driving force and $\bar{\bar{\sigma}}$ is the stress tensor, given by

$$\bar{\bar{\sigma}} = -p\bar{\bar{I}} + \mu\left(\nabla v + (\nabla v)^T\right) \qquad (5)$$

where v is the velocity field, p is a pressure term and μ is the viscosity parameter.

We now describe methods of introducing inhomogeneities into the application of the fluid algorithm [7] such that deformation is reduced or prohibited in areas specified as *passive*, *motionless* or *weakly deformable*. They are intended for use with prior estimates of the rigidity or cross-population variability of different tissue structures identified in a rough initial segmentation.

4.1   Modified Fluid 1 (MF1)

MF1 utilises prior knowledge of regions whose intensity information we do not wish to contribute to driving the registration. These regions will be *passive* in the registration. A binary array is provided whose pixels, corresponding to those in the source, are flagged as passive or active. It is subjected to the same deformations as the source image and is supplied to a Euclidean Distance Transform (EDT) which specifies the distance x from the passive regions. At each timestep in the fluid algorithm, forces at each pixel in the source are computed as in [8] from source-target intensity differences and from intensity gradients in the source. Prior to solution of the PDE, the forces are multiplied by the weighting function (6), which smoothly reduces them to zero in the neighbourhood of the passive regions.

$$
w(x; a, b) = \begin{cases} 0 & : \quad x \leq a \\ \frac{1}{2}\left(1 - \cos\left(\frac{\pi(x - a)}{b - a}\right)\right) & : \quad a < x < b \\ 1 & : \quad x \geq b. \end{cases} \tag{6}
$$

with a = 2, We used $a = 1$ and $b = 13$ and found the 4SED algorithm [9] to be an adequate approximation to the Euclidean distance.

4.2   Modified Fluid 2 (MF2)

This method allows for specified regions to remain rigid by prohibiting their pixel movements. A binary array, labelling pixels as either *motionless* or *mobile*, is passed as extra boundary conditions to the SOR function solving the fluid PDE in each timestep. Only velocities at mobile pixel locations are updated; those labelled motionless remain at zero velocity.

4.3   Modified Fluid 3 (MF3)

The third modification varies the viscosity parameter μ spatially over the image. We expand (4), ignoring p, to give the PDE for the variable viscosity fluid model:

$$
(\nabla\mu \cdot \nabla)v + \frac{\partial\mu}{\partial x_j}\nabla v_j + \mu\nabla^2 v + \mu\nabla(\nabla \cdot v) + f = 0. \tag{7}
$$

Since the partial differential operator now varies over the image, a fast solution by a basis function expansion or by convolution with filters derived from its Green's functions [10] is no longer possible; instead we use the successive over-relaxation (SOR) iterative method [11].

5   Results

5.1   Synthetic Labelled Images

We created a set of 4 artificial images of size 256×256, labelled *house, clown, house2* and *clown2*, illustrated in Fig. 1. All 4 contain 5 corresponding structures:

roof (hat) of intensity 87; shadow (hair) of intensity 39; wall (face) of intensity 127; windows (eyes and mouth) of intensity 215; and background of intensity 255.

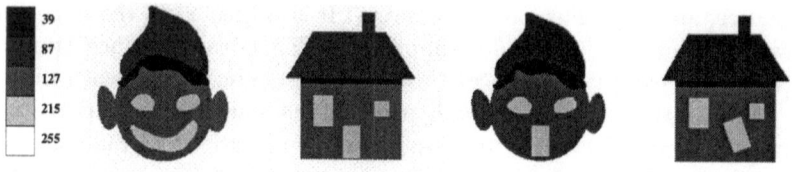

Fig. 1. Artificial images: (*left–right*) clown, house, clown2, house2

We applied unmodified (UF) and modified (MF1–3) fluid to register the house to the clown images, with the house door defined as normal, weakly-deformable, passive or motionless to compare the ability of the algorithms to reduce or prohibit deformation. Figures 2 and 3 show the results.

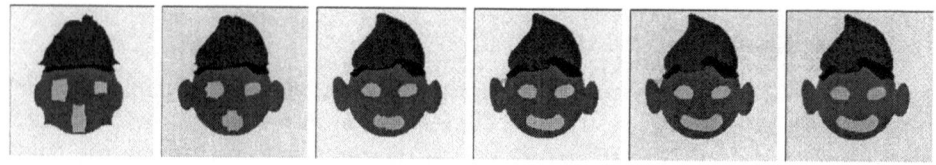

Fig. 2. Progress of the UF registration of house to clown image

To measure the deformation of the door, we applied to a grid image the same deformation as that of the source, and noted the locations of gridpoints in the door region before and after registration. For each registration, we inserted these into a thin-plate spline and computed its bending energy as given by [7]. The results were: UF (target: clown) 1.018; MF3 (target: clown) 0.065; MF3 (target: clown2) 0.058; MF1 (target: clown2) 0.045; MF2 (target: clown2) 0. Fig. 3 (bottom) shows the final deformations of the door regions in the grids.

5.2   Pre/post-operative Head Images, Rigid Scalp

The next exercise attempted to reduce deformation at an area where source-target differences are known a priori in order to highlight other areas where there are unknown differences due to abnormalities. The target and source were coronal slices of a pre-/post-operative data set exhibiting hydracephalous and coning, Fig. 4. Since these are slices through the same subject at approximately, but not exactly, the same location, they exhibit slight differences in scalp shape. To some

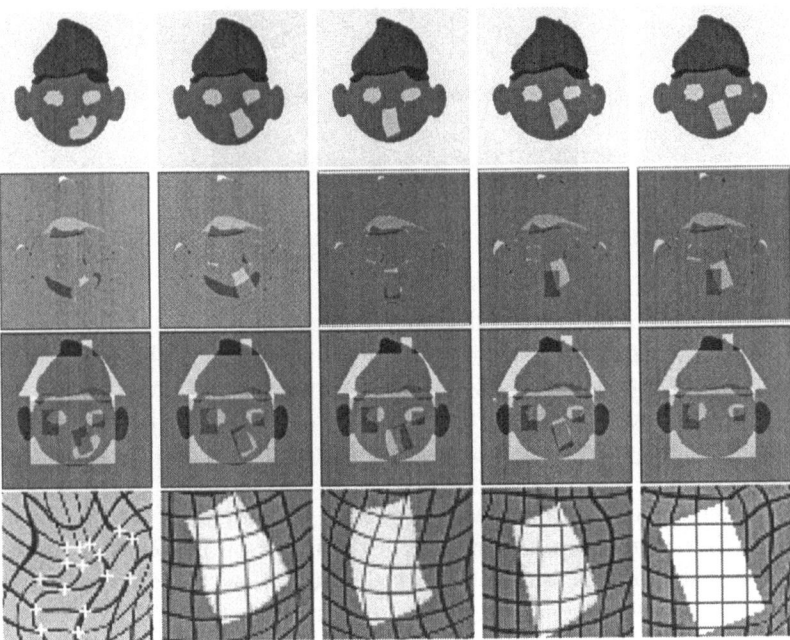

Fig. 3. Registration of S = house2 to T = clown/clown2, restricting deformation of the door. (*Columns, left–right*): UF (T = clown); MF3 (T = clown); MF3 (T = clown2); MF1 (T = clown2); MF2 (T = clown2). (*Rows, top–bottom*): Deformed S; T - deformed S; original S - deformed S; door regions of corresponding deformed grids

extent the same applies to the cortex and internal brain structures; however the main cause of their source-target differences was the surgical procedure and its after-effects. It is these differences which were to be highlighted as abnormal.

We compared registration by the UF, by MF3 and by MF2.

The target (pre-operative) image was used as an atlas, defining the normal brain shape for that subject. The scalp region was segmented manually with the aid of the display tool `xdispunc` developed by Dave Plummer of UCH Medical Physics. This prior information of known 'abnormal' scalp shape was supplied as a binary image indicating the region where deformation was to be reduced. Five sets of images were generated for each registration:

1. the deformed source image, $S(\boldsymbol{u})$ after registration to the target T.
2. the same deformation applied to a regular grid image, $G(\boldsymbol{u})$. The ideal inhomogeneous registration paradigm would exhibit no deformation in $G(\boldsymbol{u})$ in the scalp region (painted white on the grid prior to deformation).
3. local magnitudes of the resulting displacements field and local Laplacian, bending and elasticity energy metrics [12], to highlight regions of severe distortion of the source image from the normal brain shape.

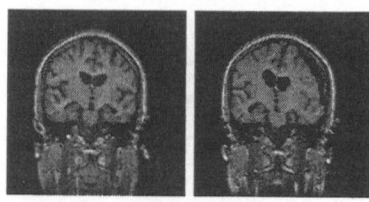

Fig. 4. Data set of (*left*) head4A and (*right*) head4B

4. the difference of the deformed source from the *undeformed source*, $S - S(u)$. Assuming registration to the target is optimal in regions where no prior information was supplied, this gives a further indication of abnormality, defined as shape difference from the target. (Known) differences in the scalp region are not highlighted if its registration to the target has been successfully suppressed.
5. the difference of the deformed source from the target, $T - S(u)$. This is to check that registration is complete in the unknown regions and suppressed in the scalp. In this case, for an ideal registration, the difference image is zero in unknown regions and non-zero in the scalp region.

The results are shown in Fig. 5. Of the three registrations, in $S - S(u)$, MF2 with motionless scalp is the clearest at highlighting only the differences in the ventricular and left-cortical areas, (Fig. 5, bottom row, far right). By inspecting the grid lines in the white regions of $G(u)$ (Fig. 5, bottom row centre left) we see it has respected the rigidity of the scalp. Finally, to check completeness of registration, Fig. 5, (bottom row centre right) shows good registration in the brain region (the difference image shows little structure) and poor registration at the scalp. In comparison, MF3 allowed the scalp to distort, shown in the grid image (Fig. 5, centre row, centre left), leaving less structure in the scalp region of $T - S(u)$ (Fig. 5, centre row, centre right); hence the known scalp shape difference shows up as an abnormality in $S - S(u)$ (Fig. 5, centre row, far right).

5.3   3D Results - Neck Images

3-dimensional versions of UF and MF3 were compared on MRI neck volumes with the vertebrae defined as weakly deformable. The original images were acquired at the Hammersmith hospital[1]. Two full-3D neck volumes were provided, neckDand neckI. NeckI was of the chin down and neckD was with the head flexed backwards within the confines of the scanner bore. Both were of the same subject. Since the imaging field of view had been the spinal column specifically, the

---

[1] The scanner was a Picker 1.0T HPQ. The acquisitions were RF spoiled volume scans with TR = 42, TE = 7, 192 x 255 matrix, 1 Nex 30 cm FoV, 38 x 2 mm slices. The final images were Fourier interpolated to a 256 x 256 matrix. A c-spin quadrature surface coil was used for reception. All 3 volumes were 16-bit, of dimension $256 \times 256 \times 38$, with the neck vertebrae as the field of view; pixel dimensions were $1.17188 \times 1.17188 \times 2$.

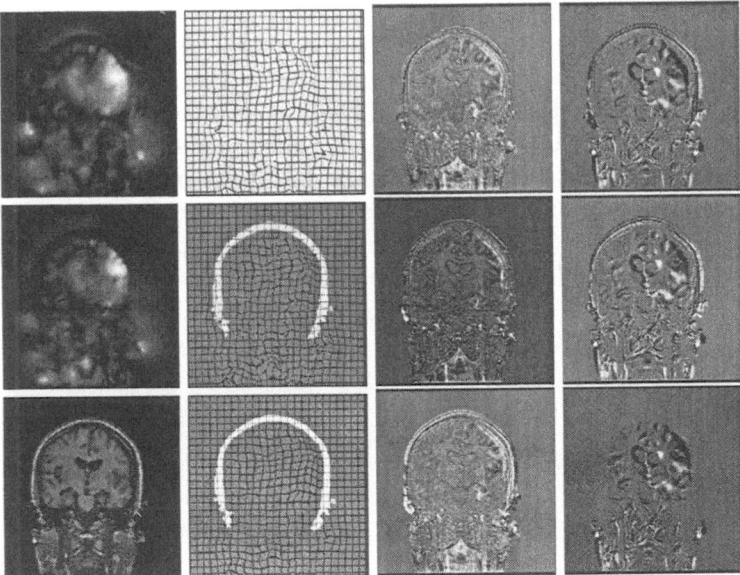

Fig. 5. Results of registering source S = head4B to target T = head4A. (*Rows, top–bottom*): UF; MF3; MF2. (*Columns, left–right*): deformed S, S(u); deformation applied to grid, G(u); T - S(u), showing completeness of registration; S - S(u), highlighting differences due to the deformation (*right 2 columns are contrast-enhanced*)

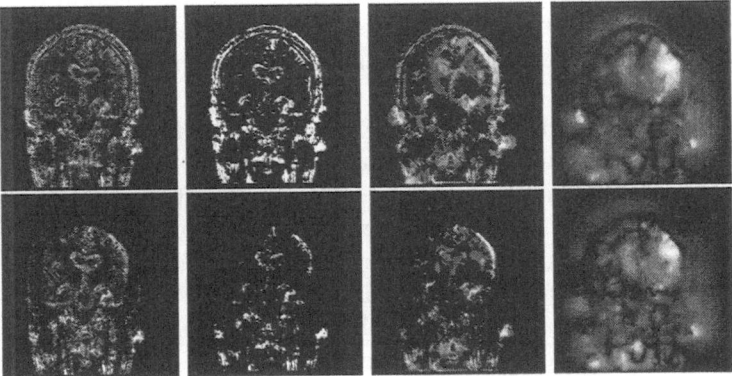

Fig. 6. Deformation metrics (*left–right*): Laplacian, bending, elastic, magnitude of transformation, of the registration by (*top*) UF and (*bottom*) MF3

volumes did not extend to include the whole neck laterally. The images exhibited a strong intensity ramp, with high values at the back of the neck and total
signal loss in the face. We pre-processed the images to give a more uniform range
of intensities in the anterior-posterior direction, using the scheme described by
Fig. 7. Due to memory capacity and time constraints, it was not feasible to
apply the fluid registrations directly to the full-resolution data sets; hence they
were downsampled, by blurring with a Gaussian of standard deviation $\sigma = 2$ and
storing alternate pixels (Fig. 7, right). Since the Gaussian blurring for downsam-
pling, and intensity gradient calculations during registration, were performed in
the Fourier domain and required image dimensions of powers of two, we used
zero padding to give full resolution dimensions $256 \times 256 \times 64$ and downsampled
volumes of $128 \times 128 \times 32$.

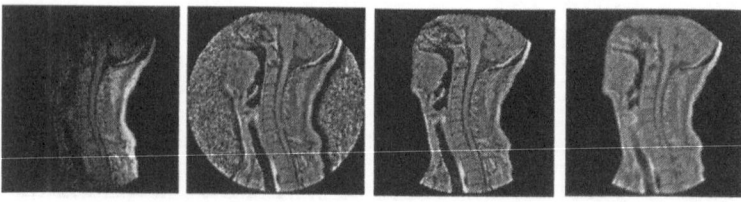

Fig. 7. Pre-processing stages shown on neckD. (*left–right*): slice 19 of the original 3D
$256 \times 256 \times 38$ volume; after division pixelwise by the same image blurred with a
Gaussian of spatial standard deviation $\sigma = 5$; masked with the aid of the automatic
contouring and manual alteration tool in xdispunc; downsampled by a half

We segmented the spinal vertebrae slice-by-slice from the full-resolution source
volumes using the xdispunc display tools. The contrast between vertebrae and
intervening tissue was variable and so segmentation was performed manually
with reference to an atlas [13]. The segmentations were converted to binary
spine volumes which were then downsampled using the same process as for the
necks.

Both fluid registration tests (UF, MF3) were applied in a six-level scale space
(Gaussian blurs of spatial standard deviation $2i$ with $i = \{5, 4, 3, 2, 1, 0\}$). Within
each scale level, the fluid was set to iterate through at least three timesteps,
with an optional extra 100 timesteps until the stopping criterion was met, the
stopping criterion being a reduction in correlation coefficient of less than 10^{-4}.
On termination, we upsampled the displacement fields obtained from both fluid
registrations of neckD to neckI and applied them to the original neckD images,
to give full-resolution deformations. These are shown in Fig. 8 (top, centre).

We applied the transformation fields produced by both fluid tests to the intial
spine volumes segmented from neckD; the results of the volume-rendered spines
are shown from two angles in Fig. 9. The UF registration shows an extension of
the upper two vertebrae of the spines on comparison to the original segmentation
from neckD (Fig. 9 far right).

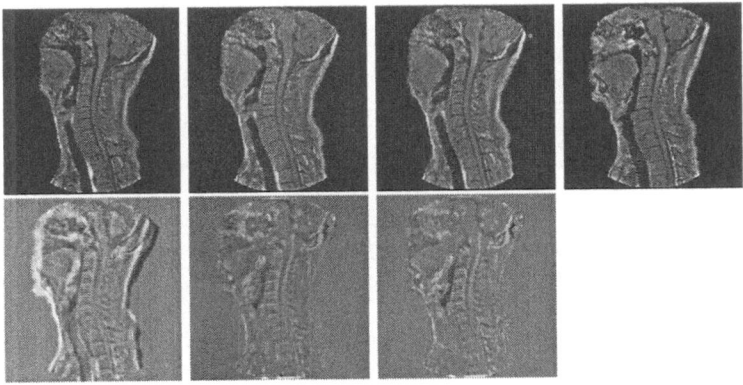

Fig. 8. (*top*) Central slices of full resolution neckD (*left*) and neckI (*right*). (*centre-left*) UF and (*centre-right*) MF3 registration of neckD to neckI. (*bottom*) Central slices of (*left to right:*) neckD - neckI; UF neckD - neckI; MF3 fluid neckD - neckI

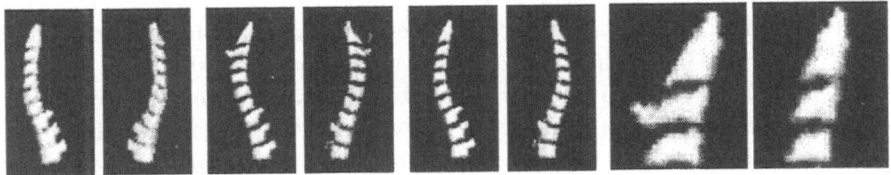

Fig. 9. (*left–right*) original spineD; spineD after UF registration of neckD to neckI; spineD after MF3 registration of neckD to neckI with vertebrae weakly deformable; (*far right*): the upper three vertebrae after (*left*) UF and (*right*) MF3 registration. The 3D images were volume-rendered using the Analyze package

Figure 10 shows logs of the Laplacian and elasticity energies as local deformation metrics computed from the displacements of both registrations of neckD to neckI. The deformation metrics clearly show dark patches in the vertebrae in MF3 indicating low distortion: compare Fig. 10 (*left*) with those of the UF (Fig. 10 right).

5.4   Computational Time

Solution of the fluid PDE in the spatial domain using finite differencing and relaxation is slow. We restricted the upper limit of the number of SOR iterations within each timestep to 4000^2 in the 2D case and to 50 in the 3D case. This provided a compromise between speed and accurate solution of the PDE, since within each timestep computation of velocities is approximate and is improved on in the next timestep. For images sized 32×128^2, 50 SOR iterations took 2 minutes 36 seconds for the constant-viscosity fluid on a Sun UltraSPARC -

---

[2] generally around 1300 were sufficient for the norms calculated from the residuals to drop to less than 0.1% of those calculated at the start of each iteration cycle.

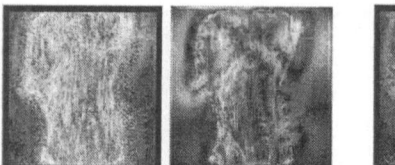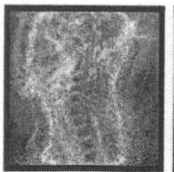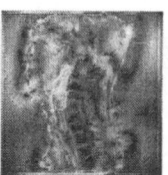

Fig. 10. Central slices of the deformation metric images, after registration of neckD to neckI (*left*) log of Laplacian, UF; (*centre left*) log of elasticity energy, UF; (*centre right and far right*) the equivalent for MF3

equivalent to 416 minutes for 4000 iterations for a 64×128^2 image. [14] have implemented full-multigrid (FMG) solution of the same PDE applied to the displacement field for elastic registration; they estimate 6,592 Jacobi relaxation iterations for a 64×128^2 grid. For a grid sized $J \times J$, SOR requires $\frac{2}{3J}$ the number of iterations compared to Jacobi relaxation [15]. [14] show that two 3D FMG cycles are sufficient for a 64×128^2 grid to solve the elasticity PDE per iteration, giving 20 minutes per iteration. Hence we estimate that replacing SOR with FMG would speed the fluid registration by a factor of 20.

MF1 additionally multiplies each pixel by (6) once per timestep, a minimal overhead compared to the SOR iterations. MF2 provides a considerable gain in speed over UF, depending on the volume percentage of rigid bodies(pixels whose velocities are not computed). The percentage of passive regions in the image is equal to the percentage speed-up in the SOR solution. For MF3, extra finite differencing computations are added to the SOR due to the extra terms in (7); we timed 3 minutes 47 seconds for 50 SOR iterations for images sized 32×128^2.

6   Conclusions and Discussion

We have presented a new fluid deformation algorithm with variable viscosity for the registration of images containing structures with variable deformability. Results show the algorithm reduces the deformation of selected regions. The hierarchical strategy (registration within Gaussian scale space) was not optimal for the 3D case since it preferred initial registration at the strongest boundaries which were the (non-homologous) outer boundaries. We suggest instead a model-based hierarchy, using initial registration by an (automated) C-MTQ with rigid vertebrae, followed by MF3 for more localised deformations.

Inhomogeneities in deformability can be extended to include *anisotropies* in the constraint parameters, such that there are preferential *directions* of deformation. Anisotropies in ease of deformation are common in physical tissue such as muscle. Adapting the mathematical representation of the deformation of a physical medium to allow anisotropies is more complex than only allowing for isotropic inhomogeneities; we leave such a possibility for future research. Another possible amendment to the fluid registration is to supply pre-determined uniform and constant but non-zero velocities within regions defined as *independently moving* to allow rigid-body transformations within an overall fluid deformation.

Acknowledgements

Hava Lester was supported by the Engineering and Physical Sciences Research Council. We thank the anonymous reviewers for their helpful criticisms.

References

1. Hava, L. and Arridge, S.R.: A survey of hierarchical non-linear medical image registration. *Pattern Recognition*, 32(1):129–149, January 1999.
2. Gee, J.C., Le Briquer, L., Barrilot, C., Haynor, D.R. and Bajcsy, R.: Bayesian approach to the brain image matching problem. In *SPIE Medical Imaging 1995*, San Diego, 1995.
3. Manduca, A., Muthupillai, R., Rossman, P.J., Greenleaf, J.F., and Ehman, R.L.. Visualization of tissue elasticity by magnetic resonance elastography. In Karl Heinz Hohne and Ron Kikinis, editors, *Visualization in Biomedical Computing*. Springer, 1996.
4. Davatzikos, C.: Spatial transformation and registration of brain images using elastically deformable models. *Computer Vision and Image Understanding*, 66(2):207–222, May 1997.
5. Edwards, P.J., Hill, D.L.G., and Hawkes, D.J.: Image guided interventions using a three component tissue deformation model. In *Medical Image Understanding and Analysis*, Oxford, UK, July 1997.
6. Little, J.A., Hill, D.L.G., and Hawkes, D.J.: Deformations incorporating rigid structures. *Computer Vision and Image Understanding*, 66(2):223–232, May 1997.
7. Bookstein, F.L.: Principal warps: Thin-plate splines and the decomposition of deformations. *IEEE Transactions on Pattern Analysis and Machine Intelligence*, 11(6):567–585, June 1989.
8. Christensen, G.E., Rabbitt, R.D., Miller, M.I., Joshi, S.C., Grenander, U., Coogan, T.A., and van Essen, D.C.: Topological properties of smooth anatomic maps. In Y Bizais et al., editors, *Information Processing in Medical Imaging*, pages 101–112. Kluwer Academic Publishers, 1995.
9. Danielsson, P.-E.: Euclidean distance mapping. *Computer Graphics and Image Processing*, 14:227–248, 1980.
10. Bro-Nielsen, M. and Gramkow, C.: Fast fluid registration of medical images. In *SPIE Medical Imaging*, pages 267–276, 1996.
11. Strikwerda, J.C.: *Finite Difference Schemes and Partial Differential Equations*, chapter 13: Linear Iterative Methods. Wadsworth and Brooks, 1989.
12. Lester, H., Arridge, S.R., and Jansons, K.M.: Local deformation metrics and non-linear registration using a fluid model with variable viscosity. In *Proceedings of Medical Image Understanding and Analysis (MIUA98)*, Leeds, UK, July 1998.
13. McMinn, R.H.M, Hutchings, R.T., and Logan, B.M.: *Color Atlas of Head and Neck Anatomy*. Mosby-Wolfe, London, 2nd edition, 1994.
14. Schormann, T., Henn, S., and Zilles, K.: A new approach to fast elastic alignment with applications to human brains. In *Lecture Notes in Computer Science*, volume 1131, pages 337–342. Springer-Verlag, 1996.
15. Press, W.H., Teukolsky, S.A., Vetterling, W.T., and Flannery, B.P.: *Numerical Recipes in C*. Cambridge University Press, 2nd edition, 1995.

Approximating Thin-Plate Splines for Elastic Registration: Integration of Landmark Errors and Orientation Attributes

Karl Rohr, Mike Fornefett, and H. Siegfried Stiehl

Universität Hamburg, Fachbereich Informatik, Arbeitsbereich Kognitive Systeme
Vogt-Kölln-Str. 30, D-22527 Hamburg, Germany
rohr@informatik.uni-hamburg.de

Abstract. We introduce an approach to elastic registration of tomo-graphic images based on thin-plate splines. Central to this scheme is a well-defined minimizing functional for which the solution can be stated analytically. In this work, we consider the integration of anisotropic land-mark errors as well as additional attributes at landmarks. As attributes we use orientations at landmarks and we incorporate the corresponding constraints through scalar products. With our approximation scheme it is thus possible to integrate statistical as well as geometric information as additional knowledge in elastic image registration. On the basis of syn-thetic as well as real tomographic images we show that this additional knowledge can significantly improve the registration result. In particu-lar, we demonstrate that our scheme incorporating orientation attributes can preserve the shape of rigid structures (such as bone) embedded in an otherwise elastic material. This is achieved without selecting further landmarks and without a full segmentation of the rigid structures.

1 Introduction

Image registration based on point landmarks plays a major role in, e.g., neuro-surgery planning and intraoperative navigation. While rigid and affine schemes can only describe global geometric differences between images, elastic schemes can additionally cope with local differences. Reasons for local geometric differ-ences are different anatomy (or pathology), scanner- or patient-induced distor-tions, as well as intraoperative deformations due to surgical interventions.

The most widely applied method for point-based elastic image registration is based on thin-plate splines. This approach has been introduced into medical image analysis by Bookstein [2]. Evans *et al.* [9] applied this scheme to 3D med-ical images. Thin-plate splines have a physical motivation, are mathematically well-founded, and are moreover computationally efficient. Alternative splines based on the Navier equation, which have been named elastic body splines, have recently been introduced by Davis *et al.* [7]. Extensions of point-based elastic schemes which allow to include additional attributes at landmarks have been proposed by Bookstein and Green [5] and Mardia and Little [11]. The combina-tion of thin-plate splines with mutual information as similarity measure for the

A. Kuba et al. (Eds.): IPMI'99, LNCS 1613, pp. 252–265, 1999.

purpose of refining initially coarsely specified landmarks has been proposed by Meyer *et al.* [16].

In all of these approaches from above the interpolation case has been treated. This means that corresponding landmarks are forced to match exactly and thus it is (implicitly) assumed that the landmark positions are known exactly. This assumption, however, is unrealistic since landmark extraction is always prone to error. Approximation schemes, on the other hand, allow to incorporate landmark errors. The error information is used to control the influence of the landmarks on the registration result, which is important in clinical applications. Also, the resulting computational scheme is more robust in comparison to an interpolation approach. However, it seems that approximation schemes have so far not been a focus of research (but see Bookstein [3], Rohr *et al.* [17], and Christensen *et al.* [6] for exceptions). A more detailed discussion of these schemes is given in Section 2 below.

This contribution is concerned with an approximation scheme for point-based elastic image registration using thin-plate splines. Central to this scheme is a well-defined minimizing functional for which the solution can be stated analytically. Therefore, we yield an efficient computational scheme for determining the transformation between two images. In earlier work, we have introduced an approach that allows to incorporate isotropic as well as anisotropic landmark errors and we have proposed a scheme for estimating landmark localization uncertainties directly from the image data (Rohr *et al.* [17,19]). In this contribution, we suggest a generalization of our work which allows to integrate additional attributes at point landmarks. By this, additional knowledge is used to further improve the registration result without the necessity of specifying additional landmarks. In our case, we consider orientation attributes at corresponding points. Generally, these attributes characterize the local orientation of the contours at the landmarks. In previous work on the incorporation of additional attributes, Bookstein and Green [5] have represented orientations by additional points close to the landmarks, thus they used a finite difference scheme. Mardia and Little [11] have proposed a scheme based on the method of kriging where exact orientations are incorporated. Their scheme requires the orientation vectors to be unit vectors. This imposes constraints which may not be desired. The approach we propose also includes exact orientations, however, in comparison to [11] the orientation vectors need not to be normalized to unit vectors. This is achieved by representing the constraints due to the orientations through scalar products. Additionally, we treat the interpolation as well as the approximation case. In particular, we propose a combined scheme that integrates isotropic as well as anisotropic errors together with orientation attributes. Also, we extend the domain of application of our scheme to the important case of preserving rigid structures (such as bone) embedded in an otherwise elastic material. It seems that this application has so far not gained much attention in previous work on point-based registration using attributes (but see Mardia and Little [11]). In comparison to other schemes such as Little *et al.* [14] a full segmentation of the rigid structures is not necessary for our approach.

The remainder of this contribution is organized as follows. In the next section, we discuss in more detail related work on approximation schemes for point-based nonrigid image registration. Then, we describe our approach based on thin-plate splines which integrates anisotropic landmark errors and orientation attributes. The applicability of the approach is demonstrated for synthetic data as well as real tomographic images of the human brain.

2   Related Work

In this section, we discuss approximation schemes for point-based nonrigid image registration. For other approaches to medical image registration we refer to a recent review by Maintz and Viergever [15].

In [3], Bookstein proposed an approach to relaxing the original interpolating thin-plate spline approach [2] by straightforward combination of different energy terms, where one term represents the bending energy of interpolating thin-plate splines and the other the distance of the landmark configurations (note, that in total four different energy terms have been proposed which may be combined). The basis of the approach is a linear regression model and the technique is referred to as 'curve décolletage' (Leamer [13]). With this approach it is possible to incorporate isotropic and anisotropic errors. However, since the approach has not been related to a minimizing functional w.r.t. the searched transformation it is generally not clear whether all solutions in the whole function space are obtained. The approach has been described for 2D datasets and experimental results have been reported for 2D synthetic data. The landmarks as well as the corresponding errors have been specified manually.

In [17], we have introduced approximating thin-plate splines for elastic image registration. Our approach is based on the mathematical work of Duchon [8] and Wahba [21] which is a different mathematical framework in comparison to that in Bookstein [3]. The basis is a minimizing functional w.r.t. the searched transformation. The solution in the whole function space can be shown to be unique and can be stated analytically. While in [17] we have treated the case of isotropic errors, in [18,19] we have recently incorporated anisotropic errors for the landmarks in both of the images to be registered. Also, we have proposed to estimate the landmark localization uncertainties directly from the image data utilizing the Cramér-Rao bound (see [19]). The approach has been applied to 2D as well as 3D tomographic images of the human brain and the landmarks have been localized semi-automatically using differential operators.

Recently, Christensen et al. [6] introduced a hierarchical approach to image registration combining a landmark-based scheme with an intensity-based approach using a fluid model. The landmark scheme is based on the linear elasticity operator, thus the resulting splines are different from thin-plate splines. Another difference to our approach is that the nonaffine part of the transformation is separated from the affine part in their functional. The approach has been applied to the registration of 3D cryosection data of a macaque monkey brain as well to MR images of the human brain. Isotropic landmark errors have been included in one of the two images to be registered. Since no further details have been given on how the errors have been determined, it seems that equal isotropic errors have been used in their application.

As already mentioned above, Bookstein and Green [5] as well as Mardia and Little [11] introduced nonrigid registration schemes incorporating orientation attributes. These schemes are based on a finite difference scheme and the method of kriging, resp. In both of these works the interpolation case has been treated only, although a generalization to approximation is principally possible.

3   Thin-Plate Splines with Landmark Errors and Additional Attributes

We now describe our approach to elastic image registration based on thin-plate splines. This approach incorporates landmark errors as well as orientation attributes at landmarks. While the landmark errors represent statistical information about the uncertainty of landmark localization, the orientation attributes represent geometric information about the contours at the landmarks. Below, we first briefly review our scheme incorporating anisotropic landmark errors and then describe an extension for incorporating orientation attributes.

3.1   Anisotropic Landmark Errors

We denote the sets of landmarks in two images by $\mathbf{p}_i$ and $\mathbf{q}_i$, $i = 1 \ldots n$, and the transformation that maps two images by $\mathbf{u}$ with components $u_k, k = 1 \ldots d$, where d is the image dimension. The bending energy of thin-plate splines can be written as a function of the order m of derivatives in the functional as well as the image dimension d as

$$J_m^d(\mathbf{u}) = \sum_{k=1}^{d} J_m^d(u_k), \tag{1}$$

where

$$J_m^d(u_k) = \sum_{\alpha_1 + \ldots + \alpha_d = m} \frac{m!}{\alpha_1! \cdots \alpha_d!} \int_{\mathbb{R}^d} \left(\frac{\partial^m u_k}{\partial x_1^{\alpha_1} \cdots \partial x_d^{\alpha_d}} \right)^2 dx \tag{2}$$

according to Duchon [8], Wahba [21]. Under the necessary and sufficient condition of $2m - d > 0$ the functional is bounded.

Anisotropic landmark errors are represented by covariance matrices $\mathbf{\Sigma}_i$. In this case the minimizing functional reads as

$$J_\lambda(\mathbf{u}) = \frac{1}{n} \sum_{i=1}^{n} (\mathbf{q}_i - \mathbf{u}(\mathbf{p}_i))^T \mathbf{\Sigma}_i^{-1}(\mathbf{q}_i - \mathbf{u}(\mathbf{p}_i)) + \lambda J_m^d(\mathbf{u}) \tag{3}$$

and consists of two terms (see Rohr et al. [18,19]). The first term measures the distance between the two landmark sets weighted by the covariance matrices

Σ_i. The second term represents the smoothness of the transformation, and the parameter λ weights the two terms. Special cases of this approximation scheme are interpolating thin-plate splines and optimal affine transformations. The approach is applicable to arbitrary image dimensions d, e.g., 2D and 3D images. For the functional in (3) there exists a unique analytic solution, which can be stated as

$$u_k(\mathbf{x}) = \sum_{\nu=1}^{M} a_{k,\nu}\phi_\nu(\mathbf{x}) + \sum_{i=1}^{n} w_{k,i}U(\mathbf{x}, \mathbf{p}_i), \qquad k = 1, ..., d, \qquad (4)$$

with monomials ϕ up to order $m - 1$ and suitable radial basis functions U (see Wahba [21,22], Wang [23]). The coefficients $\mathbf{a} = (\mathbf{a}_1^T, ..., \mathbf{a}_M^T)^T$, $\mathbf{a}_i^T = (a_{1,i}, ..., a_{d,i})$, and $\mathbf{w} = (\mathbf{w}_1^T, ..., \mathbf{w}_n^T)^T$, $\mathbf{w}_i^T = (w_{1,i}, ..., w_{d,i})$ of the transformation $\mathbf{u}$ can efficiently be computed through the following system of linear equations:

$$(\mathbf{K} + n\lambda\mathbf{W}^{-1})\mathbf{w} + \mathbf{Pa} = \mathbf{v} \qquad (5)$$
$$\mathbf{P}^T\mathbf{w} = \mathbf{0},$$

where $\mathbf{W}$ represents the landmark errors by $\mathbf{W}^{-1} = \text{diag}\{\Sigma_1, \ldots, \Sigma_n\}$ and is a block-diagonal matrix. The other matrices in (5) are given by $\mathbf{K} = (K_{ij}\mathbf{I}_d)$, where $K_{ij} = U(\mathbf{p}_i, \mathbf{p}_j)$ and $\mathbf{I}_d$ is the $d \times d$ unity matrix, and $\mathbf{P} = (P_{ij}\mathbf{I}_d)$, where $P_{ij} = \phi_j(\mathbf{p}_i)$. The vector $\mathbf{v}$ can be written as $\mathbf{v} = (\mathbf{v}_1^T, ..., \mathbf{v}_n^T)^T$, $\mathbf{v}_i^T = (q_{i,1}, ..., q_{i,d})$.

Note, that our approximation scheme using covariance matrices is also a generalization of the work in Bookstein [4], where the interpolation case is solved while the landmarks are allowed to slip along straight lines within a 2D image. Actually, this is a special case of our approximation scheme since for straight lines the variance in one direction is zero whereas in the perpendicular direction it is infinite.

3.2   Landmark Errors and Orientation Attributes

The approach described above can further be generalized for inclusion of additional attributes at landmarks. In our case, we incorporate orientation attributes. These attributes characterize the local orientation of the contours at the landmarks and represent additional knowledge for elastic image registration.

At corresponding landmarks we assume to have orientations which we want to match (note, that these landmarks are generally a subset of the overall landmarks). We denote those landmarks in the first and second image by $\mathbf{p}_{\theta_i}$ and $\mathbf{q}_{\theta_i}$ and the corresponding orientations by $\mathbf{d}_i$ and $\mathbf{e}_i$, resp. To define a matching criterion between the orientations, we need the transformed vector of $\mathbf{d}_i$. This vector can be stated as $(\mathbf{d}_i^T\nabla)\mathbf{u}(\mathbf{p}_{\theta_i})$. Now we require that this transformed vector is perpendicular to $\mathbf{e}_{i,k}^\perp$, which are the k-th orthogonal vectors to the orientation vector $\mathbf{e}_i$ in the second image. In this case, the scalar product between the vectors is zero, otherwise it is different from zero. Choosing vectors from the orthogonal space has the advantage that the corresponding scalar product is zero independently of the length of the vectors. This is an advantage over the approach in Mardia and Little [11] (see also Mardia *et al.* [12]), where the orientation vectors are required to be unit vectors and where the interpolation case has been treated only. In our work, we both treat the interpolation as well as the approximation case. Note, however, that the property of length independence only holds in the case of interpolation, but not for approximation. In general we have $d-1$ perpendicular orientations $e_{i,k}^{\perp}$ which constrain the orientation of the transformed orientation vector of the first image to lie on a line. If the number of perpendicular orientations is smaller, i.e., the number of constraints is lower, then the orientation of the transformed orientation vector is not constrained w.r.t. a line, but w.r.t. a plane, for example (see also Fornefett *et al.* [10]).

Having defined the matching criterion between orientations we can now state the generalized minimizing functional using $\epsilon_i = q_i - u(p_i)$ as

$$J_{\lambda}(u) = \frac{1}{n} \sum_{i=1}^{n} \epsilon_i^T \Sigma_i^{-1} \epsilon_i + \frac{1}{n_2'} \sum_{i=1}^{n_\theta} \sum_{k=1}^{d-1} \left((d_i^T \nabla) u^T (p_{\theta_i}) e_{i,k}^{\perp} \right)^2 + \lambda J_m^d(u), \quad (6)$$

where $n_2' = n_2/c$, $c > 0$, and $n_2 = n_\theta(d-1)$. In comparison to the functional (3) from above we have an additional term that incorporates the orientation constraints. n_θ is the total number of orientations in each of the images. The parameter c weights the orientation term w.r.t. the term representing the landmark errors and also determines (besides λ) whether we interpolate or approximate the orientations. Note, that we can incorporate an arbitrary number of orientations at each landmark. As described above, the orientation constraints are incorporated by scalar products between the transformed orientations of the first image and orientations perpendicular to the orientations in the second image. The solution to the functional in (6) can be stated as

$$u(x) = \sum_{\nu=1}^{M} \sum_{k=1}^{d} a_{k,\nu} \phi_{\nu}(x) \varepsilon_k + \sum_{i=1}^{n} \sum_{k=1}^{d} w_{1,k,i} U(x, p_i) \varepsilon_k$$
$$- \sum_{i=1}^{n_\theta} \sum_{k=1}^{d-1} w_{2,k,i} (d_i^T \nabla) U(x, p_{\theta_i}) e_{i,k}^{\perp}, \quad (7)$$

with monomials ϕ up to order $m-1$ and radial basis functions U as above. ε_k, $k = 1 \ldots d$, are the canonical basis vectors of the $\mathbb{R}^d$. The solution is analogous to (4) from above, but additionally we have a term that represents the orientation constraints. Note, that in order to obtain bounded functionals the used function space has to be constrained. Choosing $m = 2$ for the order of derivatives of the smoothness term, then for both cases of 2D and 3D images ($d = 2, 3$) incorporating orientations, we have the basis function $U(x) = |x|^3$. The parameter vectors $a = (a_1^T, ..., a_M^T)^T$, $a_i^T = (a_{1,i}, ..., a_{d,i})$, and $w = (w_{1,1}^T, ..., w_{1,n}^T, w_{2,1}^T, ..., w_{2,n_\theta}^T)^T$, $w_{1,i}^T = (w_{1,1,i}, ..., w_{1,d,i})$, $w_{2,i}^T = (w_{2,1,i}, ..., w_{2,d-1,i})$ of the transformation u can be computed by solving the linear system of equations

$$Kw + Pa = v \quad (8)$$
$$P^T w = 0,$$

with

$$\mathbf{K} = \begin{pmatrix} \mathbf{K}_1 + n\lambda\mathbf{W}^{-1} & \mathbf{K}_2 \\ \mathbf{K}_3 & \mathbf{K}_4 + n_2'\lambda\mathbf{I}_{n_2} \end{pmatrix} \quad \text{and} \quad \mathbf{P} = \begin{pmatrix} \mathbf{P}_1 \\ \mathbf{P}_2 \end{pmatrix}, \qquad (9)$$

where $\mathbf{W}^{-1} = \mathrm{diag}\{\boldsymbol{\Sigma}_1, \dots, \boldsymbol{\Sigma}_n\}$ as in (5) and $\mathbf{I}_{n_2}$ is the $n_2 \times n_2$ unity matrix with $n_2 = n_\theta(d-1)$. The other matrices in (9) are given by $\mathbf{K}_1 = (K_{1,ij}\mathbf{I}_d)$, where $K_{1,ij} = U(\mathbf{p}_i, \mathbf{p}_j)$ and $\mathbf{I}_d$ is the $d \times d$ unity matrix; $\mathbf{K}_2 = (K_{2,ij}\mathbf{F}_j)$, where $K_{2,ij} = -(\mathbf{d}_j^T\nabla)U(\mathbf{p}_i, \mathbf{p}_{\theta_j})$, $F_{j,kl} = \boldsymbol{\varepsilon}_k^T\mathbf{e}_{j,l}^\perp$, and $\mathbf{F}_j$ are $d \times (d-1)$ matrices; $\mathbf{K}_3 = \mathbf{K}_2^T$; $\mathbf{K}_4 = (K_{4,ij}\mathbf{E}_{ij})$, where $K_{4,ij} = -(\mathbf{d}_j^T\nabla)(\mathbf{d}_i^T\nabla)U(\mathbf{p}_{\theta_i}, \mathbf{p}_{\theta_j})$, $E_{ij,kl} = (\mathbf{e}_{i,k}^\perp)^T\mathbf{e}_{j,l}^\perp$, and $\mathbf{E}_{ij}$ are $(d-1) \times (d-1)$ matrices; $\mathbf{P}_1 = (P_{1,ij}\mathbf{I}_d)$, where $P_{1,ij} = \phi_j(\mathbf{p}_i)$, and $\mathbf{P}_2 = (P_{2,ij}\mathbf{F}_i^T)$, where $P_{2,ij} = (\mathbf{d}_i^T\nabla)\phi_j(\mathbf{p}_{\theta_i})$. $\mathbf{K}$ and $\mathbf{P}$ are of dimension $n' \times n'$ and $n' \times dM$, resp., with $n' = nd + n_\theta(d-1)$. The vector $\mathbf{v}$ is given by $\mathbf{v} = (\mathbf{v}_1^T, ..., \mathbf{v}_n^T, 0, ..., 0)^T$, $\mathbf{v}_i^T = (q_{i,1}, ..., q_{i,d})$, with n_2 zeros at the end.

4   Experimental Results

We demonstrate the applicability of our approach using synthetic data as well as real tomographic images of the human brain. In the first two experiments we have incorporated either anisotropic landmark errors only or orientation attributes only. For the last two experiments we have integrated both landmark errors (isotropic as well as anisotropic errors) and orientation attributes.

In the first example, we register the 2D MR brain images of different patients displayed in Fig. 1. We have used normal landmarks and quasi-landmarks. The quasi-landmarks have no unique position in comparison to normal landmarks, e.g., arbitrary edge points. The incorporation of quasi-landmarks is important since normal point landmarks are hard to define at the outer parts of the human head. For all landmarks the covariance matrices have been estimated directly from the image data by utilizing the Cramér-Rao bound

$$\boldsymbol{\Sigma}_g = \frac{\sigma_n^2}{m}\mathbf{C}_g^{-1}, \qquad (10)$$

where σ_n^2 denotes the variance of additive white Gaussian image noise, m the number of voxels in a local 3D window, and $\mathbf{C}_g = \overline{\nabla g \, (\nabla g)^T}$ is the averaged dyadic product of the image gradient (Rohr [19], van Trees [20]). Note, that the Gaussian noise model is an approximation and that we assume that the dependence of the noise on the signal can be neglected (but see Abbey et al. [1]). In Fig. 1 the landmark localization uncertainties are represented by error ellipses (note, that the ellipses have been enlarged by a factor of 7 for visualization purposes). It can clearly be seen that for the normal landmarks the localization uncertainty is small in all directions, while for the quasi-landmarks (landmarks no. 9-12) the localization uncertainty is large along the edge but small perpendicular to it. Fig. 2 on the left shows the registration result when using only the normal landmarks for elastic image registration (landmarks no. 1-6 and 8). Here, we have applied our approximating thin-plate spline approach while incorporating isotropic errors and setting $m = d = 2$ in (3). We have transformed

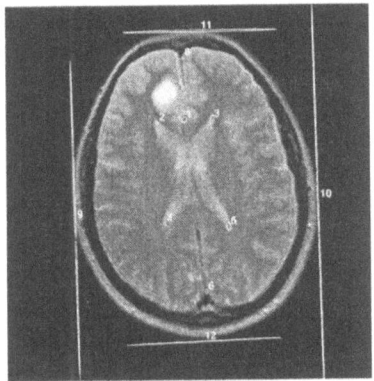 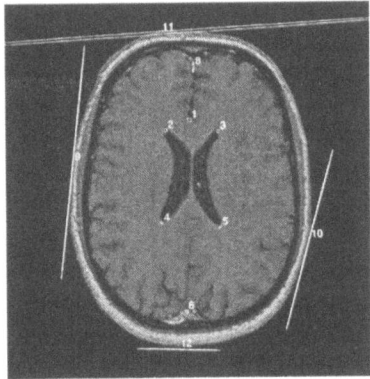

Fig. 1. MR data sets of different patients: normal landmarks, quasi-landmarks, and estimated error ellipses (enlarged by a factor of 7)

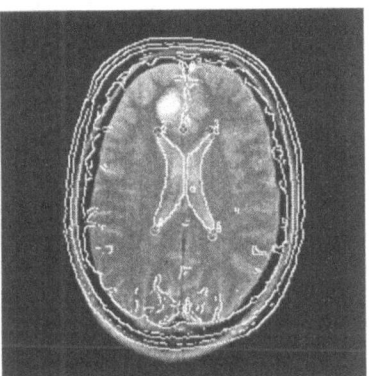 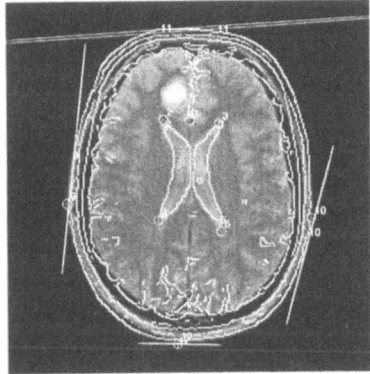

Fig. 2. Registration results: Thin-plate spline approximation using normal landmarks along with equal scalar weights (left), and using normal landmarks, quasi-landmarks and estimated covariance matrices (right)

the first image and have overlayed it onto the computed edges of the second image. While the registration accuracy within the inner parts of the brain is quite good, at the outer parts there are larger errors. If instead we use both the normal landmarks and the quasi-landmarks while incorporating anisotropic errors, then we can significantly improve the registration accuracy as shown in Fig. 2 on the right.

With the second example we demonstrate the usefulness of incorporating orientation attributes at landmarks. With the two synthetic images in Fig. 3 we simulate the rotation of a rigid structure (such as bone) embedded in an otherwise elastic material. If we use point landmarks only (four landmarks at the rigid structure and four landmarks at the image corners), then we obtain the result shown in Fig. 4 on the left. We see that the whole image including the rigid structure is elastically deformed. Next, we have incorporated orientations

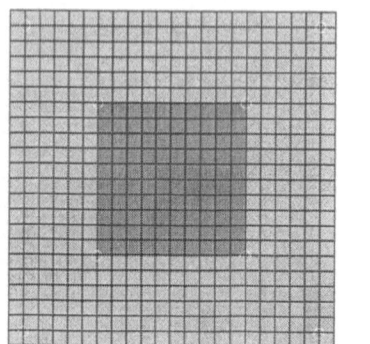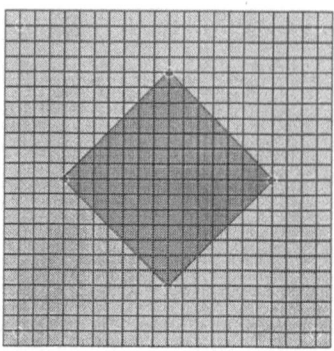

Fig. 3. Synthetic images simulating the rotation of a rigid structure in an otherwise elastic material

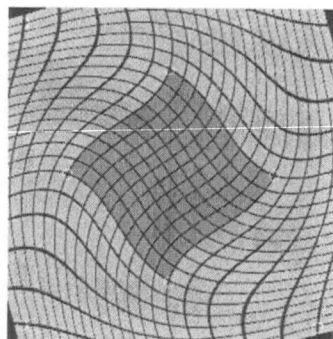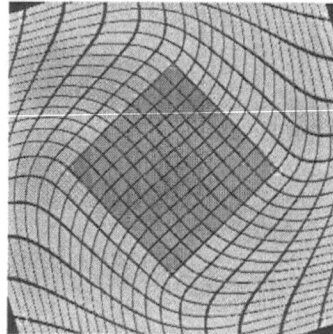

Fig. 4. Registration results: Interpolating thin-plate splines using only point landmarks (left) and incorporation of orientations at landmarks (right)

at the landmarks of the rigid structure. In all our experiments incorporating orientations we used $c = 1$ and $m = 2$ for the functional in (6). At each of the four landmarks of the rigid object in Fig. 3 we have specified two orientations which are aligned with the contours of the object. Using this additional knowledge for image registration significantly improves the result, i.e., the shape of the rigid object is well preserved (Fig. 4 on the right). Previously, Little *et al.* [14] have considered the problem of preserving rigid structures within elastic material. However, in their approach a full segmentation of the rigid structures is necessary. With our scheme we neither needed a full segmentation nor have we needed additional point landmarks.

In the third example we treat the case of several rigid structures embedded in elastic material. Fig. 5 shows two synthetic images that simulate the bending of a spine which is represented by five rigid components (see also [14]). The registration result in Fig. 6 on the left is obtained if we apply interpolating thin-plate splines while using four landmarks for each rigid component as well as four image border landmarks. In Fig. 6 in the middle the result is shown if we include two orientations at each landmark of the rigid components, while still applying an interpolation scheme. It can be seen that the shape of the rigid structures is better preserved, particularly the outer contours of the rigid components are not curved as in the case of using point landmarks only. A further improvement is obtained if we use both the point landmarks and the orientations but apply an approximation scheme (Fig. 6 on the right). Here we have used equal isotropic landmarks errors in the functional in (6). From the result it can be seen that the contours of the rigid components are straight and now also the gridlines within the rigid components are nearly straight. Thus the shape of the rigid structures is better preserved.

With the last example we show an application where we have integrated both anisotropic landmark errors and orientation attributes. In Fig. 7 two MR images of different patients are shown. We have selected normal point land-marks and quasi-landmarks, and we have estimated the error ellipses directly from the image data. If we use only the normal landmarks (9 landmarks; no. 1,2,4,7,10,11,16,17,18) and apply interpolating thin-plate splines, then we obtain the result shown in Fig. 8 on the left. Deviations can be observed in the regions where no landmarks have been specified, particularly at the upper part of the brain and at the corpus callosum. Next, we have used the normal landmarks from above together with three quasi-landmarks at the skin contour (landmarks no. 25,26,27). For all landmarks we have automatically estimated the covariance matrices and we have applied the approximating thin-plate spline approach incorporating anisotropic errors. From Fig. 8 on the right it can be seen that the registration accuracy at the upper part of the brain is now much better while at the corpus callosum there is still a larger deviation. We can further improve the result in this region if we additionally integrate orientations at landmarks. In this example, we have included one orientation at landmark no. 1 (genu of corpus callosum). In both images this orientation points to the top of the corpus callosum. From Fig. 9 we see, that we now obtain a significantly better registration accuracy of the whole corpus callosum.

5   Summary and Future Work

In this contribution, we have proposed an approach to elastic registration of medical images that is based on point landmarks and additional attributes. Our scheme is based on a minimizing functional which covers the full range from interpolation to approximation. Since the solution can be stated analytically we yield an efficient computational scheme. Central to this work is the integration of anisotropic landmark errors and orientation attributes at landmarks. By this we incorporate statistical as well as geometric information as additional knowledge in elastic image registration. We have demonstrated that this additional knowledge can significantly improve the registration result. In particular, we have shown that by incorporating orientation attributes it is possible to preserve the

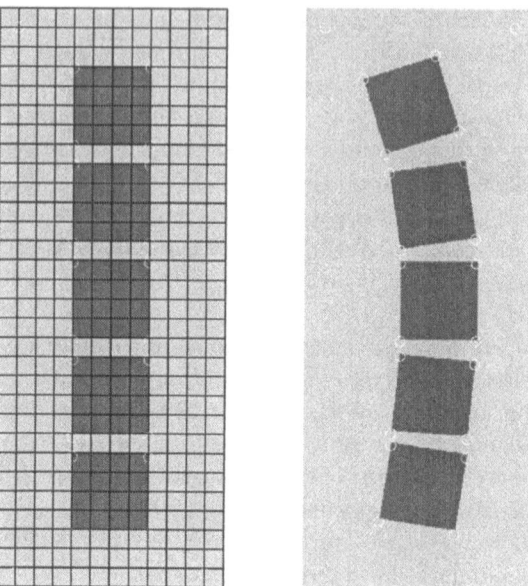

Fig. 5. Synthetic images simulating a spine that is bended

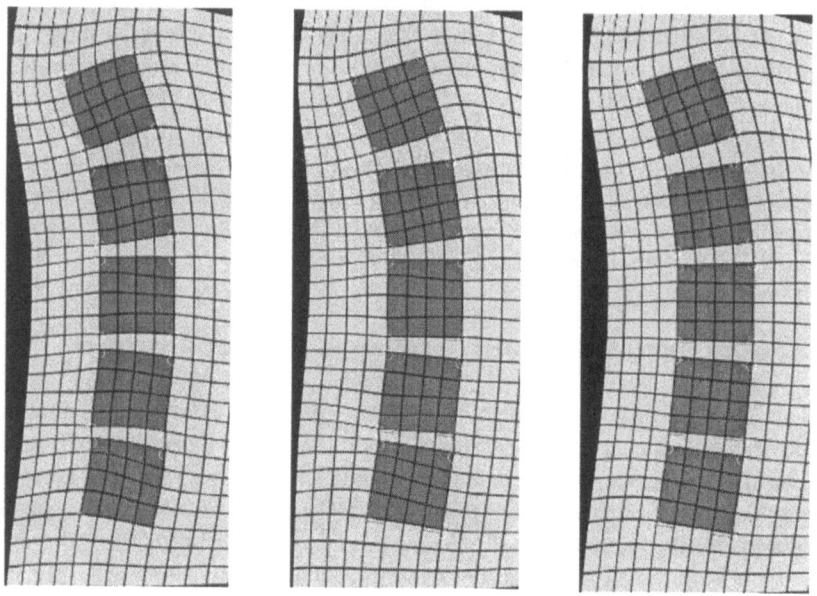

Fig. 6. Registration results: Interpolating thin-plate splines using only point landmarks (left), integration of two orientations at each object landmark (middle), and approximating thin-plate splines using point landmarks and orientations (right)

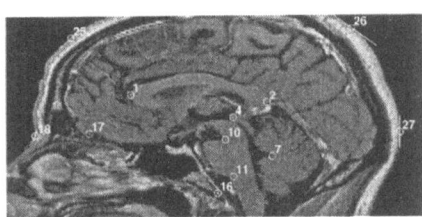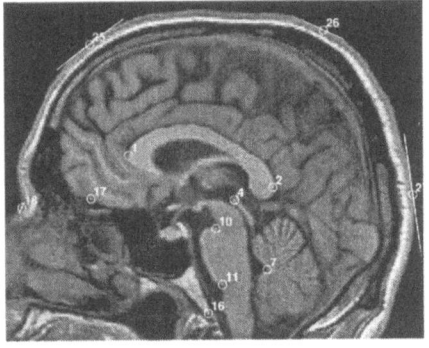

Fig. 7. MR images of different patients: normal landmarks, quasi-landmarks, and estimated error ellipses

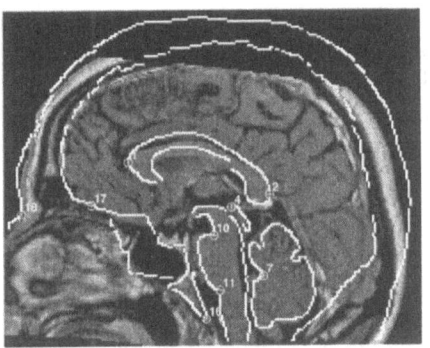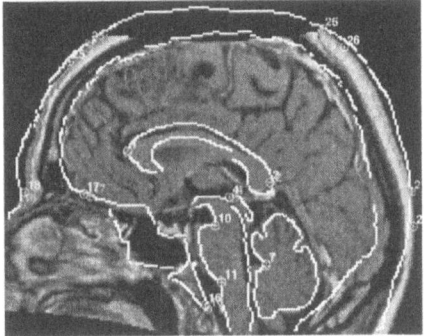

Fig. 8. Registration results: Interpolating thin-plate splines using normal landmarks (left), and approximating thin-plate splines using normal landmarks, quasi-landmarks and estimated covariance matrices (right)

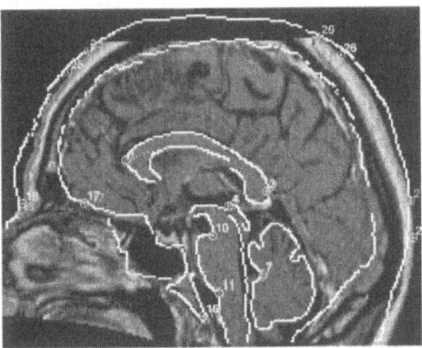

Fig. 9. Registration result: Approximating thin-plate splines using normal landmarks, quasi-landmarks, estimated covariance matrices, and orientations

shape of rigid structures (such as bone) in an otherwise elastic material. This can be achieved without selecting further landmarks and without a full segmentation of the rigid structures.

One problem with our approach is that the influence of incorporated orientations is rather global, i.e., image parts further away from the positions of added orientations are often strongly affected, which is generally not desired. This observation has already been made earlier (see Mardia *et al.* [12]). In future work, means have to be found to constrain this global influence. Another topic for further research is the automatic estimation of the orientation attributes. While for rigid structures within elastic material the local orientation of the contour seems to be quite appropriate, for elastic material other choices which rather reflect the global geometry of anatomical structures, seem to be better suited.

Acknowledgement

This work has been supported by Philips Research Hamburg, project IMAG-INE (IMage- and Atlas-Guided Interventions in NEurosurgery). We thank R. Sprengel for his contribution to this work. The original MR images have kindly been provided by Philips Research Hamburg and W.P.Th.M. Mali, L. Ramos, and C.W.M. van Veelen (Utrecht University Hospital) via ICS-AD of Philips Medical Systems Best.

References

1. Abbey, C.K., Clarkson, E., Barrett, H.H., Müller, S.P., and Rybicki, F.J.: A method for approximating the density of maximum-likelihood and maximum *a posteriori* estimates under a Gaussian noise model. Medical Image Anal. 2:4 (1998) 395-403
2. Bookstein, F.L.: Principal Warps: Thin-Plate Splines and the Decomposition of Deformations. IEEE Trans. on Patt. Anal. and Mach. Intell. 11:6 (1989) 567-585
3. Bookstein, F.L.: Four metrics for image variation. Proc. Int. Conf. Information Processing in Medical Imaging (IPMI'89), In: Progress in Clinical and Biological Research, Vol. 363, D. Ortendahl and J. Llacer (Eds.), Wiley-Liss New York, 1991, 227-240
4. Bookstein, F.L.: Landmark methods for forms without landmarks: morphometrics of group differences in outline shape. Medical Image Analysis 1:3 (1996/7) 225-243
5. Bookstein, F.L., and Green, D.K.: A Feature Space for Edgels in Images with Landmarks. J. of Mathematical Imaging and Vision 3 (1993) 231-261
6. Christensen, G.E., Joshi, S.C., and Miller, M.I.: Volumetric Transformation of Brain Anatomy. IEEE Trans. on Medical Imaging 16:6 (Dec. 1997) 864-877
7. Davis, M.H., Khotanzad, A., Flamig, D.P., and Harms, S.E.: A Physics-Based Coordinate Transformation for 3-D Image Matching. IEEE Trans. on Medical Imaging 16:3 (1997) 317-328
8. Duchon, J.: Interpolation des fonctions de deux variables suivant le principe de la flexion des plaques minces. R.A.I.R.O. Analyse Numérique 10:12 (1976) 5-12
9. Evans, A.C., Dai, W., Collins, L., Neelin, P., and Marrett, S.: Warping of a computerized 3-D atlas to match brain image volumes for quantitative neuroanatomical and functional analysis. Medical Imaging V: Image Processing, 1991, San Jose, CA, Proc. SPIE 1445, M.H. Loew (Ed.), 236-246

10. Fornefett, M., Rohr, K., Sprengel, R., and Stiehl, H.S.: Elastic Medical Image Registration using Orientation Attributes at Landmarks. Proc. Medical Image Understanding and Analysis (MIUA'98), Leeds/UK, 6-7 July 1998, E. Berry, D.C. Hogg, K.V. Mardia, and M.A. Smith (Eds.), Univ. Print Services Leeds 1998, 49-52

11. Mardia K., and Little, J.: Image warping using derivative information. In: Mathematical Methods in Medical Imaging III, 25-26 July 1994, San Diego, CA, Proc. SPIE 2299, F.L. Bookstein, J. Duncan, N. Lange, and D. Wilson (Eds.), 16-31

12. Mardia, K., Kent, J.T., Goodall, C.R., and Little, J.: Kriging and splines with derivative information. Biometrika 83:1 (1996) 207-221

13. Leamer, E.E.: Specification Searches – Ad Hoc Inferences with Nonexperimental Data. John Wiley & Sons New York Chichester 1978

14. Little, J.A., Hill, D.L.G., and Hawkes, D.J.: Deformations Incorporating Rigid Structures. Computer Vision and Image Understanding 66:2 (1997) 223-232

15. Maintz, J.B.A., and Viergever, M.A.: A survey of medical image registration. Medical Image Analysis 2:1 (1998) 1-36

16. Meyer, C.R., Boes, J.L., Kim, B., Bland, P.H., Zasadny, K.R., Kison, P.V., Koral, K., Frey, K.A., and Wahl, R.L.: Demonstration of accuracy and clinical versatility of mutual information for automatic multimodality image fusion using affine and thin-plate spline warped geometric deformations. Medical Image Analysis 1:3 (1996/7) 195-206

17. Rohr, K., Stiehl, H.S., Sprengel, R., Beil, W., Buzug, T.M., Weese, J., and Kuhn, M.H.: Point-Based Elastic Registration of Medical Image Data Using Approximating Thin-Plate Splines. Proc. Int. Conf. Visualization in Biomedical Computing (VBC'96), Hamburg, Germany, Sept. 22-25, 1996, Lecture Notes in Computer Science 1131, K.H. Höhne and R. Kikinis (Eds.), Springer Berlin 1996, 297-306

18. Rohr, K., Sprengel, R., and Stiehl, H.S.: Incorporation of Landmark Error Ellipsoids for Image Registration based on Approximating Thin-Plate Splines. Proc. Computer Assisted Radiology and Surgery (CAR'97), Berlin, Germany, June 25-28, 1997, H.U. Lemke, M.W. Vannier, and K. Inamura (Eds.), Elsevier Amsterdam Lausanne 1997, 234-239

19. Rohr, K.: Image Registration Based on Thin-Plate Splines and Local Estimates of Anisotropic Landmark Localization Uncertainties. Proc. Int. Conf. on Medical Image Computing and Computer-Assisted Intervention (MICCAI'98), Cambridge/MA, USA, Oct. 11-13, 1998, Lecture Notes in Computer Science 1496, W.M. Wells, A. Colchester, and S. Delp (Eds.), Springer Berlin 1998, 1174-1183

20. van Trees, H.L.: Detection, Estimation, and Modulation Theory, Part I. John Wiley and Sons, New York London 1968

21. Wahba, G.: Spline Models for Observational Data. Society for Industrial and Applied Mathematics, Philadelphia, Pennsylvania, 1990

22. Wahba, G.: Multivariate Function and Operator Estimation, Based on Smoothing Splines and Reproducing Kernels. In: Nonlinear Modeling and Forecasting, SFI Studies in the Sciences of Complexity, Vol. XII, M. Casdagli and S. Eubank (Eds.), Addison-Wesley 1992, 95-112

23. Wang, Y.: Smoothing Spline Models With Correlated Random Errors. J. of the American Statistical Association 93:441 (1998) 341-348

A Hierarchical Feature Based Deformation Model Applied to 4D Cardiac SPECT Data

Jacob K. Laading[1], Colin McCulloch[2], Valen E. Johnson[1],
David R. Gilland[3], and Ronald J Jaszczak[3]

[1] Institute for Statistics and Decision Sciences
Duke University, Durham, NC 27707, USA
jkl@stat.duke.edu
[2] Department of Biostatistics
Johns Hopkins School of Public Health, Baltimore, MD 21205, USA
[3] Department of Radiology
Duke University Medical Center, Durham, NC 27710, USA

Abstract. In this paper we describe a statistical model for the observation of labeled points in gated cardiac single photon emission computed tomography (SPECT) images. The model has two major parts: one based on shape correspondence between the image for evaluation and a reference image, and a second based on the match in image features. While the statistical deformation model is applicable to a broad range of image objects, the addition of a contraction mechanism to the baseline model provides particularly convincing results in gated cardiac SPECT. The model is applied to clinical data and provides marked improvement in the quality of summary images for the time series. Estimates of heart deformation and contraction parameters are also obtained.

1 Introduction

In the SPECT modality, a patient is injected with a radiotracer compound and an image is recorded based on using photons emitted from the tissue where the compound accumulates. In traditional SPECT, a single 3D volume is imaged. However, when applied to cardiac imaging, motion artifacts result in a serious degradation of the reconstructed image. To overcome this problem, gated cardiac SPECT can be used to divide the image acquisition period into n subsegments or gates based on the patient's electrocardiogram. If this is done, n SPECT images are acquired in parallel over several heart beats, one image corresponding to each gate. This imaging technique provides a useful diagnostic tool for direct evaluation of heart tissue damage, since the image artifacts due to the motion of the heart are much reduced. However, its success depends heavily on the compilation of data across gates, since each gated image is based on a relatively low number of photon counts (compared to the traditional approach). A reasonable summary of the n images can only be be obtained once the physical deformation of the heart through time is accurately modeled. The resulting summary image

A. Kuba et al. (Eds.): IPMI'99, LNCS 1613, pp. 266–279, 1999.

will then ideally have a signal-to-noise ratio (SNR) comparable to the traditional ungated SPECT images but with minimal motion blur.

We propose a method for modeling and summarizing gated cardiac SPECT data by tracking anatomical points within the heart volume through the series of gated images. Based on this tracking, a composite image can be calculated by summing each gate's image intensity at voxels dictated by the estimated path of each anatomical point through time. This procedure offers the potential of combining the benefits of better delineation of the heart walls with more accurate estimates of the tissue perfusion as measured by radiotracer compound uptake.

Several previous approaches have been taken in similar problems. Klein *et. al.* [10] have applied an approach which matches gated positron emission tomography (PET) images based on image values, smoothness of the motion field and physical incompressibility. Tagged magnetic resonance imaging has also been used to identify specific regions of heart tissue and match those through a time series [19]. There exist a variety of other approaches to modeling heart deformations in medical images based, for example, on surface matching[17,4]. Several "ground truth" studies for determining heart tissue motion have been carried out, for example by Potel *et. al.*, who [21] have performed marker-based direct measurements of the motion of surface points, and numerical phantoms of the heart have been used in dose calculations and simulations [5,20]. Similar approaches for deformation modeling to those offered here have been successfully applied to the case of finding image features, for example, using active shapes [7], snakes [8,9], and landmark-type methods[3,1,16]. The deformation method as described for a single image is comparable to the work of Collins *et. al.* [6], in which a varying-resolution grid is used to register MR brain images to an atlas by balancing constraints on grid continuity and a local feature function match. A similar multiresolution approach was applied in the work by Klein *et. al.* [10]. The multiresolution approach to maximization (and the description of images in general) is well-documented in the literature, particularly within the scalespace framework (see e.g. [12] or [22])and work in the context of optical flow[13].

Our general facet model approach, previously described in [15] and [14], is perfectly suited to gated cardiac SPECT since it provides a method for calculating the deformations required to trace a set of anatomical points through a set of images. Facet models are based on a large number of landmark-like points, termed facets, acting on a set of images drawn from a common class. Facets combine ideas from many of the approaches cited above in a framework which is intended to model observer placement of an arbitrary number of points in an image based on knowledge of those points in a reference image. This is accomplished via a probability distribution defined on facet locations and on image feature values at the facet locations.

In this paper, we extend the facet model to incorporate a gross model for heart contraction by including a set of contraction parameters in the shape portion of the probability distribution. Facet motion results are obtained by maximizing the joint distribution on facet locations for each image in the series.

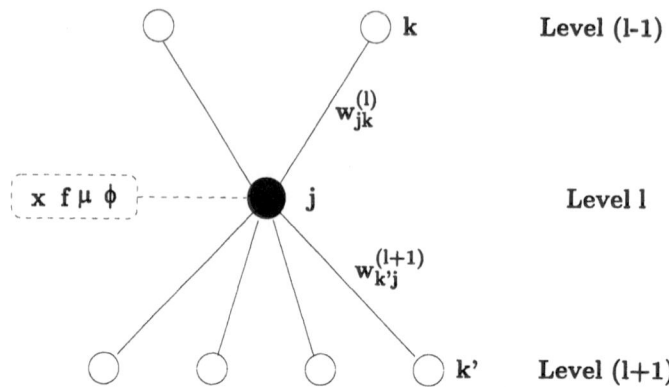

Fig. 1. Basic model element (for image dimension $d = 1$). Each facet has an associated parameter pair (μ, x); positions in the reference image and an image for evaluation, respectively. The facet can also contain the pair (ϕ, f) which represent a reference image feature and the image feature observed at the estimated facet location x, respectively. Facets are modeled jointly in a hierarchy (see Sect. 2.1), where they are influenced directly by 2^d facets one level up and in turn influence 4^d facets on the next level down

Several methods for exploring the high-dimensional results are exhibited, in order to show the utility of the method for the gated cardiac SPECT application.

2   Model and Methods

In the following subsections, the statistical model is defined. First, the general facet model is briefly reviewed. (For more details, see [14].) This model is generally applicable to a broad range of image modalities, however, we introduce several model extensions specific to the cardiac gated SPECT application based on a priori knowledge of general heart motion. Finally, the details of implementation are discussed.

2.1   General Model

The process that we wish to model is the placement of labeled points, or facets, within an image by a human observer. Facets differ from landmarks (following Bookstein[3]) in that facets do not correspond to specific pre-defined anatomical or mathematical features. Instead, each facet's label is generally inferred by its location in a reference image. A set of facets is applied hierarchically (see Fig. 1) to capture deformation on several levels of coarseness as inspired by models of vision[23]. Each facet has an associated position x, and may also have an associated feature value f, depending on its location in the hierarchy (see Sect. 2.1.1). A joint distribution is defined for all facet positions and feature values. We model the vectors x and f as conditionally independent given a parameter vector $\theta = \{\theta_x, \theta_f\}$; that is

$$p(x, f|\theta) = p_S(x|\theta_x)p_I(f|\theta_f).\qquad(1)$$

The parameter vector θ_x contains location and scale parameters $\{\mu, \kappa, \sigma^2\}$ for the facet location (shape) portion of the distribution, and θ_f similarly contains parameters $\{\phi, \tau\}$ for the feature (image) part of the distribution. These parameters are described below.

Shape Distribution Let x be the vector of facet positions. Let x_l indicate the vector of facets at level l in the hierachy and let x_{lj} refer to an individual facet j in that level. Similarly, let μ be the vector of corresponding facet locations in the reference image T. The distribution $p_S(x|\theta_x)$ is then assumed to have a hierarchical normal structure defined by (2) and (3). Each level has N_l facets, and d is the dimension of the image. For $(L+1)$ levels in the hierarchy, $l \in \{0, \dots, L\}$, define

$$p_S(x|\theta_x) = p_S(x_0|\theta_x)p_S(x_1|x_0; \theta_x)\dots p_S(x_L|x_{L-1}; \theta_x) ,\qquad(2)$$

where each factor is a density of the form

$$\begin{aligned}
p_S(x_0|\kappa, \mu) &= \mathrm{MVN}(\mu_0, \kappa\sigma_0^2 I_d)\\
p_S(x_1|x_0; \kappa, \mu) &= \mathrm{MVN}(\mu_1 + A_1\Delta x_0, \kappa\sigma_1^2 I_{N_1 d})\\
&\vdots\\
p_S(x_L|x_{L-1}; \kappa, \mu) &= \mathrm{MVN}(\mu_L + A_L\Delta x_{L-1}, \kappa\sigma_L^2 I_{N_L d}) .
\end{aligned}\qquad(3)$$

Here, $\mathrm{MVN}(a, \Sigma)$ denotes the multivariate normal density with mean a and covariance matrix Σ. The vectors x_l and μ_l have length $N_l d$, $\Delta x_l = x_l - \mu_l$, I_n is the n by n identity matrix, and A_l is an $N_l d$ by $N_{l-1} d$ design matrix for the hierarchical model. For example, in one dimension, A might be defined schematically as follows (refer also to Fig. 1),

$$A_l = \begin{bmatrix} w_{11}^{(l)} & \cdots & w_{1k}^{(l)} & \cdots & w_{1N_{l-1}}^{(l)} \\ w_{21}^{(l)} & \cdots & w_{2k}^{(l)} & \cdots & w_{2N_{l-1}}^{(l)} \\ & & \vdots & & \\ w_{j1}^{(l)} & \cdots & w_{jk}^{(l)} & \cdots & w_{jN_{l-1}}^{(l)} \\ & & \vdots & & \\ w_{N_l 1}^{(l)} & \cdots & w_{N_l k}^{(l)} & \cdots & w_{N_l N_{l-1}}^{(l)} \end{bmatrix} = \begin{bmatrix} \vdots & \vdots & \vdots & \vdots & \vdots \\ \cdots 0 & w_{(j-1)1}^{(l)} & w_{(j-1)2}^{(l)} & 0 & 0 \cdots \\ \cdots 0 & w_{j1}^{(l)} & w_{j2}^{(l)} & 0 & 0 \cdots \\ \cdots 0 & 0 & w_{(j+1)1}^{(l)} & w_{(j+1)2}^{(l)} & 0 \cdots \\ \cdots 0 & 0 & w_{(j+2)1}^{(l)} & w_{(j+2)2}^{(l)} & 0 \cdots \\ \vdots & \vdots & \vdots & \vdots & \vdots \end{bmatrix}$$

where the $w_{jk}^{(l)}$ values are set proportional to the inverse distance between μ_{lj} and $\mu_{(l-1)k}$, constrained by $\sum_k w_{jk}^{(l)} = 1$ and such that only the 2^d closest facets on level $(l-1)$ to facet lj are given non-zero weights $w_{jk}^{(l)}$. In the 3-dimensional application presented here, such entries in a row of A_l are thus kept limited to 8 by extending the above A_l in the most obvious way to 3 dimensions. Each level in the hierarchy is laid out such that μ_l forms an evenly spaced grid with $N_l = 2^{ld}$ facets per level. Finally, σ_l^2 is the conditional variance of a facet on level l given the locations of facets on level $(l-1)$. These parameters were set such that the marginal variance for bottom level facets is approximately independent of the number of levels in the hierarchy. The parameter κ is an overall scale factor to allow for adjustments in the weighting of shape (p_S) versus image (p_I) portions of the density in (1). This parameter was set empirically.

The form for p_S captures the deformation on several levels of scale, thus easing the exploration of configuration space. This means that gross deformations are modeled by upper-level facets and that lower-level facets will not be subsequently penalized for the same movement. The form chosen for A_l enforces some smoothness on the deformation, i.e., the marginal covariance between any pair of facets on a level l is a smooth decreasing function of their distance $(\mu_{lj} - \mu_{lj'})$ in the reference image [14]. This is unlike previous models in which only one non-zero term per row was used[11]. Computational tractability is ensured by the choice of a normal hierarchical model.

Feature Distribution Let f be the vector of image-derived feature values associated with the set of facets. Similarly, let ϕ be the corresponding vector of reference image feature values. Then given an image match function g, we model the facet features as drawn from the exponential family distribution given in (4). Here, we further assume that if $\{f_j, \phi_j\}$ are the corresponding jth element of the vectors $\{f, \phi\}$, then the feature distribution p_I is modeled as a product of univariate distributions with a common image match function g_I. Thus,

$$p_I(f|\tau, \phi) \propto \exp\{-g(f, \phi)\}$$

$$\propto \exp\left\{-\frac{1}{2\tau}\sum_{j=1}^{N_L} g_I(f_j, \phi_j)\right\}, \tag{4}$$

where τ is an overall scale parameter which is similar to κ defined for the shape distribution p_S. The sum extends over those facets that have associated feature values, which in this paper are the facets on the lowest level L in the hierarchy. The means ϕ_j are taken to be the image feature value calculated at the locations μ_{Lj} in the reference image T: $\phi_j = \phi(T, \mu_{Lj})$. Note that this does not necessarily imply taking the image value at μ_{Lj} directly. The derivation of $\{f_j, \phi_j\}$ from the image data can be specified in a number of ways; we have used either a quantile-rescaled image intensity or a low-scale image Laplacian. For choices of the functions g, scaled squared differences between f_j and ϕ_j (yielding independent normal distributions) have been used[15,11], and a local intensity regression, as described in the next subsection, has also been employed.

2.2 Application-Specifics

The baseline shape model (3) captures the shape changes in the general case when little prior knowledge is available about the shape change within the image class. Since we know a priori that the heart size changes during the heart beat cycle, it is sensible to build this into the model. We choose a simple scalar correction, due in part to the coarseness of the images. The left ventricular (LV) wall is approximately 3 pixels wide across in a 2D slice. Also, non-linear contractions not incorporated into the gross model can still be accommodated by the deformation model.

To define the contraction model, let γ_1 be coordinates for a center of contraction, and let γ_2 be a 3-dimensional set of contraction factors for orthogonal directions $\{1, 2, 3\}$. The full vector $\gamma = \{\gamma_1, \gamma_2\}$ transforms μ in the shape portion of the model (3) to a vector of contracted means $\mu^c(t)$ at time t in the image time series, and the shape distribution p_S is modified accordingly :

$$p_S(x_l | x_{l-1}; \kappa, \mu, \gamma(t)) = \text{MVN}(\mu_l^c(t) + A_l \Delta x_{l-1}, \kappa \sigma_l^2 I_{N_l d}),$$
$$\mu_l^c(t) = \gamma_1 \mathbf{1}_{N_l d} + (\mu_l - \gamma_1 \mathbf{1}_{N_l d}) \bar{\gamma}_2(t) , \tag{5}$$

where $\bar{\gamma}_2$ is a stacked vector of N_l replicates of γ_2 and $\mathbf{1}_n$ is the n-dimensional vector of ones. Otherwise, A_l, $\kappa \sigma_l^2$ and μ remain unchanged. A prior distribution can also be included to capture the expected contraction pattern during the beat cycle, for example

$$p(\gamma_2(t)) = \text{MVN}(\omega(t), \nu^{-1} I_3) , \quad \{\gamma_2^1(t), \gamma_2^2(t), \gamma_2^3(t)\} \in< 0, \infty > , \tag{6}$$

yielding the final form for the joint shape distribution,

$$p_S(x, \gamma_2 | \theta_x) = p_S(x | \theta_x, \gamma_2) p(\gamma_2) . \tag{7}$$

The center of contraction γ_1 is fixed in this implementation at μ_0, since having it vary for a scalar contraction only involves a non-informative translation of the reference grid. Note that the introduction of μ^c does not change the values of ϕ_j, which are still taken as the reference image feature values at μ_{Lj}. (For a graphical outline representation of the model, see Fig. 2.)

The feature function g_I found to be most effective for gated cardiac SPECT images is one based on a local intensity regression around the facet in question. A small neighborhood defined by a set of m points is placed around the facet's position in the reference image T (around μ_{Lj}) and observed image Q (around x_{Lj}). Subsequently, these points are evaluated in T and Q, respectively, to form m-vectors ϕ_j and f_j, indexed by k. A normalized regression parameter (see [14] for details) is then calculated,

$$g_I(f_j, \phi_j) = 1 - f_j^{*'} \phi_j^* \phi_j^{*'} f_j^*,$$
$$= 1 - \frac{(\sum_k \phi_{jk} f_{jk} - \frac{1}{m} \sum_k \phi_{jk} \sum_k f_{jk})^2}{(\sum_k \phi_{jk}^2 - \frac{1}{m}(\sum_k \phi_{jk})^2)(\sum_k f_{jk}^2 - \frac{1}{m}(\sum_k f_{jk})^2)} , \tag{8}$$

which is then used to define the distribution function p_I (4).

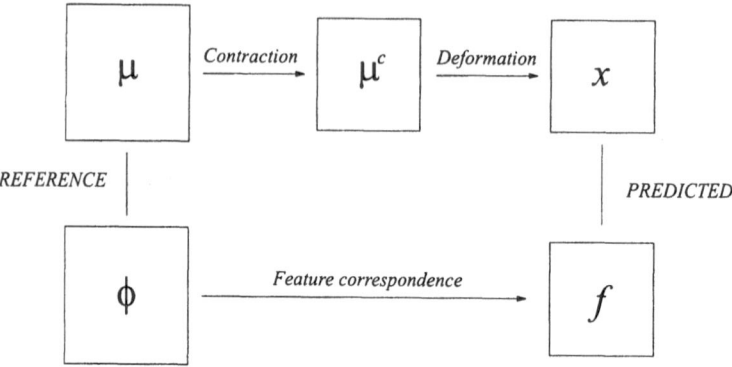

Fig. 2. Conceptual model framework. The facets at locations μ are placed in the reference image to obtain the feature vector ϕ. The deformation is then modeled as a contraction of the μ to μ^c and a deformation from μ^c to the predicted facet positions x. At the same time, the deformation is evaluated for image feature match between ϕ (fixed) and f at the facet locations x; $f = f(Q, x)$

2.3   Implementation

As described above, one goal of this methodology is to provide a computationally tractable method for estimating observed facet locations. This maximization is relatively straightforward in the framework of iterated conditional modes (ICM), in which each parameter is updated by setting it to the mode of its full conditional distribution[2].

Since our interest lies in the facet positions x, we treat the image Q which is to be evaluated as a constraint on the model, thus imposing $f = f(Q, x)$ given the image Q (details in [14], Appendix A). The resulting constrained distribution on facet locations x in an image Q is proportional to (2), namely

$$p(x|\theta) \propto p_S(x|\theta_x)p_I(f = f(Q, x)|\theta_f) \ . \tag{9}$$

Numerical maximization is required when the locations of facets on the lowest level are predicted, since the p_I factor in (9) introduces a non-standard distribution on x under this constraint. Maximization steps over the full conditional distributions for upper-level facets have closed form solutions. The full conditional mode for facet position x_{lj} on a level l in the hierarchy, for l not equal to the top or bottom level ($l \notin \{0, L\}$) is given as

$$x_{lj}^{ICM} = \mu_{lj}^c + \frac{\sigma_l^2}{\sigma_c^2} \sum_{k \in P_{lj}} w_{jk}^{(l)}(x_{(l-1)k} - \mu_{(l-1)k}^c) + \frac{\sigma_{l+1}^2}{\sigma_c^2} \sum_{k \in D_{lj}} w_{kj}^{(l+1)}\xi_{lk} \ , \tag{10}$$

$$\xi_{lk} = \{(x_{(l+1)k} - \mu_{(l+1)k}^c) - \sum_{j' \in P'_{(l+1)k}} w_{j'k}^l(x_{lj'} - \mu_{lj'}^c)\},$$

$$\sigma_c^{-2} = \sigma_l^{-2} + \sigma_{l+1}^{-2} \sum_{k \in D_{lj}} (w_{kj}^{(l+1)})^2 \ .$$

In this expression, k indexes facets on level $(l-1)$ or $(l+1)$ in the set P_{lj} or D_{lj}, respectively, of those facets which contribute to the means in the full conditional distribution on x_{lj}. The prime notation $(')$ indicates facet index or parent set relating to one of the children of facet lj. The top level $(l=0)$ facet has a similar form to (10), dropping terms relating to the set P_{lj}.

The full conditional distribution for the contraction factor γ_2 also has normal form, with the mode given in (11). Assume a normal distribution truncated at zero with mean ω and precision ν for the prior $p(\gamma_2)$. Then

$$\gamma_2^{ICM} = \frac{\sum_{l=1}^{L}\sum_{j=1}^{N_l}\{(\Delta_\mu^{lj})^{-2}(\kappa\sigma_l)^{-2}\Delta_x^{lj}\Delta_\mu^{lj}\} + \omega\nu}{\sum_{l=1}^{L}\sum_{j=1}^{N_l}\{(\Delta_\mu^{lj})^{-2}(\kappa\sigma_l)^{-2}\} + \nu} \quad , \tag{11}$$

$$\Delta_\mu^{lj} = \mu_{lj} - \sum_{k\in P_{lj}} w_{jk}^{(l)}\mu_{(l-1)k} \quad , \quad \Delta_x^{lj} = x_{lj} - \sum_{k\in P_{lj}} w_{jk}^{(l)}x_{(l-1)k} \quad ,$$

and as before, k is the index for a facet in the set P_{lj} which contribute non-zero terms to the full conditional distribution on x_{lj}.

For the ICM maximization steps involving the lowest-level facets, the Nelder-Mead simplex method is applied[18]. To enhance computational efficiency, our maximization approach involves partial maximization of the upper levels with relations between lower-level facets kept fixed, and with approximate image feature contributions calculated based on the scale-space[12] of the observed and reference image.

3   Results

The method described was applied to a dataset from Duke University Medical Center consisting of 16 images acquired during the heart beat cycle. For each gate, an image of size 64x64x16 voxels was acquired (7.1 mm voxel size). The heart was contained entirely in a 16x16x16 voxel volume. Using a 5 level facet hierarchy, each voxel in the reference heart volume contained one bottom-level facet, located at the voxel center. The entire hierarchy spans a 16^3 cube at five different resolutions ($L=4$) and has a total of 4681 facets. Gate 8 (filling phase, mid-diastole) was used as the reference image throughout. The resulting density on facet locations x was then maximized for each of the other gates individually. Typical maximization time was approximately 3 minutes per gated image on a DEC 433au workstation.

The results are summarized as follows. First, we show plots of facet movement from slices in the reference image to slices in another gated image for three orthogonal directions. Next, several individual facets are displayed on the reference and the other gated image to demonstrate the deformation achieved under the model. We then display a composite image and compare it to the traditional SPECT image and a single gated image. Difference images for the composite versus the traditional and gated image are also shown. Subsequently, estimated changes in overall size (contraction) are shown for the time series. Finally, convergence and stability relative to initial condition is examined.

3.1   Facet Motion

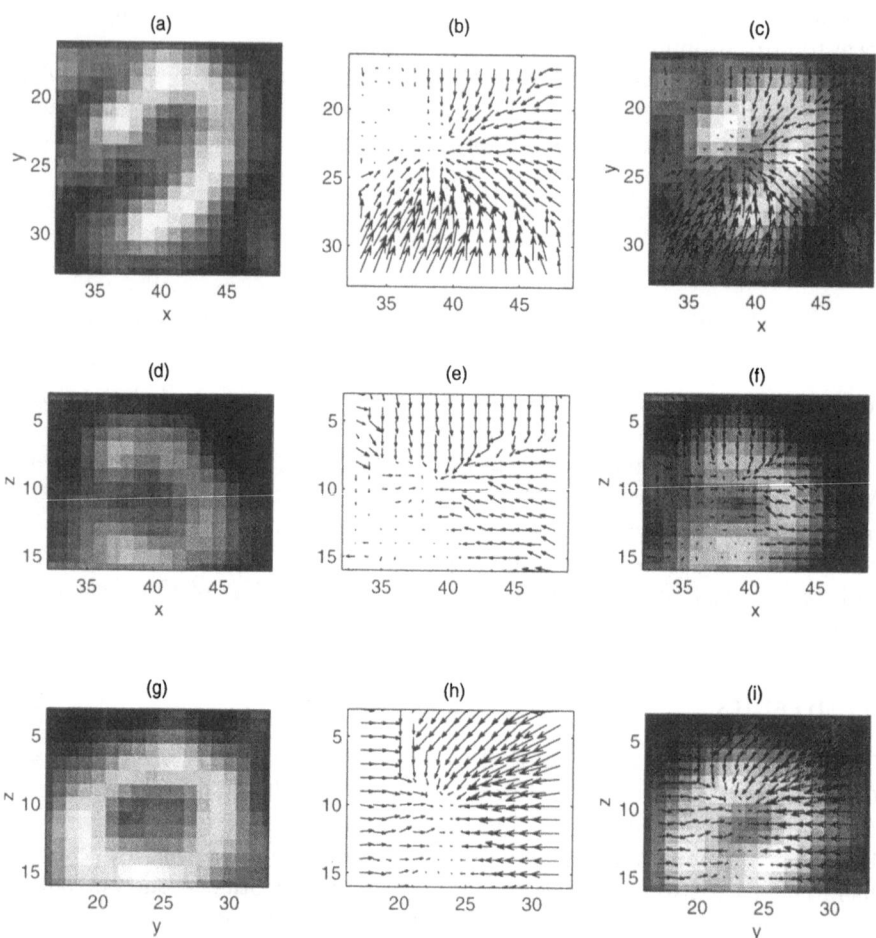

Fig. 3. Facet motion from gate 8 (reference;mid-diastole) to gate 4 (end-systole) in representative slices. Panels (a)–(c) show a transaxial plane, (d)–(f) a coronal plane and (g)–(i) a sagittal plane. The left column shows the reference image slice, the middle column shows the facet motion estimate and the right column shows that same estimate superimposed on the image slice from the gate 4 image

In Fig. 3, facet displacement vectors from gate 8 to gate 4 are shown for a representative slice in three orthogonal directions. Gate 4 corresponds to the contracted state (end-systole). The general contraction from diastole (gate 8) to systole is clearly captured by this estimated mode of the joint density on facet locations. Note also that though the grid has contracted, there are also regions on the heart which have not moved significantly. This is consistent with typical

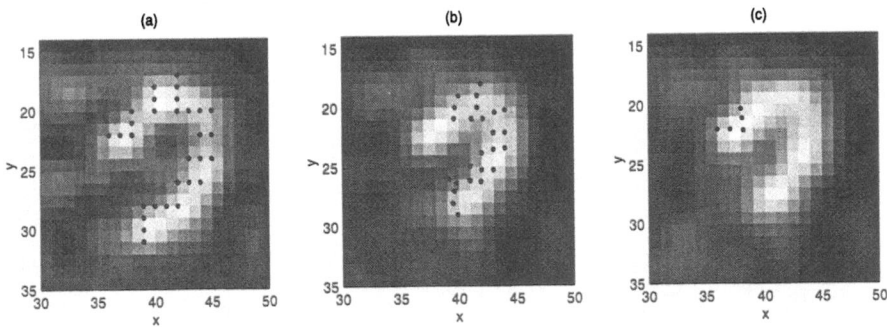

Fig. 4. Selected facet positions in transaxial slice 8 of the reference image (a), with corresponding estimated facet positions in the gate 4 image, slice 8 (b) and 9 (c). Note the contraction and deformation in relative positioning without losing relations between neighboring facets, as well as the slice-jump, indicating fully 3D deformation

heart motion. Thus, the model achieved two of the objectives stated earlier; there was an overall size correction as well as a local deformation.

The positions of several individual facets in the reference image and gate 4 are shown in Fig. 4. Points in the heart are estimated under the model to deform in a complex manner, and are consistent with the heart shape seen. Note also the fully 3-dimensional nature of the deformation as evidenced in the slice-jump of the upper leftmost section.

3.2   Summary Images

To more accurately represent the distribution of radiotracer uptake in the heart, a facet-composite (composite for short) image was calculated. The maximization for facet placement in all gated images was consolidated into this composite image by mapping the gated image intensity found at the facet position in each image to that facet's reference image position and averaging across the image sequence; $S^{comp}(\mu_{Lj}) = \frac{1}{n}(T(\mu_{Lj}) + \sum_{t \neq t_\mu} Q_t(x_{Lj}(t)))$, where Q_t is the t-th image in the time series of n images and t_μ is the gate used as the reference, i.e. $Q_{t_\mu} = T$. This image (Fig. 5(a)) compares favorably to both of the other representations of the data, the voxel-wise mean (standard SPECT equivalent, Fig. 5(b)) and the gated image alone (Fig. 5(c)). Image intensity uniformity has also been improved in the LV wall region relative to the gated image alone, while retaining image contrast. Comparing the facet-composite with the mean image shows a better delineation of the lateral wall of the left ventricle. The composite image thus represents a specific state of the heart (here, it maps to mid-diastole) rather than a time-averaged state which does not exist. The difference images shown in Fig. 6 highlight the structural differences between the summary images. The mean image minus the composite image (pixel-wise difference) shows a clear pattern (dark and bright) that corresponds to the lateral wall of the left ventricle. Again, this corresponds to known heart motion. Also, when the composite image

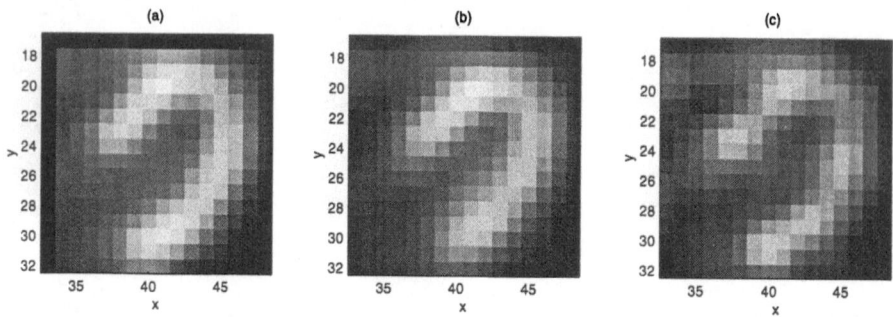

Fig. 5. Slice 9 (transaxial) : (a) Composite image mapped to gate 8, (b) mean voxel-wise image (standard SPECT), (c) gate 8 image only. The composite image was formed by computing average intensity based on the facet motion through the series of images and mapping back to the reference image (gate 8). We observe similarity between gate 8 and composite, with the composite having superior smoothness in regions of activity. Furthermore, a better spatial delineation of the heart wall in the composite image relative to the standard SPECT image is seen

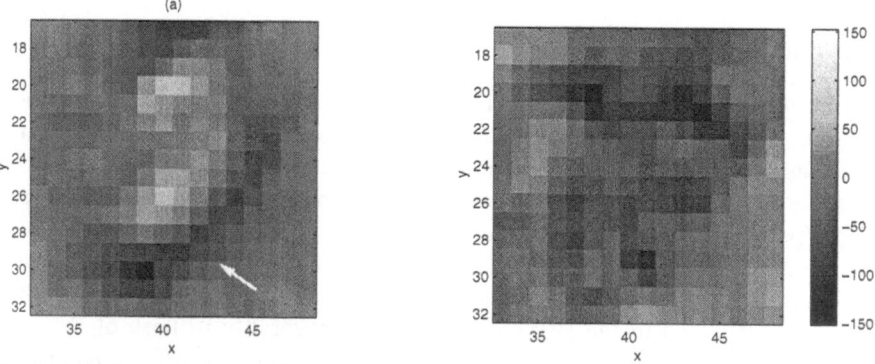

Fig. 6. Difference images corresponding to the images in Fig. 5; (a) mean minus composite (mapped to gate 8), (b) gate 8 minus composite. For detailed explanation of the composite image, see Sect. 3. Here we see clearly the structural difference between the standard (mean) image and the composite facet-based image. The regions of dark and bright indicate that the deformation model has shifted intensity outward for the lateral wall of the left ventricle (arrow). This is in accordance with the use of gate 8 (mid-diastole) as the reference. The gated versus composite comparison shows no structural differences other than an overall intensity level difference in the heart region, which is attributable to a known intensity trend discussed in the text

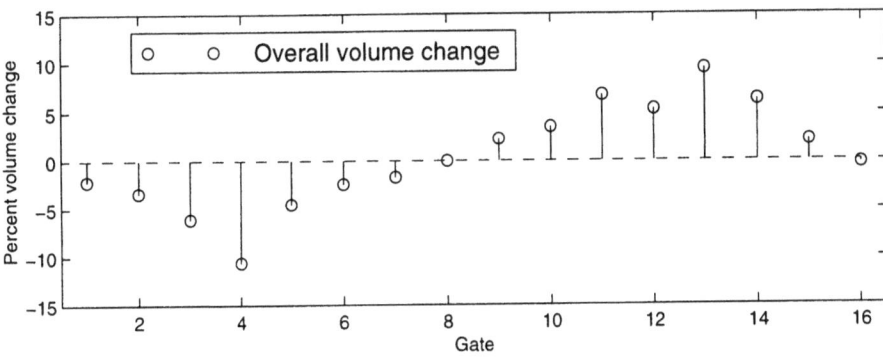

Fig. 7. Estimated overall contraction through cycle, measured in percent of total volume spanned by μ_c relative to μ. This corresponds well to the expected and observed heart contraction through the series of images. It is not interpretable as heart chamber volume, however

is subtracted from the gate 8 reference image, no pattern other than the known intensity difference between an average and any individual gate late in the time series is apparent. (Early gates tend to have more intensity due to an out-of-phase blurring effect which worsen towards the end of the beat cycle.)

3.3 Contraction

A relatively non-informative prior distribution on γ_2 (uniform on $< 0, 3 >$) was used for the results reported here. Figure 7 shows the contraction correction as a function of time (gates) when taken as an overall volume change. The parameters behave sensibly through the cycle: Gates 1–6 comprise the relatively short contraction phase (systole), while the remaining images are acquired in the expanded or dilated state (diastole) of the heart. The parameter time evolution tracks this. Since this is an overall correction, this parameter could be interpreted as a rough indicator of relative heart size, but it should not be used as a measure of particular quantities, such as LV chamber volume. The general trend shown in Fig. 7 matches well with visual inspection of changes in heart size over the image series.

3.4 Stability

Each full ICM cycle includes an iterative maximization over facet locations x, followed by a maximization for γ_2. The model was allowed to run for 200 such cycles, and did not exhibit any significant changes in parameter estimates or facet locations from the values determined with a shorter run (5 full cycles). Previous work [14] has shown fast convergence of the maximization for a model which does not incorporate contraction (γ) directly. Finally, several starting positions for the maximization routine were used without changing the final results.

4   Discussion

The model proposed in this paper improves the utility and applicability of gated cardiac SPECT data. While future modifications to the model are being investigated, current results are promising. Taken together, the set of locations for every facet in every gate constitutes a very rich representation of this image data. With further investigation of true anatomical correspondence, this representation will offer new diagnostic ways to look at heart function abnormalities via estimated deformations rather than based solely on radiotracer uptake. The facet-composite image is also a clearly improved summary of the image time series over the voxel-wise sum and offers better intensity uniformity in the heart region and from that a better SNR than the individual gated images. In the future, we plan to evaluate numerically this improvement in SNR and the accuracy of estimated facet locations using a newly developed Monte Carlo computed phantom of a beating heart in a thorax [20]. This is important since we currently have no clinical data available to evaluate the real motion of individual heart tissue elements for these time series. With such reference data, numerical evaluations of performance and subsequent educated model modifications will be possible. More advanced modeling based on known physiology of heart contraction, use of smoothness constraints on individual facet motion and the inclusion of registered and simultaneously acquired transmission computed tomography (TCT) data are current model extensions under investigation.

Acknowledgments

This work was supported by PHS grants R01-CA33541 and R01-CA76006 from the National Institutes of Health, grant DE-FG02-96ER62150 from the Department of Energy and NHLBI grant number HL52162. The first author is supported by a doctoral fellowship from the Norwegian Research Council.

References

1. Amit, Y., Grenander, U., Piccione, M.: Structural image restoration through deformable templates. Journal of the American Statistical Society **86** (1991) 376–387
2. Besag, J.: On the statistical analysis of dirty pictures. Journal of the Royal Statistical Society (series B) **48** (1986) 259–302
3. Bookstein, F.: Morphometric tools for landmark data. Cambridge University Press, Cambridge (1991)
4. Clarysse, P., Friboulet, D., Magnin, I.E.: Tracking geometrical descriptors on 3-D deformable surfaces: Application to the left-ventricular surface of the heart. IEEE Transactions on Medical Imaging **16** (1997) 392–404
5. Coffey, J.L., Cristy, M., Warner, G.: Specific absorbed fractions for photon sources uniformly distributed in the heart chambers and heart wall of a heterogeneous phantom. Journal of Nuclear Medicine (MIRD pamphlet no. 13) **22** (1980) 65–71
6. Collins, D., Holmes, C., Peters, T., Evans, A.: Automatic 3-d model-based neuroanatomical segmentation. Human Brain Mapping **3** (1995) 190–208

7. Cootes, T.F., Hill, A., Taylor, C.J., Haslam, J.: The use of active shape models for locating structures in medical images. Image and Vision Computing **12** (1994) 355–366

8. Davatzikos, C., Vaillant, M., Resnick, R.: A computerized approach for morphological analysis of the corpus callosum. Journal of Computer Assisted Tomography **20** (1996) 88–97

9. Kass, M., Witkin, A., Terzopolous, D.: Snakes: active contour models. International Journal of Computer Vision (1988) 321–331

10. Klein, G.J., Reutter, B.W., Huesman, R.H.: Non-rigid summing of gated pet via optical flow. IEEE Transactions on Nuclear Science **44** (1997) 1509–1512

11. Laading, J.K., McCulloch, C.C., Johnson, V.E.: A hierarchical object deformation model applied to the digital chest radiograph. In: The American Statistical Association Proceedings of the Section on Bayesian Statistical Science, Anaheim, California (1997)

12. Lindeberg, T.: Scale-space Theory. Kluwer Academic Publishers, Boston, MA (1994)

13. Luettgen, M.R., Karl, W.C., Willsky, A.S.: Efficient multiscale regularization with applications to the computation of optical flow. IEEE Transactions on Image Processing **70** (1994) 41–64

14. McCulloch, C.C.: High-level image understanding via Bayesian hierarchical models. PhD thesis, Duke University (1998)

15. McCulloch, C.C., Laading, J.K., Johnson, V.E.: Image feature identification via bayesian hierarchical models. In: The American Statistical Association Proceedings of the Section on Bayesian Statistical Science, Anaheim, California (1997)

16. McCulloch, C.C., Laading, J.K., Wilson, A., Johnson, V.E.: A shape-based framework for automated image segmentation. In: The American Statistical Association Proceedings of the Section on Bayesian Statistical Science, Chicago, Illinois (1996) 1–6

17. McEachen, J.C., Duncan, J.S.: Shape-based tracking of left ventricular motion. IEEE Transactions on Medical Imaging **16** (1997) 270–283

18. Nelder, J., Mead, R.: A simplex method for function minimization. The Computer Journal **7** (1965) 308–313

19. Park, J., Metaxas, D., Young, A.A., Axel, L.: Deformable models with parameter functions for cardiac motion analysis from tagged mri data. IEEE Transactions on Medical Imaging **15** (1996) 1–13

20. Peter, J., Gilland, D.R., Jaszczak, R.J., Coleman, R.E.: Four-dimensional quadric-based cardiac-thorax phantom for monte carlo simulation of radiological imaging systems. Submitted to: IEEE Transactions on Nuclear Science (1998)

21. Potel, M.J., MacKay, S.A., Rubin, J.A., Aisen, A.M., Sayre, R.E.: Three-dimensional left ventricular wall motion in man. coordinate systems for representing wall movement direction. Investigative Radiology **19** (1984) 499–509

22. terHaar Romeny, B.M., Florack, L., Koenderink, J., Viergever, M.: Scale-space: its natural operators and differential invariants. In: Lecture Notes in Computer Science **511** Springer-Verlag, Berlin, Germany (1991) 239–255

23. Young, R.: The gaussian derivative model for machine vision: I. retinal mechanisms. Spatial Vision **2** (1987) 273–293

Local Orientation Distribution as a Function of Spatial Scale for Detection of Masses in Mammograms

Nico Karssemeijer

University Hospital Nijmegen, Department of Radiology, The Netherlands
nico@radiology.azn.nl

Abstract. A method has been developed for detection masses in mammograms by analysis of local orientation patterns. Concentration of gradient and line orientation computed at a fine scale reveals the presence of masses and spiculation, respectively. In this paper a new computational approach is presented which allows efficient computation of these features as a continuous function of spatial scale. It is shown that by using these scale signatures estimates of mass size can be readily obtained. Experimentally it was found that mass size estimates can be used to improve mass detection, while full exploitation of the information represented by the scale signatures is expected lead to further improvement. Results are presented for detection of malign masses in a database of 264 mammograms representing 71 consecutive cancers found in screening.

1   Introduction

The success of breast cancer screening programs critically depends on the ability to detect non-palpable invasive cancers when they are still small, as tumor size is a very important prognostic factor [1]. Invasive cancers are visible as masses. Ideally, these should be detected when they are smaller than 1.5 cm, because then they are detected early enough to have a strong impact on overall mortality reduction. Masses smaller than 5 mm are rarely visible in mammograms. Detection of non-invasive intraductal in situ cancers, only visible by microcalcifications, is less effective as many of these do not get invasive during lifetime.

Detection of small masses in screening mammograms is difficult, because they may be hard to distinguish from normal fibroglandular tissue patterns. Moreover, in a screening population only three to six out of thousand women have breast cancer. This very large fraction of normal cases makes screening a complex visual task for radiologists. To avoid perception errors, radiologist need to be alert at a constant high level. That failures are not uncommon has been revealed by a number of studies [2,3,4]. Recently, it was found in a large multi-center study that as much as 70 percent of the cancers detected in screening were are already visible on previous screening mammograms, where up to 20 percent was obvious enough to be classified as actionable by the majority of a panel of reviewing radiologists [5]. In another recent study, findings at previous screening mammograms of 544

A. Kuba et al. (Eds.): IPMI'99, LNCS 1613, pp. 280–293, 1999.

cancers that were *not* detected in screening were reviewed [6]. In 25% of these cases the tumor was classified as overlooked or misinterpreted. An effective way to increase performance of radiologist in screening is double reading [7]. Increases of sensitivity with 5-15 percent have been reported by having two independent readers. However, implementation of double reading may be hard to organize because of cost and time limitations. As an alternative, it has been suggested that computer programs that identify suspicious regions in mammograms can be used as a second reader. This approach turned out to be successful in a few small studies [8,9,10], but its success in practice will depend on the level of performance of detection algorithms in terms of both sensitivity and specificity.

Masses in mammograms can be described as more or less compact areas that appear brighter than the tissue in which they are embedded, due to a higher attenuation for X-rays. When the tissue surrounding a mass is fatty, the detection problem is relatively easy and tumors as small as 5 mm can be detected. However, when a mass is projected in dense fibroglandular tissue it may be very difficult to recognize. Even large masses may be completely obscured by dense tissue [11]. This is one of the reasons for taking two different views of each breast, as is common practice in most screening programs. Usually, oblique and cranio-caudal (CC) projections are recorded. The appearance of masses can be circumscribed, fuzzy, or spiculated. In the latter case there is a radiating pattern of spicules surrounding the central mass area. Differentiation of masses from normal glandular tissue structures may be so difficult that one has to rely on distortion or asymmetry of the normal mammographic pattern, while sometimes a comparison with previous mammograms provides an important cue. Especially stellate patterns of straight lines are suspect, or straight retractions of the glandular tissue boundary. Bilateral asymmetry may form an important clue when a mass like area only appears in one side. Furthermore, the location of a suspect area sometimes plays a role. For instance, in a fatty area behind the glandular tissue and close to the chest wall, the presence of a mass is very suspect if it does not have a corresponding sign in the contralateral breast. Some examples of malign masses are shown in Fig. 1.

In the past decade different methods for detection of masses in mammograms have been suggested, some focusing on bilateral asymmetry [12,13,14], detection of spiculation [15], or on contrast and texture differences [16,17,18]. All these methods have some aspects in common. Usually, a first phase is executed in which local image features are calculated at each pixel or at a set of regularly spaced points across the segmented breast area. Using these features, pixels are grouped into regions by a segmentation scheme. In a second phase features are calculated for each candidate region and a classifier determines regions that are regarded as suspicious. Various methods differ in the way they address and emphasize each of the two phases. Some apply very simple procedures to form many candidate regions and rely heavily on region classification in order to remove an abundance of false positives. The approach that is taken here is to concentrate on designing features that can be computed directly from the pixel grid, e.g. without requiring a region boundary. A classifier computes the likelihood of each pixel to be part

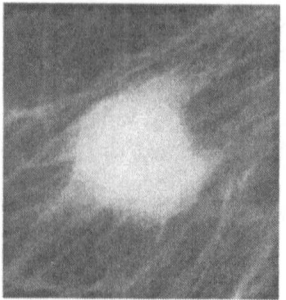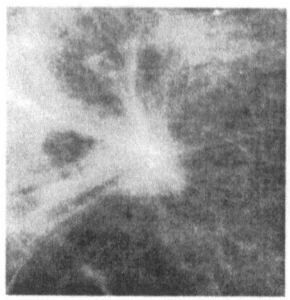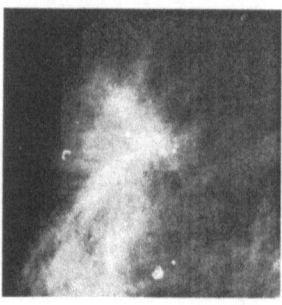

Fig. 1. Examples of malignant lesions: a circumscribed mass (left), a spiculated mass (middle), and an architectural distortion (right)

of a mass, and a simple threshold on this likelihood image is applied to segment regions marked as suspicious as the final output.

Analysis of local line and gradient direction patterns forms the basis for computation of the local features that are used. A detailed description of this method is given in Sect. 2. The method is an extension of earlier work [15,19]. The size of the neighborhood in which orientations patterns are evaluated is one of the most important parameters in the computation of these features. Variation of this size can have a dramatic effect on the detection of individual cancers, although the influence of this parameter on the overall performance measured on a large database tends to be less. In the past, the output of a local contrast operator has been used to set the size of the neighborhood adaptively. In Sect. 2 a new approach is presented, in which features are computed as a continuous function of the neighborhood size, only slightly increasing the computational load. The curves that represent the directional features as a function of the radius of the neighborhood reveal aspects of the neighborhood patterns that may be very useful for improving detection performance by removing false positives.

In Sect. 3 it is shown that the maximum of a gradient orientation feature can be used to estimate the size of a lesion. This size is used as an additional feature to improve detection performance in a scheme where various local features are combined using a neural network classifier. In Sect. 5 results are shown that were obtained using on a series of 264 mammograms, representing consecutive cases of cancer detected in screening, excluding cases which only had microcalcifications.

2   Methods

2.1   Local Orientation Distributions

It has been shown that features representing local orientation distributions are well suited for detection of masses in mammograms [20,15,19]. The fact that such features are very insensitive to changes in contrast is a major advantage when processing large datasets of mammograms of various origin, because one has to deal with unknown non-linear variation of the greyscale. Orientation maps are computed using first and second order Gaussian derivatives. When there is a concentration of gradient orientation towards a certain point this indicates the presence of a mass. A concentration of line orientations computed from second order directional derivatives indicates the presence of spiculation or architectural distortion. These concentration features will be denoted by $g1$ and $l1$, respectively for gradient and line orientations. In addition, features representing radial uniformity measure whether or not increase of pixels oriented to a center comes from the whole surrounding area or from a few directions only. These will be denoted by $g2$ and $l2$.

Previously, features for orientation concentration were computed by counting the number of pixels pointing to a center, and were defined to measure deviations of this number from the expected value in a random orientation pattern. The assumption was made that a binomial distribution of this number with mean probability $\bar{p}$ of a pixel pointing to a center can be used for normalization. As the probability p of hitting the center varies with the distance, this normalization may not be best choice. A more general definition of the features is given below, which allows to deal with varying values of p properly.

For computation of the features at a given pixel i a circular neighborhood is used. All pixels j located within a distance $r_{min} < r_{ij} < r_{max}$ from i are selected when the magnitude of the orientation operator exceeds a small threshold. This selected set of pixels is denoted by S_i. The features are based on a statistic x_j defined by

$$x_j = \begin{cases} 1 - p_j, & \text{if pixel } j \text{ oriented to center,} \\ -p_j & \text{else} \end{cases} \tag{1}$$

with p_j the probability that pixel j is oriented towards the center given a random pattern of orientations φ with a probability density $f_i(\varphi)$. In principle this density can be estimated from the image in an area around site i. However, in this work only a uniform density is used. Pixels that are oriented to the center are determined by evaluating

$$|\varphi_j - \alpha_{ij}| < \frac{D}{2r_{ij}} \tag{2}$$

with α_{ij} the direction of the line through i and j and D a constant determining the accuracy with which pixels should be directed to the center to be counted. A weighted sum X_i is computed by

$$X_i = \sum_{j \in S_i} w_j x_j \tag{3}$$

where the weight factors can be chosen as a function of the distance r_{ij}, for instance to give pixels closer to the center a larger weight. For a noise pattern, the variance of this sum can be estimated when it is assumed that all pixel contributions are independent:

$$var(X_i) = var(\sum_{j \in S_i} w_j x_j)$$

$$= \sum_{j \in S_i} w_j^2 var(x_j)$$

$$= \sum_{j \in S_i} w_j^2 p_j (1 - p_j). \tag{4}$$

Normalizing the sum X_i by the square root of the variance the value of the concentration feature f_1 is defined by

$$f_1 = \frac{\sum_{j \in S_i} w_j x_j}{(\sum_{j \in S_i} w_j^2 p_j (1 - p_j))^{\frac{1}{2}}}. \tag{5}$$

When no weight factors are used and the neighborhood S_i is subdivided in K rings around i in which the probability p_k can be considered constant, the sum X_i can be written as

$$X_i = \sum_k \sum_{j \in S_{i,k}} x_j. \tag{6}$$

These rings are circular and concentric when the probability density of the orientations $f(\varphi)$ is taken uniform. In each ring k the number of pixels hitting the center $N_{k,hit}$ can be counted, allowing the sum to be rewritten as

$$X_i = \sum_k N_{k,hit}(1 - p_k) + (N_k - N_{k,hit})(-p_k)$$

$$= \sum_k N_{k,hit} - N_k \bar{p}_k$$

$$= N_{hit} - N\bar{p} \tag{7}$$

with N_k and N the number of pixels in ring k and in total, respectively. This is identical to the definition used previously, but the normalization factor, which can be written as $(N(\bar{p} - \bar{p^2}))^{-\frac{1}{2}}$, is slightly different than the one used before, $(N(\bar{p} - \bar{p}^2))^{-\frac{1}{2}}$.

If weight factors are used that only depend on p_j, the sum X_i can be written as

$$X_i = \sum_k w_k [N_{k,hit} - N_k \bar{p}_k] \tag{8}$$

which shows that the expected value of f_1 remains zero. If the probability density $f(\varphi)$ is uniform, all choices of w_j that depend only on r_{ij} fall in this category. Results shown in this paper were obtained without using weights. Thus far no clear advantage of using a non-uniform weight function could be demonstrated experimentally.

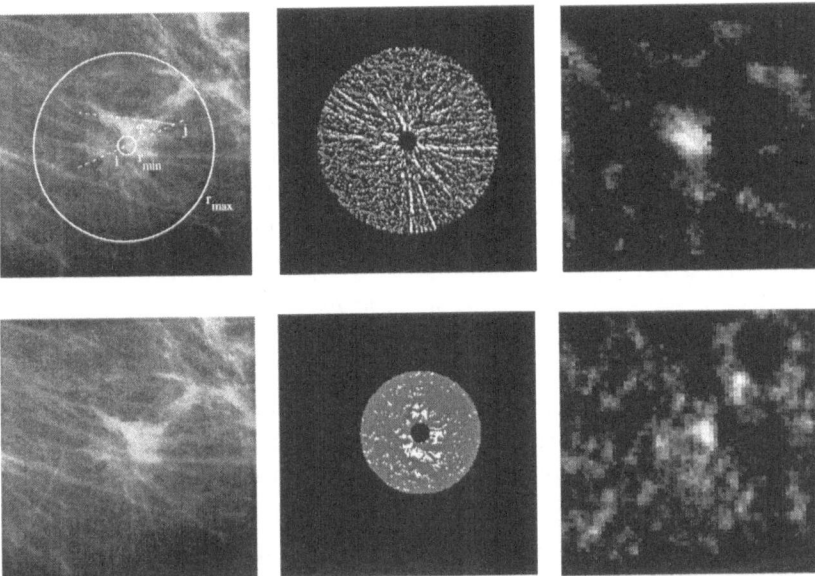

Fig. 2. Detection of a spiculated mass using line (top) and gradient orientation (bottom) maps. The figures in the central column show the labels allocated to pixels based on their orientations, when the window is centered at the tumor. The right column shows the output of line and gradient concentration filters $l1$ and $g1$. Pixels are marked white when they are oriented towards the center, or grey when they are not. For the orientation filter, pixels are marked black when their line magnitude is negative: dark linear structures do not represent spicules and are excluded

It is noted that the approximation that is made by assuming all pixels to have independent directions is clearly incorrect, even when pixels have independent random values. Orientations of neighboring pixels become correlated by the use of convolution kernels for estimation. This leads to underestimation of the variance, which becomes larger with larger kernels. However, it seems that this effect is similar for normal and abnormal areas. For the purpose of removing dependency of the size of the neighborhood and compensating unwanted effects at the breast edge boundary the method is effective.

In Fig. 2 an example is shown of a spiculated lesion. The line orientation feature $l1$ shows a peak at the center of a spiculated mass. This coincides with an increase of the gradient concentration feature $g1$, which is not very strong in this case because the mass is not very compact. By combination of the features at each pixel using a classifier and by segmentation of the result a highly suspicious region results.

Features $g2$ and $l2$ that measure radial uniformity of the orientation patterns around site i are computed by subdividing the neighborhood S_i in L directional bins, that is like a pie. The statistic X_i is computed now for each bin. When there is only noise the expected value of X_i in each bin is zero. In previous work, the number of bins was counted in which the number of pixels pointing to the center was larger than the median of a binomial distribution determined by N_l and $\bar{p}$, with N_l and $\bar{p}_l$ the number of pixels in bin l and $\bar{p}_l$ the average probability of hitting the center. This definition had some problems, as the median of a binomial distribution is not exactly defined. With the approach described here, it is sufficient to compute the number of bins n_+ in which the sum of $X_{i,k}$ is positive. The radial uniformity feature is defined by

$$f2 = \frac{n_+ - K_i/2}{\sqrt{K_i/4}},\tag{9}$$

with K_i the number of sectors at i. The standard deviation of n_+ for random noise $\sqrt{K_i/4}$ is used for normalization, which is important to avoid problems at the edge of the breast where not all sectors can be used.

2.2   Computation of Features as a Function of Scale

In multiscale methods one tries to match the scale of feature extraction to the scale of the abnormality in order to optimize detection performance. Generally, the value of features used for mass detection depend strongly on the size of the abnormality, which makes multiscale approaches attractive. However, most multiscale methods are computationally intensive, because features have to be computed repeatedly at a number of scales. Usually only a very limited number of scales are chosen, which reduces accuracy. Multiscale methods that have been proposed for detection of masses in mammograms include wavelets [21,22], maximum entropy [16], and multi-resolution texture analysis [23]. Also line concentration measured at a number of scales was used in previous work on detection of stellate lesions, where the maximum over the scales was used [15].

   In this section a method is described that allows very efficient computation of a class of local image features as a continuous function of scale, only slightly increasing the computational effort needed for computation at the largest scale considered. The non-linear features described in the previous subsection belong to this class. In the first step of the algorithm an ordered list is constructed in which each element represents a neighbor j within distance r_{ij} of the central location i. In this list, positional information of the neighbor that is needed for the computation is stored, here the x_j, y_j offset, angle φ_j and distance r_{ij} with respect to center. This list is constructed by visiting all pixels in any order, and by subsequently sorting its elements by distance to the center. In the second step the actual computation of the features takes place, at each pixel or at a given fraction of pixels using a sampling scheme. The ordered list of neighbors is used to collect the data from the neighborhood. The x_j, y_j offsets in the list are used to address the pixel data and precomputed derivatives or orientations at the location of the neighbor. The orientation with respect to i is used to compute orientation related features. Because the neighbors are ordered with increasing distance to the center, computation of the features from the collected data can

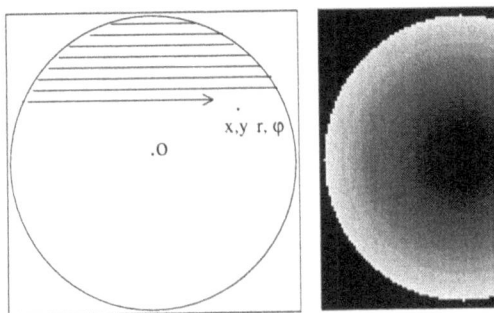

Fig. 3. Construction of an ordered list neighborhood pixels. In the right figure the grey value of each pixel represents its placement in the list, obtained by sorting with respect to distance to center

be carried out at given intervals, for instance each time the number of neighbors has increased by some fixed number. As the computational effort lies in collection of the data, this only slightly increases the computational load. We use intervals in which the number of neighbors increases quadratically. Thus, features are computed at regularly spaced distances from the center. An example is shown in Fig. 1, where line and gradient concentration are plotted as a function of the distance to the center. In a similar way, a contrast feature can be computed by collecting the sum of pixel values as a function of distance to the center, and by and subtracting the mean of the last interval from the mean of the previous intervals.

The curves that represent features as a function of the distance to the center reveal aspects of the neighborhood patterns that can be very useful for differentiation of true and false positive detections. For instance, in Fig. 4 the peak of the gradient orientation signature $g1(r)$ is reached at the edge of the mass, and coincides with the radius at which the spiculation feature $l1(r)$ reaches some kind of plateau. This observation fits with the model of a mass from which most spicules radiate from the contour, and therefore should raise more suspicion that two similar maximum values reached at radii that do not correlate.

3   Applications

By taking the maximum of the scale signature $g1(r)$ representing gradient orientation concentration the size of a mass can be estimated. In this section the accuracy of such a measurement is determined, and the use of size estimates to improve detection performance is studied.

Results are obtained on a database of 71 consecutive cancers detected in a bi-annual screening program in Nijmegen, in the period of 1993 to 1996. In total, this set consisted of 132 mammograms with a cancer. In ten cases only

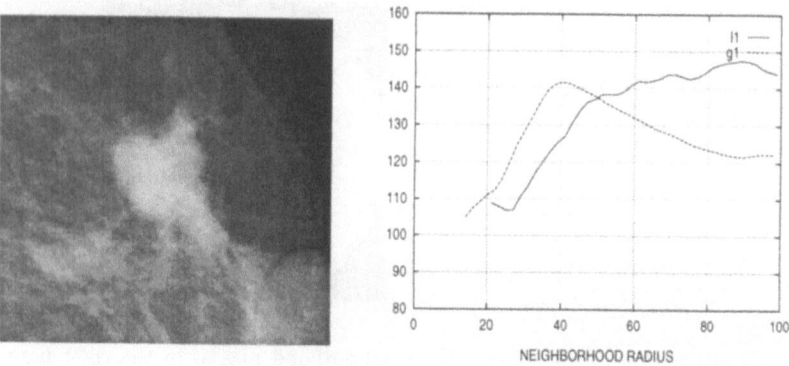

Fig. 4. Scale signatures of line and gradient concentration features, computed in the center of the tumor

oblique views had been taken at screening. All cases detected by screening in the selected period were included, with an exception to those that only showed microcalcifications. Thus, the set may be regarded as representative for cases with masses detected by screening mammography. All cancers were annotated with the help of an expert mammographer. The annotations were used as the gold standard for evaluation of estimated mass sizes and detection performance. In cases with spiculated masses or stellate lesions, only the central mass or area was annotated. The median diameter of the annotated lesions was 15.4 mm, and 72 percent of the lesions was smaller than 2 cm. This may seem somewhat large for cancers detected by screening, but one should realize that many small intraductal cancers with only microcalcifications where excluded. The images were digitized with a Lumisys-85 digitizer at 50 microns and 12 bits per pixel, and were averaged down to 200 micron/pixel prior to all further processing.

3.1   Estimation of Tumor Size

For each mammogram in the database the gradient orientation signatures $g1(r)$, were computed at sites spaced regularly at distances of 1.6 mm apart, storing the radius $r_{i,max}$ at which $g1(r)$ has its maximum for each site i. Before taking the maxima, the signatures were smoothed. Two parameters needed to be adjusted for calculation of $g1$, the scale σ at which gradient orientations are determined and the parameter D used to determine whether or not a pixel is oriented to the center. Results that are shown were obtained by using $\sigma = 0.2$ mm and $D = 4$ mm. The interval in which $g1(r)$ was computed was $r \in [2, 20]$ mm, and the maximum of $g1(r)$ was searched for in the interval $[6, 20]$ mm.

If a pixel is close to the true center of a mass, it is reasonable to use the maximum of the g1 signature to estimate the size of the mass. In the detection application we have in mind, however, the true center is unknown. Moreover, it appeared that the g1 signatures may change considerably when the central location used in the measurement is somewhat changed, especially when small values of D are used. Therefore, to estimate size all maxima of the g1(r) curves measured in a small region were taken into account, rather than relying only on the curve measured at one place. A small circular region was chosen, denoted by C. Different methods to estimate size were evaluated:

1. The radius corresponding with the highest maximum of g1 in C
2. The mean of the radii corresponding to the maxima of g1 in C
3. The minimum radius corresponding with a maximum of g1 in C

In the experiments the radius of C was 2 mm.

For validation of the size estimation methods the annotations in the database were used. It should be noted that not all the annotations in the database correspond with masses that can be clearly identified. Also architectural distortions without a clear central mass are included. Using the annotations as ground truth, the effective radius for each mass is used as size measure. This radius is defined as $\sqrt{A/\pi}$, with A the area of the annotation in mm^2. The circular measurement region C was chosen at the center of mass of each annotation.

Results are shown in Fig. 5. It appears that taking the mean of the radii in a small region yields the most accurate estimates. It is also shown that the tumor sizes are somewhat overestimated by the radius at which the maximum of $g1(r)$ occurs. This bias can be easily corrected for by subtracting a constant. In some cases, however, it appears that the estimated tumor size is far too large. Some of these are cases where a central mass is less or hardly visible. It would be interesting, if a measure could be derived from the $g1(r)$ signature that represents whether the shape of the curve is typical for a mass. Obviously, a curve with a clear maximum will more likely yield a good estimate of tumor size than a curve that is more flat. Such a measure was defined by

$$g3 = \frac{1}{2R - r_{min}} \int_{r=r_{min}}^{2R} |g1(r) - g1(r - \Delta r)| \tag{10}$$

with R the estimated size of the mass. In Fig. 5 it is shown that by using this measure a subset of mass cases can be obtained that have better size estimates, where a threshold on g3 was set as such that 60 percent of the cases was selected.

It was found that size estimates based on g1 signatures computed with a high value of σ, the gradient scale, were less accurate. Size estimates obtained by using a smaller value of D in the g1 computation were comparable to those in Fig. 5.

3.2   Mass Detection Performance

Experiments to determine detection performance were carried out using the database described earlier in this section. By adding 132 bilateral normal mammograms a set of 264 mammograms was obtained. According to the major radiologic sign, mammograms were classified as masses (68), spiculated masses (44), architectural distortions (12) and asymmetries (8). Features that were used were

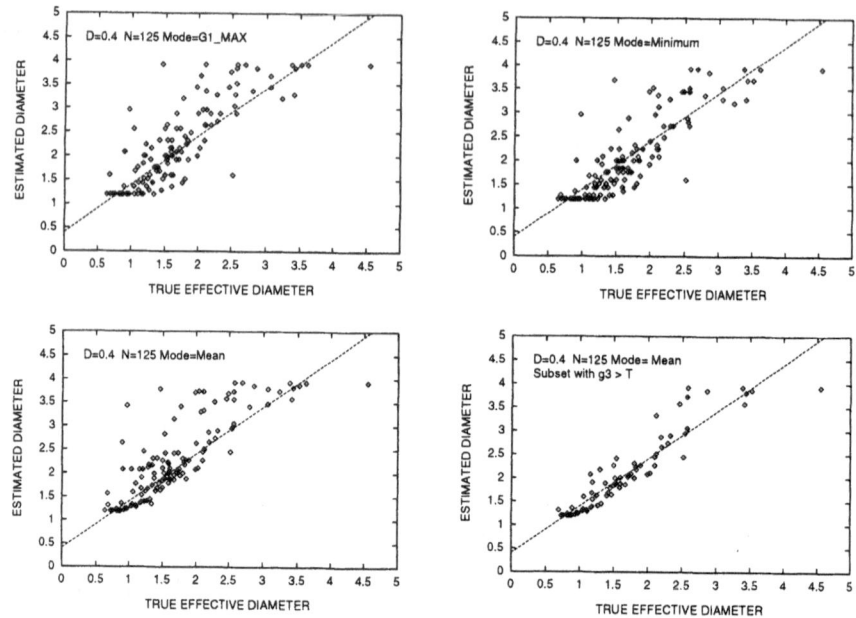

Fig. 5. Comparison of tumor size estimates with true sizes derived from annotations. The estimates are based on g1 signatures in a region of 125 pixels around the center of mass of the annotation. The g1 signatures were computed with $D = 4mm$ and $\sigma = 0.2mm$. Top row: size estimates obtained at the site with the highest value of $g1_{max}$ (left) and at the site with the smallest radius at the maximum of $g1(r)$ (right). In the bottom row the plots show estimates computed as the mean of the radii in the region, for all cases (left) and for cases with $g3 > T$, which more likely correspond to a well defined mass

the line and gradient orientation features described in Sect. 2, each computed at the scale where the orientation concentration feature reached its maximum value. In addition, features representing bilateral asymmetry and estimated size were used, where size was computed as explained in the previous section, centering a small region at each site to be classified. The asymmetry feature was computed by non-rigid registration and subtraction of the right and left breast, followed by a Gaussian smoothing to focus on large asymmetries only [24].

A neural network classifier was used to compute the likelihood of suspiciousness of individual pixels was trained on a separate dataset. All 39 mammograms with malignancies in the public MIAS database were used for this purpose [25], excluding those with only microcalcifications. It should be noted that these images were digitized using a different digitizer. Features that are used are defined in such a way that this should not make a difference.

FROC curves displaying results are shown in Fig. 6. Sensitivity is computed as the number of lesions hit divided by the total number of lesions. A hit was

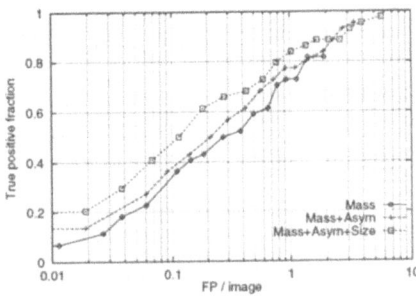 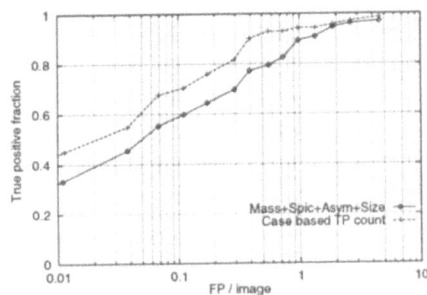

Fig. 6. Using estimated size in combination with asymmetry and mass detection features (a). The overall performance is improved when adding features for detection of spiculation (b). The case based FROC curve is obtained by counting a true positive whenever a cancer is found in either the CC or Oblique view

counted when the center of mass of a region marked by the detection program fell inside the annotation, otherwise a false positive was counted.

The results in Fig. 6 show that adding estimated size to the mass detection method based on asymmetry and gradient orientation in single views improves detection performance. The performance improves further when features to detect spiculation are added. The sensitivity that is obtained using a cases based measure is over 90 percent at a false positive rate of 0.5 FP/image. Remarkably, at a rate of 1 false positive in 50 images still 50 percent of the cases are flagged.

4   Conclusions

An efficient method to compute features representing line and gradient orientation concentration as a function of spatial scale was developed. Using such scale signatures size estimates of mammographic masses can be obtained. These estimates can be useful when regions with masses need to be segmented. Also, the radii at which the feature maxima occur can be used to select the neighborhood size adaptively. In combination with other features, including asymmetry, adding estimated size as a feature led to improved detection results.

On a consecutive sample of non-microcalcification cases from screening, most with oblique and CC views, a high case sensitivity was obtained. The use of the mass detection features gave a much larger improvement of the FROC curve on this database than on datasets biased towards spiculated masses used previously [19], as could be expected. Interestingly, this also holds for very low FP/image values. At 0.02 FP/image a case sensitivity of 50 percent was obtained. Assuming an incidence of 5 cancers per 1000 women and 4 mammograms per case this corresponds with a recall rate of 8 percent, which is quite common in the US. It may be advantageous in a prompting system to present suspicious regions that have such a high specificity in another way to the radiologists than regions only generated at lower specificity levels.

The method described in this paper is applicable to other areas in medical image analysis, for instance to lung nodule detection in CT. The features used to represent local orientation patterns are general and can be computed efficiently in 3D datasets as well.

References

1. Tabar, L., Fagerberg, G., and Day, N.E.: Breast cancer treatment and natural history: new insights from results ofscreening. Lancet **339** (1992) 412–414
2. Bird, R. E., Wallace, T.W., and Yankaskas, B.C.: Analysis of cancers missed at screening mammography. Radiology **184** (1992) 613–617
3. van Dijck, J. A. M., Verbeek, L. M., Hendriks, J. H. C. L., and Holland, R.: The current detectability of breast cancer in a mammographic screening program. Cancer **72** (1993) 1933–1938
4. Harvey, J. E., Fajardo, L. L., and Inis, C. A.: Previous mammograms in patients with impalpable breast carcinoma: retrospective vs blinded interpretation. AJR **161** (1993) 1167–1172
5. Roehrig, J., Doi, T., Hasegawa, A., Hunt, B., Marshall, J., Romsdahl, H., Schneider, A., Sharbaugh, R., and Zang, W.: Clinical results with r2 imagechecker in support of fda pma application. In N Karssemeijer, MAO Thijssen, JHCL Hendriks, and LJTO van Erning, editors, Digital Mammography, Kluwer, Dordrecht, (1998) 395–400
6. Vitak, B.: Invasive interval cancers in the Östergötland mammographic screening programme: Radiological analysis. European Radiology **8** (1998) 639–646
7. Thurfjell, E. L., Lernevall, K. A., and Taube, A. A. S.: Benefit of independent double reading in a population-based mammography screening program. Radiology **191** (1994) 241–244
8. Chan, H. P., Doi, K., Vyborny, C. J., Schmidt, R. A., Metz, C. E., Lam, K. L., Ogura, T., Wu, T., and Macmahon, H.: Improvement in radiologist's detection of clustered microcalcifications on mammograms. Inv Radiol **25** (1990) 1102–1110
9. Astley, S., Hutt, I., Adamson, S., Rose, P., Miller, P., Boggis, C., Taylor, C., Valentine, T., and Davies, J.: Automation in mammography: computer vision and human perception. SPIE **1905** (1993) 716–730
10. Kegelmeyer, W. P., Pruneda, J. M., Bourland, P. D., Hillis, A., Riggs, M.W., and Nipper, M. L.: Computer-aided mammographic screening for spiculated lesions. Radiology **191** (1994) 331–337
11. Dean, P. B.: Overview of breast cancer screening. In K Doi, M L Giger, R M Nishikawa, and R A Schmidt, editors, Digital Mammography, Elsevier, Amsterdam (1996) 19–26
12. Lau, T. K., and Bischof, W. F.: Automated detection of breast tumors using the asymmetry approach. Comp and Biomed Research **24** (1991) 273–295
13. Yin, F F., Giger, M. L., Doi, K., Metz, C. E., Vyborny, C. J., and Schmidt, R. A.: Computerized detection of masses in digital mammograms : Analysis of bilateral substraction images. Med Phys **18** (1991) 955–963
14. Miller, P., and Astley, S. M.: Automated detection of mammographic asymmetry using anatomical features. Int. Journal of Pattern Recognition and AI **7** (1992) 1461–1476

15. Karssemeijer, N., and te Brake, G. M.: Detection of stellate distortions in mammograms. IEEE Trans Med Imag **15** (1996) 611–619

16. Miller, L., and Ramsey, N.: The detection of malignant masses by non-linear multiscale analysis. In K Doi, M L Giger, R M Nishikawa, and R A Schmidt, editors, Digital Mammography, Elsevier, Amsterdam (1996) 335–340

17. Petrick, N., Chan, H. P., Sahiner, B., and Wei, D.: An adaptive density-weighted contrast enhancement filter for mammographic breast mass detection. IEEE Trans Med Imag **15** (1996) 59–67

18. Vujovic, N., and Brzakovic, D.: Establishing the correspondence between control points in pairs of mammographic images. IEEE Trans Imag Processing **6** (1997) 1388–1399

19. te Brake, G. M., and Karssemeijer, N.: Detection of stellate breast abnormalities. In K Doi, M L Giger, R M Nishikawa, and R A Schmidt, editors, Digital Mammography, Elsevier, Amsterdam, (1996) 341–346

20. Karssemeijer, N.: Detection of stellate distortions in mammograms using scale space operators. In Y Bizais, C Barrilot, and R Di Paola, editors, Information Processing in Medical Imaging, Kluwer, Dordrecht (1995) 335–346

21. Laine, A. F., Schuler, S., Fan, J., and Huda, W.: Mammographic feature enhancement by multiscale enhancement. IEEE Trans on Med Imag **13** (1994) 725–740

22. Laine, A., Huda, W., Chen, D. W., and Harris, J.: Segmentation of masses using continuous scale representations. In K Doi, M L Giger, R M Nishikawa, and R A Schmidt, editors, Digital Mammography, Elsevier, Amsterdam (1996) 447–450

23. Wei, D., Chan, H. P., Helvie, M. A., Sahiner, B., Petrick, N., Adler, D. D., and Goodsitt, M. M.: Classification of mass and normal breast tissue on digital mammograms : multiresolution texture analysis. Med Phys **22** (1995) 1501–1513

24. Karssemeijer, N., and te Brake, G.M.: Combining single view features and asymmetry for detection of mass lesions. In N Karssemeijer, MAO Thijssen, JHCL Hendriks, and LJTO van Erning, editors, Digital Mammography, Kluwer, Dordrecht (1998) 95–102

25. Suckling, J., Parker, J., Dance, D. R., Astley, S., Hutt, I., Boggis, C. R. M., Ricketts, I., Stamatakis, E., Cerneaz, N., Kok, S L., Taylor, P., Betal, D., and Savage, J.: The mammographic image analysis society digital mammogram database. In A G Gale, S M Astley, D R Dance, and A Y Cairns, editors, Digital Mammography, Elsevier, Amsterdam (1994) 375–378

Physiologically Oriented Models of the Hemodynamic Response in Functional MRI

Frithjof Kruggel and D. Yves von Cramon

Max-Planck-Institute of Cognitive Neuroscience,
Stephanstraße 1, 04103 Leipzig, Germany
{kruggel, cramon}@cns.mpg.de

Abstract. Today, most studies of cognitive processes using functional MRI (fMRI) experiments adopt highly flexible stimulation designs, where not only the activation amount but also the time course of the measured hemodynamic response is of interest. The measured signal only indirectly reflects the underlying neuronal activation, and is understood as being convolved with a hemodynamic modulation function. An approach to better allow inferences about the neuronal activation is given by modeling this convolution process. In this study, we investigate this approach and discuss computational models for the hemodynamic response. An analysis of a recent fMRI experiment underlines the usefulness of this approach.

1 Introduction

Functional magnetic resonance imaging (fMRI) has become one of the major experimental methods for analyzing cognitive processes in humans. The most common fMRI technique employs the blood-oxygen-level-dependent (BOLD) contrast [1], which is sensitive to changes of the relative local concentration of oxygenated hemoglobin (HbO_2) vs. deoxy-hemoglobin and thus reflects an indirect measure of the brain's neuronal activation. This effect is small, and data are noisy: thus, analysis of fMRI data has mostly focused on the detection and statistical quantification of functional activation.

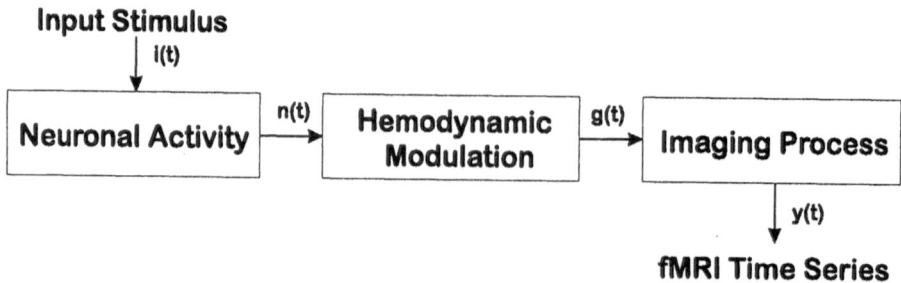

Fig. 1. Signals at various stages of the convolution model of fMRI time series

A. Kuba et al. (Eds.): IPMI'99, LNCS 1613, pp. 294–307, 1999.
© Springer-Verlag Berlin Heidelberg 1999

Understanding brain function requires information not only on the spatial localization of neural activity, but also on its temporal evolution. There is an increasing interest in the time course (i.e. the shape) of the hemodynamic response (HR) and its modulation with respect to different experimental conditions. The measured fMRI signal $y(t)$ is understood as the result from a series of convolutions of the input stimulus function $i(t)$ ([2], see Fig. 1). So the question was raised to what extent conclusions may be drawn about the neuronal activation $n(t)$ from the HR shape $g(t)$. For example, the hemodynamic modulation introduces time constants at least an order longer than the underlying functional activation; the time-to-maximum of a HR due to a transient stimulus is typically delayed by 5-8s and dispersed by 3-4s [3]. So the key to detecting changes in the neuronal activation is the adoption and deconvolution of the HR by a model function [4].

A number of heuristic functions have been proposed to describe the hemodynamic response: the Poisson function [3], the Gamma function [5,6], a linear combination of the Gamma function and its temporal derivatives [7], and the Gaussian function [8]. The evolution of these approaches follows their modeling complexity; early approaches assumed constant pre-set values for the lag [3], while current models determined HR parameters voxelwise in the time series [5,6,8], or even per stimulus period [9]. HR parameters were shown to depend on the subject, the site and the stimulation conditions [8,9,10], which underlines the usefulness of this approach. However, some issues were raised.

- With the Poisson or the Gamma functions, interesting shape characteristics like delay (time-to-maximum), rise and fall times are hard to obtain.
- While the best fits to an HR are generally found with the Gaussian function, especially responses following short stimuli were asymmetric (shorter rise than fall times).
- For a better understanding of the underlying neuronal processes, a deconvolution of the hemodynamic modulation to yield parameters of the neuronal activation directly is highly desirable.
- None of these functions is based on a physiological model. Although models of the oxygen delivery at membranes have been proposed [11], details of the neurono-vascular coupling are still under discussion and have not yet led to a comprehensive physiological model of hemodynamic modulation.

Aims of this study were: (1) to test the feasibility of introducing more complex model functions for the HR, (2) to separate parameters describing the hemodynamic modulation from parameters of neuronal activation, and (3) to find physiologically more plausible models for the hemodynamic modulation.

Recently, we described and validated a non-linear regression context [9] to model the HR per stimulation period (trial) and region-of-interest (ROI), which is briefly reviewed in the next section, along with a discussion of the three model functions studied here: (1) the Gaussian function, (2) a convolved asymmetric Gaussian function, and (3) a convolved compartment model. To compare the usefulness of these approaches, we re-analyzed a fMRI study of working memory.

2   Description of the Estimation Model

A theoretical discussion and validation of our estimation model is described elsewhere [9]. For an excellent discussion about non-linear regression procedures, see [12]. Throughout this paper, we assume that the locus of a functional activation is known. This knowledge may arise from a previous determination by well-established signal detection procedures or defined as regions of neurofunctional interest. These regions are considered as stationary in space. Note that we focus on single trial experimental designs here: a single cognitive task is given, and the hemodynamic response to this stimulus recorded.

2.1   Model Definition

We consider a subset of the fMRI data collected spatially from a ROI of k voxels and temporally from a single experimental trial at l discrete timesteps and denote this $n = k * l$-dimensional vector as $\mathbf{y}$. Timesteps are referenced by a l-dimensional vector $\mathbf{t}$. We model the hemodynamic response as a deterministic function $g(\mathbf{t}, \boldsymbol{\beta})$, where $\boldsymbol{\beta}$ denotes a p-dimensional vector of model parameters, and we require that $g(\mathbf{t}, \boldsymbol{\beta})$ is differentiable at least once with respect to $\boldsymbol{\beta}$. Data $\mathbf{y}$ are composed of $g(\cdot)$ and a stochastic part $\boldsymbol{\epsilon}$:

$$\mathbf{y} = g(\mathbf{t}, \boldsymbol{\beta}) + \boldsymbol{\epsilon}. \tag{1}$$

The stochastic part is independent of the signal and stationary with respect to time, and its elements are normally distributed with a nonsingular covariance matrix $\mathbf{V}$:

$$\boldsymbol{\epsilon} \sim N_n(0, \mathbf{V}), \qquad \text{then} \qquad \mathbf{y} \sim N_n(g(\boldsymbol{\beta}), \mathbf{V}). \tag{2}$$

This allows us to use preprocessed data where the processing has introduced (or enhanced) a correlation structure. A way to determine the covariance structure from experimental data is described later in this section.

We will now propose the model functions $g(\cdot)$ investigated in this paper. The first two are heuristic but offer a parsimonous number of parameters. The third function is complex but tries to incorporate the properties of tissue compartments involved in the BOLD effect.

Model 1: Gaussian Function The best compromise between goodness-of-fit and the number of model parameters is found with the Gaussian function [8]:

$$g(t, \boldsymbol{\beta}) = a \exp(-(t - t_0)^2/(2d_0^2)) + b. \tag{3}$$

We denote the 4 components of $\boldsymbol{\beta}$ as a: gain (the "height" of the HR), d_0: dispersion (proportional to the duration of the HR), t_0: lag (the time from stimulation onset to the HR peak), and b: baseline. Here, no distinction can be made between "neuronal" and "vascular" parameters.

Model 2: Convolved Asymmetric Gaussian Function A first approach to closer model the processes depicted in Fig. 1 is to define the HR function $g(t)$ by a convolution of a neuronal stimulation function $n(t)$ with a hemodynamic modulation function $f(t)$:

$$g(t, \boldsymbol{\beta}) = n(t) \otimes f(t) + b, \tag{4}$$

where $\otimes$ denotes the convolution operator and b is a baseline term. We simply assume a square-wave function for the neuronal stimulation $n(t)$:

$$n(t) = \begin{cases} a \text{ if } t >= t_0 \text{ and } t < t_0 + t_1, \\ 0 \text{ otherwise.} \end{cases} \tag{5}$$

A Gaussian function is introduced for hemodynamic modulation function $f(\cdot)$, here with different dispersions (d_0, d_1) for the rising and the falling edge:

$$f(t) = \begin{cases} \exp(-t^2/(2d_0^2)) \text{ if } t < 0, \\ \exp(-t^2/(2d_1^2)) \text{ if } t >= 0. \end{cases} \tag{6}$$

In this model, $\boldsymbol{\beta}$ consists of 6 parameters (d_0: dispersion on the rising edge, d_1: dispersion on the falling edge, a: gain, t_0: neuronal response onset, t_1: neuronal response duration, b: offset). Modeling of the convolution process allows us to address the meaning of a, t_0, and t_1 as "neuronal" parameters, resp. d_0, d_1 as vascular parameters.

Model 3: Convolved Compartment Model In model 3, the formulation of a stepwise defined Gaussian function for the hemodynamic modulation function $f(\cdot)$ is still heuristic. It is physiologically more plausible to model the hemodynamic modulation process by a compartment model. We define the HR model function $g(t)$ as in 4 and the neuronal stimulation $n(t)$ as in 5 and now focus on a new definition of $f(t)$.

For the BOLD contrast, as discussed in the introduction, it is viable to think of the oxygenated blood as an "endogenous tracer" of brain activation. The kinetic of external tracers such as radioactive markers or pharmaceuticals have successfully been modeled by compartment models since 1920 [13]. This modeling context is rich and well understood (for introductions, see [12,14]). Compartments correspond to a body subspaces (i.e. tissue, vasculature), in which the local concentration of a tracer (i.e. oxygenated blood) is modified by transport between compartments (i.e. by diffusion, flow) or active processes (i.e. by consumption). If we assume a linear imaging process, then the HR measured in fMRI is proportional to the HbO_2 concentration, and a compartment model should allow us to draw conclusions about the temporal oxygen flow pattern. Such a model is depicted in Fig. 2.

HbO_2 flows from the arterial into the capillary compartment at a rate γ_0, as mediated by a consumption process in the tissue compartment. The oxygen exchange between capillaries and tissue is described by rates γ_1 and γ_2. Finally,

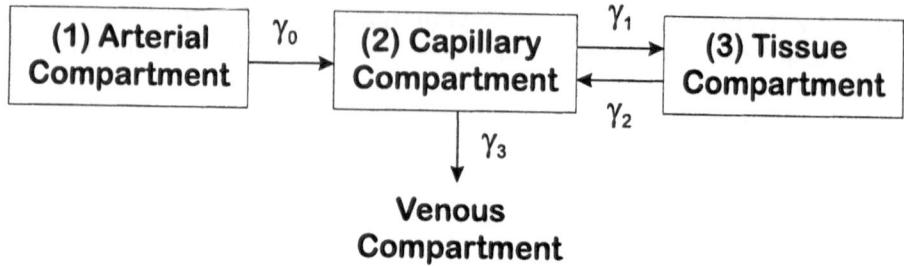

Fig. 2. Movement of oxygen in two vascular and a tissue compartments

rate γ_3 denotes the HbO_2 drainage into the venous compartment. Assuming constant rates, the kinetic equations for the compartment model in Fig. 2 are:

$$\dot{f}_1 = -\gamma_0 f_1,$$
$$\dot{f}_2 = \gamma_0 f_1 + \gamma_2 f_3 - (\gamma_1 + \gamma_3) f_2, \qquad (7)$$
$$\dot{f}_3 = \gamma_0 f_2 - \gamma_2 f_3.$$

The solution to this linear system of differential equations can be written in a *sum-of-exponentials* model for the ith compartment (see [12], p. 379ff):

$$f_i = k_{i1} \exp(-\gamma_0 t) + k_{i2} \exp(\lambda_0 t) + k_{i3} \exp(\lambda_1 t), \qquad (8)$$

where the parameters $\lambda_{0,1}$ and k_{ij} are:

$$
\begin{aligned}
\lambda_0 &= -\frac{1}{2}\left(\gamma_1 + \gamma_2 + \gamma_3 + \sqrt{(\gamma_1 + \gamma_2 + \gamma_3)^2 - 4\gamma_2\gamma_3}\right), \\
\lambda_1 &= -\frac{1}{2}\left(\gamma_1 + \gamma_2 + \gamma_3 - \sqrt{(\gamma_1 + \gamma_2 + \gamma_3)^2 - 4\gamma_2\gamma_3}\right), \\
k_{1j} &= [1, 0, 0], \\
k_{2j} &= \left[\frac{\gamma_0(\gamma_2 - \gamma_0)}{(\gamma_0 + \lambda_0)(\gamma_0 + \lambda_1)}, \frac{\gamma_0(\gamma_2 + \lambda_0)}{(\gamma_0 + \lambda_0)(\lambda_0 - \lambda_1)}, \frac{\gamma_0(\gamma_2 + \lambda_1)}{(\gamma_0 + \lambda_1)(\lambda_1 - \lambda_0)}\right], \\
k_{3j} &= \left[\frac{\gamma_0\gamma_1(\gamma_2 - \gamma_0)}{(\gamma_0 + \lambda_0)(\gamma_0 + \lambda_1)}, \frac{\gamma_0\gamma_1(\gamma_2 + \lambda_0)}{(\gamma_0 + \lambda_0)(\lambda_0 - \lambda_1)}, \frac{\gamma_0\gamma_1(\gamma_2 + \lambda_1)}{(\gamma_0 + \lambda_1)(\lambda_1 - \lambda_0)}\right].
\end{aligned}
\qquad (9)
$$

The parameter vector β for this model consists of 8 items (γ_i: 4 transfer rates, a: gain, t_0: neuronal response onset, t_1: neuronal response duration, b: offset). We attribute a, t_0, and t_1 as "neuronal" parameters, resp. the transfer rates as vascular parameters.

2.2   Stochastic Background Model

It was shown [15,16] that the stochastic part in preprocessed fMRI data may approximately be described by an Ornstein-Uhlenbeck process [17]: (1) it is stationary with respect to time, (2) its elements ϵ_i are normally distributed with a covariance matrix $\mathbf{V}$ (see 1) and (3) their correlation is described by an AR(1) model. We assume that the spatio-temporal covariance matrix $\mathbf{V}$ is separable in space and time:

$$\mathbf{V} = \mathbf{S} \odot \mathbf{T}, \tag{10}$$

where $\odot$ denotes the Kronecker product. The elements of the (spatial) covariance matrix $\mathbf{S}$ are given by the variance $s_{ii} = \sigma^2$ and the covariance $s_{ij} = cov(h)$ which depend on the distance h of the voxels i and j. Most easily, a semivariogram $\eta(h)$ [18] is used to determine the type of stationary dependence in the data:

$$\eta(h) = \sigma^2 - cov(h) \approx \frac{1}{2 * n_h} \sum_{(i,j) \in N(h)} (y_i - y_j)^2, \tag{11}$$

where $N(h)$ is the set of voxel pairs at distance h, and n_h is the number of pairs in the set. For an AR(1) process with positive correlations, an exponential function fits to the semivariogram:

$$\eta(h) = \alpha_0(1 - \exp(-\alpha_1 h)), \tag{12}$$

where h is the distance between voxel sites. From the model parameters, we can derive the variance $\sigma^2 = \alpha_0$ and the autocorrelation $\rho = \exp(-\alpha_1)$. The covariance matrix $\mathbf{S}$ of a linear array of k voxels is defined as:

$$\mathbf{S} = \sigma^2 \begin{pmatrix} 1 & \rho & \rho^2 & \cdots & \rho^{k-1} \\ \rho & 1 & \rho & \cdots & \rho^{k-2} \\ \rho^2 & \rho & 1 & \cdots & \rho^{k-3} \\ & & \cdots & & \\ \rho^{k-1} & & & \cdots & 1 \end{pmatrix}, \tag{13}$$

Similarly, a matrix $\mathbf{T}$ is formed for the temporal domain and composed as given in 10.

2.3   Estimation

We find the ML estimate $\hat{\beta}$ of our model parameters as the vector β that minimizes the quantity:

$$\arg\min_{\beta} \left\{ (\mathbf{y} - g(\mathbf{t}, \beta))^T \mathbf{V}^{-1} (\mathbf{y} - g(\mathbf{t}, \beta)) \right\}. \tag{14}$$

In the case of the Gaussian function in model 1, this problem corresponds to a 4-dimensional nonlinear minimization problem, which can easily be solved by the downhill simplex method of Nelder and Mead [19]. This method is not feasible with the more complex models 2 and 3, where the cost function (14) is expected to possess multiple local minima. Because derivatives of the model functions are only available as finite difference approximations, derivative-free optimization methods are preferable. We investigated the use of (1) a combination of simulated annealing with the downhill simplex method [19], (2) Shor's minimization method [20], and (3) an optimization using a genetic algorithm [21].

2.4   Confidence Limits and Statistical Tests

Using a first-order linear model, we can derive confidence limits for the estimation from the inverse of the Fisher information matrix $\mathbf{F}$ [22]:

$$\hat{\beta} \sim N(\beta, \mathbf{F}_\beta^{-1}), \quad \text{where} \quad \mathbf{F}_\beta = \mathbf{G}_\beta \mathbf{V}^{-1}\mathbf{G}_\beta^T, \tag{15}$$

and $\mathbf{G}_\beta$ denotes the Jacobian matrix of $g(\cdot)$ with respect to β.

A simple measure for the goodness-of-fit (GOF) is given by the χ^2-statistics:

$$\chi^2 = \epsilon^T \mathbf{V}^{-1}\epsilon, \quad \text{where} \quad \epsilon = \mathbf{y} - g(\mathbf{t}, \beta) \tag{16}$$

A more complex measure is derived for the F-statistics, following Hartley [23]:

$$\mathbf{P} = \mathbf{G}_\beta \mathbf{F}_\beta^{-1}\mathbf{G}_\beta^T \tag{17}$$

$$F_{p,n-p} \sim \frac{(n-p)}{p} \frac{\epsilon^T \mathbf{P}\epsilon}{\epsilon^T(\mathbf{I}_n - \mathbf{P})\epsilon}, \tag{18}$$

where n corresponds to the number of data points, p to the number of parameters, and $\mathbf{I}_n$ is the $n * n$ identity matrix.

3   Experiments

To study the usefulness of this modeling approach, we re-evaluated datasets acquired in a fMRI study of working memory [24].

Behavioral Experiment: Subjects learned three sets of letters (4, 6 or 8 characters) at least two days before the scanning session. A trial started with the display of a small red box (for 800ms), followed by the cue and, after a delay (0, 2 or 4 seconds), the probe. Subjects had to indicate by a button press whether the probe item belonged to the cued set. 108 randomized trials were run using an intertrial interval of 18s.

fMRI Parameters: During the behavioral experiment, 7 axial slices (64x64 voxels, 3.8x3.8x5mm voxel size, 2mm gap) were recorded on a Bruker Medspec 300 system using an EPI protocol with a repetition time of 1s. All timings were corrected for the slice acquisition delay in the EPI protocol.

Preprocessing: We randomly selected data obtained from 4 subjects. Data were preprocessed by (1) correction for in-plane movements and (2) corrected for baseline fluctuations, (3) lowpass filtered in the temporal domain to reduce the amount of system and physiological noise (see [25] for details). As a result of this preprocessing, only the fundamental frequency (corresponding to the stimulation) and its first harmonic were retained in the temporal domain of the data.

Definition of ROIs: Standard procedures were applied to detect functional activation in the datasets: (1) analysis for activated regions by Pearson correlation with a time-shifted box-car waveform ($\Delta = 6s$), (2) conversion of the correlation coefficient into z-scores and thresholding of the corresponding z-map by a score of 10, (3) assessment of the activated regions for their significance on the basis of their spatial extent [26]. Now that we detected voxels with functional activation, we defined ROIs by collecting the 6 most highly activated voxels around local maxima in the z-map. We obtained a total of 94 ROIs from 4 subjects. An illustrative map of ROIs is shown in Fig. 3.

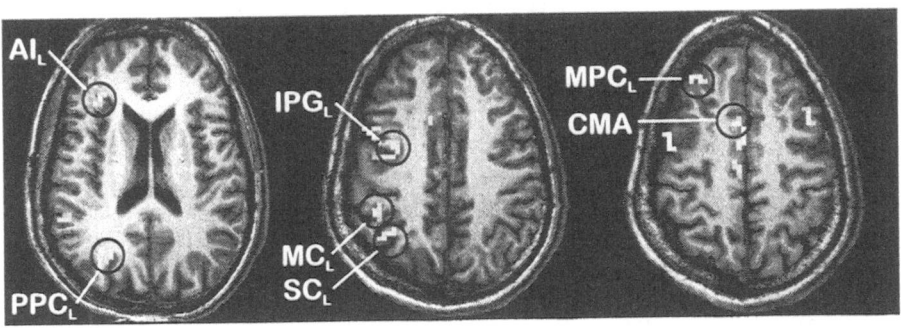

Fig. 3. An illustrative z-map overlay onto the corresponding anatomical from the working memory experiment. Neurofunctionally interesting ROIs are labeled: AI_L: superior anterior insula, MPC_L: middle prefrontal cortex, IPG_L: inferior precentral gyrus, CMA: cingulate motor area, MC_L: motor cortex, PPC_L: posterior parietal cortex, SC_L: sensory cortex

Averaging: To reduce the number of estimations, we averaged voxels within a ROI at a given timestep and across trials with the same delay time manipulation (0, 2, and 4 s). So per ROI, we obtained three different timecourses of 18 timepoints each. As a consequence of averaging in space, we simplified our estimation model by setting $\mathbf{S} = \mathbf{I}_k$, where $k = 6$.

Tests We adapted the 3 HR models defined in the preceeding section to the 3 averaged timecourses in the 94 ROIs. To achieve realistic solutions, we constrained the solution space by the following intervals:

- *model 1:* gain: $0 <= a < 5000$, dispersion: $0 <= d_0 < 10$, lag: $0 <= t_0 < 10$, and baseline: $-500 < b <= 0$,
- *model 2:* onset and duration: $0 <= t_i < 10$, dispersions, gain and offset as above.
- *model 3:* diffusion constants: $0 <= \gamma_i < 10$, onset, duration gain and baseline as above.

For model 1, the downhill simplex algorithm was applied, with computation times of less than a second per estimation. For models 2 and 3, we achieved the best GOFs using the genetic algorithm. Parameters of the genetic optimization process were: 1000 generations, 500 population members, p(exchange) = 0.2, p(mutation) = 0.01, p(crossover) = 0.2.

4   Results

To give an impression of typical waveforms and modeling results, we selected
a signal from the left motor cortex MC_L (see Fig. 3) in one of the subjects.
Averaged HRs of different experimental delay times are shown in Fig. 4.

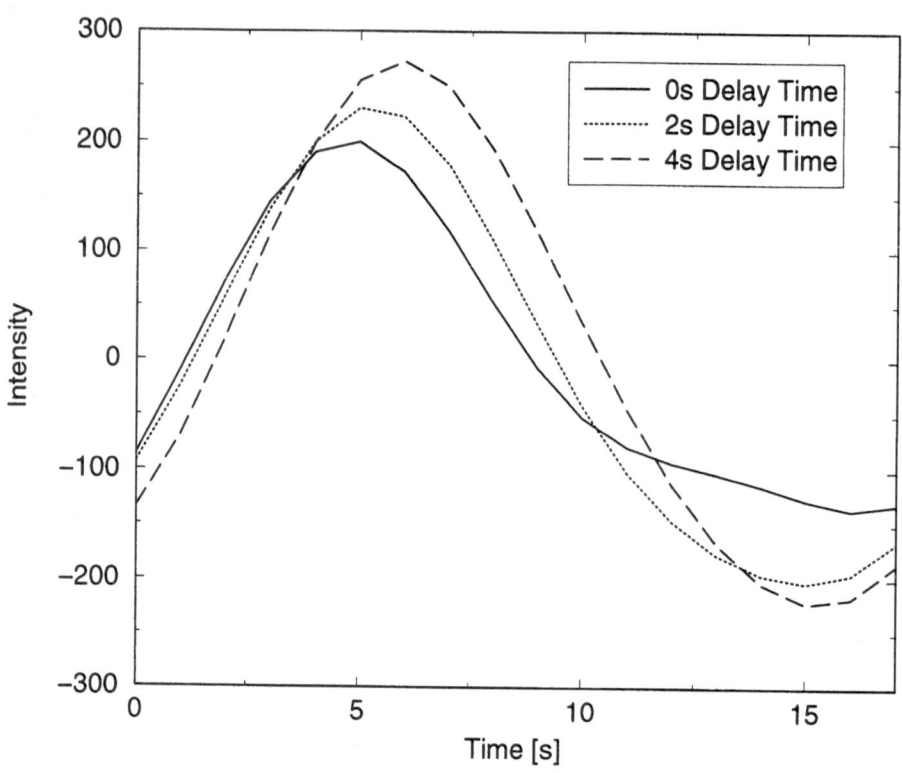

Fig. 4. HRs from region MC_L for the 3 different delay times

For longer delays, the HR in this region was higher, the time-to-maximum and
duration were longer. This was reflected in the parameters of the 3 HR models
(see Table 1). For all models, the increasing height of the HR with delay time was
found as an increase of the gain a. For model 1, the shift of the time-to-maximum
led to an increase of t_0, the increasing width to an increase in the dispersion
d_0. For model 2, the parameters attributed to the hemodynamic modulation
(d_0 and d_1) were relatively independent of the delay time manipulation. Shift
and delay were reflected in increasing values of t_0 and t_1. Finally, with the

convolved compartment model, only an increase of t_1 with the delay was found, rate constants were similar.

Table 1. HR parameters for the signals in Fig. 4 for the 3 different experimental delays

Model 1: Gaussian Function

Delay [s]	a	t_0 [s]	d_0 [s]	χ^2
0	324	3.95	2.78	2381
2	429	4.34	3.21	1270
4	496	5.05	3.34	1994

Model 2: Convolved Asymmetric Gaussian Function

Delay [s]	a	t_0 [s]	t_1 [s]	d_0 [s]	d_1 [s]	χ^2
0	2324	2.58	3.31	2.00	3.30	724
2	3420	3.45	3.55	2.94	3.07	1193
4	4062	3.36	5.05	2.78	3.04	1625

Model 3: Convolved Compartment Model

Delay [s]	a	t_0 [s]	t_1 [s]	γ_0	γ_1	γ_2	γ_3	χ^2
0	1847	0.06	5.63	0.66	6.11	4.60	1.27	770
2	2439	0.03	6.47	0.39	6.50	6.10	1.54	1934
4	3056	0.06	7.24	0.60	6.17	6.56	1.52	2161

By inspection of the waveforms, we typically found that ROIs in all subjects showed an increase of the time-to-maximum and the gain with increasing delay time, similar to the example HR in Fig. 4. A closer examination of the estimated modeling parameters by a cluster analysis revealed differences, which allowed us to group ROIs into 4 categories (see Table 2):

- *Group 1*: early rise, little dependence on the delay time manipulation. ROIs of this category were found in cortical areas, which are relevant for encoding the stimulus. Examples include the posterior parietal cortex PPC_L.
- *Group 2*: early rise, delay dependence: ROIs of this category are relevant for maintaining the stimulus. Examples include the anterior insula AI_L.
- *Group 3*: late rise, delay dependence: ROIs take part in the decision process following the delay and for generating the motor response. An ROI in the primary motor cortex (MC_L) belongs to this group.
- *Group 4*: late rise, little delay dependence. An example for this group is given with the sensory cortex (SC_L): subjects left their finger on the response button independent on the delay time.

In accordance with the observation of general delay dependence, most ROIs either belong to group 2 or group 3. It is interesting to note that most early

Table 2. Onset (t_0), duration (t_1) and end time ($t_e = t_0 + t_1$) of the neuronal activation as estimated by model 2. Examples for 4 groups defined by their different temporal behaviour are shown. ROI labels correspond to Fig. 3, all values are given in [s]

Delay	Group 1: PPC_L			Group 2: AI_L			Group 3: MC_L			Group 4: SC_L		
	t_0	t_1	t_e	t_0	t_1	t_e	t_0	t_1	t_e	t_0	t_1	t_e
0	2.90	1.74	4.64	3.27	0.71	3.98	4.02	1.46	5.48	4.04	4.26	8.30
2	2.78	2.54	5.32	2.86	1.85	4.91	3.71	4.68	8.39	4.80	4.34	9.14
4	3.90	1.64	5.54	2.92	3.61	6.53	4.92	4.89	9.81	4.98	4.93	9.91

activated areas in group 2 exhibited their delay time dependence in the duration time t_1, while late responses in group 3 showed a delay time dependence in the end time t_e. This finding may be interpreted as a pre-activation of group 3 areas during the delay phase: i.e. the motor cortex is "held active" until the response decision following the delay period.

Experiences with the 3 models were summarized as:

- *Model 1:* For the Gaussian model, 3 parameters describe the shape of the response: the lag t_0, the dispersion d_0, and the gain a. It was shown [9] that these parameters are interpretable in terms of the experimental stimulation. However, there is no distinction between parameters describing the hemodynamic modulation and neuronal activation in this model. Thus, no decision is possible whether a wide HR is due to a longer activation (i.e. a neuronal effect) or a longer dispersion (i.e. a hemodynamic effect). However, good convergence properties allowed us to use a rather simple and very efficient optimization scheme.
- *Model 2:* Fits are better in comparison with model 1, often down to $\chi^2 \approx 50$, which was a consequence of modeling the HR asymmetry by two different dispersion parameters. As it was suspected previously [9], HRs which arise early and follow short stimuli were found asymmetric with a shorter rising edge d_0 (typically 2-3s) than falling edge d_1 (typically 3-4s). Late and wide HRs tend to be symmetric with dispersions in the order of 3-4s. The attributed neuronal activation parameters, onset t_0, and duration t_1, are interpretable in the context of the fMRI experiment. A genetic algorithm was necessary to optimize this model, so there is a marked increase in the computation time (12min per estimation) in comparison with the previous model.
- *Model 3:* We adapted HRs both to model equations for the capillary compartment 2 and the tissue compartment 3. Fits for both compartments are comparable with model 1, with slightly better values for compartment 2. This is in agreement with the mechanism of the BOLD effect; the fMRI signal arises from the vascular compartment. Rates γ_0 (inflow) and γ_3 (outflow) (see Fig. 2) were found between 0.3-0.7, rates γ_1 (vessel to tissue) and γ_2 (tissue to vessel) in the order of 6-9. This is interpretable as an easy transfer

(of oxygen) between the vascular and tissue compartment, while the sluggish (active) effect of vascular dilatation and constriction was modeled by low inflow and outflow rates. Onset times t_0 were always below 1s, and the duration in the order of 4-7s. With the current formulation and optimization approach, this model needs the rather high amount of computation time of 32min per waveform.

5   Discussion

The description of the HR by a model function is considered as an advantage because it provides a compact and concise parameterization of the HR shape. Current choices for model function are arbitrary, since none is based on a comprehensive physiological model. Our preference for the Gaussian function in previous studies was only justified by the fact that we observed the best fits in a non-linear estimation procedure.

In this study we tested the feasibility of separating "neuronal" from "vascular" parameters by introducing complex HR model functions. Separating hemodynamic from neuronal factors is highly desirable in cognitive research, not only to better characterize the neuronal mechanisms of a cognitive task, but also to better understand the reasons for interindividual differences in terms of "good" and "bad" responders in fMRI experiments.

From experiences with model 2 we confirmed that asymmetries are present in HRs. By including parameters to adapt to asymmetries, marked improvements in the fits were achieved, especially with brief stimuli and early responses. The introduction of the convolution operation in the modeling context allowed us to separate parameters. However, no experimental justification yet exists for the designation as neuronal or vascular properties other than the conformance of results with the current understanding of cognitive processes involved in the example fMRI study. However, it is rather easy to design fMRI experiments better targeted towards a justification of this hypothesis.

The non-linear regression model from (1) and (14) allows the use of complex, highly non-linear functions in our problem domain. We had to resort to a costly optimization method (the genetic algorithm) and to averaged waveforms instead of using single trial data directly. From this feasibility study we learned that it is possible to derive rather narrow limits for hemodynamic modulation parameters.

An interesting reformulation of the compartment model follows from the observation that oxygen delivery to the tissue compartment obeys a Hill-type equation [11,27], i.e. transfer rates γ_i from the vascular to the tissue compartment are non-linear functions of the oxygen tension. At least in healthy subjects, this functional dependency is well described and thus may be introduced in a more complex formulation of the compartment model in 7. Since usually only a few timesteps per trial are recorded, there is an upper bound for the parameter number for any model function.

We regard HR modeling as a new tool in fMRI data analysis which will lead to a deeper understanding of the mechanisms underlying the physiological and neuronal basis of brain functioning. Models as proposed in this paper open another approach for investigating the dynamical properties of the brain.

References

1. Belliveau, J.W., Kennedy, D.N., McKinstry, R.C., Buchbinder, B.R., Weisskoff, R.M., Cohen, M.S., Vevea, J.M., Brady, T.J., Rosen, B.R.: Functional mapping of the human visual cortex by magnetic resonance imaging. Science **254** (1991) 716-719
2. Vilringer, A., Dirnagl, U.: Coupling of brain activity and cerebral blood flow: basis of functional neuroimaging. Cerebrovascular and Brain Metabolism Review **7** (1995) 240-276
3. Friston, K.J., Holmes, A.P., Worsley, K.J., Poline, J.B., Williams, C.R., Frackowiak, R.S.J.: Analysis of functional MRI time-series. Human Brain Mapping **1** (1994) 153-171
4. Kim, S.G., Richter, W., Ugurbil, K.: Limitations of temporal resolution in functional MRI. Magnetic Resonance in Medicine **37** (1997) 631-636
5. Lange, N., Zeger, S.L.: Nonlinear Fourier time series analysis for human brain mapping by functional magnetic resonance imaging. Journal of the Royal Statistical Society: Applied Statistics **46** (1997) 1-29
6. Cohen, M.S.: Parametric analysis of fMRI data using linear systems methods. Neuroimage **6** (1997) 93-103
7. Friston, K.J., Josephs, O., Rees, G., Turner, R.: Nonlinear event-related responses in fMRI. Magnetic Resonance in Medicine **39** (1998) 41-52
8. Rajapakse, J.C., Kruggel, F., von Cramon, D.Y.: Modeling hemodynamic response for analysis of functional MRI time-series. Human Brain Mapping **6** (1998) 283-300
9. Kruggel, F., von Cramon, D.Y.: Modeling the hemodynamic response in single trial fMRI experiments. Magnetic Resonance in Medicine (in press)
10. Buckner, R.L., Koutstaal, W., Schacter, D.L., Dale, A.M., Rotte, R., Rosen, B.R.: Functional-anatomic study of episodic retrieval using fMRI (II). Neuroimage **7** (1998) 163-175
11. Gjedde, A.: The relation between brain function and cerebral blood flow and metabolism. In: Cerebrovascular disease. Lippincott-Raven, Philadelphia (1997)
12. Seber, G.A.F., Wild, C.G.: Nonlinear Regression. Wiley, New York (1989)
13. Widmark, E.M.P.: Studies in the concentration of indifferent narcotics in blood and tissues. Acta Medica Scandinavia **52** (1920) 87-164
14. Rescigno, A., Lambrecht, R.M., Duncan, C.C.: Mathematical models in the formulation of pharmacokinetic models. Lecture Notes in Biomathematics Vol. 48, Springer, Heidelberg (1983) 59-119
15. Bullmore, E., Brammer, M., Williams, S.C.R., Rabe-Hesketh, S., Janoth, N., David, A., Mellers, J., Howard, R., Sham, P.: Statistical methods of estimation and inference for functional MR image analysis. Magnetic Resonance in Medicine **35** (1996) 261-277
16. Benali, H., Buvat, I., Anton, J.L., Pelegrini, M., Di Paola, M., Bittoun, J., Burnod, Y., Di Paola, R.: Space-time statistical model for functional MRI image sequences. In: Information Processing in Medical Imaging (LCNS 1230). Springer, Heidelberg (1997) 285-298
17. Neumaier, A., Schneider, T.: Multivariate autoregressive and Ornstein-Uhlenbeck processes: estimates for order, parameters, spectral information, and confidence regions. ACM Transactions in Mathematical Software (in press)

18. Cressie, N.A.C.: Statistics for spatial data. Wiley, New York (1993)
19. Press, W.H., Flannery, B.P., Teukolsky, S.A., Vetterling, W.T.: Numerical recipes in C. Cambridge University Press, Cambridge (1992)
20. Shor, N.Z.: Minimization methods for nondifferentiable optimization. Springer Series in Computational Mathematics, Vol. 3. Springer, Heidelberg (1985)
21. Goldberg, G.E.: Genetic algorithms in search, optimization, and machine learning. Addison-Wesley, Reading (1989)
22. Cox, C., Ma, G.: Asymptotic confidence bands for generalized nonlinear regression models. Biometrics **51** (1995) 142-150
23. Hartley, H.O.: Exact confidence regions for the parameters in nonlinear regression laws. Biometrika **51** (1964) 347-353
24. Zysset, S., Pollmann, S., von Cramon, D.Y., Wiggins, C.J.: Retrieval from long term memory and working memory. In: Cognitive Neuroscience Society: 1998 Annual Meeting Abstract Program, MIT Press, Harvard (1998) 83
25. Kruggel, F., Descombes, X., von Cramon, D.Y.: Preprocessing of fMR datasets. In: Workshop on Biomedical Image Analysis (Santa Barbara), IEEE Computer Press, Los Alamitos (1998) 211-219
26. Friston, K.J., Worsley, K.J., Frackowiak, R.S.J., Mazziotta, J.C., Evans, A.C.: Assessing the significance of focal activations using their spatial extent. Human Brain Mapping **1** (1994) 210-220
27. Gjedde, A., Poulsen, P.H., Østergard, L.: Model of oxygen delivery predicts deoxygenation of hemoglobin. Neuroimage **7** (1998) S248

3D Graph Description of the Intracerebral Vasculature from Segmented MRA and Tests of Accuracy by Comparison with X–ray Angiograms

Elizabeth Bullitt, Stephen Aylward, Alan Liu, Jeffrey Stone, Suresh K. Mukherji, Chris Coffey, Guido Gerig, and Stephen M. Pizer

Medical Image Display and Analysis Group, University of North Carolina, Chapel Hill, NC, USA
bullitt@med.unc.edu

Abstract. This paper describes largely automated methods of creating connected, 3D vascular trees from individual vessels segmented from magnetic resonance angiograms. Vessel segmentation is initiated by user-supplied seed points, with automatic calculation of vessel skeletons as image intensity ridges and automatic estimation of vessel widths via medialness calculations. The tree–creation process employs a variant of the minimum spanning tree algorithm and evaluates image intensities at each proposed connection point. We evaluate the accuracy of nodal connections by registering a 3D vascular tree with 4 digital subtraction angiograms (DSAs) obtained from the same patient, and by asking two neuroradiologists to evaluate each nodal connection on each DSA view. No connection was judged incorrect. The approach permits new, clinically useful visualizations of the intracerebral vasculature.

1 Introduction

Neurosurgeons and interventional radiologists must often occlude blood vessels during vascular procedures. The risk of stroke to the patient depends largely upon the collateral flow provided by other parts of the circulation. It is therefore important for the clinician to visualize vascular connections in order to make correct decisions about vessel occlusion.

Three types of medical images provide vascular information. The first is by 3D data acquisition, as computed tomographic or magnetic resonance angiography (CTA or MRA). These studies do not explicitly define vascular connections. The second method is digital subtraction angiography (DSA), which produces localized projection images of the circulation in a form that is usually difficult to interpret in 3D. Indeed, neither of these imaging methods provides the clinician direct, 3D information about vascular connections.

The third method of vascular visualization, currently under development by several commercial companies, is 3D reconstruction of a series of DSA images obtained in an arc [14]. Each contrast injection opacifies a vascular subtree that

A. Kuba et al. (Eds.): IPMI'99, LNCS 1613, pp. 308–321, 1999.

is visualized from multiple points of view. The subtree is then reconstructed into 3D using an approach similar to that used to create CT datasets. This approach still does not provide the necessary connectivity information, however. Although, in theory, one could create a connected vascular map of the entire circulation by performing hundreds of contrast injections, reconstructing each sequence into 3D, and then concatenating the results with a knowledge–based approach, the time required and the toxicity of the contrast agent preclude such methods. The fundamental problem is that, like MRA and CTA, 3D–DSA provides the clinician only visualizations based upon image intensity values.

We share this interest in 3D DSA reconstruction [3,4,5,6]. However, we believe that the utility of 3D–DSA is severely limited without an associated directed graph description of the vasculature. A symbolic representation of vascular connectivity is necessary in order to estimate collateral flow to a region, to simulate catheter motion through a 3D vascular tree, or to permit ready identification on projection images of safe occlusion points. It is exactly this kind of information that the clinician needs to know. No current imaging modality (MRA, DSA, or 3D–DSA) can provide this kind of information directly.

This paper describes methods of producing directed graphs of the intracerebral vasculature from segmented MRA data. The same approach could also be applied to 3D–DSA images. We intend these graphs for use under conditions in which errors may produce patient injury. Four requirements must be met in order for these graphs to be clinically useful. First, the segmentation must be accurate and complete in the region of interest. Second, the parent–child associations must be correct. Third, the accuracy of the construct must be evaluable. Finally, editing and display tools are required.

This paper discusses issues 2–4 above. Our MRA segmentation method is described elsewhere [2] and is only outlined here. The current report focuses upon automated methods of producing directed graphs from segmented vessels. We evaluate the accuracy of nodal connections in a final tree by comparison of projections of our construct to the "gold standard" of DSA. Finally, we describe editing and display tools. Our aim is to provide symbolic vascular descriptions that can be used effectively under clinical conditions of high risk.

2 Issues in Vascular Model Creation and Testing

This study employs both MRA and DSA images. This section outlines four important facts about the intracerebral circulation and the two imaging modalities employed. The term "vessel" refers to an unbranched, 3D, vascular segment.

First, an MRA contains vessels not seen by DSA. Human beings usually have 3 intracerebral arterial circulations arising from different parent vessels. An MRA provides a 3D image that shows all 3 circulations simultaneously. A DSA, however, provides 2D projections of child vessels opacified following focal injection of contrast. An angiogram therefore depicts flow only within a single subtree. Since an MRA visualizes all 3 circulations, it contains information a DSA does not.

Second, a DSA contains projections of vessels not seen by MRA. A DSA fills vessels of many widths. An MRA tends to contain only the larger vessels. DSA therefore provides more vascular detail than MRA. Many MRA studies also do not include the full head. A DSA therefore contains information an MRA does not.

Third, both DSA and MRA contain distortion errors that may interfere with MRA–DSA registration. DSAs contain geometrical distortions such as pincushion effects. We (and others) can largely correct such errors. The distortions produced by MR are more difficult. Although machine–specific and patient–specific flow errors can be reduced or eliminated [12,13], it is more difficult to correct distortions at a tissue–air interface. Such errors are reported to displace objects by as much as a centimeter [7,13] and tend to occur at the skull base and brain surface.

Finally, the human intracerebral circulation is complex, plethoric, and variable. Multiple vessels exist in the same region of space. The track of an individual vessel can contain tight loops. Even the 3 major circulatory groups are connected differently in different patients via the Circle of Willis at the base of the skull. It is thus impossible to create a single model applicable to all patients. Fig. 1 illustrates the circulation's complexity, the differences between DSA and MRA, and an example of MRA segmentation. The segmentation method is outlined later.

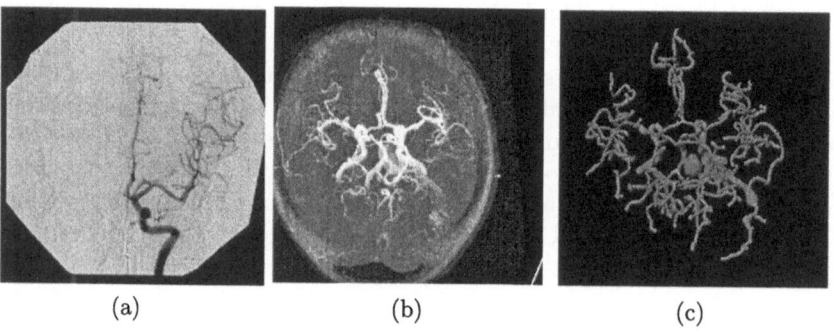

(a)   (b)   (c)

Fig. 1. DSA and MRA. (a) Left internal carotid DSA from the front. DSAs show only a portion of the circulation. No vessels fill on the right side or back of the head; these areas are supplied by different parent vessels. (b) Volume rendered MRA from below. Vessels occupy the entire head but detail is missing. (c) Vessels segmented from the MRA shown in B and projected from the same point of view. An aneurysm is at image center

This study creates a directed graph from segmented MRA vessels and tests the accuracy of nodal connections by projecting each parent–child connection against a sequence of DSA images obtained from the same patient. Evaluation is only possible for the set of vessels the two imaging modalities hold in common.

Registration is imperfect at the skull base and for some peripheral vessels close to the brain surface.

3 Methods

3.1 Image Acquisition and Image Distortion Correction

The vessel segmentation method does not require a specific image acquisition protocol, and is applicable to both CT and MR data. For this study, 3D, time of flight MRA was performed in a Siemens 1.5 T Vision unit with a quadrature head coil and with magnetization transfer suppression. Images were acquired in the axial projection over a 7.6 cm volume, using 69 contiguous 1.1 mm sections and an x and y spacing of 0.85 mm. Machine–specific distortion errors were evaluated by imaging a Siemens multi–purpose phantom. The major problem found was a 10% error in interslice spacing, which our software now corrects.

We use DSAs to evaluate the connections made by the tree creation program. The case analyzed in this report employed four 459×484 pixel DSA images (AP, lateral, LAO, and modified LAO) obtained from a portable Diasonics OEC digital angiographic unit. The field of view was variously 8 or 12 degrees. This report also includes a picture of a vessel tree created from a different patient's MRA and registered with a high resolution (1024×1024 pixel) lateral DSA obtained using a Siemens Multistar digital angiographic unit.

Major distortions in the 2D images were corrected by imaging a finely milled crosshair phantom grid placed on the image plane. Phantom images were obtained using a variety of fluoroscopic positions. Each DSA was then corrected for distortion via a landmark–based system and interpolation by triangles to adjust the spatial location of each pixel. The greyscale value at each (x,y) point in the corrected image was then determined by interpolation. For the highly distorted OEC images, the image size after correction was 476×476 pixels (pixel size 0.3 mm).

3.2 MRA Segmentation

The MRA segmentation method makes use of the geometry of blood vessels. As outlined below, extraction of a vessel involves 3 steps: definition of a seed point, automatic extraction of an image intensity ridge representing the vessel's central skeleton, and automatic determination of width at each skeleton point. Further details are provided by Aylward [2].

Extraction of each vessel begins from a user–supplied seed point. The user views a set of MRA slices and clicks on a point within a vessel, simultaneously supplying a rough estimate of that vessel's width. The method then automatically extracts the central skeleton of the indicated vessel beginning from the seed point. Vessels can be viewed as 3D tubular objects delineated from background by contrast differences. This combination of geometry and intensity means that blurring the image creates a central intensity ridge along each vessel. This intensity ridge is extracted via the height ridge definition:

Define: I as the intensity at x,

$\quad\quad\quad$ H as the Hessian of I at x,

$\quad\quad\quad$ v_i and a_i the eigenvectors and associated eigenvalues of H
$\quad\quad\quad$ where $a_1 < a_2 < a_3$.

Then for the program to classify x as being on a ridge, it must be true that:

$$a_2/\sqrt{a_1^2 + a_2^2 + a_3^2} \sim< -0.5\,, \tag{1}$$

$$v_1 \cdot \nabla I \sim= 0 \quad \text{and} \quad v_2 \cdot \nabla I \sim= 0\,. \tag{2}$$

Equation 1 states that most of the local curvature should be captured by the two principal components of the Hessian (hence 0.5) and that the curvature should be negative, corresponding to a ridge rather than to a valley.

The width of the vessel is automatically estimated at points along its central skeleton. The method takes advantage of the fact that vessels have nearly circular cross–sections. The width of a tube about a central skeleton point is proportional to the scale that produces a maximal response from a cylindrical medialness measure. Define $M(x, s)$ as the response from convolving the image at x with an extruded Laplacian of a Gaussian kernel aligned with the central skeleton and at a scale s. Then the radius r of the vessel at x is:

$$r \sim= 0.5 * \text{arg-max}_s\{M(x, s)\}\,. \tag{3}$$

3.3   Characteristics of Segmented Vessels

The output of the segmentation program is a set of unbranched, directed, 3D skeleton curves with an associated width at each point. Important characteristics of the segmentation include the following.

1) The segmentation is largely complete when compared to volume rendered images of the initial MRA [3]. Figure 1 gives an example.

2) As MRA datasets are noisy, the segmentation may include spurious vessels. One of the requirements for providing an accurate graph description is elimination of spurious curves.

3) Segmented curves representing true vessels are often long and extend past multiple branchpoints. Figure 2A shows the projection of the skeleton of a single segmented vessel.

4). The gap between the extracted vessel skeletons of a true parent–child pair is usually very short and in the order of a millimeter (Fig. 2C).

5) During segmentation, no new vessel is allowed to occupy territory previously defined by another. Segmentation therefore tends to stop at "Y" branchpoints.

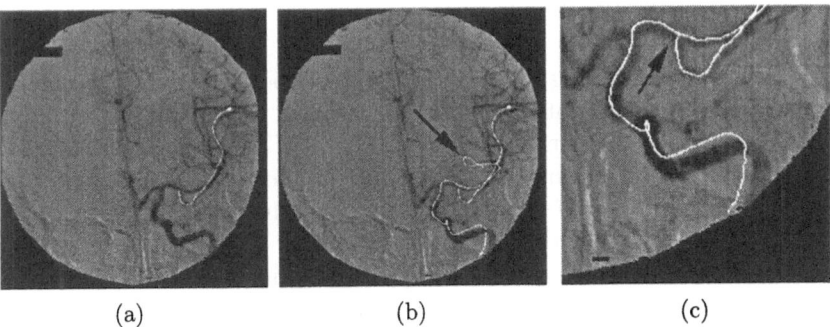

(a)   (b)   (c)

Fig. 2. Characteristics of extracted vessels. (a) An individual vessel skeleton (white) projected against a DSA. The white ball at the tip indicates flow direction. The curve is long. (b) The same vessel shown in (a) and its parent vessel. The parent begins as the carotid artery, extends into the middle cerebral trunk, and follows a path into a small middle cerebral branch (arrow). (c) Magnification of the parent–child connection region. The 1 mm distance between the segmented vessel skeletons (arrow) is so short that it cannot be seen on this projection

6) Each extracted skeleton curve consists of an ordered series of 3D points and thus has a direction. However, this direction is determined during extraction and may not correctly model the direction of blood flow. Figure 3 illustrates the three types of "Y" connections produced. For two of these three cases, the tree creation protocol must modify the child's flow direction during connection with a parent vessel.

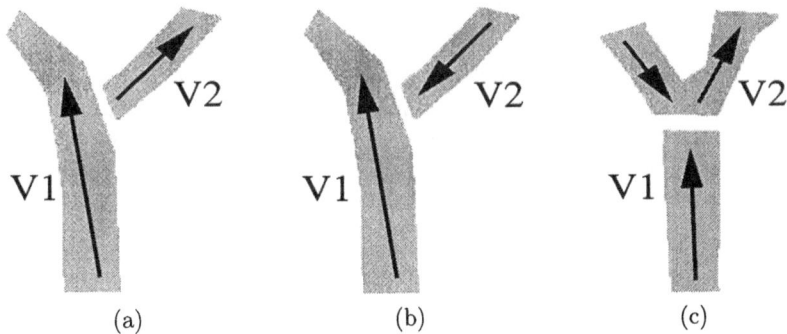

(a)   (b)   (c)

Fig. 3. "Y" connection of segmented vessels: flow redirection. Arrows indicate the direction of flow in segmented vessels prior to connection. Child vessel V2 is about to connect to parent vessel V1. (a) The direction of flow in V2 is correct. No adjustment is needed. (b) Flow direction in V2 is incorrect and must be reversed. (c) V2 must be broken and the flow reversed in the left half of the vessel

3.4 Tree Creation

The protocol for connecting segmented vessels uses both linear distance measurements and the 3D image intensity data in suspected regions of connection. Both "I" connections (connection of 2 endpoints) and "Y" connections (connection of an endpoint with an intermediate point on a segmented vessel) are permitted; "X" connections are not. All allowed connections therefore involve at least one endpoint of an extracted vessel's skeleton curve.

A version of the minimum spanning tree algorithm is employed. The user views a projection of the segmented vessels and interactively selects one or more roots. A maximum 3D–connection distance is set (default 2 mm) as is a maximum intensity ratio (default 0.75), described below. The program then automatically builds a set of trees by progressively attaching a child to the connected base until no orphan remains whose connection meets both distance and image intensity requirements.

On each iteration, the orphan is selected whose connection provides the minimum "connection value". Figure 3 shows the 3 allowed types of parent–child connection. For each orphan–parent, the program estimates the 3 pairs of possible connection points and then inspects the image data. A line is drawn between each point pair in the 3D image. A hollow, concentric cylinder of radius larger than that of the child is then constructed along this axis. The average image intensities of the cylinder and line are expressed as a ratio. A low ratio (high central intensity and low peripheral intensity) suggests a valid connection. The "connection value" is a weighted sum of this ratio (4 x ratio) with the linear distance between connection points. The orphan with the lowest connection value is added next. As noted earlier, the flow direction in segmented data may not be correct. When appropriate, the protocol therefore reverses flow in the child (Fig. 3B) or splits the child and reverses flow in one segment (Fig. 3C).

As shown later, noise in the MRA results in the extraction of multiple spurious curves that are processed along with curves representing true vessels. These spurious vessels are almost entirely eliminated during tree creation as we start from a given root, examine only connections involving an endpoint, and allow only connections involving short distances and fitting the image intensity data.

3.5 Tree Editing and Tree–Based Display

The 3 cerebral circulations are variably connected at the skull base through the Circle of Willis. Our methods cannot automatically detect the direction of flow in these connections. The program therefore provides editing tools and the ability to load a DSA as a background bitmap to help the user separate or connect major trees of interest.

During tree creation, each parent orders and marks the position of each child as the child is added, and each child marks its parent. It is therefore relatively simple to provide a set of tree–based editing tools. More specifically, the user may click on a projection point to a) delete proximal and/or distal vessel segments and associated subtrees, b) delete a vessel with associated subtrees, c) disconnect a subtree from a parent and reconnect to a user–selected parent or to a specific parent point, and d) reverse flow in a vessel with automatic recalculation of child order and position. All changes are implemented in 3D.

Similarly, a variety of display options are available. One may click on a vessel projection to view that vessel's subtree, the vessel and its parent in isolation, or the set of connections from that vessel to the root. One may even simulate passage of a catheter by progressively clicking along a desired path; only the distal vessel and its appropriate descendents will be shown.

The case analyzed in this study is that of a left carotid circulation that fills the anterior cerebral and left middle cerebral groups. Following segmentation of the left half of the supratentorial portion of an MRA, a single vascular tree was created with the left carotid as root. The editing tool was then used to delete the distal posterior communicator and right A1 segments (with simultaneous automatic deletion of all descendents of these vessels) to produce a single vascular tree that contained only the vascular groups shown by DSA.

3.6   Evaluation by DSA Images

Each 3D vascular tree may contain dozens of connections. Connection accuracy can be evaluated by the gold standard of angiography. We superimpose a projection of each 3D tree upon a series of DSA images obtained from a variety of angles. Each nodal connection can then be examined individually in light of the information provided by DSA.

Registration of segmented vessels with DSA is done as described by Liu [11]. The 3D/2D registration process uses as primitives 4–8 2D curves extracted from the DSA and an equivalent number of 3D curves extracted from the MRA. The program then optimizes a viewplane based disparity measure based on the iterative closest point paradigm between the DSA skeletons and the projections of the MRA skeletons. Newton's method on the pose parameters in 3D is used to refine the solution iteratively.

Four different DSA views of the left carotid circulation were available for the case analyzed in this paper. All four views, together with registered projections of our 3D vascular tree, were given to two neuroradiologists for evaluation. A variety of viewing options were available, including stepwise progression through the set of connections such that only one parent, child, and connection were projected (and color coded) at one time.

Each radiologist filled out a form in which each connection was judged as: 1) correct, 2) partially correct (a minor error of no clinical consequence), or 3) incorrect. A fourth category "?" indicated a miscellaneous problem, such as an extraneous vessel or indeterminable parentage.

For a vessel connection evaluable under the first 3 categories, the global rating for that connection was taken as the worst rating given. For example, a connection that was judged as incorrect on even one view was judged as globally incorrect. For vessels and vessel connections falling into the fourth category ("?"), analysis was performed in two ways: as if the vessels had been removed from analysis and as if the vessels had been judged incorrect.

Statistical analysis for this test case was summarized using confidence intervals for both the proportion completely correct and the proportion clinically acceptable (completely or partially correct). Confidence intervals were computed using StatXact, as described in Johnson et.al. [10,16]. As the confidence intervals were not independent, a Bonferroni correction was utilized so as to present a 97.5 confidence interval for each proportion.

The confidence intervals were calculated in the following manner. Suppose that p represents the true probability of success (correct or clinically acceptable, depending on the case). It follows that the distribution of the number of successes in N trials may be described as:

$$Pr\ (\ T = t \mid p\ ) = \binom{N}{t} \cdot p^t \cdot (1-p)^{N-t}. \tag{4}$$

After observing the number of successes (t) in the N trials, 97.5% confidence intervals were computed by finding (p_L, p_U), where:

$$Pr\ (\ T \geq t \mid p_L\ ) = 0.0125 \quad \text{and} \quad Pr\ (\ T \leq t \mid p_U\ ) = 0.0125\,. \tag{5}$$

If $t = 0$ it follows that $p_L = 0$. Likewise, if $t = N$ it follows that $p_U = 1$.

4   Results

Figure 4 illustrates a DSA with a superimposed projection of the constructed left carotid tree during the stages of tree creation. Figure 4A shows the skeletons of all extracted vessels prior to processing. There is an enormous amount of noise. Following automated tree creation (Fig 4B) the noise is almost entirely eliminated. Figure 4C shows the result after exclusion of connections to the posterior and right carotid circulations via point and click operations.

Two modifications to the final tree were made before giving it to the neuroradiologists for evaluation. A small branch that probably represented noise was deleted. More significantly, flow within the vessel shown in Fig. 2A was reversed. This extracted vessel terminated 0.8 mm from a peripheral middle cerebral branch and originated 1.1 mm from its proper parent. The distances involved were too short to make good use of intensity evaluations at the proposed connection point. The resultant connection error was fixed by point and click editing.

The final tree comprised 25 vessels out of the initial 140 used as input data. One of these vessels was a root with no parent. Twenty–four vessel connections were therefore available for evaluation.

On formal evaluation, not one of the nodal connections was judged as incorrect by either neuroradiologist. However, both radiologists judged 22 connections as fully correct and questioned or faulted two others. Reviewer A felt there was insufficient image data to adequately evaluate two cases. Reviewer B judged two connections as "partially correct" (containing a minor error of no clinical significance). Both reviewers agreed that one connection was questionable; they disagreed about the second connection in question with each reviewer accepting as fully correct the connection that the other reviewer queried.

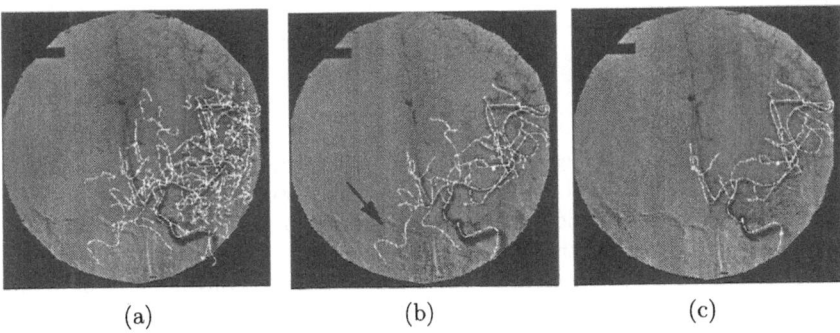

(a)   (b)   (c)

Fig. 4. Skeletons of projected 3D vessels are white. (a) Extracted vessels projected upon a DSA. There is much noise. (b) Projected vessels following tree creation with left carotid as root. Almost all noise is eliminated, but connections remain to the right carotid and posterior circulations. The arrow points to the right carotid artery, a legitimate vessel connected to the left carotid circulation, but one that does not receive flow from this patients left carotid. (c) Final tree after point and click deletions to clear the right and posterior circulations

Statistical evaluation was performed on each reviewer's response to determine the 97.5% confidence intervals for both the proportion entirely correct and for the proportion clinically acceptable. For reviewer B, who marked two connections as partially correct, these intervals were respectively (70%, 99%) and (83%, 100%). For reviewer A, who marked two connections as "?", results were calculated in two ways: with the 2 connections removed from analysis and with the 2 connections viewed as fully incorrect. For the case in which 22 of 22 connections were deemed correct, the confidence interval for both the percentage entirely correct and the percentage clinically acceptable was (82%, 100%). For the case in which 22 of 24 connections were considered correct and 2 incorrect, the confidence intervals for the proportion entirely correct and for the proportion clinically acceptable were both (70%, 99%).

Tree–based description of the vasculature permits a variety of useful viewing options not otherwise available. Figure 5 shows a sequence of images that simulate progressive passage of a catheter through a vascular tree. When this viewing mode is selected, clicking on a vessel's projection point will display only the distal portion of that vessel and its relevant descendents. The tree shown is the same as that in Fig. 4, but from a different point of view.

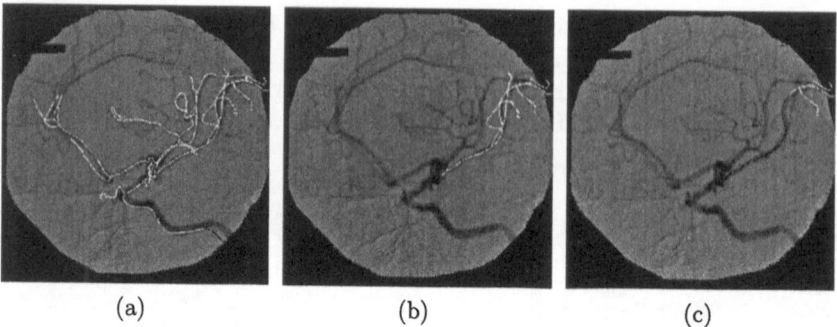

(a)   (b)   (c)

Fig. 5. Simulation of catheter passage through a tree by point and click. Projections of the skeletons of segmented vessels are in white. (a) Catheter is in the carotid artery. The anterior cerebral and middle cerebral groups fill. (b) The catheter passes into one of the three middle cerebral trunks. The anterior cerebral group and the 2 other middle cerebral trunks do not fill. (c) The catheter passes distally. Only a few small branches fill

5   Discussion

The rapid rise of interventional neuroradiology has underlined the need for individualized 3D maps of the intracranial vasculature. This paper describes creation of vascular trees from segmented MRA data.

The proposed task is made difficult by the complexity of the vasculature and because MRA datasets are noisy. Segmentation is difficult. In addition, any segmentation that includes large portions of the circulation is also likely to include spurious objects (Fig. 4A). The creation of meaningful vascular trees therefore not only requires correct determination of parent–child relationships but also the elimination of spurious vessels produced by noise.

Several groups have segmented a few vessels from MRA and have registered them with DSA [1,7,8,18]. Extraction is usually limited to large vessels, however, and no tree description is provided. Gerig and colleagues provide images that suggest more complete extraction [9,15,17]. This group also suggests graph–based description of the intracerebral vasculature [9,17]. However, the number of vessels actually included in their graph description appears small [17]. These graphs have also not been clinically tested for accuracy. It is therefore difficult to compare them with those produced by the methods described here.

5.1   Disadvantages of Our Approach

A potential disadvantage of our segmentation protocol is that it provides geometrical information alone. We do not use the MRA flow direction data used by others [9,15,17,18]. We therefore do not know flow direction in the Circle of Willis. This report employs a DSA to segregate major vascular groups. It would be preferable to eliminate this step. One solution may be to use the width information of segmented data, since arterial flow is normally directed from wider arteries into narrower ones.

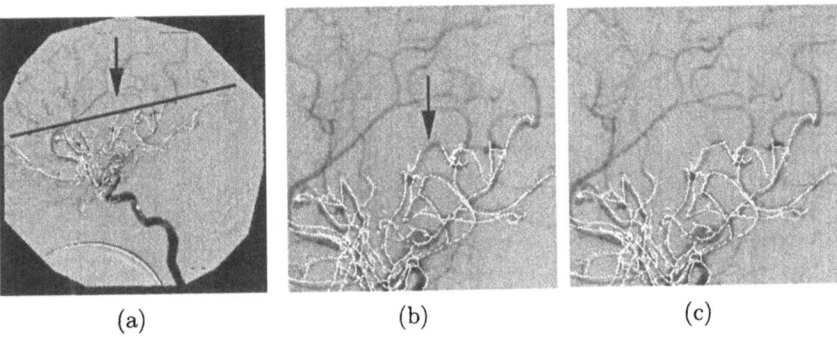

(a)   (b)   (c)

Fig. 6. Connectivity error produced by missing MR data. (a) 3D vascular tree comprised of segmented vessels (white) whose skeletons are projected upon a DSA (1024 × 1024). The topmost MR section is given by a dotted line. (b) Enlargement of the indicated region in (a). The segmentation has a gap at the top of a loop (arrow) because the MR is incomplete. A connectivity error is produced and the distal portion of the loop connects incorrectly to a nearby vessel. (c) Connectivity and flow correction by manual editing. Changes are implemented in 3D

A limitation inherent to any method of determining nodal connections is that missing data may produce connectivity errors. There are at least 3 reasons why our segmentations may contain gaps. First, if the MRA does not cover a sufficient volume of the head, vascular loops will be truncated. In such cases the graph description either fails to include the distal part of the loop or, worse, falsely connects the distal loop to a neighboring vessel. Figure 6 provides an example for a patient not included in this study.

A second reason for gaps in the data is that our segmentations require a user–supplied seed point for each vessel. If the user does not inspect the image data carefully, a faint but important vessel may be missed. A more automated approach is preferable. Our group is actively pursuing solution to this problem, and initial results from fully automated, problem specific extraction methods are promising. Finally, an MRA may fail to visualize vessels containing slow or turbulent flow. We have no solution to the connectivity problem produced by missing vessel segments other than that of manual editing.

A final disadvantage of our approach is that, for some types of surgical planning, the amount of detail provided by MRA may be insufficient. The current study analyzes only the accuracy of nodal connections and the presence of extraneous data. It does not address the issue of missing vessels except as such vessels influence the accuracy of nodal connection. We are therefore developing methods to provide a 3D map at an angiographic level of detail by reconstructing sets of DSA images and building upon the 3D base provided by MRA [3,4,5,6].

5.2   Advantages of Our Approach

Despite these limitations, our approach has several advantages, many of which are inherent to the segmentation method itself. First, our segmentation method is capable of tracking an individual vessel for long distances. Second, the extractions do not appear to jump from one vessel into another or to extend for noticeable distances into patches of noise. Third, the segmentation of each true vessel is close to complete, so that in the majority of cases the parental and child connection points are within 1–2 voxels of each other. This feature makes it possible to enforce tight connectivity requirements during tree creation and to deal effectively with the problem of spurious vessels produced by noise.

Another major advantage of our approach is that the computations are reasonably fast and inexpensive. Extraction of a full MRA takes 20–30 minutes, registration of segmented vessels with a DSA takes about 10 minutes, and tree creation is performed in seconds. All programs run well on a Pentium 220 machine under Windows. All programs require less than 64 megabytes of memory.

The ability to provide accurate graph descriptions of the vasculature will benefit both surgeons and interventional neuroradiologists. Figure 5 provides one example of how we intend to use these methods. Specifically, we intend to help guide endovascular procedures by tracking the position of the catheter and placing each vessel projection within a 3D context.

Although further testing is required before we fully know the strengths and limitations of the method, these results are highly encouraging. We have ported all programs to the Windows environment and are writing user interfaces suitable for clinicians.

Acknowledgments

Supported by R01CA67812 NIH–NCI, P01CA47982 NIH–NCI and an Intel equipment award.

References

1. Alperin, N., Levin, D.N., Pelizzari, C.A.: Retrospective registration of x–ray angiograms with MR images by using vessels as intrinsic landmarks. JMRI **4** (1994) 139–144
2. Aylward, S.R., Pizer, S.M., Bullitt, E., Eberly, D.: Intensity ridge and widths for 3D object segmentation and description. IEEE WMMBIA IEEE 96TB100056 (1996) 131–138
3. Bullitt, E., Liu, A., Aylward, S.R., Soltys, M., Boxwala, A., Rosenman, J., Pizer, S.: Methods for displaying intracerebral vascular anatomy. Am. J. Neuroradiol. **18** (1997) 417–420
4. Bullitt, E., Liu, A., Pizer, S.M.: Three dimensional reconstruction of curves from pairs of projection views in the presence of error. I. Algorithms. Med. Phys. **24** (1997) 1671–8
5. Bullitt, E., Liu, A., Pizer, S.M.: Three dimensional reconstruction of curves from projection views. II. Analysis of error. Med. Phys. **24** (1997) 1679–87
6. Bullitt, E., Liu, A., Aylward, S., Pizer, S.M.: Reconstruction of the intracerebral vasculature from MRA and a pair of projection views. Lect. Notes Comp. Sci. 1230 (1997) 537–542

7. Chapman, B.E., Sanderson, A.R., Goodrich, K.C., Alexander, A.L., Blatter, D.D., Parker, D.L.: Observer performance methodologies for evaluating blood vessel visibility in MR angiograms using accurate geometric registration to high resolution x–ray angiograms. MRM **37** (1997) 519–529

8. Feldmar, J., Malandain, G., Ayache, N., Fernandez–Vidal, S., Maurincomme, E., Trousset, Y.: Matching 3D MR angiography data and 2D X–ray angiograms. Lect. Notes Comp. Sci. 1205 (1997) 129–138

9. Gerig, G,. Koller, T., Székely, G., Brechbühler, C., Kübler, O.: Symbolic description of 3–D structures applied to cerebral vessel tree obtained from MR angiography volume data. Lect. Notes Comp. Sci. 687 (1993) 94–111

10. Johnson, N.L., Kotz, S., Kemp, A.W.: Univariate Discrete Distributions. New York, Wiley (1992)

11. Liu, A., Bullitt, E., Pizer, S.M.: 3D/2D registration using tubular anatomical structures as a basis. Lect. Notes Comp. Sci, 1496 (1998) 952–963

12. Michiels, J., Pelgrims, P., Bosmans, H., Vandermeulen, D., Gybels, J., Marchal, G., Suetens, P.: On the problem of geometric distortion in magnetic resonance images for stereotactic neurosurgery. Mag. Res. Imag. **12** (1994) 749–765

13. Michiels, J., Bosmans, H., Nuttin, B., Knauth, M., Verbeeck, R., Vandermeulen, D,. Wilms, G., Marchal, G., Suetens, P., Gybels, J.: The use of magnetic resonance angiography in stereotactic neurosurgery. J. Neurosurg. **82** (1995) 982–987

14. Navab, N., Bani–Hashemi, A., Nadar, M.S., Wiesent, K., Durlak, P., Brunner, T., Barth, K., Graumann, R.: 3D reconstruction from projection matrices in a C–arm based 3D angiography system. Lecture Notes in Computer Science 1496 (1998) 119–129

15. Sato, Y., Nakajima, S., Shiraga, N., Atsumi, H., Yoshida, S., Koller, T., Gerig, G., Kikinis, R.: Three–dimensional multi–scale line filter for segmentation and visualization of curvilinear structures in medical images. Medical Image Analysis **2** (1998) 143–168

16. StatXact: CYTEL Software Corporation, Cambridge, Mass (1995)

17. Szekely, G., Koller,T., Kikinis, R., Gerig, G.: Structural description and combined 3D display for superior analysis of cerebral vascularity from MRA. SPIE 2359 (1994) 272–281

18. Wilson, D., Noble, J.A.: Segmentation of cerebral vessels and aneurysms from MR angiography data. Lect. Notes Comp. Sci. 1230 (1997) 428–433

A Unified Framework for Atlas Matching Using Active Appearance Models

T. F. Cootes, C. Beeston, G. J. Edwards, and C.J. Taylor

Imaging Science and Biomedical Engineering,
University of Manchester,
Manchester M13 9PT, U.K.
t.cootes@man.ac.uk

Abstract. We propose to use statistical models of shape and texture as deformable anatomical atlases. By training on sets of labelled examples these can represent both the mean structure and appearance of anatomy in medical images, and the allowable modes of deformation. Given enough training examples such a model should be able synthesise any image of normal anatomy. By finding the parameters which minimise the difference between the synthesised model image and the target image we can locate all the modelled structure. This potentially time consuming step can be solved rapidly using the Active Appearance Model (AAM). In this paper we describe the models and the AAM algorithm and demonstrate the approach on structures in MR brain cross-sections.

1 Introduction

It has been recognised for some time that the ability to match an anatomical atlas to individual patient images provides the basis for solving several important problems in medical image interpretation. Once the atlas has been matched to a particular image, structures of interest can be labelled and extracted for further analysis. Matching to an atlas also defines the registration between different images of the same patient - allowing information obtained at different times or from different imaging modalities to be combined - and the non-rigid registration of images of different patients - allowing population studies to be analysed in a common frame of reference. Same-patient data fusion is sometimes approached directly as a rigid registration problem (particularly in the brain) but the atlas matching approach is more general.

Given its central importance, the atlas-matching problem has received considerable attention. Two main approaches can be identified: landmark-based - in which key points or surfaces in image and atlas are brought into alignment; and image-based - in which an atlas image is allowed to deform to achieve as close a match as possible between corresponding pixel/voxel intensity values in the deformed atlas and patient image. In either case, a dense correspondence is established between atlas and image, allowing labels and image values to be transferred between the two frames of reference. The landmark-based approach

A. Kuba et al. (Eds.): IPMI'99, LNCS 1613, pp. 322–333, 1999.

relies on extracting landmark points/surfaces on the basis of local image structure, then establishing correspondences between atlas and image landmarks. We have shown previously that this approach can be made efficient and robust if a statistical model of shape (representing the possible spatial arrangements of landmarks) is used to constrain the solution to the correspondence problem via an Active Shape Model [13]. Once landmark correspondences have been established a dense correspondence is obtained by interpolation. The image-based approach has the advantage that all the data are used in establishing the dense correspondence. To set against this is the disadvantage that shape statistics cannot easily be used in establishing the match – typically, arbitrary elastic or viscous regularisation terms are used to limit the degree of deformation allowed. Recently Wang and Staib [25] have described a method of incorporating statistical shape information into an image-based elastic matching algorithm. Although they show that this leads to more accurate results, shape and intensity matching are combined in an ad hoc way and the method is slow. In this paper we describe a unified approach to matching an atlas to patient images using both shape and intensity information. We show how a statistical appearance model (atlas), describing allowable variation in shape and intensity, can be constructed from a set of example images. We also describe an efficient Active Appearance Model (AAM) algorithm for matching the model to new images by minimising pixel/voxel intensity differences, subject to statistical constraints captured by the model. We illustrate the method applied to 2-D MR images of the brain, using an atlas containing all the important sub-cortical structures, and present quantitative results demonstrating that our method achieves accurate matching in a few seconds on a modern PC.

2   Background

The inter- and intra-personal variability inherent in biological structures makes medical image interpretation a difficult task. In recent years there has been considerable interest in methods that use deformable models, or atlases, to interpret images. One motivation is to achieve robust performance by using the atlas to constrain solutions to be valid examples of the structure(s) modelled. Of more fundamental importance is the fact that, once an atlas and patient image have been matched – producing a dense correspondence – anatomical labels and intensity values can be transferred directly. This forms a basis for automated anatomical interpretation and for data fusion across different images of the same individual or across similar images of different individuals. For a comprehensive review of work in this field there are recent surveys of image registration methods and deformable models in medical image analysis [19,18]. We give here a brief review covering some of the more important points.

Bajcsy *et. al.* describe an image-based atlas that deforms to fit new images by minimising pixel/voxel intensity differences [2]. Since this is an under-constrained problem, they regularise their solution by introducing an elastic deformation cost. Christensen *et. al.* describe a similar approach, but use a viscous flow rather than elastic model of deformation, and incorporate statistical information about local deformations [9,8]. This results in more accurate matching, but is computationally expensive. Both approaches require good initialisation to converge to a satisfactory solution since the deformations allowed are not constrained to be anatomically plausible. Landmark-based methods involve three steps: locating the landmarks, establishing correspondences, and warping the image or atlas to align the corresponded landmarks. Bookstein describes an elastic matching approach based on the use of thin plate splines [3] – he assumes that landmarks have been identified and corresponded manually. Subsol *et. al.* [23] extract crest-lines, which they use to establish landmark-based correspondence. They use these to perform morphometrical studies and to match images to atlases.

We have previously shown that a statistical deformation model can be used to simultaneously locate landmarks and establish image-atlas correspondences [12]. We obtain a parameterised statistical model of the domain of 'legal' shape variation from a set of training images. An Active Shape Model (ASM) is used to search for local image structure consistent with each of the landmarks, whilst constraining the configuration of landmarks using the statistical shape model. Typically, landmarks are closely spaced around the boundaries of structures of interest. A dense image-atlas correspondence can be established using thin plate splines. The original scheme was described in 2-D - it has been extended to 3-D by Hill *et. al.* [16] and Szekely *et. al.* [24].

None of the approaches outlined above is ideal. The use of a statistical deformation model allows rapid, reasonably robust matching and provides a principled basis for constraining deformation during matching. The ASM algorithm does not, however, use the image evidence particularly efficiently – only the intensity data in the vicinity of landmark points affects the final solution. The image-based approaches of Bajcsy *et. al.* [1] and Christensen *et. al.* [9] use the image evidence more efficiently, but allow arbitrary deformations. Wang and Staib [25] have recently attempted to incorporate statistical shape information into an image-based elastic matching approach. They do this by using a method very closely related to an ASM to find boundary landmarks in the image. An additional elastic matching term is added to the matching criterion, to encourage the image boundaries to coincide with the atlas boundaries. This is a rather *ad hoc* approach and the method is computationally expensive. In this paper we seek to unify the image-based and statistical modelling approaches in a principled way, leading to a method that is fast, robust and makes optimal use of both the image data and prior knowledge of the variability present in the class of images to be analysed.

The Active Appearance Model (AAM) approach that we describe also draws on other previous work. Cootes *et. al.* describe a model of the position-intensity surface, allowing full synthesis of the appearance of objects that are variable in shape and intensity [11]. They do not, however, describe a plausible matching algorithm. Nastar *et. al.* describe a related model combining physical and statistical modes of deformation [20]. Although they describe a matching algorithm it requires very good initialisation. Jones and Poggio use a model capable of synthesizing faces and describe a stochastic optimisation method to match the model to new face images [17]. The method is slow but can be robust because of the quality of the synthesized images. Edwards *et. al.* also describe models of the combined shape and intensity appearance of faces [14]. They describe how the models can be matched to new images using an ASM; the method is fast, but does not make full use of the image data. Our new AAM approach is an extension of this idea, using all the information in the combined appearance model to match to the image. Sclaroff and Isidoro describe Active Blobs for tracking [22]. Their approach is similar to our AAM, though an Active Blob is derived from a single image rather than a training set of images. The example is used as a template, allowing low energy shape deformations and simple intensity variation. In contrast, AAMs learn what are valid shape and intensity variations from a training set.

3   Active Appearance Models

This section describes our statistical appearance models and outlines the basic AAM matching algorithm. A more comprehensive description is given in [10]. An AAM contains two main components: A parameterised model of object appearance, and an estimate of the relationship between parameter errors and induced image residuals.

3.1   Appearance Models

An appearance model can represent both the shape and texture variability seen in a training set. The training set consists of labelled images, where key landmark points are marked on each example object. For instance, to build a model of the sub-cortical structures in 2D MR images of the brain we need a number of images marked with points at key positions to outline the main features (Fig. 1).

Given such a set we can generate a statistical model of shape variation by applying Principal Component Analysis (PCA) to the set of vectors describing the shapes in the training set (see [13] for details). The labelled points, $\mathbf{x}$, on a single object describe the shape of that object. Any example can then be approximated using:

$$\mathbf{x} = \bar{\mathbf{x}} + \mathbf{P}_s \mathbf{b}_s \tag{1}$$

where $\bar{\mathbf{x}}$ is the mean shape vector, $\mathbf{P}_s$ is a set of orthogonal *modes of shape variation* and $\mathbf{b}_s$ is a vector of shape parameters.

To build a statistical model of the grey-level appearance we warp each example image so that its control points match the mean shape (using a triangulation algorithm). We then sample the intensity information from the *shape-normalised* image over the region covered by the mean shape. To minimise the effect of global lighting variation, we normalise the resulting samples.

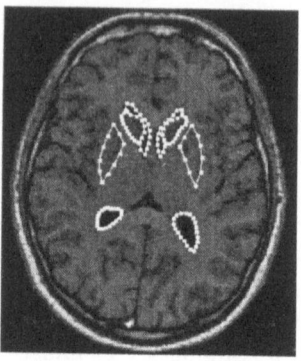

Fig. 1. Example of MR brain slice labelled with 123 landmark points around the ventricles, the caudate nucleus and the lentiform nucleus

By applying PCA to the normalised data we obtain a linear model:

$$\mathbf{g} = \bar{\mathbf{g}} + \mathbf{P}_g \mathbf{b}_g \tag{2}$$

where $\bar{\mathbf{g}}$ is the mean normalised grey-level vector, $\mathbf{P}_g$ is a set of orthogonal *modes of intensity variation* and $\mathbf{b}_g$ is a set of grey-level parameters.

The shape and appearance of any example can thus be summarised by the vectors $\mathbf{b}_s$ and $\mathbf{b}_g$. Since there may be correlations between the shape and grey-level variations, we concatenate the vectors, apply a further PCA and obtain a model of the form

$$\begin{pmatrix} \mathbf{W}_s \mathbf{b}_s \\ \mathbf{b}_g \end{pmatrix} = \mathbf{b} = \begin{pmatrix} \mathbf{Q}_s \\ \mathbf{Q}_g \end{pmatrix} \mathbf{c} = \mathbf{Q}\mathbf{c} \tag{3}$$

where $\mathbf{W}_s$ is a diagonal matrix of weights for each shape parameter, allowing for the difference in units between the shape and grey models, $\mathbf{Q}$ is a set of orthogonal modes and $\mathbf{c}$ is a vector of *appearance* parameters controlling both the shape and grey-levels of the model. Since the shape and grey-model parameters have zero mean, so does $\mathbf{c}$.

Note that the linear nature of the model allows us to express the shape and grey-levels directly as functions of $\mathbf{c}$

$$\mathbf{x} = \bar{\mathbf{x}} + \mathbf{P}_s \mathbf{W}_s^{-1} \mathbf{Q}_s \mathbf{c} \quad , \quad \mathbf{g} = \bar{\mathbf{g}} + \mathbf{P}_g \mathbf{Q}_g \mathbf{c}. \tag{4}$$

An example image can be synthesised for a given $\mathbf{c}$ by generating the shape-free grey-level image from the vector $\mathbf{g}$ and warping it using the control points described by $\mathbf{x}$.

For instance, Fig. 2 shows the effects of varying the first two shape model parameters, b_{s1}, b_{s2}, of a model trained on a set of 72 2D MR images of the brain, labelled as shown in Fig. 1. Figure 2 shows the effects of varying the first two appearance model parameters, c_1, c_2, which change both the shape and the texture component of the synthesised image.

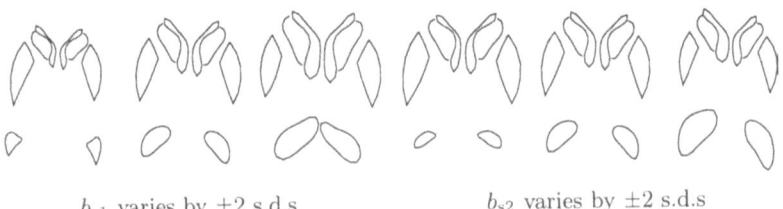

b_{s1} varies by ± 2 s.d.s b_{s2} varies by ± 2 s.d.s

Fig. 2. First two modes of shape model of part of a 2D MR image of the brain

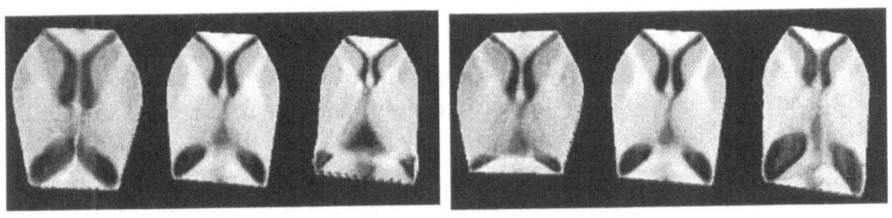

c_1 varies by ± 2 s.d.s c_2 varies by ± 2 s.d.s

Fig. 3. First two modes of appearance model of part of a 2D MR image of the brain

3.2   Active Appearance Model Matching

We treat matching as an optimisation problem in which we minimise the difference between a new image and one synthesised by the appearance model.

Given a set of model parameters, $\mathbf{c}$, we can generate a hypothesis for the shape, $\mathbf{x}$, and texture, $\mathbf{g}_m$, of a model instance. To compare this hypothesis with the image, we use the suggested shape to sample the image texture, $\mathbf{g}_s$, and compute the difference, $\delta\mathbf{g} = \mathbf{g}_s - \mathbf{g}_m$. We seek to minimise the magnitude of $|\delta\mathbf{g}|$.

This is potentially a very difficult optimisation problem, but we exploit the fact that whenever we use a given model with images containing the modelled structure the optimisation problem will be similar. This means that we can learn how to solve the problem off-line. In particular, we observe that the pattern in the difference vector $\delta\mathbf{g}$ will be related to the error in the model parameters.

During a training phase, the AAM learns a linear relationship between $\delta\mathbf{g}$ and the parameter perturbation required to correct this,

$$\delta\mathbf{c} = \mathbf{A}\delta\mathbf{g}. \tag{5}$$

The matrix $\mathbf{A}$ is obtained by linear regression on random displacements from the true training set positions and the induced image residuals (See [10] for details).

We can use (5) in an iterative matching algorithm. Given the current estimate of model parameters, $\mathbf{c}$, and the normalised image sample at the current estimate, $\mathbf{g}_s$, each iteration proceeds as follows:

- Evaluate the error vector $\delta\mathbf{g} = \mathbf{g}_s - \mathbf{g}_m$
- Evaluate the current error $E = |\delta\mathbf{g}|^2$
- Compute the predicted displacement, $\delta\mathbf{c} = \mathbf{A}\delta\mathbf{g}$
- Set $k = 1$
- Let $\mathbf{c}' = \mathbf{c} - k\delta\mathbf{c}$
- Sample the image at this new prediction, and calculate a new error vector, $\delta\mathbf{g}'$
- If $|\delta\mathbf{g}|^2 < E$ then accept the new estimate, $\mathbf{c}'$,
- Otherwise try at $k = 0.5$, $k = 0.25$ etc.

This is repeated until no improvement is made to the error, $|\delta\mathbf{g}|^2$, and convergence is declared.

We use a multi-resolution implementation, in which we iterate to convergence at each level before projecting the current solution to the next level of the model. This is more efficient and can converge to the correct solution from further away than search at a single resolution.

For example, Fig. 4 shows an example of an AAM of the central structures of the brain slice converging from a displaced position on a previously unseen image. The model could represent about 10000 pixels and had 30 parameters of $\mathbf{c}$. The search took about a second on a modern PC. Figure 5 shows examples of the results of the search, with the model points found superimposed on the target images.

4   Results of Experiments

We have applied our approach to 2D slices taken from similar positions in 28 3D MR images of the brain. The in-slice resolution is 1mm and the between slice resolution 1.5mm. A total of 72 slices were used, two or three from each brain image. Ground truth for the structures of interest (ventricles, caudate nucleus and lentiform nucleus) was annotated by hand using expert radiologist input.

A set of 'leave-one-brain-out' experiments were performed to test the performance of our approach.

We trained a model using all the examples except those from one brain, then ran the AAM to convergence on each of the excluded slices. We measured the quality of fit of the texture model, and the errors in the model point positions compared to the original labelling. We missed out each brain in turn, and averaged the results.. Table 1 summarises the results. It includes the results of 'leave-all-in' experiments for comparison, in which the model was used to search the training set. This gives an upper bound on performance.

In addition we give the errors obtained when the model is fit directly to the labelled points - the 'best fit' column. This gives a measure of the best possible model fit.

The texture difference is given as the RMS difference between the intensities synthesised by the model and those in the target image over the modelled region. The units are those of grey-level. The full range of grey-levels in the image was about 140 units, with noise of about 7 units (s.d.). Notice that in the miss-1-out

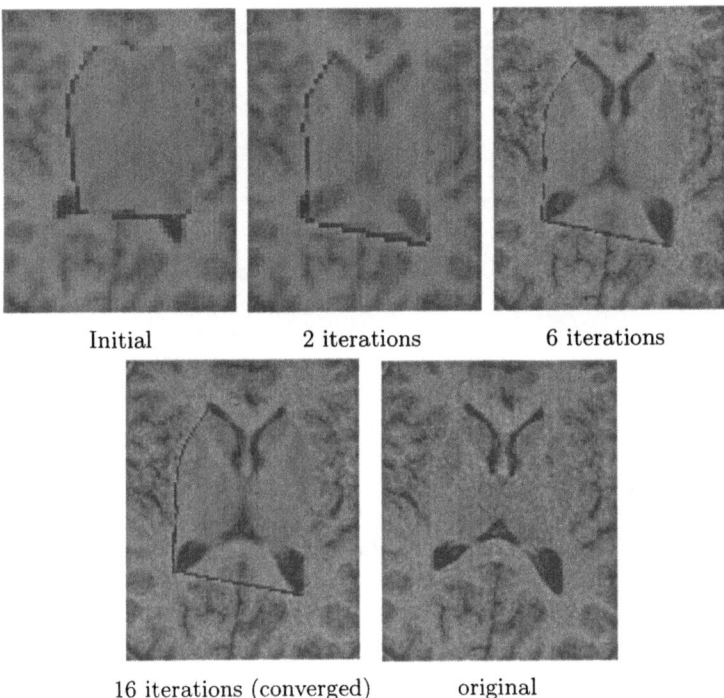

Initial   2 iterations   6 iterations

16 iterations (converged)   original

Fig. 4. Multi-resolution AAM search from a displaced position

experiments the texture error found by search is better than that when fitting to the hand labelled points. This is because the search is able to compromise point position in favour of reducing texture error.

The point error is given as the mean distance between corresponding model and image label points (Pt-Pt) and as the mean distance between model points and the labelled image boundary (Pt-Bnd). Close examination of the hand labelled points suggests there is noise in their placement which may contribute considerably to the measured results.

The code was written in C++ and run on a 166MHz Pentium II under Linux. The mean time per model match was about five seconds for a 30 parameter, 10000 pixel model. This would take around one second on a modern PC.

Table 1. Performance of AAM at matching brain model to images (± s.d.)(See Text)

Measure	Miss-1-Out		Leave-all-in	
	Search	Best Fit	Search	Best Fit
Texture Error	12.8 (±3.1)	14.6 (±2.8)	10.9 (±2.2)	8.4 (±1.5)
Pt-Pt Error (pixels)	2.4 (±0.7)	0.9 (±0.3)	1.7 (±0.4)	0.4 (±0.07)
Pt-Bnd Error (pixels)	1.2 (±0.3)	0.6(±0.2)	0.9 (±0.2)	0.3(±0.05)

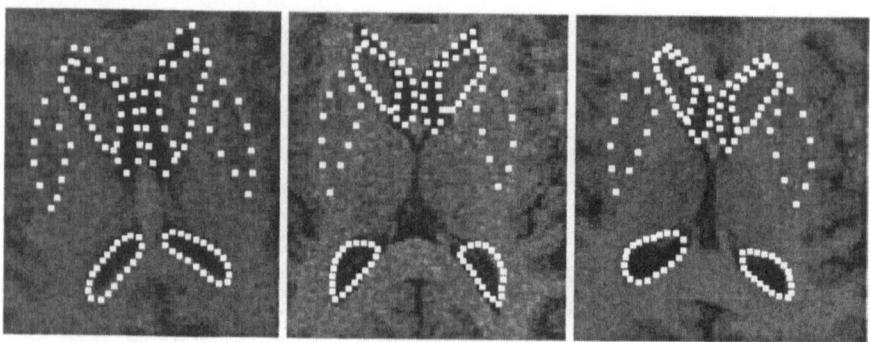

Fig. 5. Results of AAM search. Model points superimposed on target image

4.1   Examples of Failure

Figure 6 shows two examples where the AAM has failed to locate boundaries correctly on unseen images. In both cases the examples show more extreme shape variation from the mean, and it is the outer boundaries that the model cannot locate. This is because the model only samples the image under its current location. There is not always enough information to drive the model outward to the correct outer boundary. One solution is to model the whole of the visible structure (see below). Alternatively it may be possible to include explicit searching outside the current patch, for instance by searching along normals to current boundaries as is done in the Active Shape Model [12]. This is the subject of current research. In practice, where time permits, one can use multiple starting points and then select the best result (the one with the smallest texture error).

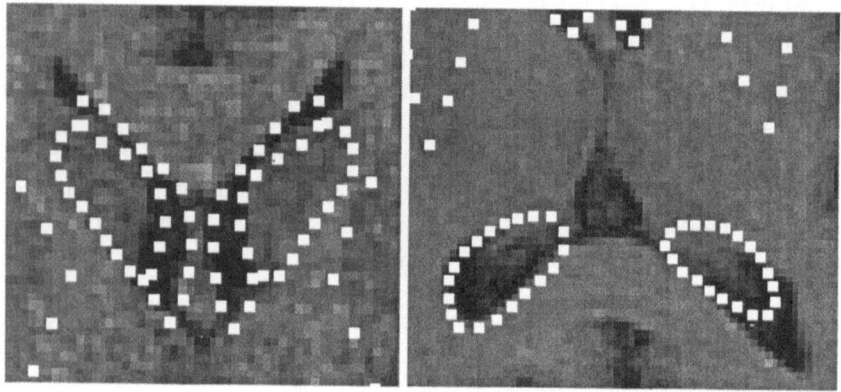

Fig. 6. Detail of examples of search failure. The AAM does not always find the correct outer boundaries of the ventricles (see text)

5   Discussion and Conclusions

We have demonstrated that a deformable anatomical atlas can be built using statistical models of shape and appearance. Both the shape and the appearance of the atlas can vary in ways observed in the training set. Arbitrary deformations are not allowed. Matching to a new image involves minimising the difference between the synthesised atlas image and the target. This can be achieved rapidly using the Active Appearance Model matching algorithm.

The AAM may not always give optimal results, but it would be straightforward to use a general purpose optimiser (e.g. Simplex or Powell [21]) to 'polish' the final fit.

Though we only demonstrated on the central part of the brain, models can be build of the whole cross-section. Figure 7 shows the first two modes of such a model. This was trained from the same 72 example slices as above, but with additional points marked around the outside of the skull. The first modes are dominated by relative size changes between the structures.

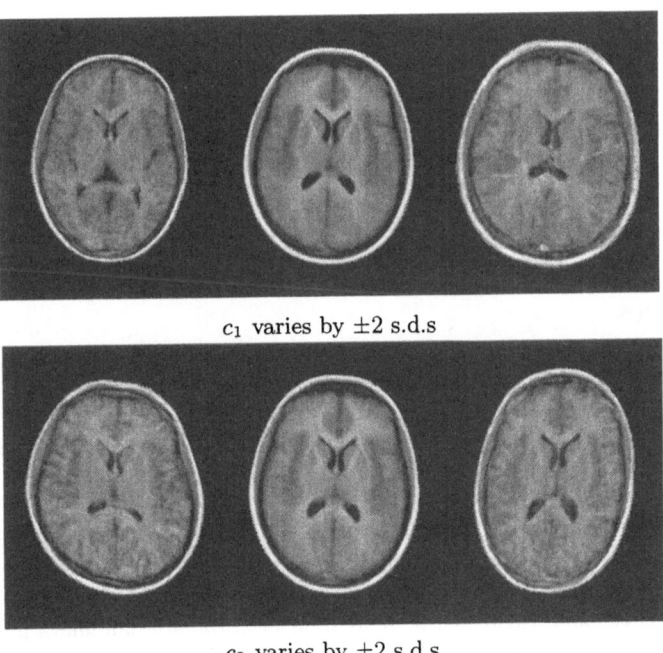

c_1 varies by ± 2 s.d.s

c_2 varies by ± 2 s.d.s

Fig. 7. First two modes of appearance model of full brain cross-section from an MR image

The appearance model relies on the existence of correspondence between structures in different images, and thus on a consistent topology across examples. For some structures (for example, the sulci), this does not hold true. An alternative approach for sulci is described by Caunce and Taylor [7,6].

The approach has been demonstrated in 2D, but is extensible to 3D. The main complications are the size of the model and the difficulty of obtaining well annotated training data. Each mode of the texture model is the same size as an image - if many modes are used, the model could be rather large. Obtaining good (dense) correspondences in 3D images is difficult, and is the subject of current research [4,5,24,15].

We hope to be able to match the models to different modalities by maximising mutual information, rather than minimising intensity errors. During search we would form an 'information difference' image, measuring the areas in the target image not well predicted by the model, and use this to update the current parameters.

We have shown how statistical models of appearance can represent both the mean and the modes of variation of shape and texture of structures appearing in medical images. Such models act as deformable anatomical atlases, in which the allowed deformation is learnt from a training set. The Active Appearance Model algorithm gives a fast method of matching the atlas to new images.

Acknowledgements

Dr Cootes is funded under an EPSRC Advanced Fellowship Grant. The brain images were generated by Dr Hutchinson and colleagues in the Dept. Diagnostic Radiology. They were marked up by Dr Hutchinson, Dr Hill and K. Davies and Prof. A. Jackson (from the Medical School, University of Manchester) and Dr G. Cameron (from Dept. Biomedical Physics, University of Aberdeen).

References

1. Bajcsy, and Kovacic, A: Multiresolution elastic matching. Computer Graphics and Image Processing **46** (1989) 1–21
2. Bajcsy, R., Lieberson, R., and Reivich, M: A computerized system for the elastic matching of deformed radiographic images to idealized atlas images. J. Comput. Assis. Tomogr. **7** (1983) 618–625
3. Bookstein, F. L: Shape and the infromation in medical images: A decade of the morphometric synthesis. Computer Vision and Image Understanding **66**, 2 (1997), 97–118
4. Brett, A. D., and Taylor, C. J: A method of automatic landmark generation for automated 3D PDM construction. In: British Machine Vison Conference **2**, (1998) 914–923
5. Brett, A. D., and Taylor, C. J: A framework for automated landmark generation for automated 3D statistical model construction. In: IPMI (1999)
6. Caunce, A., and Taylor, C: Using local geometry to build 3D sulcal models. In: IPMI (1999).
7. Caunce, A., and Taylor, C. J: 3D point distribution models of the cortical sulci. In: British Machine Vision Conference. (1997) 550–559
8. Christensen, G. E., Joshi, S. C., and Miller, M: Volumetric transformation of brain anatomy. IEEE Trans. Medical Image **16** (1997), 864–877

9. Christensen, G. E., Rabbitt, R. D., Miller, M. I., Joshi, S. C., Grenander, U., Coogan, T. A., and Essen, D. C. V: Topological Properties of Smooth Anatomic Maps. Kluwer Academic Publishers, (1995), 101–112

10. Cootes, T., Edwards, G. J., and Taylor, C. J: Active appearance models. In: ECCV (1998), 484–498

11. Cootes, T., and Taylor, C: Modelling object appearance using the grey-level surface. In: British Machine Vision Conference, (1994) 479–488

12. Cootes, T. F., Hill, A., Taylor, C. J., and Haslam, J: The use of active shape models for locating structures in medical images. Image and Vision Computing **12** (1994), 276–285

13. Cootes, T. F., Taylor, C. J., Cooper, D. H., and Graham, J: Active shape models - their training and application. Computer Vision and Image Understanding **61**, (1995), 38–59.

14. Edwards, G. J., Taylor, C. J., and Cootes, T: Learning to identify and track faces in image sequences. In: British Machine Vison Conference (1997) 130–139

15. Fleute, M., and Lavallee, S: Building a complete surface model from sparse data using statistical shape models: Application to computer assisted knee surgery. In: MICCAI (1998) 878–887

16. Hill, A., Cootes, T. F., Taylor, C. J., and Lindley, K: Medical image interpretation: A generic approach using deformable templates. Journal of Medical Informatics **19** (1994) 47–59

17. Jones, M. J., and Poggio, T: Multidimensional morphable models. In: ICCV (1998) 683–688.

18. Maintz, J. B. A., and Viergever, M. A: A survey of medical image registration. Medical Image Analysis **2** (1998) 1–36

19. McInerney, T., and Terzopoulos, D: Deformable models in medical image analysis: a survey. Medical Image Analysis **1** (1996) 91–108

20. Nastar, C., Moghaddam, B., and Pentland, A: Generalized image matching: Statistical learning of physically-based deformations. In: ECCV Vol. 1 (1996) 589–598.

21. Press, W., Teukolsky, S., Vetterling, W., and Flannery, B: Numerical Recipes in C (2nd Edition). Cambridge University Press, (1992)

22. Sclaroff, S., and Isidoro, J: Active blobs. In: ICCV (1998) 1146–53

23. Subsol, G., Thirion, J. P., and Ayache, N: A general scheme for automatically building 3D morphometric anatomical atlases: application to a skull atlas. Medical Image Analysis **2** (1998) 37–60

24. Székely, G., Kelemen, A., Brechbühler, C., and Gerig, G: Segmentation of 2-D and 3-D objects from mri volume data using constrained elastic deformations of flexible fourier contour and surface models. Medical Image Analysis **1** (1996) 19–34

25. Wang, Y., and Staib, L. H: Elastic model based non-rigid registration incorporating statistical shape information. In MICCAI (1998) 1162–1173

An Integral Method for the Analysis of Wall Motion in Gated Myocardial SPECT Studies

Michael L. Goris and Robert L. Van Uitert Jr.

Stanford University School of Medicine, Stanford California 94305-5281, USA
mlgoris@pacbell.net

1 Introduction

Our aim was to investigate and further develop a system of analysis of complex left ventricular wall kinetics. The proposed method is specifically adapted to gated myocardial perfusion SPECT data. The unique properties of gated SPECT data in this respect are the lack of fiduciary points, the relatively low spatial resolution and the conservation of total counts during the cardiac cycle

In gated blood-pool studies, contrast ventriculography and echocardiography, individual points of the ventricular wall are not immediately identified. There may be some structures (valve plane, leaflets) which can serve as fiduciary points, but generally the ventricular wall is identified by an edge, i.e. as the interface between cavity and myocardium. Wall segments are identified from one moment of the cardiac cycle to the next by the intersection between an axis and an edge defining the wall. Motion is thus defined as the displacement of this intersection. The axis can be defined in various ways: as originating at the center of the cavity, as perpendicular to the long axis of the cavity, or as the normal to the edge. In all cases the intersection between axis and edge identifies the segment and identifies the motion. Therefore, motion unrelated to the axis cannot be detected (Fig. 1).

2 Materials and Methods

The data are gated myocardial perfusion SPECT images, consisting of eight or sixteen isometric image volumes in a 64^3 format. Each image volume maps the distribution of the tracer (^{99m}Tc–Sestamibi or Tetrofosmin) in the chest of the patient as count rate densities during a segment of the cardiac cycle. The images are reconstructed from 63 or 64 projection images, obtained from a dual or triple–head scintillation camera (Anger type). Reconstruction is achieved by filtered back-projection with a restorative band-pass filter (Buttherworth). After the acquisition and prior to the reconstruction, the data are corrected for under-sampling due to slight variations in the cycle length. The reconstructed images are centered over the myocardium, zoomed and reoriented such that the long axis becomes parallel to the z–axis of the image volume. The center of the cavity is placed approximately at the pixel location 32,32,32. The final zoomed image contains the myocardium as the main structure with high count rate densities. Non-structured background has lower count rate densities, but occasional sub-diaphragmatic high densities remain (representing intra-luminal gut activity).

A. Kuba et al. (Eds.): IPMI'99, LNCS 1613, pp. 334–339, 1999.

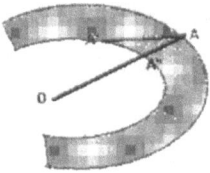

Fig. 1. Tracking Intersection of Axis and edge

At the time of the acquisition the tracer has largely left the vascular system and is located mainly in the intracellular space. The exception is that part of the tracer that is excreted into the gut through the biliary tract. In the reconstructed images this affects the sub–diaphragmatic count rate densities only, but in equal fashion and degree through the eight or sixteen image volumes. For this reason the total count rate in the images is conserved. The changes in the position of myocardial elements during the cardiac cycle therefore affect only the spatial distribution of the count rate densities.

The proposed method rests on two principles of which only the first can be derived from first principle: First, the changes in the spatial distribution of the count rate densities affect an integral function of the count rate densities computed along any axis. Second, the actual changes can be recovered from those integral function computed along congruent angles.

2.1 Integral Counts Analysis

The total image activity, $S(t)$, is constant for all values of t (and all projection directions). The integral function $P(L, 0)$ defines the percentile activity at $x = L$ in time–bin 0. The location in x of the percentile P at $t > 0$ is found by linear interpolation. The displacement vector $D(x, t)$ is the function showing the difference in location of a given percentile P between image 0 and image "t" (Fig. 3). The values of $D(x, t)$ are periodic over "t" for all values of x and the value of $D(x, 0)$ is zero for all values of x.

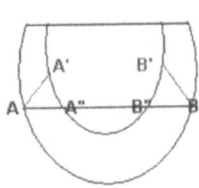

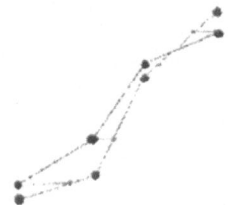

Fig. 2. Effect of out–of–plane motion on in–plane analysis

Fig. 3. Computing the displacement function

2.2 Analysis Along Multiple Congruent Angles

This derivation assumes that the analysis is performed for an integral function defined in "x". In this section we derive the same values, assuming that the image has been rotated by an angle θ. As an example let θ be an angle in the x, y planes. There is no rotation in the y, z or x, z planes. The rotated volume has a coordinate system (x', y', z'). The transformation is defined by: $z = z'$, $y = x' \sin(\theta)$, $x = x' \cos(\theta)$. The integral analysis is now performed in x'. The vector $D(x', t)$ can be decomposed in an x and an y component. In this example there is no z component. This approach can be expanded to 3 dimensions.

2.3 Reconstructing Three–Dimensional Motion Vectors

Three–dimensional image vectors X, Y, and Z are then reconstituted as follows: Consider the component $D(x, t)$ computed after the rotation θ, Φ: the vector is re–projected in a volume $D'(x', y', z', t)$ in such a way that $D'(x', y', z', t) = D(x, t)$. The volume $D'(x', y', z', t)$ is then rotated by $-\theta, -\Phi$ and added to a volume $Dx(x, y, z, t)$ which was initially set to zero. The same operation produces the vectors $Dy(x, y, z, t)$ and $Dz(x, y, z, t)$. The working hypothesis is that the vector volumes Dx, Dy, and Dz contain the x, y, and z motion components of the count rate densities, and, that the multiplicity of sampling angles provided motion resolution at a near pixel level.

The congruent sampling, and the method of sampling, makes the measures independent of orientation and makes no reference to a cardiac related coordinate system. The assumption is that all motion can thus be detected and is fully expressed in the X, Y, and Z components. Furthermore, each pixel has motion characteristics, rather than those pixels that are at the edge or the center of the ventricular wall. If a particular motion is judged to be of particular significance, it can be derived *a posteriori*. As an example we consider radial motion and rotational motion.

3 Results

Preliminary results address the following questions.

1. Can motion that is usually detected with a preset cardiac coordinate system be recovered by the integral approach, which uses *a posteriori* coordinates?
2. Does the integral approach give some regional information, or does the information remain global?
3. Can complex motion be derived?
4. Is the method insensitive to orientation?

The motion is displayed by the phase and amplitude of the derived displacement vector. From the displacement in X, Y, and Z we have derived motion toward the long axis (in plane), motion towards the center of the cavity (off plane) and angular or rotational motion (in plane). The results of the analysis are displayed by looking at the central orthogonal slices (long axis horizontal, long axis vertical and short axis as in Figs. 4–7).

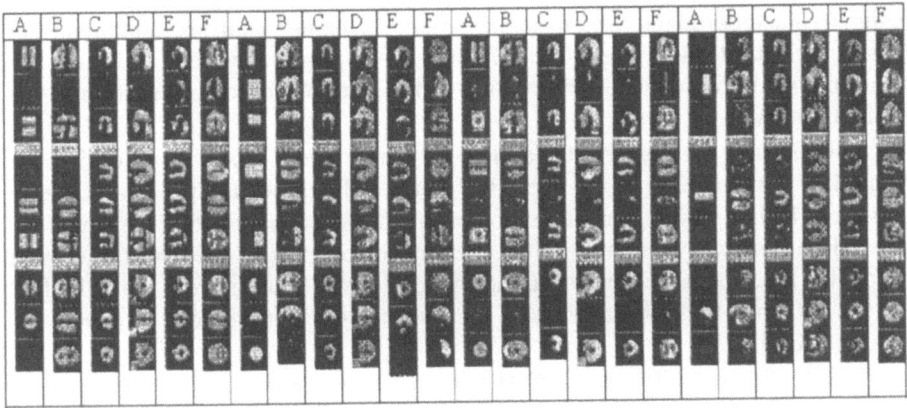

A	B	C	D	E	F	A	B	C	D	E	F	A	B	C	D	E	F	A	B	C	D	E	F

Fig. 4. X, Y, and Z amplitudes

Fig. 5. X, Y, and Z phases

Fig. 6. Cylindrical radial, Short axis Angular and spherical radial amplitudes

Fig. 7. Short axis Angular and spherical radial phases

Figures 4–7 shows the amplitudes and phases of the first harmonic of the displacement functions DX, DY and DZ, and derived motion (radial, spherical and angular). The first three rows are the representation of the central horizontal long axis slices. Next we show the central vertical and finally the central short axis slices. Case A is a mathematical phantom of a shrinking cylinder. The other columns represent 5 patient cases.

All questions can be answered positively. We can indeed recover centripetal motion, in plane and off plane, and local or regional particularities can be detected.

4 Discussion

If ventricular wall kinetics adds information to the myocardial perfusion studies or indeed yields important clinical information by itself, one can expect that any improvement in the definition of it would increase its clinical utility. One possible improvement is the inclusion of complex motion or deformation analysis. Complex motion includes off–plane motion and rotational motion. Most described methods (for the analysis of gated myocardial SPECT) cannot detect complex motion. Our proposal addresses the problem directly. The ultimate goal is not to develop a method that could effectively use all the information yielded by MRI or echocardiography, but to enrich at no or little cost the information yielded by myocardial perfusion studies.

One important feature of gated SPECT is that the data are truly three–dimensional, isotropic and that all parts of the image are recordings of the same cardiac cycles. The truly volumetric aspect of the data has generally not been fully utilized, with many authors restricting the analysis to motion or deformation in a plane [15,13,12,11] or in complex combinations of planes [6,16]. We believe that cross plane displacement makes "in plane" analysis fundamentally incomplete, that the polar 3D method is an improvement (Fig. 2), but that motion detection independently of an a–priori cardiac coordinate system is the ultimate answer.

The method is experimental and in an early phase. There is no derivation from first principle that assures that the method should work. Specifically, we do not know if the additive decomposition of the integral function, taken at different spatial angles, will yield sufficiently accurate displacement vectors at the pixel level. We are, however, able to predict which factors could have a critical effect on the outcome. In addition, we have methods to test if motion can be effectively characterized.

The basic assumption is that the unstructured background and the sub–diaphragmatic structured background remain invariant during the cardiac cycle. This assumption seems physiologically reasonable, but noise could produce regional variations, which in turn could influence the integral function. In addition, the original (centered, zoomed and reoriented) image contains non–zero pixel densities in all pixels of the cube. However, after a full rotation and mapping into another cube, some pixels (at the corners) cannot be mapped in the new volume. The effect of clipping the counts (setting all count rate densities $< T$ equal to zero, while maintaining those $> T$ at their original value) must be investigated. The level of T could be defined by the functional criterion we defined earlier [7]. Another possibility is masking. All pixels outside the largest sphere inscribed in the image volume can be set at zero, or all pixel outside of a mask surrounding the myocardium. Masking could be based on a segmentation described earlier [14,2,4,9,10].

It should be mentioned at this point that one method was described [3] which was at the same time truly three–dimensional and did not use a preset coordinate system. The method was based on a three–dimensional matching method, originally described by Besl [1] and later Feldmar [5]. The method was initially utilized to match static myocardial SPECT images [2,8,9,10]. Declerck [2] adapted the method to four dimensions. The analysis however favors some directions and works only on endo– and epicardial surfaces.

In conclusion: Our preliminary results show that we are able to extract kinetic information from gated myocardial perfusion SPECT images using prototype analysis algorithms. The results also support our hypothesis that a combined analysis of perfusion and kinetics from the same perfusion SPECT images will enable more accurate classification of patients with a variety of perfusion defects.

References

1. Besl, P.,NcKay, N.: A method for registration of 3D shapes. IEEE Transactions on Pattern Analysis and Machine Intelligence **14** (1992) 239–256
2. Declerck, J., Feldmar, J., Goris, M.L., Betting, F,: Automatic registration and alignment on a template of cardiac stress and rest SPECT images. INRIA Rapport de recherche # 2770 (1996)

3. Declerck, J., Feldmar, J., Ayache, N.: Definition of a 4D continuous polar transformation for the tracking and the analysis of the LV motion. INRIA Research Report # 3025 (1996)
4. Declerck, J., Feldmar, J., Goris, M.L., Betting, F.: Automatic registration and alignment on a template of cardiac stress and rest SPECT reoriented SPECT images. IEEE Transactions on Medical Imaging 16 (1997) 727–733
5. Feldmar, J., Ayache, N.: Rigid, affine, and locally affine registration of free-form surfaces. International Journal of Computer Vision, Accepted for publication (Also Technical Report INRIA # 2220 (1997))
6. Germano, G., Kiat, H., Kavanagh, P.B., Moriel, M., Mazzanti, M., Su, H.T., Van Train, K.F., Berman, D.S.: Automatic quantification of ejection fraction from gated myocardial perfusion SPECT. J. Nucl. Med. 36 (1995) 2138–2147
7. Goris, M.L., Briandet, P.A., Thomas, A.J., McKillop, J.H., Sneed, P., Wiklander, D.P.: A thresholding for radionuclide angiocardiography. Invest Radiology 16 (1981) 115–119
8. Goris, M.L., Malandain, G., Marque, I.: Automatic registration of myocardial perfusion studies using a potential based rigid transformation. 2nd International conference of Nuclear Cardiology April 1995, Cannes, France. J. Nucl. Cardiology 2 (1995) S81
9. Goris, M.L., Declerck, J., Feldmar, J., Ayache, N.: Elastic transformations in referential quantification of scintigraphic images. Proceedings of the International symposium on computer and communication systems for image guided diagnosis and therapy. Lemke HU, Vannier MW, Inamura K and Farman AG editors. Elsevier (1996) 298-301
10. Goris, M.L., Declerck, J., Feldmar, J., Ayache, N., Pace, W.: Elastic matching of myocardial perfusion studies to a template (abstract). J. Nuc. Med. Technology 24 (1996) 164
11. Kouris, K., Abdel–Dayem, H.M., Taha, B., Ballani, N., Hassan, I.M., Constantinides, C.: Left ventricular ejection fraction and volumes calculated from dual gated SPECT myocardial imaging with 99Tcm-MIBI. Nucl. Med. Commun. 13 (1992) 648–655
12. Marcassa, C., Marzullo, P., Parodi, O., Sambuceti, G., L'Abbate, A.: A new method for noninvasive quantitation of segmental myocardial wall thickening using technetium–99m 2–methoxy–isobutyl–isonitrile scintigraphy — results in normal subjects. J. Nucl. Med. 31 (1990) 173–177
13. Mochizuki, T., Murase, K., Fujirawa, Y., Tanada, S., Hamamoto, K., Tauxe, W.N.: Assessment of systolic thickening with thallium–201 ECG-gated single photon emission computed tomography: a parameter for focal left ventricular function. J. Nucl. Med. 32 (1991) 1496–1500
14. Monga, O., Deriche, R., Rocchisani, J.M.: 3D edge detector using recursive filtering: application to scanner images. In Computer Vision Graphics and Image Processing (1991)
15. Takeda, T., Toyoma, H., Ishikawa, N., Satoh, M., Masuoka, T., Ajisaka, R., Iida, K., Wu, J., Sugishita, Y., Itai, Y.: Quantitative phase analysis of myocardial wall thickening by technetium–99m 2–metoxy–isobutyl–isonitrile SPECT. Annals of Nucl. Med. 6 (1992) 69–78
16. Williams, K.A., Taillon, L.A.: Left ventricular function in patients with coronary artery disease assessed by gated tomographic myocardial perfusion images. Comparison with assessment by contrast ventriculography and first-pass radionuclide angiography. J. Am. Coll. Cardiol. 27 (1996) 173–181

Enhanced Artery Visualization in Blood Pool MRA: Results in the Peripheral Vasculature

Wiro Niessen[1], Alexander Montauban van Swijndregt[2], Bernard Elsman[3], Onno Wink[1], Max Viergever[1], and Willem Mali[2]

[1] Image Sciences Institute, University Hospital Utrecht
Room E.01.334, 3584 CX Utrecht, The Netherlands
wiro@isi.uu.nl
[2] Department of Radiology, University Hospital Utrecht
[3] Department of Surgery, University Hospital Utrecht

Abstract. Blood pool contrast agents for Magnetic Resonance Angiography (MRA) have a prolonged intravascular half-life and therefore have the potential for visualizing large anatomical regions with high resolution. A potential problem is that both the arteries and veins are enhanced, resulting in venous overprojection in Maximum Intensity Projections (MIPs), which are most widely used for inspecting MRA datasets. In this paper a novel approach for improved arterial visualization is introduced. It is based on suppressing the major overlapping veins in MIPs. The approach is illustrated on MRA images of the peripheral vasculature acquired using the blood pool agent NC100150. The resulting visualizations are compared to Digital Subtraction Angiography (DSA) images.

1 Introduction

Conventional noninvasive MRA is an accepted clinical technique which facilitates high quality depiction of the cerebral vasculature. For abdominal and peripheral imaging, the effectiveness of conventional MRA is limited owing to some intrinsic limitations of the technique. Especially complicated flow patterns and in-plane flow may result in signal voids which can lead to an overestimate of a stenosis [1].

The introduction of Gadopentetate dimeglumine as a T1 shortening contrast agent [2] has considerably increased the clinical applicability of MRA. Since the shortened T1 of blood provides contrast, rather than the flow dynamics, the technique is less sensitive to flow conditions. Moreover, high contrast can be obtained in shorter examination times, enabling breath hold sequences which reduce motion artifacts. A shortcoming of Gadopentetate dimeglumine is its rapid diffusion in extracellular space. This limits the imaging window to a few minutes since the background signal increases as well.

Ultra-small SuperParamagnetic Iron Oxide (USPIO) particles are a new class of MRI contrast agents. They were primarily designed for their T2* relaxation properties, but also exhibit strong T1 shortening properties in blood [3], and can therefore also be used for Contrast Enhanced (CE) MRA. The primary

A. Kuba et al. (Eds.): IPMI'99, LNCS 1613, pp. 340–345, 1999.

advantage of these blood pool agents is their long intravascular half-life, which paves the way for steady state MRA. Longer examination times enable coverage of larger anatomical regions at higher spatial resolution.

An important drawback of blood pool agents is the simultaneous enhancement of arteries and veins. This can significantly hamper diagnosis of *e.g.* the main arterial branches [4,5,6]. An anatomical region in which this is certainly the case is the leg, which is highly vascularized and has arteries and veins running close to each other. Either the acquisition should be modified in order to construct selective arterial and venous angiograms, which is nontrivial, or retrospective image processing is required. In this paper we introduce one possible approach for enhanced arterial visualization, which is based on the idea of removing the most important overlapping veins, prior to performing a MIP.

2 Image Acquisition

Patients were included as a part of a Phase II study of NC100150 injection (Nycomed Imaging AS, Oslo). Imaging was performed on a 1.5 T system (Gyroscan NT, Powertrak 6000, Philips Medical Systems, Best, The Netherlands), using a gradient echo technique. Images showed strong vascular enhancement, both in the arteries and veins. In Fig. 1 we show a coronal slice of the upper leg/abdominal region and a corresponding MIP. Owing to the adjacency of the major arteries and veins, the status of the arteries can not be determined from these images, even if MIPs from different angles are reconstructed. Therefore, enhanced arterial visualization is considered an important step towards the clinical use of MRA blood pool agents [4,5,6].

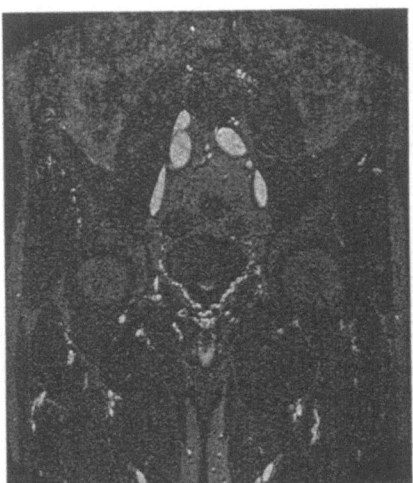 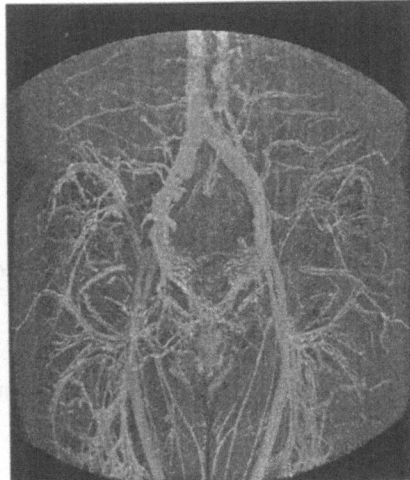

Fig. 1. Coronal slices in the abdominal/upper leg region (left) and the corresponding MIP (right)

3   Enhanced Arterial Visualization

Existing techniques for vessel enhancement and segmentation cannot straightfor-
wardly be used for blood pool MRA images. The adjacency of a large number of
small arteries and veins makes segmentation more complicated than in conventional MRA images. To overcome these problems, we devised a relatively simple
technique which is limited to the automated segmentation of a small number of
the main overlapping veins, which are selected by an operator. This approach has
two main advantages. First, the algorithm is fast since it only uses local computations. This distinguishes the method from approaches that first compute
all features in the image that have a vessel-like shape, which are subsequently
grouped. Results from our procedure are readily available, which is important for
clinical use. Secondly, the segmented veins are removed rather than performing
a segmentation of the arteries. Thus, the status of the arteries is judged from the
original data, which limits the chance of introducing errors in diagnosis, owing
to imperfections in the segmentation. The procedure is schematically drawn in
Fig. 2.

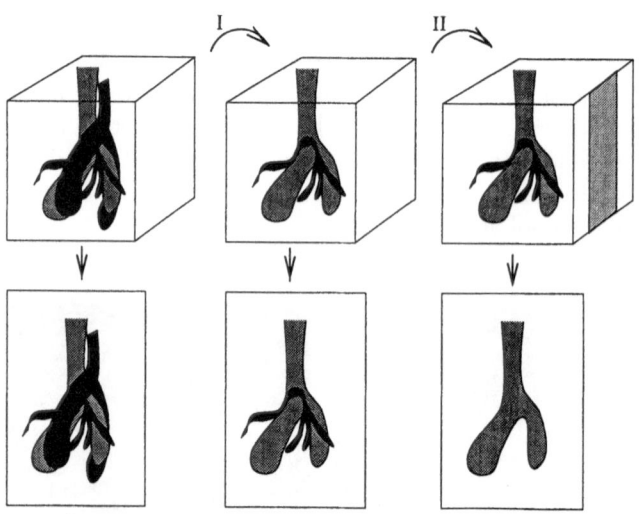

Fig. 2. Outline of the algorithm to enhance arterial visualization in MIP images. In
the images the main arteries (grey), the major veins (black) and other overlapping
venous structures (dark grey) are shown. First (I), the major venous structures are
segmented and suppressed in the MIP. Subsequently (II), a targetted MIP (grey band)
is performed, which removes most remaining overlapping vessels

The tools which are required for this procedure are (i) a reliable segmentation
tool for the veins, and (ii) an interactive tool to perform targetted MIPs in
arbitrary directions. The procedure for vessel segmentation is adapted from an
algorithm to determine the central vessel axis for the preoperative evaluation of

patients who are scheduled for minimally invasive treatment of an abdominal aneurysm [7] and is illustrated in Fig. 3.

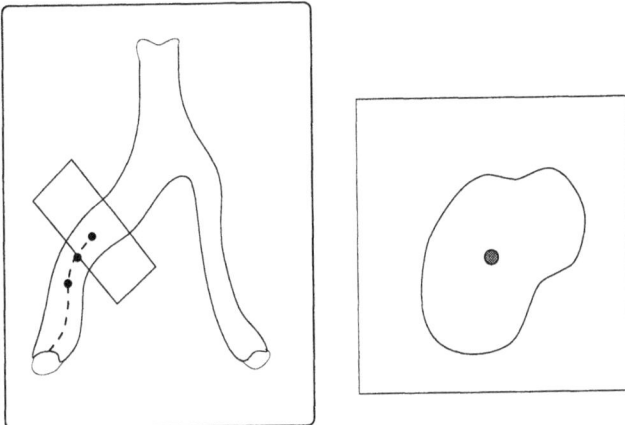

Fig. 3. Schematic of vessel segmentation. The user initializes two starting points on the central vessel axis. Segmentation is performed in a plane perpendicular to the vessel segment which is defined by these points. The gravity point of the segmentation becomes the new point on the vessel axis. A next point is predicted by extrapolation, and the procedure iterates until the desired vessel segment is tracked

First, two points are selected which define a first segment of the central vessel axis. A plane perpendicular to this segment is constructed, where the boundary of the vessel is determined using dynamic programming. Here a transformation into polar coordinates is made with the point on the central vessel axis as origin. A minimal cost path is found based on the image gradient magnitude in the direction of a ray originating from the origin:

$$\frac{\partial L}{\partial \boldsymbol{r}}(\boldsymbol{x}, \sigma) = \frac{|\boldsymbol{r}.\nabla L(\boldsymbol{x}, \sigma)|}{|\boldsymbol{r}|}. \tag{1}$$

Using the gradient in the direction of the ray assures that only transitions from high signal (vessel) to low signal (background) are considered being part of the lumen boundary. The gradient is computed by convolving with a Gaussian of scale $\sigma = 2$ in order to be more robust to noise. Based on the estimated contour a new point on the central vessel axis is defined by the gravity point. Based on this point and the previous point a new point is estimated by extrapolation. The procedure is iterated until the desired vessel segment is tracked.

4   Results

The algorithm to enhance arterial visualization has been applied to six patients included in the study. In the left image of Fig. 4 we show a typical result of venous segmentation using the semi-automated tracking procedure. In this case, no user interaction other than the initialization of the first two points was required.

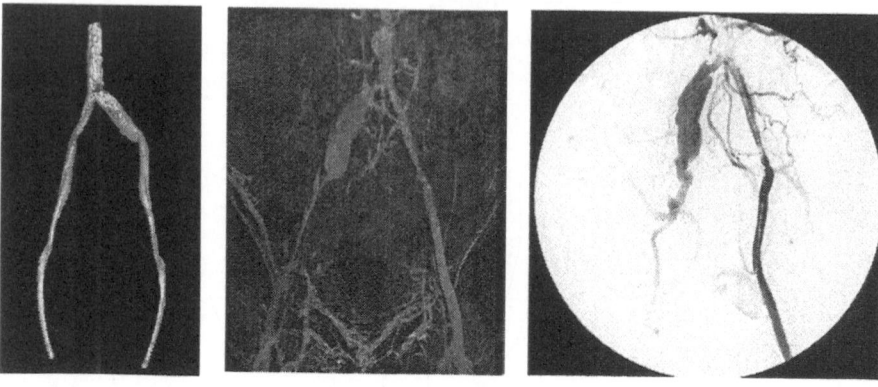

Fig. 4. Venous segmentation in the upper leg and abdominal region (left), a targeted MIP after venous suprression (middle) and the corresponding DSA image (right)

In the middle of Fig. 4 we show a MIP after the major venous structures adjacent to the important arteries have been removed. Since other overlapping venous structures are now relatively distant (in the original 3D data) from the main arterial branches remaining overprojection is reduced by a targeted MIP. Both in the DSA image and the processed MRA image a large dissection in the right ilic artery and a stenosis can be seen, which were not visible in the unprocessed MIP.

5   Discussion

MRA using blood pool agents has the potential for covering large anatomical regions of interest at high resolution. However, the simultaneous enhancement of veins and arteries hampers a quick interpretation of the images using MIPs, and possibly limits the clinical utility of these agents.

A possible strategy, which is advantageous for a number of applications, is the segmentation of the entire venous structure. For certain anatomical locations with a small number of vessel structures, or for sufficiently reduced regions of interest, this seems possible without excessive user interaction. For the entire leg, however, it is a difficult procedure. In this paper, we investigated whether a relatively simple procedure, which only segments the major veins which are adjacent to the arterial branches of interest, and subsequently removes other structures by performing targetted MIPs, yields satisfactory arterial visualization. The method is fast, allows for user supervision and does not influence the original data around the arteries, so that the anatomical context can still be assessed interactively. Results in the aortoiliac region show that the procedure aids in diagnosis from MIPs.

There are a number of points that could be improved. Simultaneously tracking arteries and veins which run close along each other will avoid the chance of including arterial voxels in the venous segmentation. Second, additional information can be obtained during the MRA acquisition, *e.g.* using first pass imaging or flow information. Developments in this area will be crucial to the clinical applicability of blood pool agents.

References

1. Ekelund, L., Sjöqvist, K.-A., Asberg, B.: MR angiography of abdominal and peripheral arteries. Acta Radiologica **37** (1996) 3–13
2. Prince, M.R.: Gadolinium-enhanced MR aortography. Radiology **191** (1994) 155–164
3. Weissleder, R., Elizondo, G., Wittenberg, J., Rabito, C.A., Bengele, H.H., Josephson, L.: Ultrasmall superparamagnetic iron oxide: characterization of a new class of contrast agents for MR imaging. Radiology **175** (1990) 489–493
4. Marchal, G., Bosmans, H., Hecke, P.V., Jiang, Y., Aerts, P., Bauer, H.: Experimental Gd-DPTA polylysine enhanced MR angiography: Sequence optimization. Journal of Computer Assisted Tomography **15** (1991) 711–715
5. Stillman, A.E., Wilke, N., Li, D., Haacke, M., McLachlan, S.: Ultrasmall superparamagnetic iron oxide to enhance MRA of the renal and coronary arteries: Studies in human patients. Journal of Computer Assisted Tomography **20** (1996) 51–55
6. Engelbrecht, M.R., Saeed, M., Wendland, M.F., Canet, E., Oksendal, A.N., and Higgins, C.B.: Contrast-enhanced 3D-TOF MRA of peripheral vessels: Intravascular versus extracellular MR contrast media. Journal of Magnetic Resonance Imaging **8** (1998) 616–621
7. Wink, O., Niessen, W.J., Viergever, M.A.: Fast quantification of abdominal aortic aneurysms from CTA volumes. Medical Image Conference and Computer Assisted Interventions (1998) 138–145

Four–Dimensional LV Tissue Tracking from Tagged MRI with a 4D B–Spline Model

Jiantao Huang and Amir A. Amini

CVIA Laboratory, Campus Box 8086, 660 S. Euclid Ave.
Washington University Medical Center
St. Louis, MO 63110, USA
{huang, amini}@cauchy.wustl.edu
http://www-cv.wustl.edu/

Abstract. Accurate delineation of the volumetric motion of left ventricle (LV) of the heart over time from tagged MRI is an important area of research. We have built a system that takes tagged short-axis (SA) and long-axis (LA) image sequences as input, fits a 4D B-spline model to the LV of the heart by simultaneously fitting knot solids to the SA and LA frame sequences via matching 3 sequences of model knot planes to LV tag planes for 4D tracking. The advantage of the 4D model is that 3D material point localization and displacement reconstruction is achieved in a single step. The generated 3D displacement fields are validated with a cardiac motion simulator, and 3D motion fields capturing *in-vivo* deformations in a parcine model of a LV with postero-lateral myocardial infarction are illustrated.

1 Introduction

Noninvasive techniques for assessing the dynamic behavior of the human heart are invaluable in the diagnosis of ischemic heart disease, as abnormalities in the myocardial motion sensitively reflect deficits in blood perfusion [9]. In MR tagging, the magnetization property of selective material points in the myocardium are altered in order to create tagged patterns within a deforming body such as the heart muscle. The resulting pattern defines a time-varying curvilinear coordinate system on the tissue. During tissue contractions, the grid patterns move, allowing for visual tracking of the grid intersections over time. The intrinsic high spatial and temporal resolutions of such myocardial analysis schemes provide unsurpassed information about local deformation in the myocardium which can be used to derive strain and deformation indices from different myocardial regions.

Previous research in analysis of tagged images includes [1,2,5,6,7]. Among various approaches which have been proposed in the literature for analysis of tagged images, our previous work in [4] is most closely related to this paper. In our former paper, we proposed a B-spline solid model to concurrently track tag lines in different image slices by implicitly defined B-spline surfaces which align themselves with tagged points. The primary contribution of this paper is in utilizing a knot solid to represent each pair of SA and LA frame of data and

A. Kuba et al. (Eds.): IPMI'99, LNCS 1613, pp. 346–351, 1999.

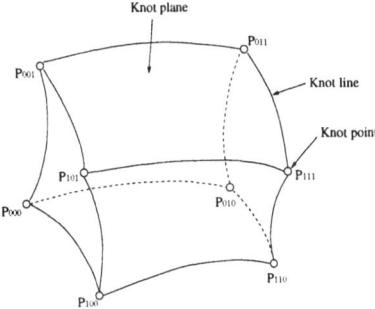

Fig. 1. A hyperpatch representing a small deforming cuboid enclosed by 6 tag planes

using 3 sequences of model knot planes to detect 3 sequences of LV tag planes. Once the 4D model is able to generate a B-solid which varies continuously over time, a 3D motion field between any two time instants is immediately available. The advantages of the B-spline approach over previous approaches to tagged MR image analysis are: (1) B-spline interpolation is performed over 3D space and time. (2) The movement of each myocardial point over time can be captured very accurately by setting the three parameters u, v, w of the model to any fractional value. (3) Intersections of three orthogonal tag planes and their motions are immediately available. (4) Change of strain over time can easily be computed at all myocardial points.

2   4D B-spline Representation

The simplest and most direct geometric element to model a time-varying solid is a **hyperpatch** [3]. A hyperpatch (Fig. 1) is a patch-bounded collection of points whose coordinates are given by continuous, four-parameter, single-valued mathematical functions of the form: $\{x = x(u, v, w, t), y = y(u, v, w, t), z = z(u, v, w, t)\}$ where t is the time variable. The parametric variables u, v, and w are constrained to the interval $u, v, w \in [0, 1]$ in a hyperpatch. A point (x, y, z) inside the hyperpatch is represented by $\mathbf{S}(u, v, w, t)$ and at a time instant $t = t^*$, fixing the value of one of the parametric variables results in an **isoparametric surface** within or on the boundary of the hyperpatch in terms of the other two variables, which remain free. Many hyperpatches tightly placed together, form a solid, and each hyperpatch shares its six faces with six neighboring hyperpatches. In the solid representation, ranges of u, v, w are from 0 to some integer value. For instance, $u \in [0, 1]$ denotes the first array of hyperpatches in terms of the v, w parameters; $u \in [1, 2]$ denotes the second array of hyperpatches, and so forth. The surface determined by setting one of u, v, w to a constant integer value is called a **knot surface** or a **knot plane** which are the delimiting surfaces of these hyperpatches. In a 4D B-spline model, knot planes become temporal functions, and the 3D solid captured at each knot time instant is called a **knot solid**. A tensor product 4D B-spline model is expressed as:

$$\mathbf{S}(u,v,w,t) = \sum_{i=1}^{I}\sum_{j=1}^{J}\sum_{k=1}^{K}\sum_{l=1}^{L}\mathbf{p}_{ijkl}N_i(u)N_j(v)N_k(w)N_l(t) \qquad (1)$$

where $(I \times J \times K \times L)$ is the total number of model control points; $N_i(u)$, $N_j(v)$, $N_k(w)$, and $N_l(t)$ are B-spline basis functions which blend control points $\mathbf{p}_{ijkl}$. By changing the order of B-spline summation, a more efficient approach to computing a multi-dimensional B-spline model results. Given any time instant t^*, a 3D grid of control points is specified that determines the 3D solid at t^*. To compute the solid at t^*, let us start with calculating the $u = u^*$ isoparametric planes. This is implemented in two steps: first we calculate all points with $u = u^*$ value along the B-spline curves, specified by each thread of control points in the u direction. We then calculate each B-spline surface by taking these $u = u^*$ points from the first step as control points, obtaining the $u = u^*$ isoparametric planes. This procedure may be mathematically stated as:

$$\mathbf{S}(u^*,v,w,t^*) = \sum_{l=1}^{L}\left(\sum_{k=1}^{K}\sum_{j=1}^{J}N_j(v)N_k(w)\left(\sum_{i=1}^{I}\mathbf{p}_{ijkl}N_i(u^*)\right)\right)N_l(t^*). \qquad (2)$$

Once we are able to compute the isoparametric plane, $\mathbf{S}(u^*,v,w,t^*)$, we can obtain the entire model at time instant t^* by continuously varying u^*. The advantage of this method over the tensor product method in (1) is its efficiency in speed, bypassing the need for multiplication of large matrices whose majority of elements are zeros (due to B-spline bases having limited spatial extent).

3   B-spline Fitting

The tag lines on LA and SA images are formed by intersecting image slices with one or two sequences of tag planes, respectively. From the tag lines on SA and LA frames, the B-spline model can fit each knot solid to each frame of data by matching 3 orthogonal sequences of knot planes to 3 orthogonal sequences of tag planes (Fig. 2). Since these tag planes deform with the myocardial tissue, the 4D model will then automatically interpolate the volumetric deformations of the LV over time and 3D space. We employ the Chamfer distance to build an objective function for fitting the tag planes. The total energy for the model, which is to be minimized, is defined as the sum of the energy of each knot solid which is defined by the sum of the energy of each knot plane. The energy of each knot plane is further defined as the integral of the corresponding potential over the knot plane surface. Thus the total energy for the model can be expressed as:

$$E = \sum_{t=1}^{T_m}\left(\sum_{u=1}^{U_m}\int\int C_u(\mathbf{S}(u,v,w,t))dvdw + \sum_{v=1}^{V_m}\int\int C_v(\mathbf{S}(u,v,w,t))dudw + \right.$$
$$\left.\sum_{w=1}^{W_m}\int\int C_w(\mathbf{S}(u,v,w,t))dudv\right) \qquad (3)$$

Tag data from frame: 1   2   3   ......   N

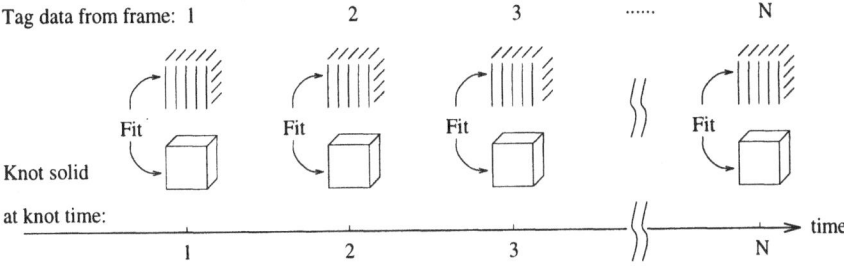

Fig. 2. Knot solids fit temporal frames of data, each including 3 orthogonal sequences of tag lines

where we have used $\mathcal{C}_u, \mathcal{C}_v, \mathcal{C}_w$ to denote the split 4D potentials (a separate one for each tag plane) and U_m, V_m, and W_m are the maximum knot values.

Our model is based on a 4D grid of control points and the total energy of the model is a function of all control points. Every control point is related to frames of data and 3 sets of tag planes. Although the potential functions are split, all knot planes are simultaneously optimized. For energy minimization, we used the adaptive conjugate gradient descent method which shortens the step length prior to taking a step in the search direction that passes over the minimum point. The process halts if the step length becomes smaller than a threshold.

4   Application to Tagged Images of the LV

We adopted a quadric-quadric-quadric-quadric B-spline model to perform validations. We utilized a cardiac motion simulator [2,8] to generate a sequence of deformed prolate spheroidal models of the LV. The tag lines in the simulated SA and LA images were first extracted. Then the system grouped tag lines by each tag plane and separate 4D Chamfer distance potentials were created for each tag plane.

The simulated data included 6 frames. Each frame included 8 SA image slices, 7 LA image slices, 14 tag planes (7 horizontal and 7 vertical) intersecting SA image slices, and 8 tag planes intersecting LA image slices. The fitting iteration for all frames took about $4.86\,ms$ per control point on a Sun Ultra 30/300 platform. We used an $8 \times 8 \times 9 \times 7$ grid of control points. The fitting algorithm converged in about 30 iterations. Therefore, the total fitting process approximately took 588 seconds for 6 frames of data.

An important byproduct of our approach is that at the conclusion of fitting knot solid to frames of data, a 4D model $\mathbf{S}(u,v,w,t)$ is determined. Given two solids $\mathbf{S}(u,v,w,t_0)$ and $\mathbf{S}(u,v,w,t_1)$, a 3D B-spline interpolated motion field is immediately generated by employing the computation in (2):

$$\mathbf{V}(u,v,w) = \mathbf{S}_1(u,v,w,t_1) - \mathbf{S}_0(u,v,w,t_0) \qquad (4)$$

The cardiac motion simulator was used to validate the accuracy of the generated motion fields. True 3D motion fields were first generated by the simulator. The

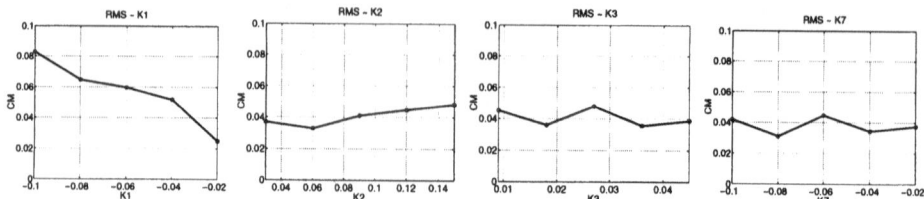

Fig. 3. RMS error plots between 3D ground-truth and 3D computed motion fields for a range of parameters of k_1: Radially dependent compression, k_2: torsion, k_3: Ellipticalization in LA plane, and k_7: Shear in z direction

computed $\mathbf{V}$ by (4) was then strictly compared with the ground-truth. Figure 3 shows RMS error plots between true and computed motion fields for a range of deformation parameters of the simulator. The method was also applied to images collected from a parcine model of a LV at baseline and after induction of a postero-lateral myocardial infarction (MI). Results from this experiment are illustrated in Fig. 4. The motion fields displayed were computed from the knot solid at frame 11 and the knot solid from frame 0 (see (4)). The akinetic areas of the myocardium can readily be recognized from the post-MI motion fields.

5   Conclusions

We have built a system to fit and track tagged MRI data by the 4D deformable B-spline model. The presented framework for fitting model knot solid to frames of data by matching three orthogonal sequences of knot planes to three sequences of tag planes for volumetric tracking is the primary contribution of this article. After the tag lines were extracted and grouped by tag planes, 4D Chamfer distance potentials were computed and used in fitting B-spline knot solids to frames of data. The generated 3D motion fields were validated with a cardiac motion simulator, and methods were applied to *in-vivo* data sets.

Acknowledgements

This work was supported in part by grant HL-57628 from the NIH.

References

1. Amini, A., and et al.: Energy-minimizing deformable grids for tracking tagged MR cardiac images. Computers in Cardiology, Durham, North Carolina (1992) 651-654
2. Amini, A., Chen, Y., Curwen, R., Mani, V., Sun, J.: Coupled B-Snake Grids and Constrained Thin-Plate Splines for Analysis of 2-D Tissue Deformations from Tagged MRI. IEEE-TMI **17** (1998) 344–356
3. Mortenson, M.: Geometric Modeling. John Wiley & Sons (1985)
4. Radeva, P., Amini, A., Huang, J.: Deformable B-Solids and Implicit Snakes for 3D Localization and Tracking of SPAMM MRI Data. Computer Vision and Image Understanding **66** (1997) 163–178

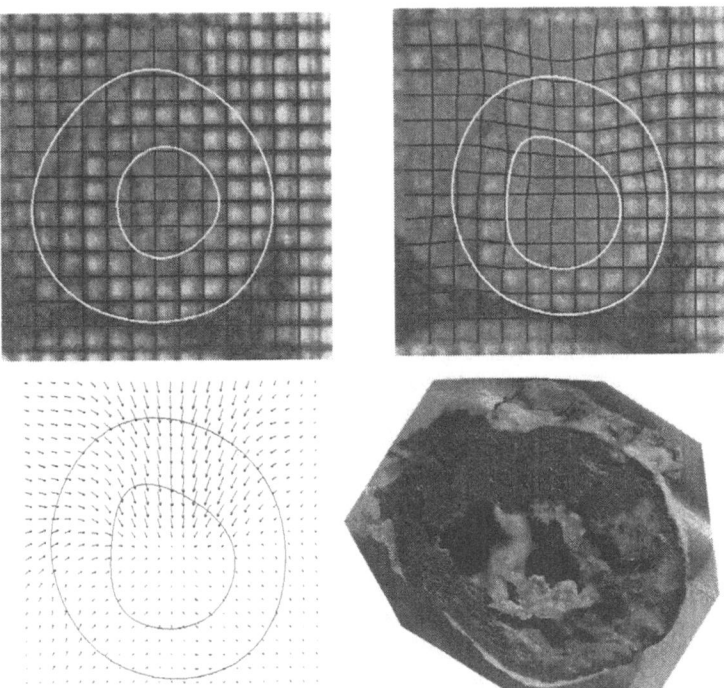

Fig. 4. The parcine model of a LV in short-axis orientation with a postero-lateral myocardial infarction. The top left image is the undeformed slice (slice 0, frame 0). The corresponding deformed slice (slice 0, frame 11) is shown on top right. The projected motion field (slice 0, frame 11) is shown in lower left. Please note that the motion field is truly 3D, and that it was projected into the plane of its respective image slice at frame 0 for display purposes. The lower right area of motion field (between 3 and 8 o'clock positions) indicates akinesis. The picture of the histochemically stained tissue slice, roughly corresponding to the same MR image slice location is shown in lower right. Brighter myocardial areas correspond to necrotic zones with no dye uptake, and darker areas correspond to normal zones where dye is taken up by the tissue.

5. Young, A., and et al.: Tracking and finite element analysis of stripe deformation in magnetic resonance tagging. IEEE-TMI **14** (1995) 413–421

6. Park, J., Metaxas, D., Axel, L.: Volumetric deformable models with parameter functions: A new approach to the 3d motion analysis of the LV from MRI-SPAMM. International Conference on Computer Vision (1995) 700–705

7. Gupta, S., Prince, J.: On variable brightness optical flow for tagged MRI. Information Processing in Medical Imaging (1995) 323–334

8. Waks, E., Prince, J., Douglas, A.: Cardiac Motion Simulator for Tagged MRI. Mathematical Methods in Biomedical Image Analysis (1996) 182–191

9. Zerhouni, E., Parish, D., et al.: Human heart: Tagging with MR imaging – a method for noninvasive assessment of myocardial motion. Radiology **169** (1988) 59–63

Recovery of Soft Tissue Object Deformation from 3D Image Sequences Using Biomechanical Models

Xenophon Papademetris[1], Pengcheng Shi[4], Donald P. Dione[3],
Albert J. Sinusas[23], R. Todd Constable[2], and James S. Duncan[12]

[1] Departments of Electrical Engineering, [2] Diagnostic Radiology, and
[3] Medicine, Yale University New Haven, CT 06520-8042
papad@noodle.med.yale.edu
[4] Department of Computer and Information Science,
New Jersey Institute of Technology.

Abstract. The estimation of soft tissue deformation from 3D image sequences is an important problem in a number of fields such as diagnosis
of heart disease and image guided surgery. In this paper we describe a
methodology for using biomechanical material models, within a Bayesian
framework which allows for proper modeling of image noise, in order to
estimate these deformations. The resulting partial differential equations
are discretized and solved using the finite element method. We demonstrate the application of this method to estimating strains from sequences
of in-vivo left ventricular MR images, where we incorporate information
about the fibrous structure of the ventricle. The deformation estimates
obtained exhibit similar patterns with measurements obtained from more
invasive techniques, used as a gold standard.

1 Introduction

There is a class of medical image analysis problems where the goal is the estimation of the displacement field of an object or a group of objects. Examples
of such problems are left ventricular (LV) wall motion estimation [9,10,11] and
image guided surgery[4]. In most of these applications, only a relatively sparse
set of points, often called *landmarks,* can be reliably followed on the object from
the image data and the estimation of the displacements of remainder of the estimation task can be thought of as *interpolation,* in other words our problem is:
given the displacements of such landmarks, find the best displacements for the
rest of the region of interest. Often, however, the displacement estimates of the
landmarks are corrupted by noise. In this case, the task becomes an *approximation* problem, where now the goal is to estimate a displacement field that is close
to the originally estimated displacements at the landmark points, and provides
reasonable values elsewhere.

A. Kuba et al. (Eds.): IPMI'99, LNCS 1613, pp. 352–357, 1999.

2   Methods

We will pose this general problem in a Bayesian-Estimation framework where the goal is to find the displacement field $\hat{u}$ which maximizes the posterior probability:

$$\hat{u} = \begin{array}{c} \arg\max \\ u \end{array} p(u|u^m) = \begin{array}{c} \arg\max \\ u \end{array} \left(\frac{p(u^m|u) \times p(u)}{p(u^m)} \right) \tag{1}$$

where u is the output displacement field and u^m are the original sparse displacement estimates. The prior probability of the measurements $p(u^m)$ is a constant once these measurements have been made and therefore drops out of the minimization process. The first term $p(u^m|u)$ will be derived from the noise model assumed in estimating the landmark positions and the second term $p(u)$, the prior probability of the displacement, will be derived from a mechanical model. For a more detailed discussion see[8].

2.1   Mechanical Model-based priors

As previously demonstrated by Christiansen *et al.* [2] there is a correspondence between an internal energy function and a Gibbs-Prior. If the mechanical model is described in terms of an internal energy function $W(C, u)$, where C represents the material properties and u the displacement field, then we can write an equivalent prior probability density function $p(u)$ (see equation 1) of the Gibbs form:

$$p(u) = k_1 \exp(-W(C, u)). \tag{2}$$

We will derive the model term W by a biomechanical model; this can be described in terms of an internal or strain energy function which depends on the deformation of the object and its intrinsic material properties. There are different classes of such models depending on the application; in the case of the left ventricle we will use an anisotropic linear elastic model which will allow us to incorporate information about the preferential stiffness of the tissue along fiber directions[5]. If this method were to be applied to model brain deformation, one could use a model adapted from [6].

Deformation and Strain: Consider a body $B(0)$ which after time t moves and deforms to body $B(t)$. A point X on $B(0)$ goes to a point x on $B(t)$ and the transformation gradient F is defined as $dx = FdX$. The deformation is expressed in terms of the strain tensor ϵ. Because the deformations to be estimated in this work are bigger than 5%, we use a finite strain formulation, the logarithmic strain ϵ^L, which is defined as: $\epsilon = ln\sqrt{F.F'}$. Since the strain tensor is a 3×3 symmetric 2nd-rank tensor (matrix), we can re-write it in vector form as, $e = [\epsilon_{11} \ \epsilon_{22} \ \epsilon_{33} \ \epsilon_{12} \ \epsilon_{13} \ \epsilon_{23}]'$. This will enable us to express the tensor equations in a more familiar matrix notation.

Strain Energy Function: The mechanical model can be defined in terms of a strain energy function. The simplest useful continuum model in solid mechanics is the linear elastic one which is of the form: $W = e'Ce$ where C is a 6×6 matrix and defines the material properties of the deforming body. The left ventricle of the heart is specifically modeled as a transversely elastic material to account for the preferential stiffness in the fiber direction, using the matrix C:

$$
C^{-1} = \begin{bmatrix}
\frac{1}{E_p} & \frac{-\nu_p}{E_p} & \frac{-\nu_{fp}}{E_f} & 0 & 0 & 0 \\
\frac{-\nu_p}{E_p} & \frac{1}{E_p} & \frac{-\nu_{fp}}{E_f} & 0 & 0 & 0 \\
\frac{-\nu_{fp}E_f}{E_p} & \frac{-\nu_{fp}E_f}{E_p} & \frac{1}{E_f} & 0 & 0 & 0 \\
0 & 0 & 0 & \frac{2(1+\nu_p)}{E_p} & 0 & 0 \\
0 & 0 & 0 & 0 & \frac{1}{G_f} & 0 \\
0 & 0 & 0 & 0 & 0 & \frac{1}{G_f}
\end{bmatrix}
\tag{3}
$$

where E_f is the fiber stiffness, E_p is cross-fiber stiffness and ν_{fp}, ν_p are the corresponding Poisson's ratios and G_f is the shear modulus across fibers. ($G_f \approx E_f/(2(1+\nu_{fp}))$. If $E_f = E_p$ and $\nu_p = \nu_{fp}$ this model reduces to the more common isotropic linear elastic model. Alternatively a different form of W altogether could be used such as the one from a Rivlin-Mooney Material Model[6].

2.2   Landmark displacement estimation

In our work, the original displacements on the outer surfaces of the myocardium were obtained by using the shape-tracking algorithm whose details where presented in [11]. We note that other displacement data, including that from magnetic resonance tagging [9,10], could also be used.

The shape-tracking algorithm also produces a set of confidence measures for each match. We model these estimates with a Gaussian noise model and generate the term $p(u^m|u)$ of equation (1) to be

$$
p(u^m|u) = \frac{1}{\sqrt{2\pi\sigma^2}} e^{\frac{(u-u^m)^2}{2\sigma^2}}
\tag{4}
$$

where σ^2 is set to be the reciprocal of the confidence of the particular displacement estimate. Where no displacements estimates are available the confidence is set to zero.

2.3   Solution using the Finite Element Method

Having defined both the model $p(u)$ and data $p(u^m|u)$ portions of the problem, we can now minimize equation (1) to find the optimal displacement field $\hat{u}$. Taking logarithms and differentiating with respect to the displacement field u results in a system of partial differential equations, which we solve using the Finite Element Method[1]. The first step in the finite element method is the division or tessellation of the body of interest into elements; these are commonly tetrahedral or hexahedral in shape. Once this is done, the partial differential equations are written down in integral form for each element, and then the integral of these equations over all the elements is taken to produce the final set of equations. For more information one is referred to standard textbooks such as Bathe[1]. The final set of equations is then solved to produce the output set of displacements.

3 Results

In this section we present results from the application of this methodology to ten sets of cardiac MR sequences acquired from anesthetized dogs. The resulting 3D image set consists of sixteen 2D image slices per temporal frame, and sixteen temporal 3D frames per cardiac cycle. First the dogs were positioned in the magnet for initial imaging under baseline conditions. The left anterior descending coronary artery was then occluded and a second set of images was acquired. The images were pre-segmented to extract the endo- and epi-cardial boundaries surfaces and interactively corrected using a platform specially developed for this purpose[7]. Then points on the corresponding surfaces were tracked to generate the input displacement data using shape-based algorithms described in [11]. The myocardium was modeled as an anisotropic linear elastic material which was stiffer in the fiber directions[5]; shown in figure 1. The tissue was assumed to be 3.3 times stiffer along the fiber direction, obtained by linearization of the non-linear model from [5], and approximately incompressible.

For each frame between end-systole (ES) and end-diastole (ED), a two step problem is posed: (i) solving equation (1) normally and (ii) adjusting the position of all points on the endo-and epi-cardial surfaces so they lie on the endo- and epi-cardial surfaces at the next frame using a modified nearest-neighbor technique and solving equation (1) once more using this added constraint. This ensures that there is no bias in the estimation of the radial strain. Figure 2 shows a contour map of radial strain (thickening) in a long-axis section of a normal left ventricle and in the same animal after occlusion.

Table: Radial and Circumferential Percentage Strain Changes for Normal and Infarcted Regions.

Percentage change	Radial normal	Radial Infarct	Circum. Normal	Circum. Infact
Our Method (Average)	-16.4 %	-135.1%	+18.9%	+77.2%
Sonomicroemeters[3]	+5.6 %	-150.0%	+15.4%	+73.3%

The validation measures used were the percentage end-systolic strain change for the radial and circumferential components between the baseline and post-occlusion measurements. The normal and infarcted regions where defined by post-mortem measurements. These results are compared to measurements made by using implanted sonomicrometers, work performed by members of our research team and reported in[3], which provide highly accurate strain measurements by calculating relative Doppler-based displacements, and are used as a

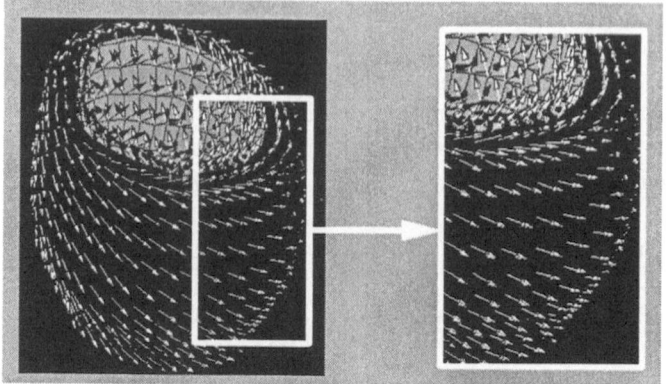

Fig. 1. Fiber direction in the left ventricle as defined in Guccione *et al.* [5]

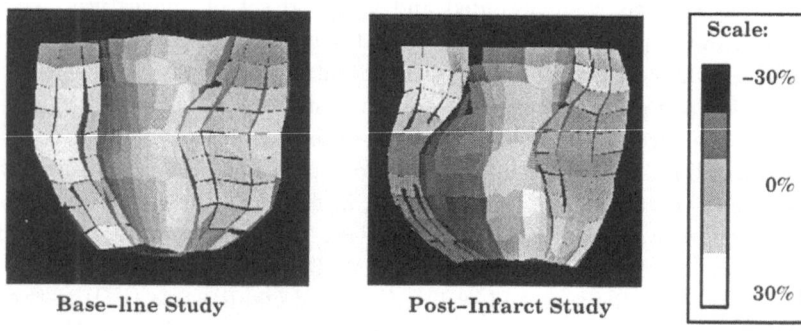

Base–line Study   **Post–Infarct Study**

Fig. 2. Radial Strain at end-systole in a section normal left-ventricle (left) and post-occlusion(right) shown in an a long-axis sectional view. Normal behavior is thickening (positive). Note the infarct region on the right which is in darker color

gold standard. The results are summarized in the table and are consistent with the observation that in the case of infarction the tissue thins instead of thickens, hence there is a negative change in the radial strain and it bulges out instead of contracting, explaining the positive change in the circumferential strain. For a more detailed discussion see a related technical report[8].

4   Conclusions

In this paper we have described a methodology for the estimation of deformation from sequences of 3D images of individual objects, using the left ventricle of the heart as a key example. We believe that the best approach to this problem involves the modeling of the mechanical properties of the object explicitly in the language of continuum mechanics, as this makes possible the incorporation of existing theoretical and experimental research in biomechanics, and it provides a growth path for solving more difficult problems by naturally invoking more sophisticated/appropriate models. In this cardiac work for example, we were able to easily take advantage of knowledge of fiber orientation to create a model of the heart that is anisotropic and accounts for more of the actual properties of the tissue. In the future, we hope to use a non-linear mechanical model which will capture the 'hardening' of the tissue as it is stretched. We also note that the only part of this work that is specific to the left ventricle is the particular strain-energy function. By substituting an appropriate matrix C in the case of a linear elastic material or an altogether different form of W in equation (2) altogether, this method can be used to estimate the deformation of other objects.

Acknowledgments

The first author would also like to thank professors Turan Onat and Gary Povirk from the Department of Mechanical Engineering at Yale University for their help.

References

1. Bathe. K. *Finite Element Procedures in Engineering Analysis.* Prentice-Hall, New Jersey, 1982.
2. Christiansen G. E., Rabbitt R. D., and Miller M. I. 3D Brain mapping using deformable neuroanatomy. *Physics in Medicine and Biology*, 39:609–618, 1994.
3. Dione D. P., Shi P., Smith W, De Man P., Soares J., Duncan J.S., and Sinusas A.J. Three-dimensional regional left ventricular deformation from digital sonomicrometry. In *19th Ann. Int. Conf. of the IEEE Engineering in Medicine and Biology Society*, pages 848–851, Chigago, IL, March 1997.
4. Edwards P. J., Hill D.L.G., Little J.A., and Hawkes D.J. Deformation for image guided interventions using a three component tissue model. In *Information Processing in Medical Imaging*, pages 218–231, Vermont, USA, June 1997.
5. Guccione J. M. and McCulloch A. D.. Finite element modeling of ventricular mechanics. In Hunter P.J., McCulloch A. D., and Nielsen P., editors, *Theory of Heart*, pages 122–144. Springer-Verlag, Berlin, 1991.
6. Mendis K.K., Stalnaker R.L., and Advani S.H. A constitutive relationship for large deformation finite element modeling of brain tissue. *Journal of Biomechanical Engineering*, 117(3):279–85, 1995.
7. Papademetris X., Rambo J., Dione D.P, Sinusas A.J., and Duncan J.S. Visually interactive cine-3D segmentation of cardiac mr images. *Suppl. Journ. of the American College of Cardiology Volume 31, #2 (Supplement A)*, February 1998.
8. Papademetris X. and Shi P. and Dione D.P. and Sinusas A.J. and Constable R.T. and Duncan J.S. Recovery of Soft Tissue Object Deformation from 3D Image Sequences using Biomechanical Models Technical Report 1999-01, Image Processing and Analysis Group, Dept. of Diagnostic Radiology, Yale University, March 1998.
9. Park J., Metaxas D., and Axel L.. Volumetric deformable models with parameter functions: a new approach to the 3D motion analysis of the LV from MRI-SPAMM. In *Fifth International Conference on Computer Vision*, pages 700–705, 1995.
10. Prince J. L. and McVeigh E. R. Motion estimation from tagged mr image sequences. *IEEE Transactions on Medical Imaging*, 11:238–249, June 1992.
11. Shi P., Sinusas A.J., Constable R.T., Ritman E., and Duncan J.S. Point-tracked quantitative analysis of left ventricular motion from 3D image sequences. *IEEE Transactions on Medical Imaging*, in-press.

Forward Deformation of PET Volumes Using Non-uniform Elastic Material Constraints

Gregory J. Klein

Lawrence Berkeley National Laboratory, Berkeley, CA 94720, USA
GJKlein@lbl.gov

Abstract. A method for non-rigidly deforming 3D PET datasets is described. The method uses a Lagrangian motion field description and a forward deformation mapping. To regularize the deformation, an anisotropic strain energy function is used that separately models the material properties of cardiac and background tissues. The method is applied to motion compensation in PET so that different time frames of a cardiac sequence may be combined.

1 Introduction

In gated acquisition of cardiac Positron Emission Tomography (PET), motion of the heart is stopped in the images by dividing the data obtained during each cardiac cycle into a number of different time frames, or gates. An unfortunate effect of distributing the data into many time frames is that the statistical quality of each reconstructed volume suffers, and the individual images appear to be very noisy. Ideally, one would like to correct the images for cardiac motion, then add them back together to obtain a composite image with less motion blur and better contrast to noise properties.

We describe here a deformable motion technique that allows motion compensation for subsequent combination of PET datasets. A source volume representing the heart at end systole will be deformed to match a reference volume representing the heart at end diastole. The deformed source will then be summed with the reference to produce a composite volume with better contrast to noise characteristics. Though a gated cardiac study typically results in some 10 - 15 gates, each representing a short portion of the cardiac cycle, this paper will just focus on the combination of two time frames. Unique in the approach are two aspects. First, a non-uniform regularization constraint incorporating anisotropic strain energy is used to model the underlying cardiac tissue. Second, a forward deformation mapping is used which insures that each voxel in a source dataset contributes to the calculation of a deformed volume. The work is most closely related to 3D deformable motion work based on optical flow algorithms [1,2] and material elastic models [3,4].

2 Motion Estimation

As is the case with most 3D deformable algorithms, this algorithm is based on two general criteria. An image matching constraint first attempts to find

A. Kuba et al. (Eds.): IPMI'99, LNCS 1613, pp. 358–363, 1999.

a motion field that warps a source volume to best match a reference volume. Because numerous image matching transformations exist which equally satisfy the image matching constraint, the solution is regularized by imposing an additional criterion constraining motion field smoothness. This latter requirement treats the volume as a continuously stretching and bending medium that can only deform as is consistent with elastic material models. In our smoothness constraint formulation, we use a pre-segmented volume which masks the heart. This enables smoothing of the motion field to be carried out differently in cardiac tissue than is done in the adjacent tissue and blood pool.

The motion estimation framework is described as follows. Define two 3D density fields, a source volume, $f_1(\mathbf{r})$, and a reference volume, $f_2(\mathbf{r})$, where $\mathbf{r} = (x, y, z)$ represents the voxel index. A dense Lagrangian motion field is defined as $\mathbf{m}(x, y, z) = (u(x, y, z), v(x, y, z), w(x, y, z))$ and the deformed volume of f_1 is defined as $\hat{f}(\mathbf{r}) = f_1(\mathbf{r} + \mathbf{m})$. With these definitions, we can express an image matching error term, $e_I(\mathbf{r})$, and an anisotropic material strain energy term [5], $e_S(\mathbf{r})$, at each voxel location $\mathbf{r}$, as follows:

$$e_I(\mathbf{r}) = \gamma_I (f_2(\mathbf{r}) - \hat{f}(\mathbf{r}))^2 \tag{1}$$

and

$$e_S(\mathbf{r}) = \frac{\lambda}{2}(u_x + v_y + w_z)^2 + \mu(u_x^2 + v_y^2 + w_z^2) +$$
$$\frac{\mu}{2}(u_y^2 + u_z^2 + v_x^2 + v_z^2 + w_x^2 + w_y^2 + 2u_y v_x + 2u_z w_x + 2v_z w_y) \tag{2}$$

where γ_I is a global scalar used to alter the balance between the two error terms, λ and μ are elasticity terms called the Lamé constants, and where derivatives of the motion field are denoted as $u_x = du/dx$.

It can be seen that the λ term in equation (2) penalizes non-zero divergence and the μ term penalizes sharp discontinuities in the motion field. For highly incompressible fields, the Poisson ratio, $\nu = \lambda/(2(\lambda + \mu))$, approaches a maximum of 0.5, which yields a divergence term, λ, that approaches infinity. The Lamé constants used in equation (2) are global constants for isotropic materials. Obviously, the elastic properties of the myocardium are drastically different from the blood pool inside the ventricle, and from the adjacent lung tissue and air space. In this formulation, we implement an anisotropic elastic model by using a segmented voxel mask to delineate voxels representing cardiac tissue, and represent λ and μ by vector fields instead of just two global scalars. The vector fields for each term take on two values, one value in the region labeled cardiac tissue, and another value in the background regions. As such, separate elastic properties can be ascribed to cardiac tissue and to adjacent regions. We assume here that a technique is available to obtain a reasonably correct segmentation of the cardiac tissue from the background, though it is noted that this may not always be a trivial task, and may itself be a formidable research question in some cases.

Though the motion field describing the volume deformation is a one-to-one mapping in a continuous domain, implementation in a discrete domain involves some subtleties that are important to recognize in the deformation of PET datasets. Past efforts [2,3,4] have used a reverse transformation to calculate voxel values in the deformed volume. In this Eulerian formulation, the motion vectors describe a particle's motion with respect to its final position. To obtain the value of each voxel in the deformed volume, $\hat{f}(\mathbf{r}) = f_1(\mathbf{r} - \mathbf{m})$, eight voxels from the deformation volume are sampled at the location, $\mathbf{r} - \mathbf{m}$, and weighted according to trilinear interpolation. Such *backward* sampling does not guarantee that each voxel in the source volume will contribute to the deformed volume. We use a Lagrangian forward sampling technique which distributes each voxel value of the source volume using normalized Gaussian weighting in a single-pass calculation of the deformation. Though the forward sampling scheme does not guarantee absolute conservation of total voxel intensities, it does guarantee that every voxel in the source volume contributes to the deformation volume. Also, the normalized Gaussian weighting of the displaced voxels prevents artifacts in the non-uniformly sampled deformation.

The overall minimization problem is to find a motion field consistent with elastic material properties that best matches the deformed volume to the reference volume via a minimization of:

$$E_{tot} = \sum_{\mathbf{r}} [e_I(\mathbf{r}) + e_S(\mathbf{r})] \qquad (3)$$

We invoke a minimization technique similar to the approach proposed by Zhou [2], which linearizes the calculation of an optimal deformed volume by using a Taylor series approximation. Assuming the true motion field is $\mathbf{m}$, and the current estimate is $\tilde{\mathbf{m}}$, then a Taylor series approximation of $\hat{f}(\mathbf{r})$ can be expressed in terms of a delta motion field, $(\delta u, \delta v, \delta w) = \delta \mathbf{m} = \tilde{\mathbf{m}} - \mathbf{m}$, as $\hat{f}(\mathbf{r}) = f_1(\mathbf{r} + \tilde{\mathbf{m}}) - \nabla f_1(\mathbf{r} + \tilde{\mathbf{m}}) \delta \mathbf{m}$. Substituting the expression, $\tilde{\mathbf{m}} - \delta \mathbf{m}$, for $\mathbf{m}$ in the constraint equations results a quadratic functional in $\delta \mathbf{m}$ that can be minimized via the calculus of variations [6]. The resulting Euler-Lagrange equations are solved using finite differencing techniques and a conjugate gradient method. At each step, $\hat{f}(\mathbf{r})$ is calculated and the conjugate gradient algorithm is used to find the best $\delta \mathbf{m}$ satisfying the equations. This delta motion field is added to the current total motion field and the procedure is repeated. For the results presented in this paper, ten to fifteen iterations of this outer loop were typically required to reach a overall solution. Each conjugate gradient step usually converges quickly, and also requires some ten to twenty iterations.

3   Results

Two cardiac phantoms were used to test the algorithm. The first is a simple model of gated emission PET consisting of a ellipsoidal building blocks forming the human torso [7]. The second is a finite element model (FEM) based on a parametric prolate spheroid description of a left ventricle which has been fitted to MRI data acquired from a canine heart [8]. Included in the model is the

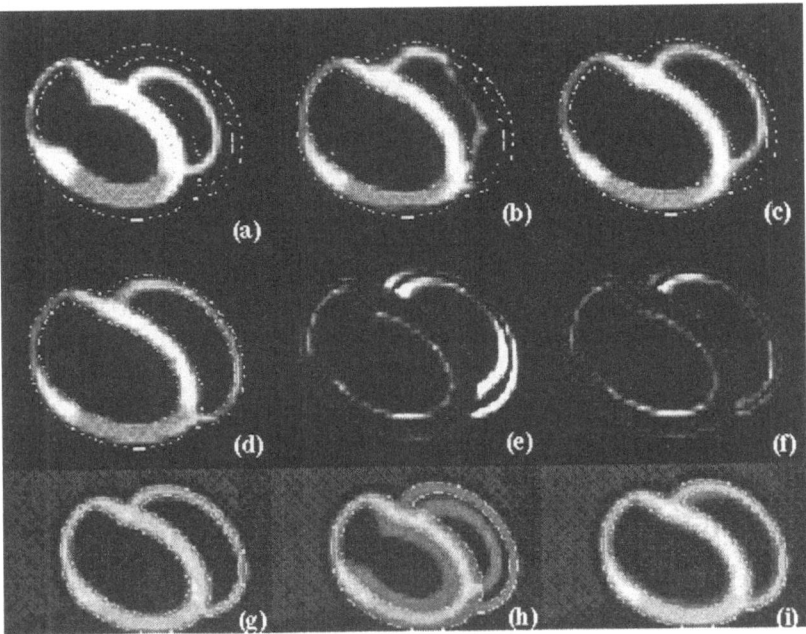

Fig. 1. Ellipsoidal phantom results

incompressible nature of cardiac tissue and non-symmetric cardiac muscle fiber orientation.

Figure 1 shows the results on the simple model. The source volume representing end systole is seen in (a). The reference volume representing end diastole is seen as an edge map overlaid on (a). An attempt at deforming the source volume using an isotropic strain energy function penalizing non-zero divergence (Poisson ratio = 0.46) shows in (b) that the non-zero divergence in the blood pool makes it difficult for the algorithm to find the correct deformation. Relaxing the divergence penalty allows a better match, seen in (c). However, the best match is obtained using an anisotropic strain energy function penalizing non-zero divergence and smoothness only in the cardiac tissue (d). Mean squared error (MSE) values between the reference volume and cases (b), (c) and (d) are 1727, 1234 and 555 respectively. Image difference maps between the reference and cases (c) and (d) are shown in (e) and (f). These further demonstrate that the anisotropic strain energy function produces the warped volume best matching the reference. It is noted that in order to find a suitable deformation in case (c), the image weighting term needed to be double the value that was used for the anisotropic case. This is troublesome, since one would not like to weight the image matching criteria so much that physically implausible motions are estimated.

As a display of the utility of this algorithm, (g), (h) and (i) show a comparison of noisy versions of the phantom summed with and without motion compensation. Obviously, if no motion compensation is done, as seen in (h),

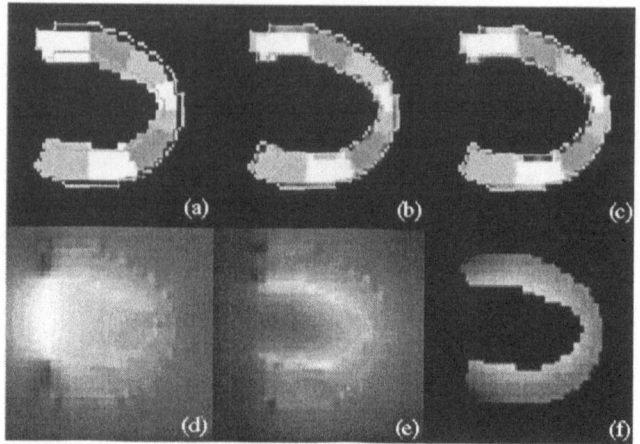

Fig. 2. Parametric FEM results

then blur due to the motion is induced which severely obscures image features. By first deforming the systole volume to match the heart shape at end diastole, and then summing (i), the contrast to noise ratio is improved over the reference volume alone (g). This is the desired result which allows us to combine gated PET datasets and increase image quantification without loss of resolution.

Results using the FEM are seen in Fig. 2. A 16 element model was used to determine the shape of the left ventricle as it was passively inflated. Here the inflated state is used as a reference volume, and the deflated state is the source volume. Because a parametric description of the two states is available, the "ground truth" motion vectors may be calculated which bring any two points into correspondence. The source volume and an edge map of the reference are seen in (a). To better visualize performance of the deformation algorithm, texture was added to the model by giving each of the 16 elements a slightly different voxel value. Deformed volumes using isotropic strain (b) and anisotropic strain (c) look similar; both match the reference fairly well. MSE values with respect to the reference are 1117 and 1002 respectively, so the anisotropic model performs only slightly better with respect to this measure. Comparing motion field magnitudes of the isotropic (d) and anisotropic (e) results verses the true motion field magnitude (f) reveals that the anisotropic model is considerably more accurate with respect to this measure. MSE values of the true magnitude volume (f) compared to (d) and (e) are 36661 and 17481 respectively. The motion magnitude images point out how the isotropic strain model falters in the region where image divergence is present (in the blood pool). Since there was a zero background in this case, the motion field error in the background region does not induce much error in the deformed volume for the isotropic case. This would not be true in general for real PET data where voxel intensities in the blood pool would be small, yet not negligible.

4   Concluding Remarks

When deforming a volume to match a reference dataset, there is always a balance between the weight of the image matching constraints and the regularization constraints. Because numerous motion fields can produce identical deformed images, it is the function of the regularization constraints to prevent physically unrealizable motion fields. In the deformation of real PET datasets, where considerable statistical noise is present, there is always the danger of weighting the image matching terms too greatly so that uncorrelated "hot spots" in the datasets are matched even though they do not originate from the same segment of cardiac tissue. The motivation for this work was to incorporate a more realistic, nonuniform elastic model into the regularization constraint so that this term could be weighted more heavily, and thus would prevent solutions with physically implausible motion fields. Though the technique required a prior segmentation step, because the segmentation was only used during the regularization process, and not during the final image warping calculation, the algorithm should not be sensitive to minor segmentation errors. The improvements shown in this paper by the anisotropic model over the isotropic strain model indicate that this more realistic model can be worth the added expense of the requirement for a segmented cardiac volume.

Acknowledgment

Supported by NIH grant HL25840 and DOE contract DE-AC03-76SF00098.

References

1. Song, S.M., Leahy, R.M., Boyd, D.P., Brundage, B.H., and Napel, S. Determining cardiac velocity fields and intraventricular pressure distribution from a sequence of Ultrafast CT cardiac images. IEEE Trans. Med Imag, 13 (1994) 386–397
2. Zhou, Z., Synolakis, C.E., Leahy, R.M., and Song, S.M. Calculation of 3D internal displacement fields from 3D X-ray computer tomographic images. Proc. R. Soc. Lond. A, 449 (1937) 537–555, 1995
3. Bajcsy, R., Kovacic, R. Multiresolution elastic matching. Comput. Vision, Graph., Image Proc. 46 (1989) 1-21
4. Christensen, G.E., Rabbitt, R.D., and Miller, M.I. 3d brain mapping using a deformable neuroanatomy. Phys Med Biol. 39 (1994) 609-618
5. Washizu, K. Variational Methods in Elasticity and Plasticity. Pergamon Press, Oxford, 1982
6. Horn, B.K.P. Robot Vision. The MIT Press, Cambridge, Massachusetts, 1986
7. Terry, J.A., Tsui, B.M.W, Perry, J.R., and Gullberg, G.T. A three-dimensional mathematical phantom of the human torso for use in SPECT imaging research studies. J Nucl Med. 31 (1990) 868
8. Costa, K.D., Hunter, P.J., Wayne, J.S., Waldman, L.K., Guccione, J.M., and McCuloch, A.D. A three-dimensional finite element method for large elastic deformations of ventricular myocardium: II - prolate spheroidal coordinates. Trans. ASME bf 118 (1996) 464-472

Brain Morphometry by Distance Measurement in a Non-Euclidean, Curvilinear Space

Martin Styner[1], Thomas Coradi[2], and Guido Gerig[1]

[1] Dept. of Computer Science, University of North Carolina at Chapel Hill, USA
{styner, gerig}@cs.unc.edu
[2] Communication Technology Lab, Image Science, ETH-Zurich, Switzerland
tcoradi@vision.ee.ethz

Abstract. Inspired by the discussion in neurological research about the callosal fiber connections with respect to brain asymmetry we developed a technique that measures distances between brain hemispheres in a non-Euclidean, curvilinear space. The technique is a generic morphometric tool for measuring minimal distances within and across 3-D structures. We applied the technique for distances from the cortical gray/white matter boundary to the cross-section of the corpus callosum. The method uses a 3-D extension of the F*-algorithm. The algorithm uses a cost matrix determined by the image data. The resulting distances are mapped to the cortical surface and differences on the two hemispheres can be visually compared. Distances were also projected back to the corpus callosum to represent asymmetry by comparing left and right measurements. We can present results obtained by processing 11 3-D magnetic resonance data sets representing a normal control group.

1 Introduction

Image analysis has become a common component to study diseases of the human body by obtaining anatomical and functional information. Since the advent of non-invasive magnetic resonance imaging, morphometry has become increasingly important. The new analysis methods described here are fully 3-D processing techniques and overcome limitations of conventional slice-by-slice analysis.

This project is driven by studying schizophrenia. In schizophrenia, changes in the morphology of various brain structures are thought to provide important clues to the disease related brain abnormalities, but the changes are subtle and can barely be detectable with current interactive segmentation techniques [1,2]. Quantitative measurements on postmortem brains and on anatomical structures segmented from magnetic resonance image data corroborate the hypothesis that the asymmetry between the brain hemispheres is reduced at first episodes of schizophrenia [4,8]. To date, the errors in measurements are often larger than the effect to be studied, and interesting findings often could not be confirmed by other research groups. Therefore, it becomes necessary to provide more accurate measurements of brain asymmetry. Bullmore *et al.* [3] proposed a measurement called *radius of gyration* to assess cerebral asymmetry. This measurement has

A. Kuba et al. (Eds.): IPMI'99, LNCS 1613, pp. 364–369, 1999.

been only applied to 2-D coronal slices. Prima *et al.* [12] used non-linear elastic registration to find corresponding regions in the two hemisphere. Differential operators applied to the deformation field result in measures of lateral asymmetry.

Symmetry of structures under a class of spatial transformations is a well-defined mathematical property. However, dealing with biological structures and the inherent variability, the mathematical approach to exact symmetry is too strict and has to be modified. Guillemaud *et al.* [8] segmented the manifold of the interhemispheric fissure and determined length between the cortical surface and the fissure along perpendicular lines emanating from the midplane. Measures from the left and right cortical surface result in estimates of local asymmetries and in a quantitative 2-D asymmetry map. This paper also suggested the use of a curvilinear coordinate system of the brain directly related to brain morphology. The encouraging results inspired the research work presented in this paper. A more realistic simulation of white matter fiber connections, however, would have to include information about local fiber directions, as nicely presented in [10] and [11], for example. The search for minimum cost paths is an 3-D extension of the F* algorithm [5] and has similarities to the interactive live-wire segmentation in [9]. In the context of analyzing the white matter structure of the brain we also would like to refer to Mangin *et al.* [7] who proposed a discrete implementation of conservative flow systems to analyze the white matter, in particular to detect the corpus callosum. Due to lack of space, details of implementations are generally omitted here, but are described in [13] (full color version).

2   Optimal Path Algorithm and Asymmetry Measurement

In our proposed approach, callosal fibers are simulated by curvilinear paths of minimal distance running inside the white matter from the white matter boundary to the interhemispheric cut through the corpus callosum. We use distance measurements propagated along trajectories determined by the graph search algorithm F*, extended to fit our specific needs. The distances at the white matter boundary are projected back onto the corpus callosum for a comparison of asymmetry between the two hemispheres.

The F*-algorithm used in our implementation is based on the approach of Tenenbaum [5], where pixels or voxels of a dataset are represented by nodes of a graph. The edges of the graphs are defined as the 8-neighborhood in 2-D space and as the 26-neighborhood in 3-D space. The F*-algorithm enables the calculation of a distance map from a certain point of reference ('seed') to any other point in the graph. This distance map assigns a distance-value to each node in the graph which is based on a cost function that determines the point-related cost of a path.

To fit our needs we have implemented several extensions of the original F* algorithm: 1) extension to 3-D space, 2) use of a seed region instead of a single seed point to allow multiple seed regions (see Fig. 1), 3) calculation of accurate costs for paths running along diagonals, but each dimension needs additional

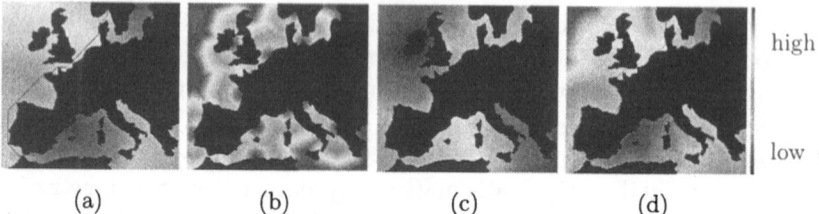

(a)   (b)   (c)   (d)

Fig. 1. 2-D F* distance maps representing the distance of the sea route to the closest seed point: (a) single seed point (at Barcelona) with highlighted optimal path running to Stockholm, (b) multiple seed points, (c) seed region (border of Ireland), (d) single seed, cost matrix penalizing optimal paths running far off the coast

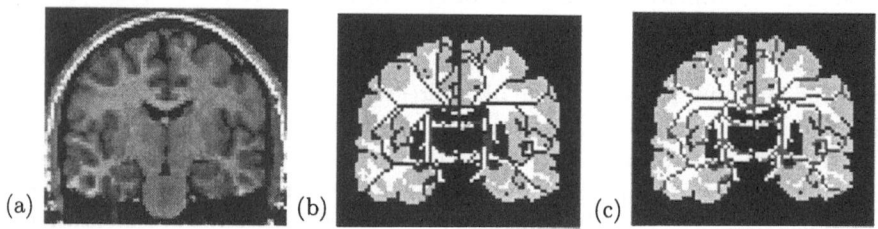

Fig. 2. Visualization of arbitrary optimal paths based on a constant cost matrix (b) and based on an a-posteriori probability cost matrix (c) on an 2D MRI image (a)

correction if voxel dimensions are non uniform, 4) propagation of additional information and measurements from the seed region to all points.

The F* algorithm needs the cost function to be stored as a matrix which represents the point-related costs for each point. The cost matrix was modeled to force optimal paths to run less likely through certain regions using two terms a constant distance term and a penalty-term. The penalty term assigns high costs to points where paths should be less likely to run through (see Fig. 1). The resulting path lengths are not measured in unit size, requiring a modification of the F* algorithm to additionally calculate the unit size distances.

The optimal path is not an explicit result of the F* algorithm, but they are extracted from the distance map using a steepest descent approach to trace trajectories back to the seed points (see Figs. 2 and 3).

So far, we have calculated distances at the white matter boundary. However such a visualization is rather unusual and requires training. More common is a projection of attributes to the cortical surface, which also allows a comparison between multiple brain surfaces. We have developed a method to project the calculated distances from the gray/white matter boundary outwards to the cortex through gray matter using the F* algorithm. The projection runs along the optimal path from the white matter boundary to the cortex (see Fig. 3).

The main problem in defining asymmetry measurements is to determine correspondence. Establishing correspondence between brain hemispheres is not well defined since the brain is not strictly symmetric and depicts structures which

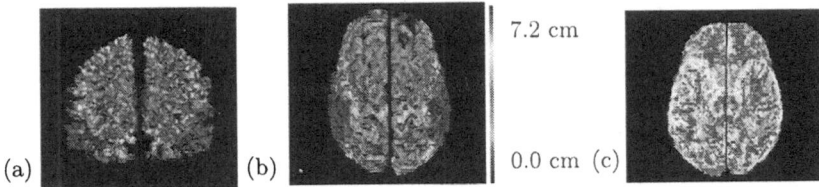

Fig. 3. Application on a 3-D brain atlas. Visualization of calculated distances on the white matter boundary (a) and as projection to the cortex (b). Visualization (c) of arbitrary paths and corpus callosum

appear only in one hemisphere. The approach chosen in our application is to compare the distances projected back to the corpus callosum along optimal paths. Measurements projected from both sides to one point of the corpus callosum can therefore be compared directly for asymmetry.

We define our asymmetry measurement as the difference of the mean of the distances after averaging the distance values separately for each side. These differences can be visualized as a 2-D difference graph or can be projected back to the cortex for visualization.

3   Results

The proposed algorithm has been applied on 2-D datasets without symmetry axis like maps (see Fig. 1) and mazes to test and extend the functionality of the F* algorithm. Further 2-D tests involved datasets with symmetry axis at the seed region, like artificial images, images of butterflies, bats, plants and 2-D-slices of a brain atlas. The mean distance asymmetry measure was shown to be superior to extrema or median measures. Corresponding catchment areas on the symmetry axis showed high variability in cases when areas were hidden behind obstacles. In such cases the asymmetry measurement turned out to be poor.

The first 3-D test has been performed on an isotropic brain atlas. Distances and paths were calculated and visualized (Figs. 2(a-c), 3). There were significant visual differences observed between the two hemispheres. The difference graph of the mean was determined from asymmetry measurement and visualized (Fig. 4). Both the asymmetry graph and the distance visualization on the cortex demonstrated that the left hemispheric paths were longer for most parts of the brain. Compared to 2-D, we observed a lower variance of the size of catchment areas, but the correspondence was still not solved to our satisfaction. One reason is that the corpus callosum is small compared to the the white matter, so rather large areas are projected onto a single point on the corpus callosum.

As further 3-D tests, datasets of 10 control patients of an Organic Amnesia study, varying in age and sex, have been processed. Both the corpus callosum and the brain hemispheres were segmented manually. The segmentation of the brain tissues has been performed using statistical classification with the Bayes-classifier. The a posteriori probabilities were used to calculate the cost matrix.

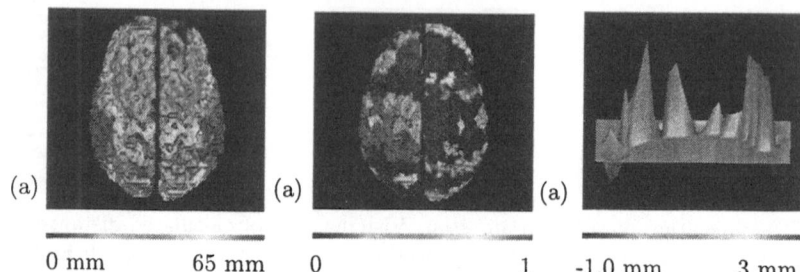

0 mm   65 mm   0   1   -1.0 mm   3 mm

Fig. 4. Application on a 3-D brain atlas. Visualization of distances (a) and of normalized asymmetry measurement (b) as a projection on the cortex. Areas of smaller distance are displayed in blue. (c) Visualization of the difference graph (left minus right) projected on the corpus callosum

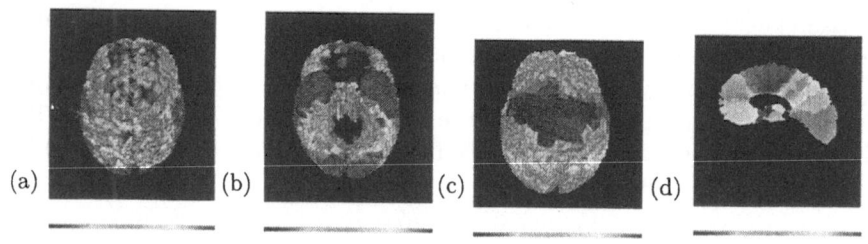

42 mm   65 mm   37 mm   84 mm

Fig. 5. Application on real 3-D datasets: Visualization of distances projected on the cortex from superior (a) and inferior (b) viewpoints. Visualization of the correspondence as projection on the cortex (c) and of the color-coded labels on a slice (d)

Distances have been visualized (see Fig. 5) and there were again significant visual differences between the two hemispheres in all datasets. The asymmetry measurements have not yet been calculated. We observed that manual segmentation of the corpus callosum is rather poor resulting in displacements from the interhemispheric fissure as large as a few millimeters. These displacements are of equal size as the mean differences of the distances for the atlas.

4   Conclusions and Discussion

In this paper, we have presented a new approach to measure minimum cost paths in a non-Euclidean curvilinear space. We use such paths as a simulation of callosal white matter fiber tracts which are of interest in current neurological research. We also proposed a technique to calculate a rough correspondence and an associated asymmetry measurement. Results are promising, but the correspondence especially needs improvement. The method has been applied to 11 3-D datasets so far, and the implementation is stable and reliable.

The distances determined with our method are based on the city-block metric with the inherent disadvantages of showing large deviations from Euclidean distance measurements and of non-isotropic propagation of distances in space. Kiryati *et al.* [6] have addressed this issue and have proposed a correction of the calculated distances. We plan to incorporate this correction in a future method. Future directions of our research include the generation of a more robust measurement of asymmetry, combining curvilinear distances with explicitly established lateral correspondence between brain hemispheres.

Acknowledgments

This work was supported by the EC-funded BIOMORPH project 95-0845, a collaboration between the Universities of Kent, Oxford, ETH Zurich, INRIA Sophia Antipolis and KU Leuven. Project funding is provided by the Swiss Federal Office for Education and Science (BBW Nr 95.0340).

References

1. Shenton, M.E.: Psychopathology: The Evolving Science of Mental disorders, chapter Temporal lobe structural abnormalities in schizophrenia: A selective review and presentation of new MRI findings. Cambridge University Press (1996)
2. Shenton, M.E.: Brain Imaging in Clinical Psychiatry chapter MRI studies in schizophrenia. Marcel Decker Inc. (1997)
3. Bullmore, E., Brammer, M.,Harvey, Murray, R., Ron, M.: Cerebral hemispheric asymmetry revisited. Psych. Medicine,**25** (1995) 249–363
4. Crow, T., Colter, N., Frith, C., Johnstone, E., Owens, D.: Developmental arrest of cerebral asymmetries in early onset schizophrenia. Psych. Res. **29** (1989) 247–253
5. Fischler, M., Tenenbaum, J., Wolf, H.: Detection of roads and linear structures in low-resolution aerial imagery using a multisource knowledge integration technique. Computer Graphics and Image Processing **15** (1981) 201–223
6. Kiryati, N., Székely,G.: Estimating shortest paths and minimal distances on digitized three-dimensional surfaces. Pattern Recognition (1993)
7. Mangin, J., Régis, J., Frouin, V.: Shape bottlenecks and conservative flow systems. Proc. MMBIA (1996) 319–328
8. Marais, P.C., Guillemaud, R., Sakuma, M., Feldmar, J., Crow, T., Zisserman, A., Brady, M.: Visualising cerebral asymmetry (1996) **1131** 411–416, 1996
9. Mortensen, E.N., Barret, W.A.: Fast, accurate, and reproducible live-wire boundary extraction. Proc. Visualization in Biomedical Computing (1996), 183–192, 1996
10. Peled, S., Gudbjartsson, H., Westin, C., Kikinis, R., Jolesz, F.A.: Magnetic resonance diffusion tensor imaging demonstrates direction and asymmetry of human white matter fiber tracts. Brain research (1998) **780** 27–33
11. Poupon, C., Mangin, J., Frouin, V., Régis, J., Poupon, F., Pachot-Clouard, M., Bihan, D.L., Bloch, I.: Regularization of mr diffusion tensor maps for tracking brain white matter bundles. Proc. Medical Image Computing and Computer-Assisted Intervention (1998) 489–498
12. Prima, S., Thirion, J., Subsol, G., Roberts, N.: Automatic analysis of normal dissymmetry of males and females in mr images. Proc. Medical Image Computing and Computer-Assisted Intervention (1998) 770–779
13. Styner, M., Coradi, T., Gerig, G.: Brain morphometry by distance measurement in a non-euclidean, curvilinear space. Tech. report - UNC-CS Department (1999)

Learning Shape Models from Examples Using Automatic Shape Clustering and Procrustes Analysis

Nicolae Duta[1], Milan Sonka[2], and Anil K. Jain[1]

[1] Department of Computer Science and Engineering, Michigan State University, USA
[2] Department of Electrical and Computer Engineering, The University of Iowa, USA,
dutanico@cse.msu.edu

Abstract. A new fully automated shape learning method is presented. It is based on clustering a shape training set in the original shape space and performing a Procrustes analysis on each cluster to obtain a cluster prototype and information about shape variation. As a direct application of our shape learning method, a 17-structure shape model of brain substructures was computed from MR image data, an eigen-shape model was automatically derived. Our approach can serve as an automated substitute to the tedious and time-consuming manual shape analysis.[1]

1 Motivation

Automated learning of shape models has direct implications in medical image interpretation. We and others have previously demonstrated the utility of incorporating shape in medical image segmentation and interpretation [1]. However, training a shape-based segmentation system is mostly done manually following a tedious and therefore impractical process. We report a novel approach to automated learning of shape models from examples and demonstrate its utility.

We have developed a novel solution to the problem of shape reparameterization–alignment–averaging problem. The main difference from previously reported methods [2,3] is that the training set is first automatically clustered and those shapes considered to be outliers are discarded. The second difference is in the manner in which registered sets of points are extracted from each shape contour.

2 Background and Notation

A *shape instance* $A = \{s_i^A\}_{i=1..n} = \{(x_i^A, y_i^A)\}_{i=1..n}$ is a set of points in the 2-D Euclidean space. A shape instance B is called *aligned* to a shape instance A if the *sum of squares* $SS(A,B) = \sum_{i=1}^{n} \left[(x_i^A - x_i^B)^2 + (y_i^A - y_i^B)^2 \right]$ cannot be decreased by scaling, rotating or translating B. In this case $SS(A,B)$ is called *Procrustes sum of squares* $PSS(A,B)$.

---

[1] See http://web.cse.msu.edu/~dutanico for a complete paper and a set of results.

A. Kuba et al. (Eds.): IPMI'99, LNCS 1613, pp. 370–375, 1999.
© Springer-Verlag Berlin Heidelberg 1999

The *Procrustes average shape* of a set of shapes $\{A_k\}_{k=1..m}$ is a shape instance near the center of the empirical distribution of A_k's in the shape space. For a detailed definition, properties and ways of computing an average shape see [2].

Let $A = \{(x_j^A, y_j^A)\}_{j=1..p}$ and $B = \{(x_k^B, y_k^B)\}_{k=1..r}$ be two shape instances. A *match matrix* $M = \{M_{j,k}\}_{k=1..r}^{j=1..p}$ is defined by:

$$M_{j,k} = \begin{cases} 1, & \text{if point } a_j \text{ corresponds to point } b_k, \\ 0, & \text{otherwise.} \end{cases}$$

We consider 0-1 match matrices M corresponding to symmetric one-to-one links (point correspondences); that is, a point $a_j \in A$ can have at most one corresponding point $b_k \in B$, in which case the correspondence is symmetric. The points from both sets that have no correspondence are called *outliers*. Let A_M and B_M be the subsets of A and B matched by M and $PSS(M) = PSS(A_M, B_M)$. We define a search criterion to be minimized over the match matrices space as: $f(M) = [PSS(M)/n + K]/n$, where n is the number of links in M and K is a constant. This functional encodes the fact that we are willing to trade a $q\%$ increase in average PSS for a $p\%$ increase in the number of correspondences. It also helps avoid the *shrinking effect* described in [4].

3   Problem Definition and Solution Outline

Mathematically speaking, we present a solution to the following problem: Given a set of m shape instances $S_k = \{(x_i^k, y_i^k)\}_{i=1..n_k}^{k=1..m}$, partition it into a set of clusters and, for each shape cluster, compute a *prototype* (Procrustes mean shape). The set of shape prototypes will be used as models for detection of object instances in new images by means of deformable template segmentation. Our shape learning method consists of the following main steps:

Algorithm 1: Shape Learning Outline

1. For each (evenly sampled) shape S_k in the training set compute a polygonal approximation S_k'.
2. For each $j, k = 1..m$ perform a flexible one-to-one registration (mapping) of S_k' to S_j. If the registration succeeds, define a set $T_{j,k}$ as the subset of S_j that corresponds (was matched) to the points of S_k', otherwise set $T_{j,k} = \emptyset$.
3. Compute a pseudo-distance matrix $\mathcal{D} = \{d_{j,k}\}_{j,k=1..m}$ where $d_{j,k} = PSS(T_{j,k}, S_k')/|T_{j,k}|$ if $T_{j,k} \neq \emptyset$ or $d_{j,k} = \infty$ otherwise.
4. Set the current training set equal to the original set of m shapes: $CTS = \{S_k\}_{k=1..m}$. While $CTS \neq \emptyset$ do
   (a) Find the shape approximation S_{i_0}' that has the least average distance to the shapes $S_j \in CTS$ (the *best fit shape* to the current training set).
   (b) Extract from CTS and put in a cluster all the shapes $S_{i_1},..,S_{i_p}$ to which S_{i_0}' can be fit ($d_{i_k,i_0} < \infty$).
   (c) The cluster prototype is defined as the *Procrustes average* of $T_{i_1,i_0},...,T_{i_p,i_0}$. The shape variance inside the cluster is defined as the covariance matrix of the aligned set $\{T_{i_k,i_0}\}_{k=1..p}$.

The shape approximations computed in Step 1 of the learning algorithm have about three times fewer points than the original shapes in order to smooth small shape artifacts, noise and quantitation effects and are only used to extract subsets of *corresponding* points from the *original* shapes, providing an *easier* task for the registration algorithm and *implicitly* bringing together the extracted subsets into a *common parameterization frame*. Indeed, if a point s_{i_0} on a polygonal approximation S' is registered to $s_{i_1} \in S_1$, $s_{i_2} \in S_2$, ..., $s_{i_m} \in S_m$ ($S_1, ..., S_m$ are original shapes that form a cluster), then by transitivity, $s_{i_1}, s_{i_2}, .., s_{i_m}$ are correspondents on $S_1, .., S_m$ of *one vertex* of an average shape. This also ensures that the shape variation present in the original data is *completely* preserved if the registration process is precise.

The employed shape registration method consists of two stages: (i) Similarity registration of two arbitrary sets of points and (ii) Non-linear registration based on local similarity of two curves:

Algorithm 2 (Global similarity registration)

1. Set $V_{min} = \infty$.
2. For every pair of points $(a_{j1}, a_{j2}) \in A \times A$
   For every pair of points $(b_{k1}, b_{k2}) \in B \times B$ do steps (a) through (e)
   (a) Find the similarity transformation ψ that aligns the sets $\{a_{j1}, a_{j2}\}$ and $\{b_{k1}, b_{k2}\}$.
   (b) Apply ψ to all the points in B to obtain B'.
   (c) For every point b_k of B', find its nearest neighbor $NN(b_k)$ in A. If the distance between b_k and $NN(b_k)$ is smaller than a threshold T (automatically set equal to 10% of the scale of B) then set a correspondence between the two. A match matrix M between A and B is constructed in this way. Since two points from B' can have the same nearest neighbor in A, we enforce on M a one-to-one correspondence requirement. That is, allow a point to be linked to its second to fifth nearest neighbor if the first one can be assigned to a closer point in B', and the length of the link does not exceed T.
   (d) Compute $f(M)$.
   (e) If $f(M) < V_{min}$ then $V_{min} = f(M)$, $\psi_{min} = \psi$.
3. Apply ψ_{min} to all the points in B to obtain B'.
4. For every point b_k of B', find its nearest neighbor $NN(b_k)$ in A. If the distance between b_k and $NN(b_k)$ is smaller than T then set the correspondence between the two. A match matrix M' between A and B is constructed in this way and enforced to correspond to one-to-one links.
5. Find the linear transformation ψ_{final} that aligns the sets $A_{M'}$ and $B_{M'}$.

We are interested not only in computing an average shape (which is robust to slight misregistrations) but also the shape variation present in the data set which is best described by the set of high curvature points. Since a *global* linear registration does not necessarily perform a good local registration (see [4]), we need to locally refine the results of the global registration such that corresponding points of high curvature from the two data sets are matched together. However, some high-curvature points in A may not correspond to high curvature points in B, therefore we do not enforce this requirement explicitly, but rather through *local similarity registration* and *monotonicity*. We define the term "local" in a topological sense according to the natural point ordering along curves A and B. A good registration should be *monotonic*, that is, preserve the topologies (point ordering) on the two shapes.

Algorithm 3 (Monotonic, local similarity-based registration)

Input: two sets of points A and B and a set $\mathcal{M}$ of one-to-one links between some subset A' of A and a subset B' of B obtained by global similarity registration.

1. Cyclically reorder the points of A, B and the links in $\mathcal{M}$ such that point a_1 corresponds to point b_1.
2. If the number of inversions (pairs of points a_i and a_j corresponding to b_k and b_l -in this order- such that $i < j$ and $k \geq l$) exceeds $|\mathcal{M}|/2$, reverse the ordering of the points in A.
3. Break the smallest number of links in $\mathcal{M}$ such that there are no more inversions. (Note that we are left with a monotonic registration).
4. For $i = 1..|B|$ do
   (a) Find a topological neighborhood of b_i, $[b_l, b_{l+1}, ..., b_i, ...b_{r-1}, b_r]$ (the actual size of the neighborhood depends on the curvature at b_i, the larger the curvature the smaller the neighborhood) such that both b_l and b_r have correspondences in A, let them be $a_{l'}$ and $a_{r'}$ with $l' < r'$.
   (b) Perform a similarity registration between the sets $[a_{l'}, a_{l'+1}, .., a_{r'}]$ and $[b_l, b_{l+1}, .., b_r]$.
   (c) If b_i is linked to a different point in A than it was before, then record this change in $\mathcal{M}$.
5. Break the smallest number of links in $\mathcal{M}$ such that there are no more inversions.

The third step of Algorithm 1 defines a pseudo-distance matrix $\mathcal{D}$ of *normalized Procrustes sum of squares* between an *approximation of a shape* and an *original shape* from the training set. A convenient way for obtaining shape clusters based on $\mathcal{D}$ and at the same time helpful for cluster prototype computation is a *k-means* type clustering algorithm:

1. Find a seed which is closest to the data. This is done in Step 4a of Algorithm 1 by finding the *shape approximation* S'_{i_0} that *best fits* the current training set (based on the average distance to the rest of the shapes). S'_{i_0} is going to be used as a common ground for extracting corresponding sets of points of the same size from as many training shapes as possible.

2. Extract from the training set and put in a cluster all shapes S_j that fit to S'_{i_0} (Step 4b).

This cluster extraction procedure continues until all shapes from the training set have been assigned to a cluster. For each cluster, the cluster prototype is the Procrustes Average of the subsets of registered points extracted from each shape in the cluster. The cluster variation is defined as the $2n \times 2n$ covariance matrix of the subsets of points used to compute the prototype (n is the number of cluster prototype points). This variation is used by the segmentation method to reject shape deformations that have not been seen in the training set [1].

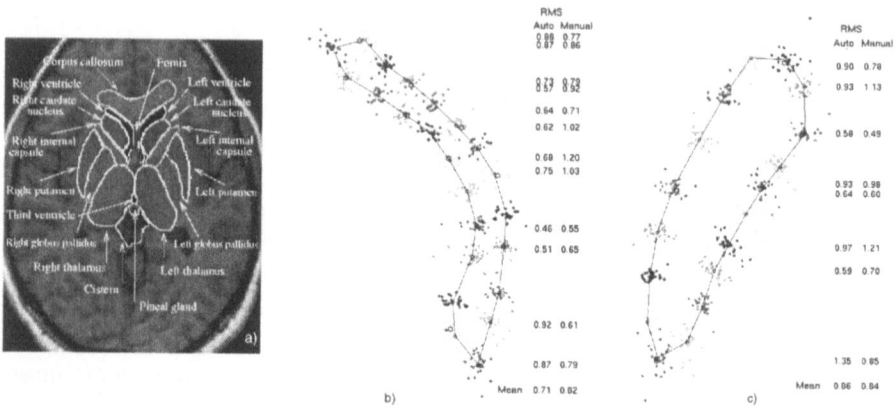

Fig. 1. The 17 neuroanatomical structures of interest (a). Procrustes average of 25 right-ventricle shapes (b) and 28 right-globus pallidus shapes (c) with the scatter of fits overlaid. The fits of consecutive points are drawn in different shades of gray to show the accuracy of the registration: consecutive clouds are non-overlapping

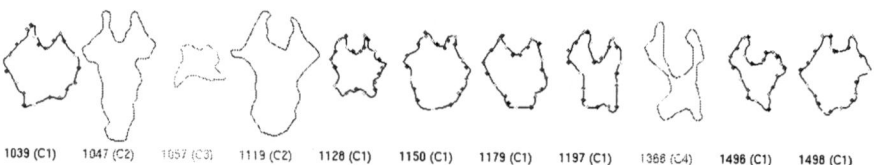

1039 (C1)   1047 (C2)   1057 (C3)   1119 (C2)   1128 (C1)   1150 (C1)   1179 (C1)   1197 (C1)   1366 (C4)   1496 (C1)   1498 (C1)

Fig. 2. A set of 11 cistern training shapes from different patients was automatically divided into clusters (main cluster (C1) and three secondary clusters). The registration of the *best fit shape* (1179) to cluster C1 is overlaid

4   Experimental Results

The shape learning method presented above was employed to design a shape model for 17 brain structures (shown in Fig. 1a) and its performance was assessed by a quantitative comparison to a manually-identified independent standard. The training set consisted of observer-defined contours identified by a neuroanatomist in 28 individual T1-weighted contiguous MR images of the human brain. Figure 2 shows the original manual tracings and clustering results for cistern together with the *best fit shape* registration to the main cluster (the sets $T_{i_1,i_0}, ..., T_{i_p,i_0}$ as defined in Algorithm 1). Figures 1(b) and (c) show the Procrustes averages for the right ventricle and globus pallidus with the *scatter of fits* overlaid.

In order to obtain a quantitative validation of our results we used the method employed in [3]. From each shape model, we manually selected several points that were considered most important in defining its shape (the points with the highest curvature) and we manually registered them to the training images. We defined the *ground truth* position of these points as the Procrustes average of the manually registered points. We computed and compared the *root-mean-square* (rms) distance of manually placed points from the independent standard and the rms distance of the automatically registered points from the independent standard, respectively. The *rms* distances for the right ventricle and globus-pallidus are also shown in Figs. 1(b) and (c): for every point selected on each shape, each distance is displayed on the same y coordinate as the ground truth point it corresponds to. As a rule, the very high curvature points (the extreme upper or lower points) are somewhat better registered manually while the intermediate points are better placed automatically. This was expected, since it is very difficult for a human to exactly place a point if there are no curvature or other anatomical cues. On average, *all* rms errors are between $0.7 - 1.5$ pixels.

5   Conclusion

A new fully automated shape learning method was presented. It is based on clustering a shape training set in the original shape space and performing a Procrustes analysis on each cluster to obtain a cluster prototype and information about shape variation. A quantitative analysis of our shape registration approach demonstrated results well comparable to those obtained by manual registration; achieving an average *rms error* of about 1 pixel. Our approach can serve as a fully valid automated substitute to the tedious and time-consuming manual shape analysis.

Acknowledgments

This work was supported by Siemens Corporate Research, Princeton, NJ.

References

1. Cootes, T., Hill, A., Taylor, C., Haslam, J.: Use of active shape models for locating structures in medical images. Image & Vision Computing **12** (1994) 355–366
2. Bookstein, F.L.: Landmark methods for forms without landmarks: Morphometrics of group differences in outline shape. Medical Image Analysis **1** (1997) 225–244
3. Hill, A., Brett, A., Taylor, C.: Automatic landmark identification using a new method of non-rigid correspondence. Proceedings of IPMI'97 (1997) 483–488
4. Feldmar, J., Ayache, N.: Rigid, affine and locally affine registration of free-form surfaces. Int. J. of Comp. Vision **18** (1996) 99–119

A Framework for Automated Landmark Generation for Automated 3D Statistical Model Construction

A. D. Brett and C. J. Taylor

Imaging Science & Biomedical Engineering
University of Manchester, Manchester M13 9PT, UK
{a.brett, c.taylor}@man.ac.uk

Abstract. We describe a method of pairwise 3D surface correspondence for the automated generation of landmarks on a *set* of examples from a class of shape. We show how the pairwise corresponder can be used in an extension of an existing framework for establishing dense correspondences between a set of training examples to build a 3D statistical model. The framework relies upon additional algorithms for the production of surface paths between vertices on a polyhedral mesh, and these are described. An example statistical model is shown for the left lateral ventricle of the brain.

1 Introduction

We describe a framework and a set of algorithms which may be used for the automated landmarking of a class of shapes in 3D. These landmarked shapes constitute a set of training examples which may be used to construct a flexible template model, an Active Shape Model (ASM) [4]. A previous publication [2] has described possible solutions to parts of the problem of automatic 3D model building. Here we describe a completely automated approach which involves extending the previous work and improving the accuracy and robustness of some of the algorithms.

Currently, the construction of an ASM involves the manual identification of a set of L *landmarks* $\{\mathbf{x}_i; 1 \leq i \leq L\}$ for each of N training examples of a class of shapes. Manual definition of landmarks on a shape has proved to be both time-consuming and subjective. Hill *at al* have previously described a method of non-rigid correspondence in 2D between a pair of closed, pixellated boundaries [5]. This pair-wise corresponder was used within a framework for automatic landmark generation. A similar framework is the basis of the approach to 3D automatic landmark generation described here, and consists of the the construction of a binary tree of merged shapes. Once such a tree has been produced, a set of L_t landmark points may be identified on the root (mean) shape of the tree and the positions of these landmarks propagated out to the N_t leaf (example) shapes.

A. Kuba et al. (Eds.): IPMI'99, LNCS 1613, pp. 376–381, 1999.

2   Background

Kambhamettu and Goldgof [6] and Benayoun *et al.* [1] both propose methods of surface correspondence based on the minimisation of a cost function which involves the difference in the curvature of the surfaces. As pointed out by Tagare *et al.* [9], curvature is a rigid invariant of shape and its applicability to general non-rigid correspondence is problematic.

Christensen *et al.* [3] propose a method of non-rigid registration by fluid deformation for the matching of brain anatomy in 3D. However, this technique is computationally expensive. Szekely *et al.* [8] parameterise surfaces by a heat diffusion model and further optimisation. Correspondence may then be established between surfaces but relies upon the choice of an origin position on each surface mapping and registration of the coordinate systems of these mappings by the computation of a rotation.

3   Polyhedral—Based Correspondence

The pair-wise correspondence algorithm comprises two stages:

1. Generation of sparse polyhedral approximations $\mathbf{A}''$ and $\mathbf{B}''$ of the input shapes $\mathbf{A}$ and $\mathbf{B}$ by triangle decimation, for which $\{\mathbf{A}_i''\} \subset \{\mathbf{A}_i\}$ and $\{\mathbf{B}_i''\} \subset \{\mathbf{B}_i\}$.
2. Generation of a corresponding pair of sparse polyhedra $\mathbf{A}'$ and $\mathbf{B}'$. This is accomplished using a global Euclidean measure of similarity between both the sparse polyhedron $\mathbf{A}''$ and a subset of labelled vertices from $\mathbf{B}$ and between $\mathbf{B}''$ and a subset from $\mathbf{A}$.

The sparse polygon generation algorithm makes use of a decimation method described by Schroeder *et al.* [7]. However, we use a distance metric which preserves sharp edges and thin structures. The distance metric, D, is computed using Schroeder's distance to mean plane measure as:

$$D(\mathbf{v}_0) = |d(\mathbf{v}_0) - d'(\mathbf{v}_0)| \tag{1}$$

where $d(\mathbf{v}_0)$ and $d'(\mathbf{v}_0)$ are the *signed* distances of the vertex $\mathbf{v}_0$ to the mean plane of the triangle loop before and after decimation i.e. $d(\mathbf{v}_0) = \hat{\mathbf{u}} \cdot (\mathbf{v}_0 - \overline{\mathbf{x}})$, see Fig. 1.

We have used a *symmetric* version of the Iterative Closest Point (ICP) algorithm to establish correspondences of the sparse pointset $\{\mathbf{A}_i''\}$ with the dense pointset $\{\mathbf{B}_i\}$ and of the sparse pointset $\{\mathbf{B}_i''\}$ with the dense pointset $\{\mathbf{A}_i\}$. Various metrics can be used to define the *closest* distance between point pairs. We weight the squared distance between points $|\mathbf{X}_i - \mathbf{Y}_j|^2$ by a factor of $2/(\hat{\mathbf{n}}_{\mathbf{X}_i} \cdot \hat{\mathbf{n}}_{\mathbf{Y}_j})$ where $\hat{\mathbf{n}}_{\mathbf{X}_i}$ is the unit surface normal on $\mathbf{X}$ at point i. This encourages the correspondence of points on the surfaces which are topographically equivalent. We label the closest points to $\mathbf{A}_i''$ from $\mathbf{B}$ as the pointset $\{\mathbf{B}_i'\}$, and the closest points to $\mathbf{B}_i''$ from $\mathbf{A}$ as the pointset $\{\mathbf{A}_i'\}$.

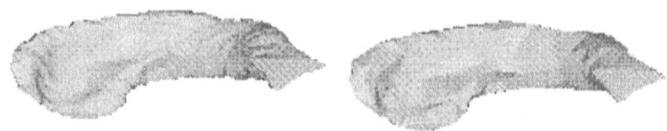

Fig. 1. Result of applying the decimation algorithm to a triangulated surface of the left ventricle of the brain. On the left is a shaded representation of the original dense triangulation with approximately 2000 vertices. On the right the same surface represented by 200 vertices (decimated by 90%)

A single corresponding pair of sparse polyhedra must be established from the two polyhedron/pointset pairs, $(\mathbf{A}'', \{\mathbf{B}_i'\})$ and $(\mathbf{B}'', \{\mathbf{A}_i'\})$. We choose the connective description which produces the lowest error in *representation*, E_R, of the sparse decimated polyhedron of each shape by the sparse reconstructed corresponding polyhedron of that shape, where

$$E_R^2 = \frac{1}{n_{\mathbf{A}''}} \sum_{i=1}^{n_{\mathbf{A}''}} \min_j |Q(\mathbf{A}_i'') - Q(\mathbf{A}_j')|^2 + \frac{1}{n_{\mathbf{B}''}} \sum_{k=1}^{n_{\mathbf{B}''}} \min_l |Q^{-1}(\mathbf{B}_k'') - Q^{-1}(\mathbf{B}_l')|^2.$$

(2)

The reconstruction is produced by combining the connectivity description of $\mathbf{A}''$ or $\mathbf{B}''$ with the pointset $\{\mathbf{B}_i'\}$ or $\{\mathbf{A}_i'\}$ to produce a pair of matching polyhedra with a one-to-one mapping $(\mathbf{A}' \mapsto \mathbf{B}')$.

4   Merging Shapes

Given a pair of corresponding sparse polyhedra $\mathbf{A}'$ and $\mathbf{B}'$, a local surface parameterisation is used to interpolate a dense set of vertices on each. The local surface parameterisation is of a single sparse triangle, and is produced by a parameterisation of the three surface paths corresponding to its three edges.

A 'brushfire' type distance transform algorithm is used to march the path across the surface between dense edges of the triangulation. At each stage, the minimisation of a cost $C_i(\mathbf{y}_0)$ locates the best next point, $\mathbf{x}_i$, for the surface path on a dense triangle edge $\{\mathbf{y}_i; 1 \leq i \leq 4\}$ attached to $\mathbf{y}_0$, see Fig. 2. We consider not just the path $(\mathbf{a}, \mathbf{b})$ which is a sparse polyhedral edge, but also the dense polyhedral triangles $\mathbf{t}_1$ and $\mathbf{t}_2$ connected to the dense edge under consideration, see Fig. 3.

We construct a plane normal to the surface defined by the reference point $\mathbf{c} = (\mathbf{a} + \mathbf{b})/2$ and by the unit normal $\hat{\mathbf{n}}_c$, where $\hat{\mathbf{n}}_c \cdot (A_1 \hat{\mathbf{n}}_1 + A_2 \hat{\mathbf{n}}_2) = 0$, in which A_1 and A_2 are the areas of the triangles $\mathbf{t}_1$ and $\mathbf{t}_2$ respectively, and $\hat{\mathbf{n}}_1$ and $\hat{\mathbf{n}}_2$ are the unit normals to these triangles. The cost function of igniting an

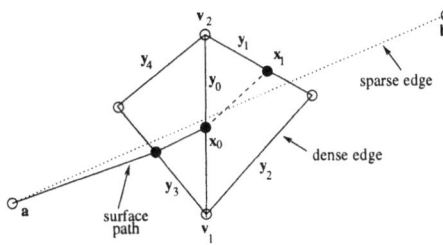 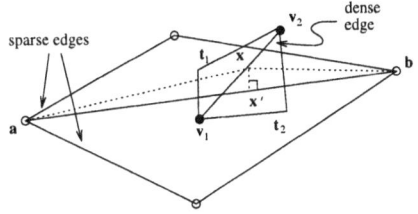

Fig. 2. Surface paths are defined on the dense triangulation of the surface by the parameterisation of triangle edges

Fig. 3. The cost function used to produce surface paths is defined in terms of a pair of dense polyhedral triangles connected to the dense edge under consideration

edge y_i from edge y_0 is defined for the intersection, x_i, of the line segment of a dense triangle edge with the plane:

$$C_i(y_0) = (|a - x_i'|^2 + |b - x_i'|^2)/|a - b|^2 \qquad (3)$$

where x_i' is the projection of x_i on the sparse edge $(a - b)$. This cost constrains the surface path to lie within the line defined by a and b, thus preventing it from looping back around the entire surface of the shape.

The connectivity of A' and B' are identical. Therefore, we can correspond the individual sparse triangles of the polyhedra. These sparse traingles are split recursively using surface paths to some *depth* to produce the dense triangulation A_d' and B_d'. Now a densely triangulated mean shape may be generated by averaging the geometric information of these dense triangulations to produce a pointset $\{C_i\}$ and this is combined with the connectivity from A_d' to produce a densely triangulated polyhedron C.

5   Automated Landmarking

The pairwise corresponder described above is used to build a binary tree of merged shapes with a single mean shape at the root and the examples from the training set at the leaves. We produce a set of landmarks $\{C_{1,i}\} \subset \{C_i\}$ on the mean shape. The connectivity of these points is defined by the sparse polyhedron C_1. These landmark points are then propagated down the branches of the tree.

At each branch of the tree, each of the landmark points can be projected onto a triangle of the sparse version of the mean shape C' which is the mean of A' and B'. The sparse triangle is then parameterised along a baseline and a vector between the baseline and opposite vertex, see Fig. 4. The projection e on the triangle (a, c, b) is now uniquely defined by the parameter pair (t, u). There is a correspondence between the vertices of this sparse triangle (a, c, b) on C' and the vertices of a pair of sparse triangles on A' and B'. Call the sparse corresponding vertices on A', (a', c', b'). The projection point e can therefore be mapped onto the sparse triangle $(\mathbf{a'}, \mathbf{c'}, \mathbf{b'})$, by parameterising it in t at u to give $\mathbf{e'}$.

We must now reconstruct a point on the *surface* of $\mathbf{A}$ which corresponds to the projection point $\mathbf{e'}$ mapped onto a sparse triangle. We do this by constructing surface paths using the method of section 4, again see Fig. 4. Finally we choose the landmark on the dense surface as the vertex with smallest Euclidean distance to the reconstruction of $\mathbf{e'}$.

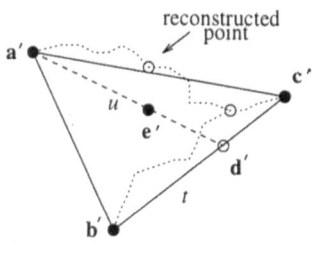

Fig. 4. Projected points are reconstructed on dense surfaces by the parameterisation of surface paths constructed across the baseline and from the opposite vertex of a sparse triangle

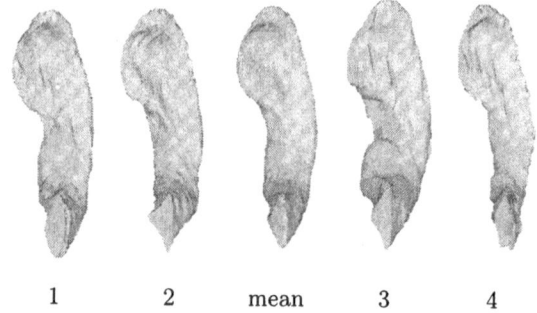

1   2   mean   3   4

Fig. 5. A group of four left brain ventricle examples and their densely triangulated mean at the third level of the tree of merged pairs used to generate a set of eight landmarked examples

6   Results

We have generated a 3D statistical model from eight complex biological shapes - left ventricles of the brain. These have been defined by hand as contours on a series of 2D slices from 3D Magnetic Resonance images. A grouping of four of the eight examples and their mean at the third level of the tree of merged shapes are illustrated in Fig. 5. The example shapes consisted of ≈ 2000 vertices, upon which were placed 200 landmark points. The first two modes of variation of this model are illustrated in Fig. 6, b_1 explains 43 % of the total variation, and b_2 explains 16 %.

7   Conclusions

We have presented a novel method for the correspondence of two faceted (triangulated) surfaces. The method is based on the production of a sparse polyhedral representation of one shape and matching this to a sparse pointset representation of the other. No curvature estimation of either surface is required. The only control parameter of the algorithm, the target number of vertices during decimation,

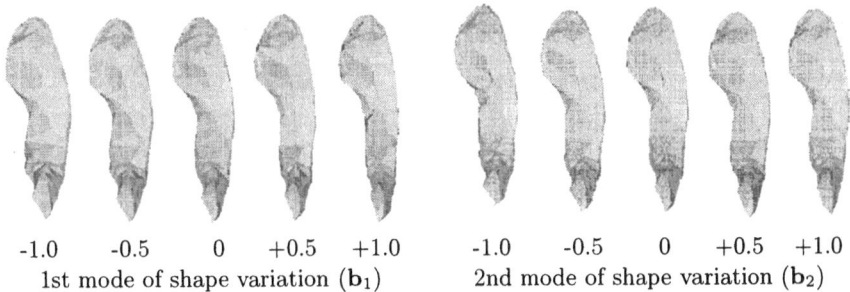

-1.0   -0.5   0   +0.5   +1.0   -1.0   -0.5   0   +0.5   +1.0
1st mode of shape variation ($\mathbf{b}_1$)   2nd mode of shape variation ($\mathbf{b}_2$)

Fig. 6. Shape instances generated using a 3D PDM of eight left brain ventricles showing the number of s.d.s (-1.0 to +1.0) from the mean shape. The model consists of 200 points

is not critical and be automated at the cost of decimating each surface twice. The use of this algorithm to produce of a binary tree of merged shapes, and the method we describe for accurate propagation of landmarks from the root to the leaf shapes of the tree, provides a framework for the automated landmarking of the input example shapes necessary for the production of a 3D statistical model.

References

1. Benayoun, A., Ayache, N., and Cohen, I.: Adaptive meshes and nonrigid motion computation. In 12th International Conference on Pattern Recognition (1994) 730–732
2. Brett, A. D., Hill, A., and Taylor, C. J.: A method of 3D surface correspondence for automated landmark generation. In 8th British Machine Vison Conference (1997) 709–718
3. Christensen, G. E., Joshi, S. C., and Miller, M.: Volumetric transformation of brain anatomy. IEEE Trans. Medical Image **16** (1997) 864–877
4. Cootes, T. F., Taylor, C. J., Cooper, D. H., and Graham, J.: Active shape models - their training and application. Computer Vision and Image Understanding **61** (1995) 38–59
5. Hill, A., Brett, A. D., and Taylor, C. J.: Automatic landmark identification using a new method of non-rigid correspondence. In 15th Conference on Information Processing in Medical Imaging (1997) 483–488
6. Kambhamettu, C., and Goldgof, D. B.: Point correspondence recovery in non-rigid motion. In IEEE Conference on Computer Vision and Pattern Recognition (1992) 222–227
7. Schroeder, W. J., Zarge, J. A., and Lorensen, W. E.: Decimation of triangle meshes. Computer Graphics **26** (1992) 65–70
8. Székely, G., Kelemen, A., Brechbühler, C., and Gerig, G.: Segmentation of 2-d and 3-d objects from mri volume data using constrained elastic deformations of flexible fourier contour and surface models. Medical Image Analysis **1** (1996) 19–34
9. Tagare, H. D., O'Shea, D., and Rangarajan, A.: A geometric criterion for shape-based non-rigid correspondence. In 5th International Conference on Computer Vision (1995) 434–439

Statistical Shape Analysis Using Fixed Topology Skeletons: Corpus Callosum Study

Polina Golland[1], W. Eric L. Grimson[1], and Ron Kikinis[2]

[1] Artificial Intelligence Laboratory, Massachusetts Institute of Technology,
Cambridge, MA 02139, USA
{polina, welg}@ai.mit.edu
[2] Surgical Planning Laboratory, Brigham and Women's Hospital,
Boston, MA 02115, USA
kikinis@bwh.harvard.edu

Abstract. The goal of this work is to develop an approach to shape representation and classification that will allow us to detect and quantify differences in shape of anatomical structures due to various disorders. We used a robust version of skeletons for feature extraction and linear discriminant analysis (the Fisher linear discriminant and the linear Support Vectors method) for classification. We propose a way to map the classification results back into the image domain, interpreting shape differences as a deformation required to bring a shape from one class to the other. An example of analyzing corpus callosum shape in schizophrenia is reported, as well as the results of the study of the statistical properties of the classifier using cross validation techniques.

1 Introduction

Our goal is to build a framework for statistical shape analysis using classification techniques applied to feature descriptors. We perform shape feature extraction using skeletons. To make the process of skeleton extraction robust to noise and quantization effects of segmentation, we have developed a new variation of the traditional skeletons: *fixed topology skeletons*.

In this paper, we limit ourselves to linear discriminant analysis, comparing performance of two different linear classification methods: the Fisher linear discriminant and the linear Support Vectors methods. Then we present the shape differences between the groups by constructing the shape deformation in the image space that corresponds to the discriminant vector in the feature space.

We tested the approach on corpus callosum data for schizophrenia patients. The results are reported in Sect. 3.

Related Work. Statistical shape modeling combines shape representation with statistical information on how the features vary across population. Principal Component Analysis (PCA) has been used by several authors for capturing statistical properties of the model [3,9]. It was well suited for applications in segmentation and object localization, where the statistical properties of the model

A. Kuba et al. (Eds.): IPMI'99, LNCS 1613, pp. 382–387, 1999.

were used to restrict the space of possible deformations of the model. It has also been used in shape analysis [4,8] to reduce the dimensionality of the model and find a decision boundary between the classes. Bookstein [2] used the shape features to align the outlines, but then the features (points along the outline) were analyzed independently of each other. We attempt to use traditional classification methods directly (without going through the dimensionality reduction step) to find the decision boundary.

We use a novel approach to robust skeleton estimation for feature extraction. Skeletons have been introduced in general computer vision several decades ago [1] and have been used extensively for object recognition and localization. In medical image analysis, a scale-space variation of skeletons was introduced and used in various applications by Pizer and colleagues [6].

2   Shape Representation: Fixed Topology Skeletons

Skeletons provide a compact, intuitive representation of a shape that can be used for segmentation, tracking, object recognition, etc. Their major drawback is their high sensitivity to noise in the boundary. There have been proposed many ways to stabilize the skeleton extraction, most of which concentrated on heuristics for pruning the original, noisy skeleton.

For shape analysis of anatomical structures, the general shape of the object is well known ahead of time and the deformations of interest are very small and do not change the global shape of the structure. *Fixed topology skeletons* take advantage of this fact: we fix the structure of the skeleton graph (the skeleton topology) and optimize for the accuracy of the original shape representation over all skeletons of that fixed structure.

Skeleton extraction. For computing the fixed topology skeleton of a shape, we use a distance map, a function that for every point in the image is equal to the distance from the point to the closest point on the boundary of the object. It can be shown that the skeleton is the set of ridge points of the distance map.

We use a snake-like approach for computing the fixed topology skeleton of a shape. The set of skeleton points defines a continuous curve that represents the skeleton. We initialize the snake at the end-points of the traditionally defined skeleton [1,6], and then use the distance map gradient to "drive" the snake. Additional regularization is required to keep the curve smooth. Formally, the update rule is

$$\mathbf{x}^{t+1} = \sigma(\mathbf{x}^t + \nabla D(\mathbf{x}^t)),$$

where $\mathbf{x}^t$ is the set of point coordinates on the curve at time t, ∇D is the gradient of the distance map computed at the locations corresponding to the points of the curve, and σ is the smoothing operator. The curve has to be resampled every few iterations to maintain uniform distribution of the points along the curve. We stop the iterations when the curve starts oscillating around the ridge.

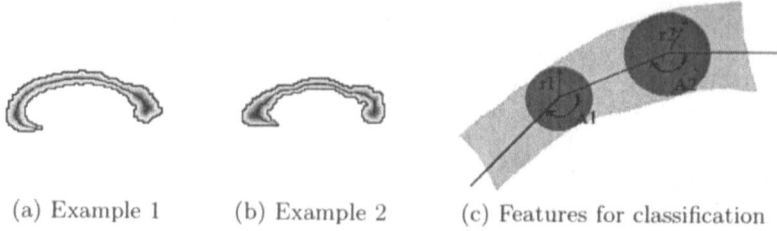

(a) Example 1   (b) Example 2   (c) Features for classification

Fig. 1. Skeleton extraction. (a) and (b) show the distance map (darker color corresponds to higher distance from the boundary) and the skeleton extracted for two different cases from the data set; (c) features used for classification: curvature angle and shape width

To find the best skeleton, we estimate skeletons for different initial pairs of points and chose the one that describes the shape the best ([7] contains more details on the algorithm). Figs. 1(a) and (b) show corpus callosum skeletons computed for two different cases in our data set.

Feature extraction. Once the skeleton is computed, we sample the skeleton curve uniformly by arc length and measure two values at every sample point (Fig. 1c): the angle between two adjacent segments in the sampled skeleton and the shape width at the sample point. These two features are invariant under rigid transformations and are therefore well suited for shape description. The number of sampling points on the skeleton determines the level of detail captured by the feature vector.

3   Classification Results

Classification methods. We tested two different linear discriminant techniques on the same data set, namely the Fisher discriminant function [5] and the linear Support Vectors classifier [10]. Given two classes of feature vectors $\{\mathbf{x}\}$, any linear learning method searches for weight vector $\mathbf{w}$ that maximizes 'spread' between the *projected* points $x = \mathbf{w}^T\mathbf{x}$. The difference between different linear techniques is in how they define spread, or separation, between the classes.

To find an optimal number of features, we use cross-validation. Since our data set is small, we had to resort to *leave-one-out* cross-validation: one case was left out of the training set and then used as a test set. Repeated for all the cases in the data set, this yields an estimate of the generalization accuracy of the method. We report cross-validation results later in this section.

Data. We tested our approach on corpus callosum images for two groups: schizophrenia patients and normal controls. We used two data sets, combined into one in our experiments (see Acknowledgments for more info). The combined data set contains scans of 30 schizophrenia patients (SZ) and of 36 normal controls (NC). We also performed testing on those data sets separately with results very similar to those obtained with the combined data set.

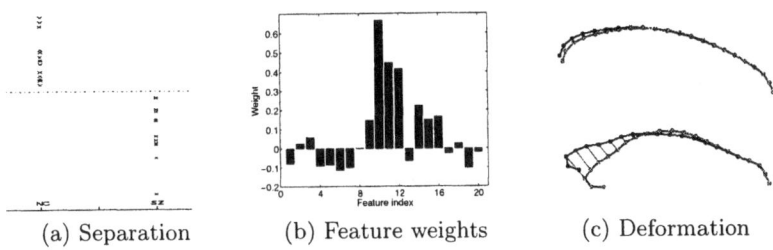

(a) Separation	(b) Feature weights	(c) Deformation

Fig. 2. Classification results based on 20 feature points: (a) separation between the two groups when projected onto **w** and (b) weights (components of **w**) for the features along the curve, in the posterior-to-anterior order; (c) deformation implied by the discriminant vector, applied to the mean of NC group (top) and to an individual case (bottom). Black corresponds to the original shape, gray indicates the result of the deformation

Classification results. Figure 2(a) shows the results of Support Vectors classification using 20 points along the skeleton. We can see that for this number of features, a perfect separation between the two classes was achieved. Figure 2(b) shows the weights corresponding to the angle features (ordered from posterior to anterior). The weights change smoothly as we move along the skeleton, and most of the weight is concentrated in the middle part of the skeleton. This suggests that the middle ridge is where most of the shape differences take place in this case.

We can also provide a direct interpretation of this result in the image domain. Since projecting onto weight vector **w** separates the two classes, negating the component of any feature vector $\mathbf{x}_i$ from the original data set along **w** should bring that vector over the threshold into the other class:

$$\mathbf{x} = \mathbf{x}_\perp + (\mathbf{w}^T \mathbf{x})\mathbf{w},$$
$$\tilde{\mathbf{x}} = \mathbf{x}_\perp - (\mathbf{w}^T \mathbf{x})\mathbf{w}.$$

We can apply this operation to any data point $\mathbf{x}_i$ in one of the classes and then reconstruct the skeleton using the resulting feature vector $\tilde{\mathbf{x}}_i$. Thus linear classification in the feature domain can be mapped into a shape deformation in the image domain.

Figure 2(c) shows the deformation applied to two different skeletons. The first example (top) shows a 'mean' normal control skeleton. It was constructed by averaging the features at the 20 points along the skeleton and reconstructing a skeleton from the resulting feature vector. The second example (bottom) shows a skeleton for one of the normal control subjects with the deformation implied by the classifier. We can see that the corpus callosum shape is more 'bent' for schizophrenia group. In other words, we would have to bend the normal corpus callosum further to make it look more like corpus callosum of a schizophrenia patient.

Cross-validation. Figure 3(a) shows learning accuracy, that is the classification accuracy, when the test set was the same as the training set. We can see that

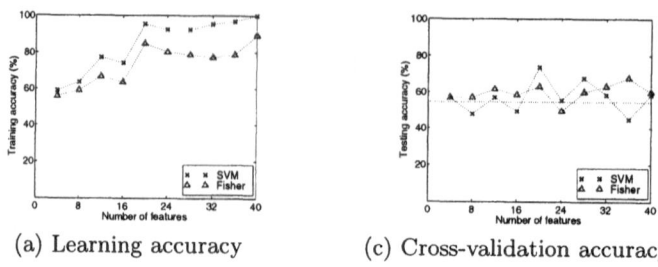

(a) Learning accuracy   (c) Cross-validation accuracy

Fig. 3. Cross-validation results

the Support Vectors method outperforms the Fisher linear discriminant, which we believe is because it makes fewer assumptions on the underlying distributions of the classes. As the number of feature points used for classification grows, the data becomes more separable and the accuracy improves.

Cross-validation is used to find the optimal number of feature points for be used for shape description of corpus callosum, as well as to test the generalization power of the classifier. Figure 3(b) shows the classification accuracy for leave-one-out cross-validation experiment. The dotted line shows the 'baseline', or the classification accuracy one would get by guessing. We can see that both methods achieve better than guessing accuracy. The best accuracy was achieved by Support Vectors method for 20 feature points. Thus that was reported as the best number of points.

The classification accuracy for cross-validation is significantly lower than for learning. There are several reasons for that. As the number of feature points grows, the data becomes more sparse in the feature space, and thus it is easier to separate between the classes, but we get poor generalization, as new examples fall into previously empty regions of the feature space. Another reason for lower testing accuracy could be that the classes are not truly separable[1].

Another question that should be addressed is the number of features. It seems that the optimal number of features is comparable with the number of cases in the data set. But it does not mean that we are fitting a model with that many *independent* parameters to the data. In fact, the features highly correlate with their neighbors along the skeleton. Another point to confirm this is the fact that adjacent points on the skeleton get similar weights (Fig. 2b).

4   Conclusions & Acknowledgments

We presented an approach for shape based classification of anatomical structures. It uses statistical learning techniques for investigating the differences between two groups of examples of the same anatomical structure. In this work,

---

[1] Implying that one could not provide a reliable diagnosis of schizophrenia based on the shape of corpus callosum alone, but only about 70% accurate estimate. But combined with analysis of other structures, it might provide a significant improvement in detecting and quantifying shape pathologies in the brain of schizophrenia patients.

we limited ourselves to using linear classifiers. We tested two different linear classification techniques: the Fisher linear discriminant and the linear Support Vectors classification.

The shape representation is also a crucial component of the system. It maps the images into points in the feature space in which the classification is performed, and also provides an interpretation of the classification results in terms of the shape deformation. We use skeletons for extracting the shape features. They provide a robust, intuitive representation of the shape, and are capable of capturing shape variations between the groups reported in the paper.

Based on the experimental results, we conclude that the shape of corpus callosum is different in schizophrenia with higher curvature of the shape. The cross-validation provided the optimal number of the feature points, as well as an estimate of the classification accuracy on the new examples.

Acknowledgments. The authors would like to thank M. Frumin and M. E. Shenton of Harvard Medical School and Brigham and Women's Hospital for providing DataSet1 and G. Gerig of University of North Carolina for providing DataSet2.

This work was supported by Mitsubishi Electric Research Laboratories and NSF IIS-9610249 grant. The project of acquisition and segmentation images for DataSet1 at Brigham and Women's Hospital was supported by Veterans Administration Psychiatric Research/Neuroscience Fellowship, Dupon Warren Fellowship from the Consolidated Department of Psychiatry, NIH grants MH 50740 and MH 01110.

References

1. Blum, H.: Biological shape and visual science. Journal of Theoretical Biology **38** (1973) 205-287
2. Bookstein, F.L.: Landmark methods for forms without landmarks: morphometrics of group differences in outline shape, Medical Image Analysis **1** (1996) 225-243
3. Cootes, T.F., and Taylor, C.J. Active Shape Models - 'Smart Snakes', In Proc. British Machine Vision Conference, Springer-Verlag (1992) 266-275
4. Csernansky, J.G. *et al*, Hippocampal morphometry in schizophrenia by high dimensional brain mapping. Proc. Nat. Acad. of Science **95** (1998) 11406-11411
5. Duda, R.O. and Hart, P.E.: Pattern Classification and Scene Analysis, John Wiley & Sons, 1973
6. Fritsch, D.S. *et al*, Stimulated Cores and their Applications in Medical Imaging. In Proc. IPMI'95 (1995) 365-368
7. Golland, P., and Grimson, W.E.L.: Fixed topology skeletons, AI Lab Memo, Massachusetts Institute of Technology, Submitted to ICCV'99, 1999
8. Martin, J., Pentland, A., and Kikinis, R.: Shape Analysis of Brain Structures Using Physical and Experimental Models, In Proc. CVPR'94 (1994) 752-755
9. Székely, G. *et al*, Segmentation of 2D and 3D objects from MRI volume data using constrained elastic deformations of flexible Fourier contour and surface models. Medical Image Analysis **1** (1996) 19-34
10. Vapnik, V.N.: Statistical Learning Theory, John Wiley & Sons, 1998

Model Generation from Multiple Volumes Using Constrained Elastic SurfaceNets

Michael E. Leventon and Sarah F. F. Gibson

[1] MIT Artificial Intelligence Laboratory,
Cambridge, MA 02139, USA
leventon@ai.mit.edu
[2] Mitsubishi Electric Research Lab
Cambridge, MA 02139, USA
gibson@merl.com

Abstract. Three dimensional models of anatomical structures are currently used to aid in medical diagnosis, treatment, surgical guidance, and surgical simulation. Limitations on the resolution of medical scans can cause artifacts to appear in the models that do not exist in the patient's anatomy. The most severe artifacts occur due to the low sampling rate between image slices of a scan. This paper describes a method of combining two orthogonal scans to generate a model with higher resolution than models created from either of the scans alone. The two scans are first registered to each other and then a net of linked surface nodes is initialized for each of the scans. The nodes from the two nets are then merged and relaxed, subject to constraints set by the resolution of each scan. This generates a smooth surface representation which stays faithful to the original binary data.

1 Introduction

The generation of three-dimensional models of anatomical structures from medical imagery is important for applications such as surgical simulation, planning, and image-guided surgery. An internal scan typically consists of high-resolution data in the imaging plane and significantly lower resolution between imaging slices. The lack of high-resolution information along the scanning direction causes aliasing or terracing artifacts in anatomical surface models, which can be distracting or misleading to surgeons. For surgical simulation, the terraces subtract from the realism of the visualization and create very noticeable ridges when using haptics to feel the object's surface. These terracing artifacts can be reduced by increasing the resolution of the scan. However, for CT scans, higher resolution between imaging planes subjects patients to a higher dose of radiation. For MR scans, longer scan times are necessary to achieve higher resolution, which is more costly and is more difficult for the patient, who must remain absolutely still during image acquisition.

For clinical practice, scans are usually acquired in more than one orthogonal direction. For example, instead of acquiring a single very high resolution sagittal MR scan, lower resolution sagittal and axial scans may be acquired (see

A. Kuba et al. (Eds.): IPMI'99, LNCS 1613, pp. 388–393, 1999.

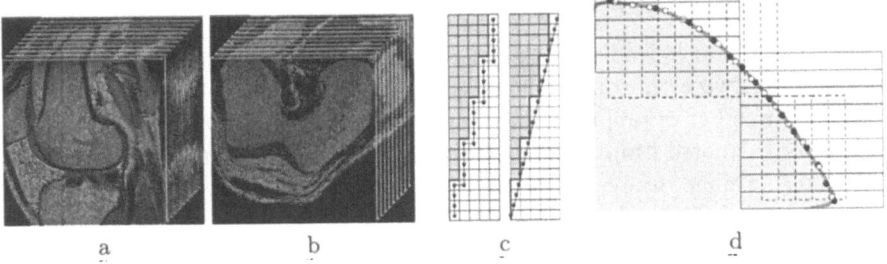

Fig. 1. (a, b) Two MR scans of a person's knee. Both images have high resolution in-plane, but have about one quarter the resolution between planes. (c) A single SurfaceNet is built around an object and then relaxed, producing a smooth surface, free of terracing. (d) Two nets are built from two orthogonal scans and relaxed

Fig. 1a,b). Surgeons and radiologists use information from both acquisitions for diagnosis, surgical guidance, and treatment. Similarly, we are interested in combining the information from two scans to produce three dimensional models of internal structures that have higher resolution than models created from either of the scans alone. The method proposed here is an extension of the Constrained Elastic SurfaceNet described in [2], which generates models from a single scan.

2   Previous Work

Two basic methods are commonly used to fit surfaces to binary data. In the first, the binary data is low-pass filtered, and an algorithm such as Marching Cubes is applied, where the surface is built through each surface cube at an iso-surface of the grey-scale data [4]. To remove terracing artifacts and reduce the number of triangles in the model, surface smoothing and decimation algorithms can be applied. However, because these procedures are applied to the surface without reference to the original segmentation, they can result in loss of fine detail.

In the second general method for fitting a surface to binary data, the binary object is enclosed by a parametric or spline surface. Control points on the surface are moved towards the binary data in order to minimize an energy function based on surface curvature and distance between the binary surface and the parametric surface [5]. This approach has two main drawbacks for general applications. First, it is difficult to determine how many control points will be needed to ensure sufficient detail in the final model. Second, this method does not handle complex topologies easily.

Recently, Gibson [2] introduced Constrained Elastic SurfaceNets which fit an elastic net of nodes over the surface of a binary segmented dataset and moved the node positions to reduce the surface curvature while constraining the net to remain within one voxel of the binary surface. This approach produces smooth surface models from binary segmented data that are faithful to the original segmentation.

3   Dual SurfaceNets

Dual SurfaceNets extend the original SurfaceNet approach by combining information from two orthogonal volume image scans. The use of Dual SurfaceNets requires a number of preprocessing steps [3]. First, the object of interest is segmented or extracted from each of the scans. The scans are then registered into a common coordinate frame by finding the pose that minimizes the sum of squared differences of the smoothed segmented images.

Once segmentation and registration are performed, a SurfaceNet is initialized for each of the models. The first step in generating a SurfaceNet is to locate cells that contain surface nodes. A cell is defined by 8 neighboring voxels in the binary segmented data, 4 voxels each from 2 adjacent planes. If at least one of the voxels has a binary value that is different from its neighbors, then the cell is a surface cell. The net is initialized by placing a node at the center of each surface cell and linking nodes that lie in adjacent surface cells. Figure 1c illustrates the creation of a net from a binary image.

Once defined, the SurfaceNet can be relaxed to reduce terracing artifacts while remaining faithful to the input segmentation [2]. To relax the net, each node is repositioned to reduce an energy measure in the links. In the examples presented here, SurfaceNets were relaxed iteratively by considering each node, $p[i]$, in sequence and moving that node towards the midpoint of its linked neighbors.

$$\hat{p}[i] = \frac{1}{\#\{\mathcal{N}(i)\}} \sum_{j \in \mathcal{N}(i)} p[j] \qquad (1)$$

where $\mathcal{N}(i)$ is the set of linked neighbors of point i. Defining the relaxation in this manner without constraints will cause the net to shrink to a single point. To remain faithful to the original segmentation, each node is constrained to lie inside its original surface cell. This constraint favors the original segmentation over smoothness and forces the surface to retain thin structures and cracks.

Relaxing a single SurfaceNet of an object significantly reduces the artifacts contained in the model. However, if the resolution in the scan is low in one direction, there may not be enough information in one scan to fully constrain the model and remove the terraces. We therefore consider using two scans, where one has higher resolution along the direction where the other has lower resolution, as illustrated in Fig. 1d. To relax two models of an object together, the individual SurfaceNets are built as described above. The two SurfaceNets, once aligned in the same coordinate frame, are iteratively relaxed towards one another with the constraint that each node much lie within its surface cell. In one relaxation step, each point $p[i]$ in the first net is updated by taking an average (weighted by distance) of the points $q[j]$ in the other net.

$$\hat{p}[i] = \frac{\sum_j w(p[i], q[j]) q[j]}{\sum_j w(p[i], q[j])} \qquad \text{where} \qquad w(u, v) = e^{\frac{-1}{2\sigma^2}||u-v||^2}. \qquad (2)$$

The point $\hat{p}[i]$ could violate its constraint by lying outside its cell, $c[i]$. The new position of the point, $p'[i]$ is $\hat{p}[i]$ if it lies inside the cell and the closest point on the cell boundary if $\hat{p}[i]$ lies outside the cell. In the next iteration, the second net is relaxed towards the first. After each full dual relaxation step, the nets are each relaxed individually for one iteration. The individual relaxation keeps each net smooth as they merge. The iteration progresses until the positions of some user-defined fraction of the nodes have converged, at which time one of the two nets is chosen to generate the final triangle model.

If the segmentation and registration were ideal, then the true surface would always lie in the intersection of the surface cells of the two images. In this case, the two nets would converge on the identical surface with all surface cell constraints satisfied. Figure 1d shows a 2D example of a surface passing through the surface cells of two nets. In general, the surface cells of the two scans do not overlap perfectly due to imaging, segmentation, and registration errors. We therefore provide a means of relaxing the constraints to allow the nets to merge more closely. After a few iterations, any point that is pulled outside its constraining cell cannot meet a corresponding point in the other net. This signifies discrepancies between the two models. In these instances, the constraining cell of every such point is dilated (preserving aspect ratio) by a small amount at the end of the iteration, allowing those points to move closer to the other net in the next iteration. Although the resultant net can move more than one voxel from the segmentations, the final model is guaranteed to be between the two initial models.

4   Results

Results of the dual relaxation are shown in Fig. 2. One scan of a femur was acquired axially at a resolution of $0.27\,\text{mm} \times 0.27\,\text{mm} \times 1.00\,\text{mm}$. The other scan (of the same person) was acquired sagittally (one year later) at a resolution of $0.25\,\text{mm} \times 0.25\,\text{mm} \times 1.40\,\text{mm}$. The femur was segmented manually from both images[1]. Figures 2(a) and (b) shows the results of running Marching Cubes [4], individual SurfaceNets [2], and Dual SurfaceNets on the images. No decimation was performed on any of the models. Notice the terracing artifacts in the models generated with Marching Cubes and individual SurfaceNets along the direction that the scans were acquired. The model generated using Dual SurfaceNets on both scans preserves the fine details in the original scans well but does not contain the terraces.

In the second example, we consider building a model from extremely low resolution scans. Figure 2(c) shows results of model generation from subsampled versions of the original segmentations. The axial and sagittal scans were subsampled by a factor of 4 to resolutions of $1.09\,\text{mm} \times 1.09\,\text{mm} \times 4.00\,\text{mm}$ and $1.00\,\text{mm} \times 1.00\,\text{mm} \times 5.60\,\text{mm}$ respectively. The model generated using Dual SurfaceNets at the low resolution contains slightly less detail than the high resolution version, but it is remarkably smooth and free of terracing artifacts, while

---

[1] These datasets were provided by the Surgical Planning Lab of Brigham and Women's Hospital.

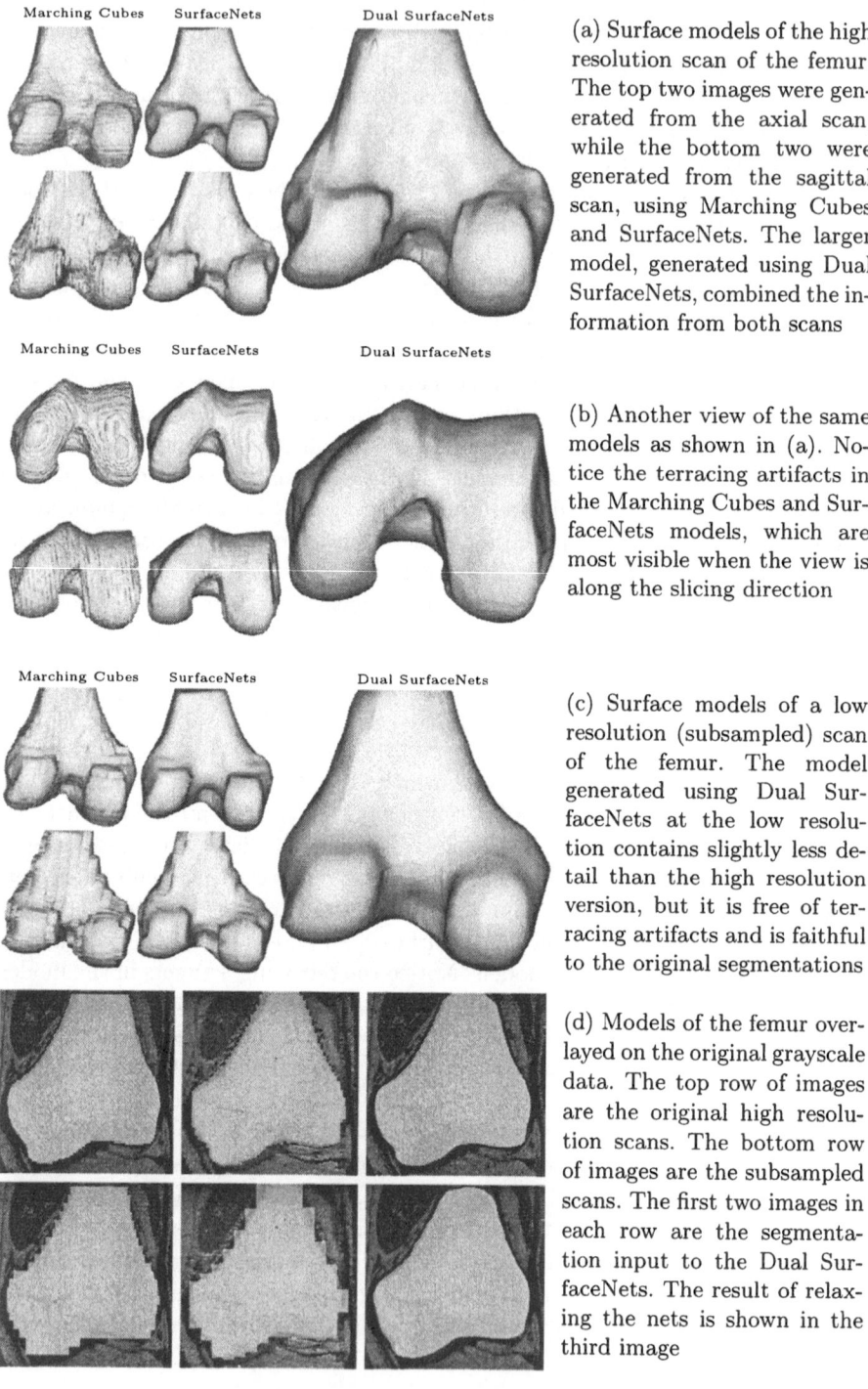

(a) Surface models of the high resolution scan of the femur. The top two images were generated from the axial scan, while the bottom two were generated from the sagittal scan, using Marching Cubes and SurfaceNets. The larger model, generated using Dual SurfaceNets, combined the information from both scans

(b) Another view of the same models as shown in (a). Notice the terracing artifacts in the Marching Cubes and SurfaceNets models, which are most visible when the view is along the slicing direction

(c) Surface models of a low resolution (subsampled) scan of the femur. The model generated using Dual SurfaceNets at the low resolution contains slightly less detail than the high resolution version, but it is free of terracing artifacts and is faithful to the original segmentations

(d) Models of the femur overlayed on the original grayscale data. The top row of images are the original high resolution scans. The bottom row of images are the subsampled scans. The first two images in each row are the segmentation input to the Dual SurfaceNets. The result of relaxing the nets is shown in the third image

Fig. 2. Results of Model Generation

remaining faithful to the original segmentations. The surface models can be visually verified by superimposing the relaxed net on the image data. Figure 2d shows the input segmentations to the Dual SurfaceNet algorithm and the final result of the net. Despite the blockiness evident in all the input segmentations, the final models are very smooth and capture the details of the femur.

5 Validation

Since three dimensional models of anatomical structures are now routinely used by surgeons, there is a clear need to validate the process by which such models are generated. One method of validating the result of relaxing Dual SurfaceNets is by visual inspection. The 3D model can be superimposed onto the original grayscale image, as shown in Fig. 2d. The borders of the model can be confirmed by examining each slice of the image.

In SurfaceNets, each node of the model is guaranteed to lie within one voxel of the original binary segmentation. Dual SurfaceNets can uphold the same constraints, but in practice these constraints need to be relaxed slightly to effectively combine the information in both nets. The distance that a node strays from its initialization point (the center of its cell) can be constrained during the relaxation. Furthermore, upon convergence, the distribution of displacements can be analyzed to determine the goodness of the fit. For both nets of the femur data set, over 97% of the points lie within one voxel of their starting position. Therefore, the final model is not only very smooth, but also faithful to the input segmentation (see [3] for more details).

The validation process is often hindered by the difficulty in obtaining ground truth. While we do not have explicit ground truth, we generated the low resolution femur model and then compared the result with the high resolution femur segmentation. Ideally, each point of the low resolution model should fall near the high resolution surface. Even though the voxel extents of the axial and sagittal scans used in generation of the nets are 4.28 mm and 5.78 mm respectively, the majority of model points fall within one millimeter of the high resolution model. Furthermore, 98% lie within one sub-sampled voxel of the original data [3]. The model produced by Dual SurfaceNets on the low resolution scans is a good estimate of the high resolution model, while true to the input images.

References

1. Gibson, S., Fyock C., Grimson E., *et al.*: Volumetric object modeling for surgical simulation. Medical Image Analysis **2** (1998) 121–132
2. Gibson, S.: Constrained Elastic SurfaceNets: generating smooth surfaces from binary segmented data. In: MICCAI. Springer-Verlag, Berlin (1998)
3. Leventon, M., Gibson, S.: Generating Models from Multiple Volumes using Constrained Elastic SurfaceNets MERL Tech Report TR99-09 (1999)
4. Lorensen, W., Cline, H.: Marching cubes: a high resolution 3D surface construction algorithm. SIGGRAPH (1987) 163–169
5. McInerney, T., Terzopoulos, D.: Deformable models in medical image analysis: a survey. Medical Image Analysis **1** (1996) 91–108

An Intelligent Interactive Segmentation Method for the Joint Space in Osteoarthritic Ankles

S.D. Olabarriaga[1,4], A.W.M. Smeulders[1], A.C.A. Marijnissen[2], and K.L. Vincken[3]

[1] Computer Science Dept., Univ. of Amsterdam, The Netherlands
{silvia, smeulders}@wins.uva.nl
[2] Rheumatology and Clin. Immunology Dept. and
[3] Image Sciences Institute, Univ. Hospital Utrecht, The Netherlands
[4] Instituto de Informática, UFRGS, Brazil

Abstract. Clinical reality is full of complex images that cannot be segmented automatically with current computer vision technology, requiring intensive user intervention. In [1] and [2] we proposed a framework for the systematic development of intelligent interactive segmentation techniques that aim at repeatable and predictable results obtained via efficient interaction. In this paper we apply this framework to segment the joint space boundary of osteoarthritic ankles. The solution is based on a heterogeneous boundary representation implemented with a new piecewise deformable model. User intervention is necessary only when this model fails, being performed via specialized interactive tools. Results obtained by a non-medical user are presented, indicating improvement over the manual practice in terms of accuracy and repeatability.

1 Introduction

In many clinical applications, to *segment* means to isolate a part *(object)* from the remainder of the image *(background)*. Segmentation techniques here aim at precise, predictable and reproducible delineation of objects of interest, being based on prior knowledge about how these are *expected* to be depicted in terms of image and geometric features. Unfortunately objects might be represented in the image differently than expected due to conditions intrinsic to medical applications, e.g. noise, pathology and low contrast. Segmentation methods fail in these cases, with the consequence that human intervention is often needed to manually enhance the results obtained with automatic techniques. With current technology, the automatic and manual parts are performed as two different and independent procedures with possibly inconsistent outcome. [1] and [2] propose a systematic approach, called *intelligent interactive segmentation* (IIS), based on the following conception: *(1)* Automatic and interactive parts are unified into one segmentation process; *(2)* The backbone is a steerable automatic segmentation method with prior knowledge about image and geometric features; *(3)* Situations when this method fails are limited and attributed to cases where the image deviates from the prior knowledge in the segmentation model, which can

A. Kuba et al. (Eds.): IPMI'99, LNCS 1613, pp. 394–399, 1999.

be *locally* reconfigured to avoid or recover from failure; and *(4)* User intervention is needed in case of failure to provide information used for reconfiguration, establishing a *user* ↦ *model* feedback mechanism called *intelligence*.

Here we describe how this framework was used to develop an IIS method for a complex clinical application. Sect.2 presents the application, Sect.3 describes the new method, and Sect.4 contains an evaluation with a non-clinical experiment.

2   Clinical Application

Osteoarthritis (OA) is a joint disorder characterized by the destruction of the articular cartilage, subchondral sclerosis, and secondary inflammation. An experimental treatment called *joint distraction* is currently applied at the University Medical Centre Utrecht, The Netherlands, to patients with OA in the ankle joint (Fig.1-a), consisting of a temporary distraction of talus and tibia using an Ilizarov external ring fixation [3]. Evaluation is done based on radiographs of the control and OA ankles taken at fixed time intervals before and after treatment. X-ray images of the ankles are acquired in *standardized mortise view*[1] and digitized with 256 grey levels and variable size (Fig.1-b).

A current project at the Image Sciences Institute Utrecht aims at the quantification of the ankle joint space (AJS) width, amount of subchondral sclerosis and angle of the joint to evaluate this treatment. Here manual segmentation consists of delineating the central part of the upper and lower boundaries of the AJS, a task that requires medical knowledge due to very low image quality resulting from the projection of concave or overlapping structures (Fig.1-b). Currently, the boundaries are approximated by two lines connecting ten points indicated by the user via a semi-automated procedure; we call this procedure *manual* because no automatic segmentation method takes part in the process. More accurate measurements can be obtained with a more precise boundary, and a reduction of variation and bias can be achieved by using image data for segmentation.

3   Intelligent Interactive Segmentation Method

The method is based on four main components: a heterogeneous model of the AJS boundary, a piecewise deformable model (DM) implementing this model, a list of cases when this method can fail and the appropriate user corrections, and a visual language used for interaction (see details in [5]).

Heterogeneous Boundary Model. The AJS boundary sketched in Fig.1-c is modeled by two open and non-intersecting curves divided in five pieces (Fig.1-d). A study of manually segmented images and anatomical information showed that these pieces are characterized by different combinations of image and geometric features, leading to the segmentation model in Table 1. This model is valid for most images, but it admits local modification as a consequence of interaction.

---

[1] The patient stands with foot turned 20° inwards; acquisition with standard settings.

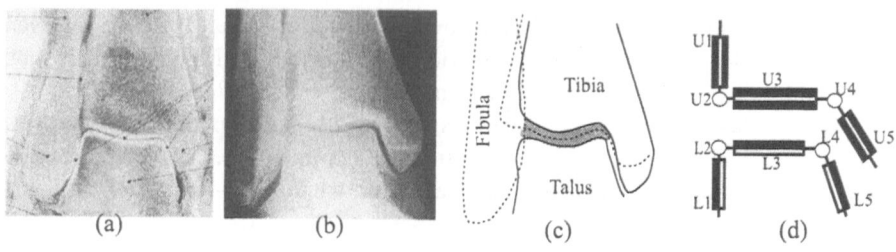

Fig. 1. The ankle joint space. *(a)* Coronal dissection of a normal ankle (from [4]). *(b)* Digital image of a control ankle in standardized mortise view (642 × 840 pixels). *(c)* Scheme showing the boundaries of interest (plain lines), the joint space (shaded area), and the misleading boundaries (dotted lines). *(d)* Model for the AJS boundary, where circles indicate corners and rectangles indicate the edge type: white or step edges

Table 1. Segmentation model for the AJS. Image features computed with scale-normalized local image structure detectors [6], using special versions for horizontal edges (ω is the scale for derivatives L_x, L_y, etc.). Shape features measured by the change of the curve's turning angle φ' [8], with v_i determined from examples

Boundary Part	Upper Boundary Features		Lower Boundary Features	
	Image	Shape (φ')	Image	Shape (φ')
lateral stretch	$\omega\lvert L_{xx} + L_{yy}\rvert$	≈ 0	$\sqrt{\omega}\sqrt{L_x^2 + L_y^2}$	≈ 0
lateral corner	$\omega\lvert L_{xx} + L_{yy}\rvert$	$\approx -2v_1$	$\sqrt{\omega}\sqrt{L_x^2 + L_y^2}$	$\approx +2v_3$
central stretch	$\lvert Min(0, \sqrt{\omega}\frac{L_{yy}}{\sqrt{L_x^2+L_y^2}})\rvert$	$\approx \pm v_2$	$\sqrt{\omega}\lvert L_y\rvert$	$\approx \pm v_4$
medial corner	$\omega\lvert L_{xx} + L_{yy}\rvert$	$\approx +v_1$	$\sqrt{\omega}\sqrt{L_x^2 + L_y^2}$	$\approx +v_3$
medial stretch	$\omega\lvert L_{xx} + L_{yy}\rvert$	≈ 0	$\sqrt{\omega}\sqrt{L_x^2 + L_y^2}$	≈ 0

Piece-DM. The upper and lower boundaries are implemented as two independent DMs initialized by curves sketched by the user. Since each boundary piece is characterized by different image and shape features, homogeneous techniques known from the literature [7] are not suited for this application. The current implementation is based on a new DM, *Piece-DM*, with the following features: *(1)* The boundary is represented by a cubic B-Spline curve to ensure geometric continuity, local control, and compact representation; *(2)* Optimization is performed with the conjugate gradients method, affecting only the position of the B-Spline control points; and *(3)* The objective function (1) is implemented as a sum of K terms with localized influence on the boundary, called *pieces*:

$$\Theta[C] = \oint_t \sum_{j=1}^{K} \mathcal{W}_j(t)\, \Theta_j[C](t)\, dt, \tag{1}$$

where $\mathcal{W}_j(t)$ is the weight of piece j at curve position t, and Θ_j is the objective function associated with piece j, implemented as a weighted sum of terms measuring the deviation of a curve segment from prior knowledge. This deviation is

Table 2. Cases in which the model fails, the possible causes, and the corresponding segmentation model correction or tuning to obtain the desired result

Failure	Cause	Model Correction
1. Wrong curve	Wrong initial. or deformation	Modify curve
2. Unseen visual evidence	Image intensity profile is different from expected	Locally replace the image feature detector
3. Low or absent visual evidence	Flat image intensity profile	Keep the curve locally near the position indicated by the user
4. Wrong visual evidence	Another structure disturbs the correct boundary identification	Locally reduce the weight of the image feature
5. Deviation from local shape	Corners are wider/narrower, or stretches are smoother/rougher	Locally modify expected turning angle values.

computed with the Mahalanobis distance [9], i.e., it is normalized to the range of expected values obtained from a sample data set, providing intuitive and predictable behavior. This *Piece-DM* is heterogeneous and flexible to accommodate local corrections resulting from interaction, by adding or replacing pieces and locally tuning the weights and range of expected feature values.

Cases of Failure. Failure happens when the contour deviates from expectations in terms of image features (*visual evidence*) and/or local shape features. A limited number of cases were identified as a result of the systematic analysis proposed in [2] – see Table 2, where these are presented together with the causes for failure and the corresponding DM correction. These cases are detected as a consequence of interaction (see Table 3).

User-Computer Interaction. Interaction is limited to three situations: initialization, model correction or confirmation, and acceptance of the final result. During initialization, the user adjusts a template to the image which is used to build a *Piece-DM* based on the segmentation model in Table 1. The DM is then displayed using an intuitive abstraction (Fig.2-a): an open curve for the boundary, and arrows for the "deformation forces," indicating the preferred direction of local boundary motion resulting from optimization. The boundary is also displayed in separate windows using other image detectors as background (e.g. Fig.2-b), to help the identification of failure case #2 in Table 2.

This visual information enables the user to plan the next action (see Table 3), essentially confirming or indicating the need for correction of current DM settings. Confirmation activates the optimization process (if forces are still large) or ends segmentation (if forces are small). In other situations, a case of failure from Table 2 is determined based on the internal status, and the model is corrected accordingly (see Table 3). Example: in Fig.2-a the boundary position is wrong, but the forces roughly point to the right orientation; the user therefore confirms the model, and the program optimizes it until the forces are very small (Fig.2-c).

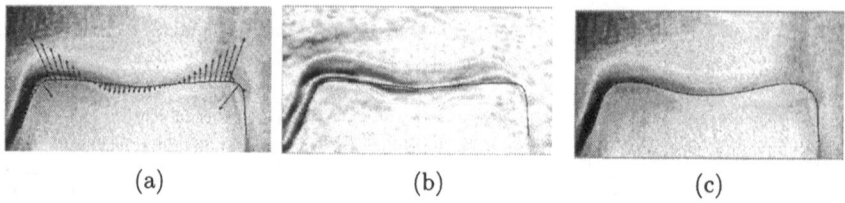

(a)   (b)   (c)

Fig. 2. Visual information showing the lower boundary and forces. *(a)* Boundary and deformation forces after initialization, with the grey image as background *(b)* Boundary after initialization, with the horizontal step-edge detector as background (dark areas correspond to high response). *(c)* Boundary after deformation (invisible forces)

Table 3. Summary of visual conditions observed by the user (boundary position and orientation of deformation forces), the corresponding user actions, internal conditions analyzed automatically, and the interpretation by the program in terms of Table 2

Visual Status		User Action	Internal Status	Program
Boundary Pos.	Forces Orient.		(Force Mag.)	Action
wrong	wrong	drag curve	-	Failure 1
right	wrong detector	point new detector	-	Failure 2
right	wrong	"freeze" curve	small image force	Failure 3
			large image force	Failure 4
			large shape force	Failure 5
wrong	right	confirm	large	Optimize
right	unseen		very small	End

4   Results and Discussion

An evaluation of intra-operator variation was performed as follows. Ten images were segmented by a non-medical user, three times each, with one day and one week interval among sessions - see qualitative results in Fig.3-a/b. The intra-operator variation was quantified by the distance in pixels from all points in the central piece of one curve to all the other curves. Results show agreement within one pixel for most images, with smaller variation for the lower boundary ($\mu_{up} = 1.56 \pm 1.62$,[2] $\mu_{low} = 0.55 \pm 0.37$). This represents a significant improvement ($> 50\%$) over the results obtained with the manual method ($\mu_{up} = 3.24 \pm 1.68$, $\mu_{low} = 2.19 \pm 1.29$).

It is difficult to validate the correctness of results in this application because the truth is not exactly known; for this purpose, evaluation with medical users is essential. For a qualitative assessment of correction, we compared results of the IIS method (non-medical user) to those obtained manually (medical user), obtaining the following conclusions: *(1)* Interactive results agree with manual boundaries to a large extent (e.g. Fig.3-c); *(2)* Agreement is bad under low visual evidence (Fig.3-d); and *(3)* Agreement is better for lower boundaries ($\mu_{up} = 5.93 \pm 4.47$, $\mu_{low} = 3.34 \pm 2.11$).

---

[2] μ_{up} refers to the upper boundary, and μ_{low} to the lower. Values in pixels.

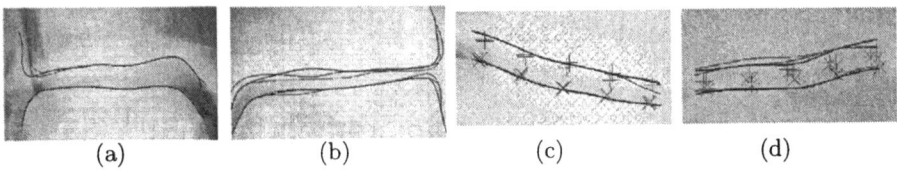

(a)   (b)   (c)   (d)

Fig. 3. Best and worst cases for (a,b) intra-operator variability and (c,d) matching between interactive and manual results. Lines refer to interactive results and crosses correspond to points indicated with the manual method. *(a)* Best agreement ($\mu_{up} = 0.46, \mu_{low} = 0.13$). *(b)* Worst agreement ($\mu_{up} = 5.51, \mu_{low} = 1.29$). *(c)* Best match ($\mu_{up} = 2.09, \mu_{low} = 2.34$). *(d)* Worst match ($\mu_{up} = 15.21, \mu_{low} = 9.22$)

5   Conclusions

Results indicate that the interactive method described here provides repro-ducible and precise delineation of the ankle joint space boundary by means of an efficient interaction process, with significant improvement over the manual practice. This method was developed in four months from a strategy [2] that can be adopted in other situations in which the segmentation task is too complex to rely completely on an automatic method. We conjecture that interactive-steered segmentation will be helpful in the majority of clinical applications.

Acknowledgments

We thank the Brazilian Council of Research and Development (CNPq) for fi-nancial support, grant #200146/95.5.

References

1. Olabarriaga, S., Smeulders, A.: Setting the mind for intelligent interactive segmen-tation: Overview, requirements, and framework. In: Proceedings of IPMI, LNCS **1230**, Springer-Verlag (1997) 417–422
2. Smeulders, A., Olabarriaga, S., Boomgaard, R., Worring, M.: Design considerations for interactive segmentation. In: Visual Conference, San Diego (1997) 5–12
3. Valburg, A.: Ilizarov joint distraction in treatment of osteoarthritis. PhD Thesis, Utrecht University (1997)
4. McMinn, R., Hutchings, R., Logan, B.: The concise handbook of human anatomy. Manson Publishing, London (1998)
5. Olabarriaga, S.D., Smeulders, A., Marijnissen, A., Vincken K.: SAIDA-I: Project Development. ISIS Tech. Report, Univ. Amsterdam (1998)
6. Lindenberg, T., Ten Haar Romeny, B.M.: Linear scale-space II: Early visual oper-ations. In: Geometry-Driven Diffusion in Computer Vision. Kluwer (1994) 39–71
7. McInerney, T., Terzopoulos, D.: Deformable models in medical image analysis: a survey. Medical Image Analysis **1** (1996) 91–108
8. Gray, A.: Differential Geometry of Curves and Surfaces with Mathematica. CRC Press, Boca Raton (1997)
9. Duda, R., Hart, P.: Pattern Classification and Scene Analysis, Wiley & Sons (1973)

Anatomical Modeling with Fuzzy Implicit Surfaces: Application to Automated Localization of the Heart and Lungs in Thoracic MR Images

Boudewijn P. F. Lelieveldt[1], Milan Sonka[2], Lizann Bolinger[3],
Thomas D. Scholz[4], Hein W. M. Kayser[5], Rob J. van der Geest[1],
and Johan H. C. Reiber[1,5]

[1] Dept. of Radiology, Leiden University Medical Center, Leiden, The Netherlands,
{hreiber, blelie}@lkeb.azl.nl
[2] Dept. of Electrical and Computer Engineering, University of Iowa, Iowa City, USA,
[3] Dept. of Radiology, University of Iowa Hospitals and Clinics, Iowa City, USA,
[4] Dept. of Pediatrics, University of Iowa Hospitals and Clinics, Iowa City, USA,
[5] Interuniversity Cardiology Institute of the Netherlands, Utrecht, The Netherlands

Abstract. In this paper a novel model driven segmentation approach for thoracic MR-images is presented. The goal of this work is to coarsely, but fully automatically localize the boundary surfaces of the heart and lungs in thoracic MR sets. The major organs in the thorax are described in a three–dimensional analytical model template by combining a set of fuzzy implicit surfaces by means of Constructive Solid Geometry, and formulating model registration as an energy minimization. The method has been validated on 20 thoracic MR volumes from two centers (patients and normal subjects). On average 90 % of the contour length of the heart and lung contours was localized with sufficient accuracy (average 6 mm positional error) to automatically provide the initial conditions for a subsequently applied locally accurate segmentation method.

1 Introduction

Though many automated segmentation methods for thoracic Magnetic Resonance image data have been described, many of these methods require at some point user interaction in the form of a seed point, volume of interest or initial boundary model. To further automate this initial image interpretation step, integration of prior knowledge in the form of an anatomical model is essential.

The goal of this work is to develop a hybrid anatomical knowledge representation suitable to *coarsely*, but *fully automatically* localize the heart and lung surfaces in thoracic MR images. The model described here combines the context-preserving properties of volume-based methods (e.g. [1]) with the compactness of surface-based (e.g. [2,3]) models by modeling multiple organs in their spatial context as a set of 3D fuzzy implicit surface templates. This template-based approach provides a number of key benefits, which can be summarized as follows:

- though limited in flexibility, it is intrinsically three-dimensional without requiring point-correspondence,

A. Kuba et al. (Eds.): IPMI'99, LNCS 1613, pp. 400–405, 1999.

- it simultaneously captures the 3D shapes and spatial context of multiple (in this application 6) organs in a single, closed-form energy function,
- it enables a fast, fully automatic image registration by integrating prior knowledge about local image gradient polarity in the matching criterion.

2 Methods

2.1 Implicit Solid Modeling

Let a regular implicit surface be given in the form $f(x, y, z) = c$. An approximation of the Euclidean distance $d(x, y, z)$ of a point (x, y, z) near the surface is given by:

$$d(x, y, z) = \frac{f(x, y, z) - c}{\|\nabla f(x, y, z)\|}. \tag{1}$$

From this signed distance estimate $d(x, y, z)$, a scalar field $v(x, y, z)$ can be derived which expresses the implicit surface as a fuzzy membership function:

$$v(x, y, z; w) = \begin{cases} 1, & \text{if } d(x, y, z) < -w, \\ \left(\frac{1}{2} - \frac{d(x,y,z)}{2w}\right), & \text{if } |d(x, y, z)| \leq w, \\ 0, & \text{if } d(x, y, z) > w. \end{cases} \tag{2}$$

When traversing the surface along the surface normal vector, $v(x, y, z; w)$ describes a gradual, approximately linear transition (width $2w$) between the state 'inside' ($v(x, y, z; w) = 1$) to 'outside' ($v(x, y, z; w) = 0$).

However, single implicit object models are intrinsically limited in their descriptive shape range. To extend the descriptive power of single implicit surfaces, a well established framework is provided by Constructive Solid Geometry (CSG) [4], which allows the description of a 3D object shape by decomposing it into a Boolean combination of simpler shapes. CSG is often implemented as a tree structure, in which the leaf nodes contain a shape descriptor of the shape primitives and the internal nodes implement the Boolean set operators. All nodes contain a transformation, which translates, rotates and scales the shape modeled in that particular node with respect to the other objects in the tree.

Classically, CSG is implemented in the form of a Boolean point classification function, which classifies a point to inside or outside of the object. By replacing the crisp Boolean set operators by fuzzy set equivalents, CSG is applicable to express a composite shape as a membership function. The following fuzzy set operators were adopted from [5]:

- Complement: $\sim v(x, y, z) = 1 - v(x, y, z)$
- Union: $v_1(x, y, z) \cup v_2(x, y, z) = \max(v_1(x, y, z), v_2(x, y, z))$
- Intersection: $v_1(x, y, z) \cap v_2(x, y, z) = \min(v_1(x, y, z), v_2(x, y, z))$

Note that for two primitives with equal surface gradient polarity (e.g. pointing outward), the combined shape's polarity is pointing outward as well.

From $v(x, y, z; w)$ a boundary membership functional $b(x, y, z; w)$ can be derived, which is maximal exactly on the boundary surface (see Fig. 1):

$$b(x, y, z; w) = 1 - 2|v(x, y, z; w) - \frac{1}{2}|. \qquad (3)$$

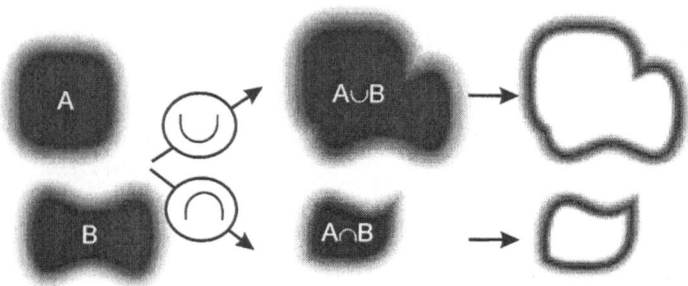

Fig. 1. Examples of the application of fuzzy set operators to two fuzzy implicit curves

2.2   Anatomical Thorax Model Construction

By combining a number of fuzzy implicit surfaces with continuous CSG, a coarse, 3D shape description of a moderately complex scene can be constructed in the form of a potential function $b(x, y, z; w)$. A set of such implicit shape templates of the major organs in the thorax has been constructed in the following steps:

1. Data acquisition: a gated transverse MR image volume of a normal thorax was acquired, in which the contours of the heart, both lungs, thoracic wall, liver and spleen were drawn manually. Contours were subsampled to form regularly tesselated 3D point meshes, which were manually subdivided into approximately convex surface patches.
2. Implicit surface fitting: the overall shape of these point grids was modeled by fitting an implicit surface to the point data. In this work the hyperquadric shape models [6] of six terms were selected, mainly because hyperquadrics compactly describe a large range of non-symmetric 3D shapes.
3. Organ model construction: for each organ the fitted primitives were grouped into small CSG-trees, forming a three-dimensional shape template for each organ. In the top node of each organ CSG-tree, a polarity direction was defined for the organ surface normal based on the three-dimensional image gradient direction of that particular organ in a typical thoracic MR volume. For organs containing air (both lungs), the model normal vector was defined as pointing inwards. For all other organ models (heart, liver, spleen and thoracic surface), the model polarity was defined as pointing outwards.
4. The separate organ templates were hierarchically grouped into two scene trees: a tree describing the lungs, heart, cardiac ventricles, liver spleen and the thoracic outer surface and a separate tree merely describing the tissue-air surfaces in the thorax (both lungs and the exterior thorax wall).

2.3 Model Matching

The model–image registration is based on the transitional boundaries between air and other tissues in thoracic volume scans for two reasons. Firstly, air is relatively robustly automatically separable from other tissues in a thoracic MR volume. Secondly, in a thoracic MR scan the image gradient vector in tissue-air surfaces can be defined to point towards the air, i.e. for the lungs as pointing inwards, and for the torso as pointing outwards.

Given a set of N points located on the transitions between tissue and air in a thoracic MR dataset. By combining the model-contained distance information with the image gradient direction, the following energy functional can be formulated, which has a strong minimum when the tissue–air model is registered to a feature pattern congruent to the model template shapes:

$$E(\vartheta_{node}) = \sum_{i=1}^{N} (1 - q_i(x_i, y_i, z_i)b(\vartheta_{node}; x_i, y_i, z_i))^2 . \tag{4}$$

$\vartheta_{node} = (s_x, s_y, s_z, t_x, t_y, t_z, r_x, r_y, r_z)$ represents the affine scaling $(s_{x,y,z})$, translation $(t_{x,y,z})$, and orientation $(r_{x,y,z})$ parameters in a CSG node, and (x_i, y_i, z_i) is a candidate boundary point. The weighting function $q_i(x_i, y_i, z_i)$ is defined as a switch selecting feature points in which the local hyperquadric gradient $\nabla_{model}(x_i, y_i, z_i)$ and the image gradient $\nabla_{image}(x_i, y_i, z_i)$ point in the same direction, within a margin φ.

$$q_i(x_i, y_i, z_i) = \begin{cases} 1, \text{ if } \nabla_{image}(x_i, y_i, z_i) \bullet \nabla_{model}(x_i, y_i, z_i) > \cos \varphi, \\ 0, \text{ if } \nabla_{image}(x_i, y_i, z_i) \bullet \nabla_{model}(x_i, y_i, z_i) < \cos \varphi. \end{cases} \tag{5}$$

The actual model-image matching is performed in the following steps:

1. Feature point detection. To detect points on the tissue–air boundaries, a simple adaptive thresholding was implemented, based on a characteristic 'air' peak in the lower gray value range in the histogram of a thoracic MR volume.
2. Initial model positioning. To initialize the matching, a fixed initial parameter set for the top node pose and scale parameters was selected. This parameter set positions the model in the middle of the scanner bore, aligned with its long axis. Angle parameter φ in (5) was set to 60 degrees.
3. Energy minimization. The energy minimization can be formulated as a hierarchical pose and scale estimation. First, $E(\vartheta_{node})$ is minimized for the top node affine parameters ϑ_{node} using a gradient descend method, therefore simultaneously translating, rotating and scaling the whole model until a minimum is reached. Subsequently, the top node parameters are frozen, and $E(\vartheta_{node})$ is further minimized with respect to ϑ_{node} of one of the subtrees for a single organ or a combination of organs. By repeating this procedure throughout a number of tree levels, the match is refined in each matching step. In the top node matching step, boundary width parameter w was set to 50 mm, whereas in all subsequent refining steps for lower tree levels w was set to 20 mm. In Fig. 2, an example is given of a matching result.

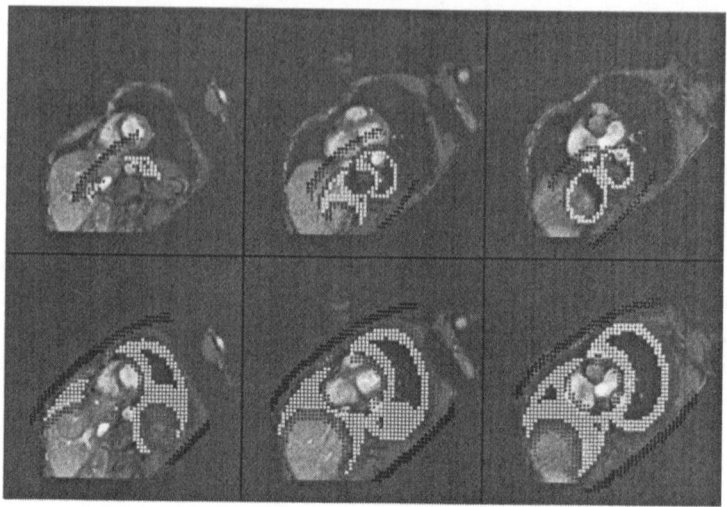

Fig. 2. A matching result for a gated short-axis cardiac MR-set. In the top row, the initial model is projected on three slice levels, whereas the bottom row shows the model after matching. The displayed boundaries are 2D cross-sections through a 3D model

3   Clinical Validation and Discussion

The model matching procedure was validated on 20 thoracic volume scans routinely acquired from 17 patients with various cardiac pathologies and 3 normal subjects. To assess the accuracy of the method for both lungs and the heart, image volumes were acquired containing all these organs, in this study the so–called localizers or scout views. To investigate the method's dependency on the MR imaging system, the studies were acquired at two centers using different MR–scanners: a GE Signa-LX real-time CVMR scanner[1] and a Philips Gyroscan NT 5[2]. Image sets consisted of 27 images (9 sagittal, 9 coronal, 9 transverse). On each image set, the model-image registration was performed fully automatically.

To quantitatively assess the accuracy of the matching results, 9 frames were selected from each image volume by an independent observer. In all these images, two observers manually traced the contours of the left lung, right lung and the epicard. Two quantitative measures were calculated to express the accuracy of the model-predicted contours. Since the model only coarsely describes thoracic anatomy, it was expected that local details possibly drawn by the observers (vessels, small local shape variations) are missed by the model. Therefore, for each organ contour a quality measure was defined as the percentage of the contour length correctly predicted by the model within a 20 mm margin on each side of the organ surface. Second, for the correctly localized contour parts, the average distance of the contours to the corresponding model surface was calculated.

---

[1] University of Iowa Hospitals and Clinics, Iowa City, USA
[2] Leiden University Medical Center, Leiden, The Netherlands

The results of this validation study can be summarized as follows:

- In all 20 cases, the automated matching converged to a semantically correct solution, demonstrating matching robustness with respect to initial position under clinically realistic circumstances. The influence of large amounts of spurious feature points generated in the low-level boundary detection step was negligible, since only feature patterns congruent to the model template shapes influenced the matching energy function. Furthermore, the matching was found to be scanner- independent for image sets acquired with the body coil of the scanner.
- On average, 90 % of the contour length of the manually drawn lung and epicardial contours was localized within a 20 mm margin (worst case: 79%). As expected, in cases where the observers had drawn a structure not present in the model, these contour parts were missed by the model. A large part of the failure rate for a contour (0-21%) could be attributed to vessel structures in the cardiac in- and outflow tract, which were not included in the model.
- The average distance of the contour parts contained within 20 mm of the automatically identified surfaces ranged from 4-8 mm.
- In general the results from both observers for the entire study corresponded well, though in some cases there was a slight discrepancy.

The computation time required to match the model increases approximately linearly with the number of images. For a scout view consisting of 27 images, the matching procedure took 4-6 minutes on a Sun Ultrasparc 2 workstation. Initial experiments were also performed where the model was matched to three images (1 sagittal, 1 coronal and 1 transverse), and qualitatively only minor differences in the matching results were visible. In these cases the matching procedure took less than 30 seconds. Based on the presented validation, it can be concluded that with the described anatomical modeling and matching method, a robust estimate of the approximate location of the heart and lung surfaces in a thoracic MR image set can be obtained fully automatically. Though the modeling method lacks local detail, on average 90% of the contour length of the lung- and epicardial contours was localized within 20 mm, with an average positional error of 6 mm.

References

1. Christensen, G.E., Joshi, S.C., Miller, M.I.: Volumetric Transformation of Brain Anatomy. IEEE Trans. Med. Imag. **16** (1997) 864–877
2. Székely, G., Kelemen, A., Brechbühler, C., Gerig, G.: Segmentation of 2-D and 3-D Objects from MRI Volume Data using Constrained Elastic Deformations of Flexible Fourier Contour and Surface Models. Med. Imag. Anal. **1** (1996) 19–34
3. Hill,A., Brett,A.D., Taylor,C.J.: Automatic Landmark Identification Using a New Method of Non-rigid Correspondence. Proc. IPMI 1997, Poultney, USA 483–488
4. Requicha, A.A.G., Voelcker, H.B.: Solid Modeling: A Historical Summary and Contemporary Assessment. IEEE Comp. Graph. & Applic. **2** (1982) 9–24
5. Zadeh, A.L.: Fuzzy sets. Information Control **8** (1965) 338–353
6. Kumar, S., Han, S., Goldgof, D., Bowyer, K.: On Recovering Hyperquadrics from Range Data. IEEE Trans. PAMI **17** (1995) 1079–1083

Detection of the Central Mass of Spiculated Lesions - Signature Normalisation and Model Data Aspects

Reyer Zwiggelaar[1], Christopher J. Taylor[2], and Caroline M. E. Rubin[3]

[1] Division of Computer Science, University of Portsmouth, Portsmouth, UK
reyer@sis.port.ac.uk
[2] Wolfson Image Analysis Unit, University of Manchester, Manchester, UK
[3] Breast Screening Unit, Royal South Hants Hospital, Southampton, UK

Abstract. We describe a method for labelling image structure based on non-linear scale-orientation signatures which can be used as a basis for robust pixel classification. The effect of normalisation of the signatures is discussed as a means to improve classification robustness with respect to grey-level variations. In addition, model data selection and scale normalisation are investigated as a means to improve the robustness of detection with respect to the scale of structures.

1 Introduction

We are interested in the detection of structures in images. We assume that the position of these structures is unpredictable and that they will be embedded in a background texture. We describe an approach based on the construction of a non-linear scale-orientation signature at each pixel. This provides a very rich description of local structure which is robust and locally stationary. Given this description, standard statistical classification methods can be used - we give results for a linear classifier. To improve detection with respect to local grey-level variation and scale change intensity and scale normalisation are investigated. The effects of different strategies for selecting training data are also explored.

2 Scale–Orientation Signatures

A Directional Recursive Median Filter (DRMF) performs a smoothing operation that removes (sieves) image peaks or troughs of less than a chosen size [1]. By applying sieves of increasing size to an image and taking the difference between the output image from adjacent size sieves, it is possible to isolate image features of a specific size. Signatures at different positions on the same structure are similar (local stationarity) and the interaction between adjacent structures is minimised. The signature, $\Psi(\sigma, \theta)$, is a 2-D array in which the columns represent measurements for the same orientation and the rows represent measurements for the same scale. For typical synthetic examples of signatures see Fig. 1.

A. Kuba et al. (Eds.): IPMI'99, LNCS 1613, pp. 406–411, 1999.

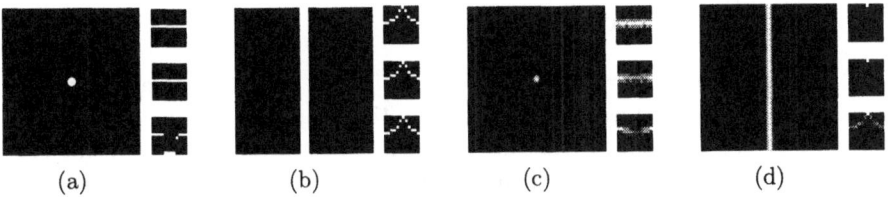

Fig. 1. Some synthetic examples of multi-scale DRMF signatures, where the larger four images show (a) a binary blob, (b) a binary linear structure, (c) a Gaussian blob, and (d) a Gaussian linear structure. The twelve smaller images are the scale-orientation signatures for the centre pixel (top), for a pixel at the extreme edge of the structure (bottom) and for a pixel in between these two extremes (middle). In the scale-orientation signature images, scale is on the vertical axis (with the finest scale at the bottom) and orientation on the horizontal

3 Statistical Methods

The objective of the work is to classify pixels, that is to label each pixel as belonging to a certain type of image structure. Since any method is likely to be imperfect it is useful to explore a range of compromises between false negative errors (poor sensitivity) and false positive errors (poor specificity). Detection can be performed by thresholding a class probability image. The probability density for an observation vector $\mathbf{x}_j$ for a pixel of class i which is given by

$$p(\mathbf{x}_j|i) = \frac{1}{(2\pi)^{n/2}|\mathbf{C}_i|^{1/2}} \exp\left(\frac{-\delta_{ij}}{2}\right) \qquad (1)$$

where δ_{ij} is the Mahalanobis distance to the class mean and $\mathbf{C}_i$ is the the covariance matrix of class i. Applying Bayes theorem a probability image for class i (e.g. blob) out of η classes is found by calculating, for each pixel

$$p(i|\mathbf{x}_j) = \frac{p(\mathbf{x}_j|i)\,p(i)}{\sum_\eta p(\mathbf{x}_j|\eta)\,p(\eta)}. \qquad (2)$$

4 Signature Preprocessing

Principal component analysis can be used to obtain data generalisation and efficiency for classification purposes, by reducing the dimensionality of the data, instead of using the full signature information [2].

We intensity normalise signatures since there is no reason to believe that high-contrast features are more important than those of low contrast. Indeed, it is particularly important to detect small, low contrast lesions of characteristic appearance. Each column in each signature is normalised independently.

We would like to treat different size features equally. A change in scale appears in the signatures as a vertical shift. The effects of such a shift can be reduced by taking the FT of each column and using the amplitude term.

5   Mammographic Data

The mammographic data we have used consists of 54 mammograms, of which 27 contain a spiculated lesion and the other 27 are normal mammograms from a sequential set. The outlines of all the lesions have been annotated by an expert radiologist. The sizes of the abnormalities range from 5 to 30 mm (mean=13.4 mm).

We build statistical models based on a subset of all the signatures in the dataset. The first approach is based on a subset of the data which uses all the signatures within the abnormalities and an equal number (150 per mammogram in this case) randomly selected from the normal images (this will be referred to as the basic signature dataset). This means that the subset contains a larger number of signatures from the larger sized lesions than from the smaller ones. In a second approach, to remove bias towards signatures from larger lesions only 150 signatures were selected from each abnormal mammogram.

6   Signature Classification — Training Data

The ROC results for the basic signature dataset are shown in Fig. 2a. These indicate that the PCA based model has an overall better performance regardless of the normalisation approach used. A second observation is that the $\mathcal{FT}$ based normalisation on its own does not do better than classification on the original data, but that normalisation or normalisation in combination with the $\mathcal{FT}$ approach provides overall better classification results. Finally, if we compare the 85% PCA based model results with the 100% based model results an overall better classification performance is achieved by the former.

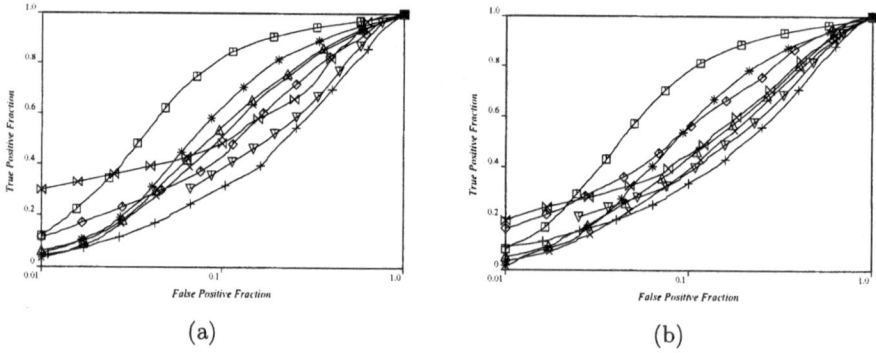

Fig. 2. ROC results for signatures based on: (a) the basic signatures model, (b) the 150 signatures model. Here ⋈: 85% PCA data, △: normalised 85% PCA data, □: $\mathcal{FT}$ of the normalised 85% PCA data, ◇: $\mathcal{FT}$ of the 85% PCA data, ▽: 100% data, ×: normalised 100% data, ∗: $\mathcal{FT}$ of the normalised 100% data, and +: $\mathcal{FT}$ of the 100% data

The ROC results for the model based on the data containing 150 signatures from each mammogram are shown in Fig. 2b. Again, the 85% PCA data based model provides superior classification results when compared with the 100% data based model. Also, the best classification is based on the 85% PCA based model for which the signatures have been normalised and subsequently a $\mathcal{FT}$ was taken.

7   Probability Images

Based on the results presented in Sect. 6, we have applied the derived models for the basic signatures dataset, the 150 signature dataset, and the $\mathcal{FT}$ of the normalised signatures of both these datasets to all the pixels in all the mammograms. Some typical examples of probability images (see Sect. 3) are shown in Fig. 3.

When comparing the 85% PCA and 100% models the probability images based on the 85% PCA data produce clearer results with fewer disconnected regions. The lesion is detected with a high probability in the models based on the $\mathcal{FT}$ of the normalised signature data (with a high level of small false positive regions).

8   Classification

Pixel classification results based on the probability images were a general confirmation of those results presented in Sect. 6.

Instead of performing pixel classification, the probability images can be used for region classification which is more appropriate for the envisioned prompting environment. Normally, probability images are thresholded and regions are grown based on the resulting binary images [1]. This is done for a number of thresholds to obtain points on a FROC curve. However, one drawback of such an approach is that for low threshold values large regions of the breast are detected which are non-localised and produce misleading results.

To improve upon this approach we have segmented the probability images prior to thresholding and the resulting regions are preserved in the subsequent classification results. To obtain the segmentation we have found convex regions (peaks) in the probability images (after applying a morphological smoothing).

In Fig. 4 the FROC results for the basic signature model are shown. Results for detected lesions larger than 4 mm in diameter (Fig. 4a) and larger than 8 mm in diameter (Fig. 4b) are shown. The first observation is that the method performs better for the larger lesions. Again there is an improved performance for the $\mathcal{FT}$ of the normalised data versus the basic signature data, and for the 85% PCA data versus the 100% data.

The FROC results for the 150 signature data are shown in Fig. 5. In this case there is a larger distinction between the detected lesion size. This means that the performance for the larger lesions was not as good as for the smaller lesions, whilst the results shown in Fig. 4 show not as much size dependence. These unexpected results (as the 150 signature models were expected to be less

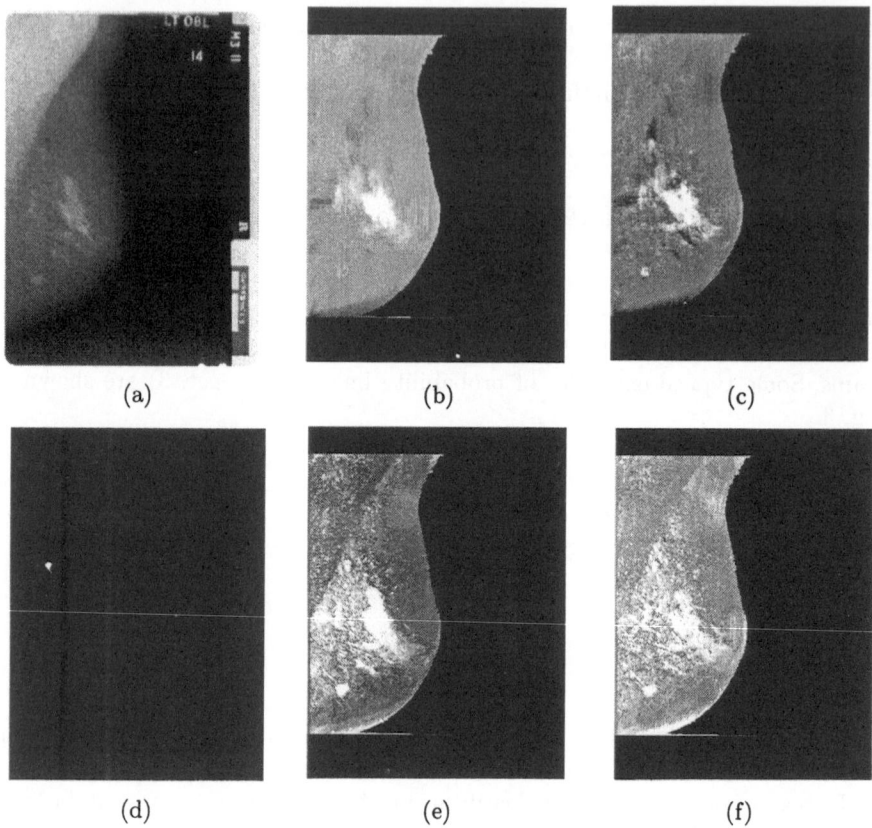

(a)   (b)   (c)

(d)   (e)   (f)

Fig. 3. Example of applying the classification approach to a mammogram. (a) original mammogram, (b) 85% PCA model based probability image, (c) 100% model based probability image, (d) lesion annotation, (e) $\mathcal{FT}$ of normalised 85% PCA model based probability image, (f) $\mathcal{FT}$ of normalised 100% model based probability image. The probability images are displayed on log-scale, with the white representing 1.0 and black representing 2×10^{-9}

size dependent) might be an artifact of our new approach to obtaining FROC curves and will need further investigation.

9   Conclusions

We have described a number of methods to improve detection of mammographic lesions based on scale-orientation signatures. These methods involve the normalisation of the scale-orientation signatures. A method incorporating both intensity and scale normalisation proved to be most successful in the classification of mammographic data.

It seems that the results presented are fairly independent of the choice of data on which the models are based (the best results are obtained for models based on taking all signatures within the lesions into account).

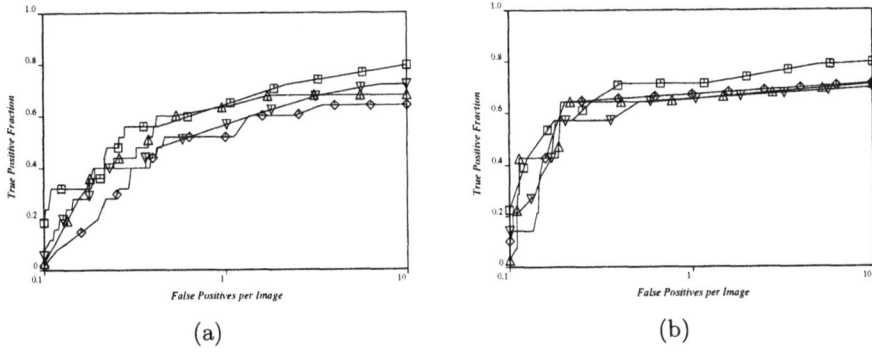

(a)   (b)

Fig. 4. FROC results for mammograms based on the basic signatures model: (a) 4 mm and (b) 8 mm detection area, where $\triangle$: 85% PCA data, $\square$: $\mathcal{FT}$ of the normalised 85% PCA data, $\diamond$: 100% data, and $\triangledown$: $\mathcal{FT}$ of the normalised 100% data

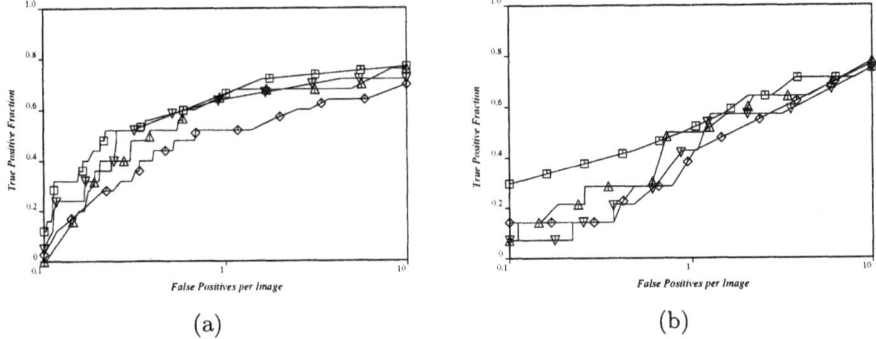

(a)   (b)

Fig. 5. FROC results for mammograms based on the 150 signatures model: (a) 4 mm and (b) 8 mm detection area, where $\triangle$: 85% PCA data, $\square$: $\mathcal{FT}$ of the normalised 85% PCA data, $\diamond$: 100% data, and $\triangledown$: $\mathcal{FT}$ of the normalised 100% data

Basicly, the approach described so far is a method for the detection of blob-like structures in mammograms (or other images). However, to reduce the number of false positive detections we are investigating a reclassification approach. With such an approach a second statistical model would be build based on the data which has a high probability of being a blob. This would result in a two-class blob-model representing blobs in normal and abnormal mammograms.

References

1. Zwiggelaar, R., et al.: Model-based detection of spiculated lesions in mammograms. Medical Image Analysis **3** (1999) 39–62
2. Jolliffe, I.T.: Principal Component Analysis. Springer Verlag (1986)

Noise Estimation and Measures for Detection of Clustered Microcalcifications

Márton Csapodi[1], Ágota Petrányi[2], György Liszka[2], Ákos Zarándy[1], and Tamás Roska[1]

[1] Analogic and Neural Computing Laboratory, Computer and Automation Institute, Hungarian Academy of Sciences, P.O.B.63, H-1502, Budapest, Hungary
Csapodi@sztaki.hu
[2] Department of Diagnostic Radiology, National Institute of Oncology, Kékgolyó u. 13, H-1126, Budapest, Hungary

Abstract. Image transforms used to preprocess mammogram images and highly selective microcalcification feature extraction are analyzed in this paper. It is demonstrated that the results obtained by the proposed method (especially at high true positive rates) exceed the specificity levels of other measures for which FROC analysis is provided using the same public (Nijmegen) database.

1 Introduction

We have based our research on the results of N. Karssemeijer, who has described in [1,2] a method for an iso-precision scale transform of mammograms and the clusterization of individual microcalcifications using an iterated statistical model. During development of our algorithms we employed the images used in [2] and made available for public use (Nijmegen database), but we have also tested them on a larger set of mammograms digitized using our system at the National Institute of Oncology (Budapest, Hungary).

We have found that the preprocessing step has a major impact on the detection results as is also stated in [2]. Therefore we have first compared different image transforms in terms of their effect on the detectability of individual microcalcifications. We also investigated whether the iso-precision scale transform can be further improved by a subsequent locally adaptive noise equalization transform. We report on our experiments and findings in Sect. 2.

With respect to the detection of individual microcalcifications, several methods have been proposed and studied so far. In this paper we propose one single feature which we have found to be very selective for the detection of microcalcifications. This is based on a local contrast measure we have specifically designed to characterize microcalcifications. By using two additional measures (a compactness measure and the result of a line detector) the results can be improved even further, but we have found that the effectiveness of our algorithm is primarily based on the high selectivity of the contrast measure with respect to microcalcifications. The proposed contrast measure is defined in Section 3. In the same

A. Kuba et al. (Eds.): IPMI'99, LNCS 1613, pp. 412–417, 1999.

section we compare our results to the results of N. Karssemeijer and others' who have provided FROC (free-response receiver operating characteristics) analysis of their methods based on the Nijmegen image database. We did not implement the statistical clusterization process described in [2]. This facilitates comparison because most detection methods do not utilize spatial interaction models and also in [2] the FROC analysis for the detection of individual microcalcifications is provided.

Due to the reduced scale of this publication we only mention that the presented method for microcalcification detection and other image processing functionalities are integrated into a complex system called Analogic Mammogram Diagnostic Workstation [3] which is fully equipped for mammogram digitization, archiving, processing and display. The system is based upon a database handling program for handling patients' personal and clinical data, which has been used in everyday practice for more than 3 years at the National Institute of Oncology (Budapest, Hungary). The system was made suitable for automated film digitization, archiving on CDs and indexing. We have developed a general purpose graphical interface which can be accessed from the database program for image display, and hosts the image processing algorithms.

Our ultimate object is to integrate with our system a specific hardware tool, the CASTLE chip [4], which is expected to be a very high-speed image processor and is now under development at our laboratory. The chip will operate on the principle of cellular neural networks [5].

2   Space-variant Noise Equalization

Processing or display of digitized mammogram images is usually preceded by some transformation. A logarithmic transform of intensity values is general for digitized film images, but several other transforms (global or adaptive) have also been investigated so far. The iso-precision transform demonstrated by N. Karssemeijer in [1] and applied for noise equalization and microcalcification detection in mammograms [2] means that the noise level is estimated as a function of the gray-scale intensity of the original image, and a transformation is applied which equalizes the specific noise measure. In this section we evaluate the effect of different image transforms on the performance of microcalcification detection. We compare a global linear transform (LIN), logarithmic transform (LOG), adaptive histogram equalization (AHE) [6], iso-precision transform (IPA), adaptive noise equalization (ANE), and the succession of iso-precision transform and adaptive noise equalization (IPA+ANE).

The difference between IPA and ANE is that while IPA uses a global estimate of noise level for each mammogram to normalize image features, the noise level is computed locally in case of ANE. Therefore the noise estimate for ANE has to be chosen carefully. It has to be avoided that areas where microcalcification clusters are to be found produce a higher noise measure only because of the presence of microcalcifications. We have found that a statistical filter is very little correlated with the presence of microcalcifications which replaces only local minimum values with the closest (higher or equal) intensity value in their neighborhood. The noise estimate is then computed from the filtered and original image difference averaged over a 21-by-21 window.

The comparison of the different transforms is performed by determining the number of detections made inside the marked clusters at a fixed number of total detections for each image. This can be adjusted by the proper setting of a contrast threshold. Here we used the local contrast measure defined in [2]. False negative clusters (i.e., in which less than two detections were made) are also considered in the comparison.

The comparison results for 500 detections per image are shown in Table 1. It is clear from this list that there is no significant difference between the IPA, ANE and IPA+ANE noise estimation techniques. Indeed, more detailed analysis shows that some of the images perform better with the IPA transform, others with ANE noise estimation. This is true for higher contrast thresholds (i.e., fewer objects detected) as well. The logarithmic transform is found to be least appropriate for microcalcification detection with the highest number of false negatives and the lowest in-cluster/out-cluster detection ratio. The AHE transform may radically increase contrast in darker areas of the images. Therefore the threshold level has to be set relatively high in order to detect only 500 objects per image, and some clusters will be missed at places where the contrast stretching was not so extensive. The LIN transform gives the highest in-cluster/out-cluster detection ratio, which can be explained by the fact that all the other transforms tend to increase the contrast of darker areas, while microcalcification clusters are most often to be found in brighter regions. However, some clusters in darker regions will hardly be detected after this transform. If we want to obtain low false negative rates, the best choice seems to be one of the methods based on noise equalization (IPA, ANE, IPA+ANE). Because the look-up tables of the IPA transform are publicly available for the images in the Nijmegen database, in the following the IPA-transformed Nijmegen images are analyzed.

Table 1. Comparison of different preprocessing transforms using the 40 images in the Nijmegen database. Results for linear (LIN), logarithmic (LOG) transforms, adaptive histogram equalization (AHE), the iso-precision transform (IPA), adaptive noise equalization (ANE) and the combination of the latter two (IPA+ANE) are shown. For a fixed number of detections per image (500), we calculated the average detections inside marked clusters and the number of missed clusters among the 104 clusters marked in the images

	LIN	LOG	AHE	IPA	ANE	IPA+ANE
detected objects in each image	500	500	500	500	500	500
in-cluster detection average	95	61	76	75	72	75
total number of FN clusters	4	7	2	0	0	0

3 FROC Analysis of a Contrast Measure for Microcalcification Detection

The local image feature we propose for measuring the contrast of a candidate microcalcification is computed as follows. Starting from the 'center' of the microcalcification, we apply a region growing algorithm which adds one pixel to the actual set of pixels in every iteration. The 'center'is the brightest pixel of the region, and at each turn, the brightest pixel is added in the neighborhood of the actual set.

During the growing process, the average gray level of pixels within the region (m_{in}) is calculated along with the average gray level of pixels in the neighborhood of the region (m_{out}). The contrast measure is defined to be the maximum difference m_{in}-m_{out} during the iteration. Because the shape of microcalcifications vary a lot, this single measure may describe the contrast of this amorphous object better than a set of standard spatial and spectral domain measures. The quality of the proposed measure is demonstrated by FROC analysis in the next section.

The power of the proposed local contrast measure in its ability to detect individual microcalcifications can be analyzed by constructing FROC (free-response receiver operating characteristic) curves [7]. We calculate the true positive fraction (TPF) and false positive (FP) clusters as defined by N. Karssemeijer [2]. However, we mention that a cluster is expected to have at least 5 microcalcifications over a 1 cm^2 area in [8], and others apply even higher limits.

We have found that – besides the local contrast – it is convenient to characterize the microcalcifications with a normalized second order central moment computed over a 9-by-9 window around the object, and a binary output line detector. These measures depend on the spatial distribution of intensity levels rather than on their contrast. In Fig. 1 we show the detection results of experiments for all 40 mammograms in the Nijmegen database. The results were obtained by using the local contrast measure (cont) and its combinations with the second order moment (m) and the binary output of the line detector (l). The following combined measures were formulated heuristically:

1. cont/m
2. cont-l
3. cont/m-l

As we have stated before, we did not take into consideration spatial distribution of microcalcification candidates. Therefore, comparisons have to be performed at the level of the detection of individual microcalcifications. In Fig. 2 we compare our results to the results of N. Karssemeijer [2], D. Meersman et al. [9], and Strickland et al. [10]. It is clear from the comparison of FROC curves that at high true positive rates our measures for microcalcification detection are superior to the measures used by the other three methods. In the same figure we also provide detection results if images from our own database are used. We have digitized 315 images of 114 patients using a Cobrascan CX-312T (RDI Inc.) X-ray film scanner at 300dpi spatial and 12 bit intensity resolution, of which 59 images contained 75 microcalcification clusters. The FROC curve

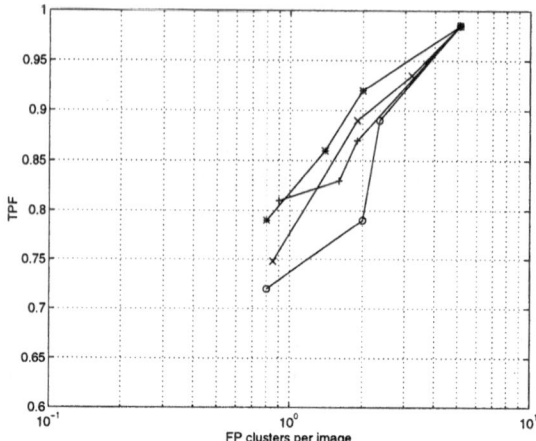

Fig. 1. FROC analysis. The four curves show results obtained by different combinations of our measures: cont (o), cont/m (+), cont-l (x) and cont/m-l (*)

shown applies to these positive cases. The FP rate changes only slightly if the rest of the images are also processed. Intensity resolution was reduced to 8 bits after the ANE transform.

4   Conclusions

We have analyzed a set of preprocessing transforms with respect to their efficiency in microcalcification detection. Based on the results shown in Table 1, we may conclude that the iso-precision transform of intensities and the estimation of local noise (adaptive noise equalization) have very similar effects, even if they are performed one after the other. We have defined three local image features, a contrast measure, a second order moment (compactness), and a line detector. We have designed these measures specifically for characterizing microcalcification candidates, and our results demonstrated in Figs. 1 and 2 show that they perform better than other methods which were tested using the same image database. The quality improvement is most striking at high true positive rates. We also provide test results using a larger set of mammograms.

Acknowledgments

The Analogic Mammogram Diagnostic Workstation was developed in the framework of the 'Secondary Prevention' component of the ESzM Project (3597-HU) financed by a World Bank loan. Images were provided (partly) by courtesy of the National Expert and Training Center for Breast Cancer Screening at the Department of Radiology at the University of Nijmegen, the Netherlands.

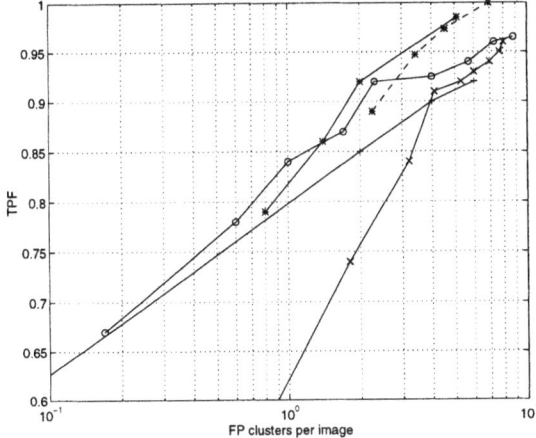

Fig. 2. Comparison of FROC curves obtained for the detection of individual microcalcifications. Our results and other three results are shown based on the same image database: Karssemeijer (o), Meersman (+), Strickland (x) and our results (*). Broken lines show results obtained using our database

References

1. Karssemeijer, N. and van Erning, L.J.Th.O.: Iso-precision scaling of digitized mammograms to facilitate image analysis. Medical Imaging, Proc. SPIE-91: Image Processing, (1991) 166–177
2. Karssemeijer, N.: Adaptive noise equalization and recognition of microcalcification clusters in mammograms. Int. Journal of Patt. Recognition and Artificial Intelligence **7/6** (1993) 1357–1376
3. Kék, L., Liszka, Gy., Petrányi, Á., Zarándy, Á., Bölöni, L.: Mammográfiás szűrőállomásokhoz telepített analogikai munkahely adatkezelése (in Hungarian). Magyar Onkológia **42** (1998) 109–120
4. Zarándy, Á., Keresztes, P. Roska T. and Szolgay, P.: CASTLE: an emulated digital CNN architecture; design issues, new results. in Proc. 5th International Conference on Electronics, Circuits and Systems, ICECS-98 (1998) 199–202
5. Chua, L.O.: CNN - a vision of complexity. Int. Journal of Bifurcation and Chaos **7** (1997) 2219–2425
6. Russ, J.C.: The Image Processing Handbook. CRC Press (1995)
7. Chakraborty, D.P. and Winter, L.H.L.: Free response methodology: alternate analysis and a new observer–performance experiment. Radiology **174** (1990) 873–881
8. Chapman, S. and Nakielny, R.: Aids to Radiological Differential Diagnosis. 3rd edition, W.B. Sanders Co. Ltd. (1995) p.350
9. Meersman, D., Scheunders, P. and VanDyck, D.: Detection of microcalcifications using neural networks. in Proc. Int Workshop on Dig. Mammography (1998)
10. Strickland, R.N. and Hahn, H.I.: Wavelet transforms for detecting microcalcifications in mammograms. IEEE Trans. on Medical Imaging **15/2** (1996) 218–229

Measuring the Spatial Homogeneity in Corneal Endotheliums by Means of a Randomization Test

M. E. Díaz[1] and G. Ayala[2]

[1] Instituto de Robótica
[2] Departamento de Estadística e Investigación Operativa
Universidad de Valencia
Avda. Vicent Andrés Estellés, s/n. 46100-Burjasot, Spain
{Elena.Diaz, Guillermo.Ayala}@uv.es

Abstract. Quantification of regularity of cell sizes and the spatial arrangement of cells in corneal endotheliums becomes of a great importance associated to stress situations such as cataract surgery, corneal transplantation or implantation of intra-ocular lenses. A new index of regularity of the spatial distribution of cell sizes in corneal endotheliums is proposed. The corneal endothelium is described by means of a spatial marked point pattern (the cell centroids marked with the cell areas). The hypothesis of no dependency between mark and locations is tested by a Monte Carlo test. The new index is the p-value of the test validating the hypothesis.

Pairs of endotheliums from different eyes of the same person are compared in terms of the traditional measures (density, hexagonality and coefficient of variation) and the new index. Results show how the index proposed can discriminate subtle morphological changes that cannot be detected by the commonly used indices.

1 Introduction

The deepest part of the human cornea is a single layer of $400,000$ to $500,000$ cells called the *corneal endothelium*. Cells are $4-6$ μm in height and 20 μm in width, and their posterior surfaces are predominantly hexagonal when viewed under *specular microscopy*. This technique is used to study 'in vivo' the size, shape and number of endothelial cells [8]. The normal endothelial cell density is 3000 to 3500 cells per mm^2 in young adults. This number decreases by about two thirds in elderly patients. The endothelial cell population also decreases following stress situations such as cataract surgery, corneal transplantation and implantation of intra-ocular lenses. When endothelial loss occurs through aging or trauma, the endothelial response is enlargement and sliding of the existing cells to cover the area previously occupied by the lost cells. As a result of the spreading of the cells, their diameters double their normal size and cells lose their hexagonal appearance. When a critical cell density is lost corneal edema results, which leads to a pain and poor vision. Some geometrical cell models have been proposed which contribute to the study of tissue morphogenesis. Interesting general references are [2,5,7].

A. Kuba et al. (Eds.): IPMI'99, LNCS 1613, pp. 418–423, 1999.

Three quantities are commonly used to describe the corneal endothelium: cell density, hexagonality (percentage of cells with 6 neighbors) and the coefficient of variation of cell areas. Cell density is a size parameter (number of cells per unit area) meanwhile the other two are measures of variability (spatial regularity and variation of the cell areas). The goal of this paper is to analyze the spatial distribution of cell sizes and to propose a new index that quantifies its variability.

One specular image per eye has been obtained with a specular microscope (Topcon). A software tool provided by Topcon (Imagenet) was used in order to process the original images. Figure 1 shows some examples. A color CCD camera (charge coupled device, XC-711P, Sony, Tokyo, Japan) captured these photographs of cells. The output of the camera was fed into a PIP-512/1024 video digitizer (Matrox Electronic Systems Limited, Quebec, Canada). All images were acquired at the same scale. Preprocessing of the original grey level images was designed in order to obtain a labelled binary image in which each cell corresponds with a different connected component so that they can be analyzed separately. A software tool was developed by using Vista version 2.1. [1]

Section 2 proposes a new index that measures the spatial homogeneity of the cell areas based on the theory of marked spatial point processes. In Sect. 3 this new index is compared with the three usual indices. Finally, conclusions are discussed in Sect. 4.

2 Describing the Corneal Endothelium

The aim of this work is to analyze the cell size distribution by taking into account the spatial arrangement of cells. We know N cells completely (i.e., non touching the frame). The n-th cell is located by its centroid, s_n, and its size is measured by its area, $Z(s_n)$. The part of corneal endothelium under study is described by means of the points s_n's *marked* with the areas $Z(s_n)$'s. The set $\{(s_n, Z(s_n))\}_{n=1}^N$ is a marked point pattern. Different parts of the same corneal endothelium produce different marked point patterns. From a probabilistic point of view, it can be considered as a realization of a marked point process, i.e., a random mechanism that produces a random set of points marked with random values. A very good introduction to this subject can be found in [3]. Regular areas uniformly located within the tissue means from a statistical point of view that the (random) areas are independent of the (random) locations. A Monte Carlo test of this null hypothesis (random locations are independent of the random marks) is used [1,4,6].

A marked spatial point process is stationary and isotropic if its distribution is invariant against translations and rotations of the locations s_n's. See [3]. It has been assumed that the observed marked point patterns are realizations of a stationary and isotropic marked point process. It can be justified by noticing that the images are a small part of the whole endothelium (only 100 to 300 cells of the total 400000 to 500000 are observed) and the relative position of the

---

[1] Vista is a public domain library for image processing applications developed by Art Pope at the Department of Computer Science, University of British Columbia

microscope and the eye is unknown. In other words, similar results would have been obtained by taking any other portion (possibly with a different orientation) of the endothelium. By taking this into account, it is natural to choose the mark variogram as the functional descriptor of each marked spatial point pattern. The mark variogram is defined as [3]:

$$\gamma(\| h \|) = \frac{var(Z(s) - Z(s + h))}{2}, \tag{1}$$

where $var(.)$ denotes the variance, h is a point of the 2-D Euclidean space and $\| h \|$ is its modulus.

Let $\gamma_1(t)$ ($t = 0, \ldots, t_{max}$) be the mark variogram estimated from the observed marked point pattern, $\{(s_n, Z(s_n))\}_{n=1,\ldots,N}$. Under the above null hypothesis, a similar marked point pattern should be expected when the observed areas are randomly interchanged among the given locations. If $(\pi_i(1), \ldots, \pi_i(N))$ is a random permutation of $(1, \ldots, N)$ then a randomized marked point pattern corresponds to $\{(s_n, Z(s_{\pi_i(n)}))\}_{n=1,\ldots,N}$. S permutations are generated ($S = 99$ in our examples). Let γ_i be the estimated mark variogram for the i-randomized pattern ($i = 2, \ldots, S + 1$). The question is now: Is $\gamma_1(t)$ similar to $\gamma_i(t)$ with $i > 1$ and $t = 1, \ldots, t_{max}$? Let

$$\bar{\gamma}_i(t) = \sum_{j \neq i} \frac{\gamma_j(t)}{S}, \text{ and } d_i = \int_0^{+\infty} (\gamma_i(t) - \bar{\gamma}_i(t))^2 dt, \tag{2}$$

for $i = 1, \ldots, S + 1$. All rankings of d_1 are equiprobable under the above null hypothesis. If $d_{(j)}$ denotes the jth largest amongst d_i, with $i = 1, \ldots, S + 1$, then under the hypothesis of independence:

$$P(d_1 = d_{(j)}) = \frac{1}{S + 1}, \quad j = 1, \ldots, S + 1, \tag{3}$$

and rejection of the null hypothesis on the basis that d_1 ranks kth largest or higher gives an exact, one-sided test with $p - value$ $k/(S + 1)$. The extension to two-sided tests follows directly. The two-sided $p - value$ is then given by the expression:

$$P_V = \frac{2k}{S + 1} \text{ if } k \leq \frac{S + 1}{2} \text{ and } \frac{2(S - k)}{S + 1} \text{ otherwise.} \tag{4}$$

From now on, P_V is called randomized variogram index. If γ_1 is similar to the γ_i's with $i = 2, \ldots, S$ then a high value $p - value$, P_V, is expected. Lower values of P_V means that the original and the randomized spatial marked point patterns are clearly different.

The mark variogram (equation 1) has been estimated by using:

$$\hat{\gamma}(t) = \frac{\sum_{i,j=1,\ldots,N; i \neq j} I(t - \delta < \| s_i - s_j \| \leq t + \delta)(Z(s_i) - Z(s_j))^2}{\sum_{i,j=1,\ldots,N; i \neq j} I(t - \delta < \| s_i - s_j \| \leq t + \delta)}. \tag{5}$$

An edge correction was not necessary to compare the estimated variogram from the original and the randomized marked spatial point patterns, since the same bias is introduced for all estimations.

3   Results

How is P_V related to cell density, hexagonality and the coefficient of variation? A population of 133 endotheliums were analyzed: 49 endotheliums correspond to normal control cases and the other 84 images correspond to potentially patho-logical eyes. The lowest correlation coefficients are between the density and the other three parameters (first row of the Table 1), since it is simply the ratio between the number of cells and the total area and does not reflect any kind of variability of shape, size or regular spatial disposition of cells. It is important to note the high correlation between hexagonality and the coefficient of variation of areas, what means that these two parameters describe to some extent similar aspects of the image. In contrast, the new index P_V has lower correlations with the hexagonality and CV.

Table 1. Correlations between density, hexagonality, CV and P_V index

	Hexagonality	CV	P_V
Density	0.1269723	-0.08751652	-0.009889984
Hexagonality	-	-0.61856124	0.248192071
CV	-	-	-0.134639198

Table 2. Density, hexagonality, CV and P_V corresponding to the selected pairs of corneal endotheliums. Rows labeled R (respectively L) correspond to right eye (respec-tively left eye)

Pair	Density (sq.mm)	Hexagonality (%)	CV (%)	P_V
1 (R)	3084.3	34	36.3	0.08
1 (L)	3179.8	65	35.3	0.78
2 (R)	2657.1	43	42.6	0.06
2 (L)	2527.9	44	36.8	0.00
3 (R)	3002.8	64	35.0	0.58
3 (L)	2881.7	52	31.9	0.02
4 (R)	1695.5	35	47.7	0.5
4 (L)	1927.3	37	52	0.00

A detailed analysis of 8 endotheliums presenting different pathologies is pre-sented. These correspond to 4 patients (4 pairs of eyes). Remember that age has a clear influence on the endothelium status.

In Fig. 1 (a and b) the endotheliums of a male aged 31 with two intraocular lenses are shown. Table 2 (the two first rows) shows that for both right and left eye neither densities nor CV's are different. Only the hexagonality and the P_V index show that the left eye's status is better that the right eye's one.

Figure 1 (c and d) correspond to a 36 year-old patient. Both eyes have un-dergone an intervention. Table 2 (third and fourth rows) shows similar densities,

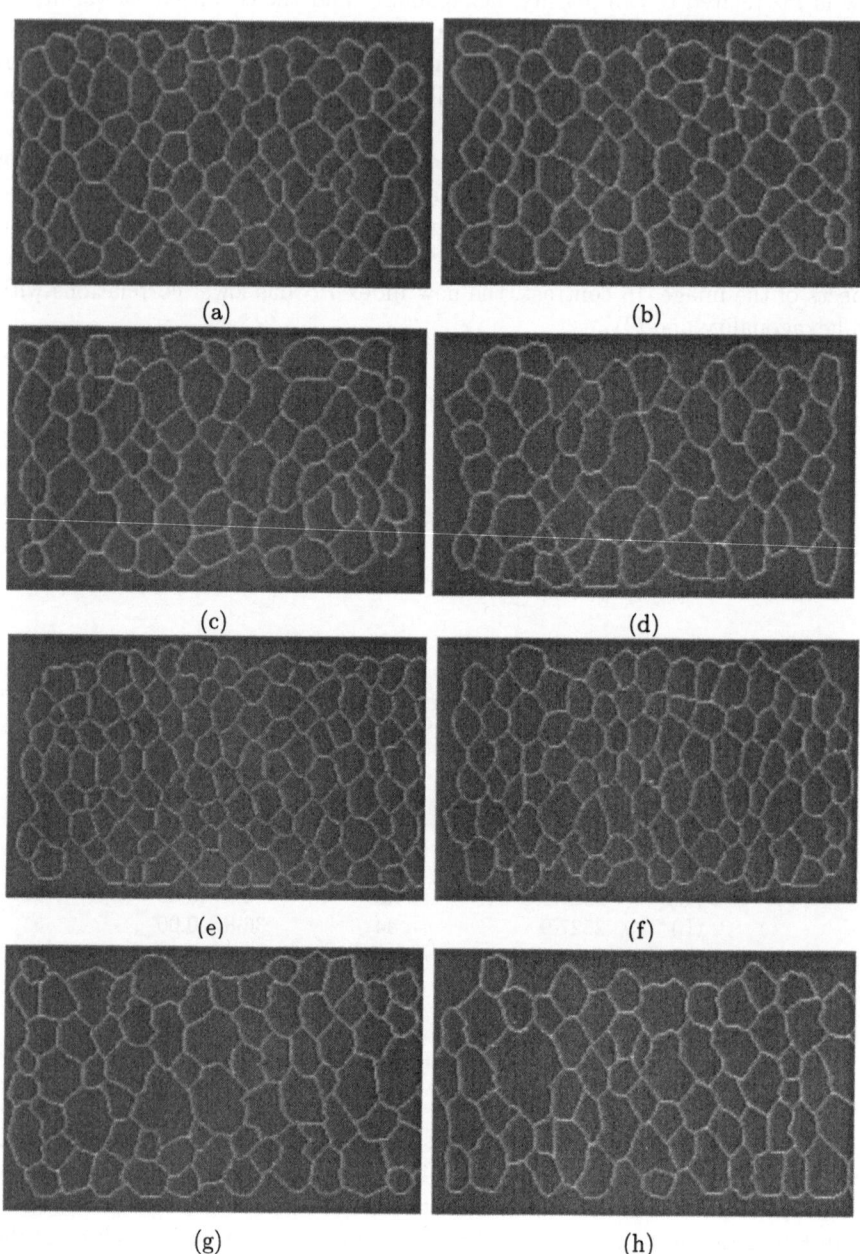

(a)　　　　　　　　　　　　(b)

(c)　　　　　　　　　　　　(d)

(e)　　　　　　　　　　　　(f)

(g)　　　　　　　　　　　　(h)

Fig. 1. Pairs of corneal endotheliums. Each row corresponds to a different patient

hexagonalities and CV's. These values reflect an irregular status of the endothelium, that is also confirmed by the P_V index.

The third patient (Fig. 1 e and f) has a right eye considered as normal and an intraocular lens in the left eye. The three usual indexes show that the status of the right eye is lightly better, the value of P_V shows clearly this difference.

The last patient (eighty four years old) is shown in Fig. 1 (g and h) whose both eyes have had cataract surgery. The three commonly used parameters do not permit to discriminate these two situations (Table 2). However, a visual inspection shows that the cell patterns are quite different. This difference is detected by the P_V index (Table 2).

4 Conclusions

A new index of spatial homogeneity of endotheliums has been proposed, the randomized variogram index, P_V. Results show how this is able to detect subtle morphological changes of cell dispositions that can not be detected by the usual indices. The P_V index is invariant against scale changes, translations and rotations (in fact, robust against image distortions) and it is defined based on a Monte Carlo test.

Acknowledgement

We are indebted to Dr. M. Maldonado from the Hospital La Fe (Valencia, Spain) for the original images and to Dra. L. Martínez-Costa from the Hospital Lluis Alcanyis (Xàtiva, Spain) for the technical comments. This work was supported in part by GV98-14-125 (first author) and TIC98-1019 (second author).

References

1. Barnard, G.A.: Contribution to the discussion of professor Bartlett's paper. Journal of Royal Statistical Society B **25** (1963) 294
2. Bourne, W.M., Hodge, D.O., Nelson, L.R.: Corneal endothelium five years after transplantation. Am. J. Ophthalmol **118** (1994) 185–196
3. Cressie, Noel A.C.: Statistics for Spatial Data. Revised Edition, John Wiley and Sons, New York (1993) 708
4. Diggle, P.J.: Statistical Analysis of Spatial Point Processes. Academic Press, London (1983)
5. Honda, H.: Geometrical models for cells in tissues. International Review of Cytology **81** (1981) 191–247
6. Manly, B.: Randomization, Bootstrap and Monte Carlo Methods in Biology. Chapman and Hall, second edition (1997)
7. Schultz, R.O., Glasser, D.B., Matsuda, M., et al.: Response of the corneal endothelium to cataract surgery. Arch. Ophthalmol **104** (1986) 1164–1169
8. Tasman, W., Jaeger, E.A.: Duane's Clinical Ophthalmology. J.B. Lippincott Company, East Washington Square, Philadelphia, Pennsylvania 19105 (1995)

The Assessment of Chronic Liver Diseases by Sonography

M.–H. Horng[1], Y.–N. Sun[2], and X.–Z. Lin[3]

[1] Department of Information Management, Shih Chien University, Taiwan, R.O.C.
horng@kh.scc.edu.tw
[2] Department of Computer Science and Information Engineering,
National Cheng Kung University, Taiwan, R.O.C.
ynsun@mail.ncku.edu.tw
[3] Department of Internal Medicine, National Cheng Kung University, Taiwan, R.O.C.
linxz@mail.ncku.edu.tw

Abstract. This paper describes a new ultrasonic scoring system based on the texture characteristics of ultrasonic liver images. This system generates an ultrasonic disease severity (UDS) score that is highly correlated with the computer morphometry (CM) score obtained from the evaluation of liver fibrosis based on the biopsy specimens. Essentially, UDS score is very similar to the CM score in the statistical presentation. Therefore, UDS score is defined mathematically referring to CM score as the scoring basis. As a result, UDS can faithfully reflect the disease progression that is determined conventionally based on the evaluation of liver fibrosis. Promising results have been obtained in experimental studies, and it will currently undergoes extensive clinical experiments.

1 Introduction

B–mode liver sonogram, the most frequently used diagnostic ultrasonic modality, produces gray–scale images from echo signals arising from pulsed ultrasound beams propagating through soft tissues. The ultrasonic scans are highly operator and instrument dependent because the characteristics of ultrasonic image are closely related to the attenuation and scattering properties. Therefore, current liver sonography is still a qualitative, or at best semi–quantitative image modality. It depends on the physician to observe certain echotexture characteristics, such as texture coarseness, echogenicity and smoothness of inferior edge, from the liver images and to compare them in order to diagnose the liver states [1]. For some liver diseases, the diagnostic result does not yet produce a conclusive diagnosis. Therefore, physicians have to further examine with other invasive methods, typically liver needle biopsies. Liver biopsy is the standard clinical routine for diagnosing chronic liver diseases and for guiding and monitoring treatment, but, there is associated morbidity (3%) and mortality (0.03%). Therefore, developing a reliable, non–invasive and quantitative ultrasonic scoring system for evaluating histological changes in ultrasonic liver images is highly promising in diagnosing and monitoring chronic liver diseases.

A. Kuba et al. (Eds.): IPMI'99, LNCS 1613, pp. 424–429, 1999.

The key to establishing the ultrasonic scoring system is to find powerful texture features that can reflect the progression of liver disease. From the histological view, the progression of liver disease mainly reflects in the amount of fibrosis of the liver specimens. In the last decade, Knodell's score was widely used to measure liver fibrosis [2]. It used only five numerical scores for staging liver fibrosis based on the physicians observation. Obviously, it was not enough to develop a quantitative progression index for liver disease. In [3,4], we proposed a quantitative index, called computer morphometry (CM) score, that was more reliable and effective than the conventional Knodell's score for evaluating the amount of liver fibrosis. Thus, the CM scores are used here as the criteria for selecting powerful texture features from texture descriptors. As mentioned previously, the CM score is closely related to the progression of liver disease. Thus, it is a good indicator to develop the ultrasonic scoring system for assessing the ultrasonic liver images.

A powerful ultrasonic scoring system should generate the disease severity score that matches the corresponding CM score as closely as possible. To establish the correlation between the selected texture features and the corresponding CM score, the quadratic equations of the selected texture features are defined mathematically based on the CM scores in the training stage. The scoring criterion of assessing the ultrasonic liver image is the minimization of variation between the observed texture features and the texture features estimated by quadratic equations. The severity scores generated here are called ultrasonic disease severity (UDS) score. The intervals of UDS scores in different liver states are also determined as the standard for classification. Experiments with forty test images demonstrate that the UDS scores generated from this system are significantly correlated with the CM scores of corresponding biopsy specimens. In addition, one hundred and twenty ultrasonic liver images are used to test the classification capability. The resulting correct classification rate was as good as 86.7%. These results reveal the possibility of replacing the invasive needle biopsy examination by the system presented here.

2   Materials and Methods

The major morphological change of the progression of chronic liver diseases is that collagen fibers are increasingly presented in liver specimens. Therefore, the amount of liver fibrosis is a powerful index for quantitatively assessing chronic liver diseases. In the literature, echotexture was also reported to be very powerful for evaluating diffuse liver disease [5]. Thus, if we can establish the correlation between the measurements of echotexture and the amount of fibrosis in liver specimens, sonography will become an effective and non–invasive tool in the systematic assessment of chronic liver diseases. In [5], we found that the co–occurrence matrix method and texture feature coding method are powerful texture descriptors for classifying the chronic liver diseases. Therefore, these two texture descriptors are used to establish the correlates with the pathological fibrosis measurement.

The disease severity of chronic liver disease is reflected by the amount of liver fibrosis of the biopsy specimens. Therefore, it is necessary to develop an objective system for measuring the amount of liver fibrosis. In [3], we developed an automatic image analysis system, which consisted of a microscope, a computer–driven slide–driver, and the software for image acquisition, processing and data analysis. The image analysis procedures included color model selection, histogram–based normalization, clustering, moment–preserving thresholding and a ranking filter for tissue characterization. The computerized motor driver and the x–y directional stage were designed and installed to move specimens on an optical microscope and to compute the fibrosis index. The system was capable of computing the ratio of fibrous area to the complete liver tissue area as an index for assessing the amount of liver fibrosis. This index is called the computer morphometry (CM) score. In [4] we found that the CM score was superior to the conventional Knodell's score for evaluating the liver fibrosis. The pathological CM score is used for selecting powerful texture features.

In [6], we found that the changes of ultrasonic liver texture in disease are more sensitive with features of the co–occurrence matrix being 3 or 4–pixels apart along the angular directions of degree 0 or 90. Thus, we use the two displacements along the two directions to obtain four co–occurrence matrices. Sixteen texture features can be extracted from these matrices. In addition, four texture features by texture feature coding methods are also adopted. Four texture features, that are significantly correlated to CM scores are selected as the most powerful features for establishing the ultrasonic disease scoring system. They are based on grey-level resolution similarity, entropy, correlation, and angular second moment. Experimental results with forty samples show that the resulting severity scores generated from this system are highly correlated with CM score more than the ones designed by other texture features.

2.1   Ultrasonic Disease Scoring System

In the literature, the texture features were only used to construct a classification system for clustering the three liver states. Widely used texture classification methods including the minimum–distance classifier, Bayesian estimation, k–nearest neighboring classifier and neural network have been reported to be useful in these studies. However, they only classified test samples into three disease states. No quantitative measurement of disease severity has yet been generated for assessing the progression of the chronic liver disease. As mentioned above, liver disease progression can be perceived and evaluated based on the amount for liver fibrosis. Among conventional methods for liver fibrosis measurement, the CM score is most reliable and accurate method [3]. Therefore, the proposed scoring system was designed, using the corresponding CM scores. For this purpose, a system of quadratic equations is used to define the correlation between the texture features and the corresponding CM scores. The design details are described as follows.

Forty training samples, including the ultrasonic images and corresponding needle specimens, were used to establish the ultrasonic scoring system in the training stage. The selected texture features and its corresponding CM score of the i–th training sample are evaluated and defined as $\langle f_{1,i}, f_{2,i}, f_{3,i}, f_{4,i} \rangle$ and t_i. The quadratic equations of selected texture features with respect to the corresponding CM score are defined in (1).

$$
\begin{aligned}
f_{1,i} &= a_1 t_i^2 + b_1 t_i + c_1 \\
f_{2,i} &= a_2 t_i^2 + b_2 t_i + c_2 \\
f_{3,i} &= a_3 t_i^2 + b_3 t_i + c_3 \\
f_{4,i} &= a_4 t_i^2 + b_4 t_i + c_4
\end{aligned}
\qquad (i = 1, 2, \ldots, 40). \tag{1}
$$

These coefficients a_j, b_j, c_j are determined using least square estimation based on (2).

$$
X = (T^t T)^{-1} T^t F \tag{2}
$$

where

$$
X = \begin{bmatrix} a_j \\ b_j \\ c_j \end{bmatrix}, \qquad
T = \begin{bmatrix} t_1^2 & t_1 & 1 \\ t_2^2 & t_2 & 1 \\ \vdots & \vdots & \vdots \\ t_{40}^2 & t_{40} & 1 \end{bmatrix}, \qquad
F = \begin{bmatrix} f_{j,1} \\ f_{j,2} \\ \vdots \\ f_{j,40} \end{bmatrix} \qquad (j = 1, 2, 3, 4).
$$

The quadratic equations defined in (2) are used to derive a disease severity score for assessing the ultrasonic liver image. The resulting score is called ultrasonic disease severity (UDS) score. The assessment criterion of image X is based on the minimization of the square error between the texture features of X and the estimated texture features obtained by the quadratic equations. The square error term is defined as (3).

$$
SE = \sum_{j=1}^{4} [g_j - (a_j u^2 + b_j u + c_j)]^2 \tag{3}
$$

where the $\langle g_1, g_2, g_3, g_4 \rangle$ are the texture features of X.

Differentiating of (3) with respect to the variable u, we obtain the root u of (4) to determine UDS such that the square error term is minimized.

$$
\begin{aligned}
& 2 \left(\sum_{j=1}^{4} a_j^2 \right) u^3 + 3 \left(\sum_{j=1}^{4} a_j b_j \right) u^2 + \\
& \left(\sum_{j=1}^{4} a_j c_j + \sum_{j=1}^{4} b_j^2 - 2 \sum_{j=1}^{4} g_j a_j \right) u + \\
& \left(\sum_{j=1}^{4} b_j c_j + \sum_{j=1}^{4} + \sum_{j=1}^{4} g_j b_j \right) = 0.
\end{aligned} \tag{4}
$$

3   Experimental Results and Conclusion

In this study, we have successfully developed an ultrasonic scoring system to assess the severity of the chronic liver disease. The system integrates the techniques of texture analysis with pathological CM score measurement. In this system, all programs are coded in Visual C++ version 4.0 with a Pentium personal computer under MS–Windows 95. The system provides user–friendly interfaces and efficient computation for real–time clinical evaluation. Forty training samples with ultrasonic images and corresponding needle specimens were collected from forty patients in whom thirteen of them are normals, nineteen are chronic hepatitis and eight are with liver cirrhosis. These training samples were used to select powerful texture features, and then to establish the quadratic equations for texture features based on CM scores in the ultrasonic scoring system. The resulting quadratic equations are used to derive the UDS scores of liver images for sequential assessment. Additionally, in the conventional clinical diagnosis, physicians always classify the ultrasonic liver image into one of three liver states. To provide the standards for classification, the forty training images are also used to determine the severity intervals of UDS score for different liver states according to their medical records. The intervals of UDS scores in different liver states are determined by ANOVA and correlation analysis. The results are: normal 2.8832 ± 1.668, hepatitis 5.9296 ± 1.554 and liver cirrhosis 13.8257 ± 2.632. The thresholds of UDS for three different disease states are 4.54 (normal $\sim$ hepatitis) and 9.62 (hepatitis $\sim$ cirrhosis) based on normal distributions with equal standard deviation.

Forty ultrasonic images and their corresponding needle specimens are used as test samples to analyze the stability and accuracy of the proposed scoring system. The accuracy of the UDS score is verified by comparing with the pathological CM scores. The Pearson correlation coefficient between the UDS scores and CM scores is 0.8843 ($p < 0.001$) This significant correlation shows that the proposed UDS scores can faithfully reflect CM scores which is an important factor in assessing the progression of chronic liver disease. In other words, the UDS score is a powerful and stable index for assessing the ultrasonic liver images. The results also reveal that the system of quadratic equations is an appropriate method for correlating the selected texture features and the corresponding CM scores. It is still an interesting topic to define the best correlation between texture features and CM scores in the future such that the resulting ultrasonic system is most effective.

In clinical diagnostic practice, the ultrasonic liver images are usually classified into three disease states. The effective scoring system should avoid misclassification, especially false–negative misclassification. The false–negative rate is the probability of a misclassification such that the patients are classified as being normal or having mild disease while the actual diagnosis is a more severe disease. High false–negative rate represents a danger to the patients when physicians use this scoring system. One hundred and twenty ultrasonic liver images, verified by needle biopsy, are used to test the discrimination capability. The classification results are listed in Table 1. From the experimental results we find that the negative–false rate is only 8.33% and the correct classification rate is 86.7%. It is superior to the conventional method utilized by the co–occurrence matrix or texture feature coding method [5].

In this paper, a quantitative ultrasonic scoring system is proposed based on the characteristics of echotexture of liver. The system not only generates quantitative indices to assess disease progression but also to classify the ultrasonic liver images. It is shown that the proposed system has potential to become a valuable clinical tool for liver diagnosis in the future. Several characteristics of liver tissues have been used to evaluate the degree of diffuse parenchyma liver disease, including the smoothness of liver surface, echogenicity, echotexture and backscattering parameters. However, the system proposed here only uses echotexture information. In further studies, it is an interesting topic if one can enhance this system's performance by integrating other features of tissue characteristics.

Table 1. The confusion matrix of forty test patients is shown. The left column indicates the true liver states of the test samples while the upper row indicates the corresponding classification results. Correct classification rate is 86.7%. The false–negative rate is only 8.33%

	Normal	Hepatitis	Cirrhosis
Normal	37	2	1
Hepatitis	5	32	3
Cirrhosis	1	4	35

References

1. Simon G.J.W., Jane E.E., Nigal B., Margaret E.H., Joe E.B., David W.: An ultrasound scoring system for the diagnosis of liver disease in cystic fibrosis. Journal of Hepatology **22** (1995) 513–521
2. Knodell G., Ishak K.G., Black W.C., et al: Formulation and application of numerical scoring system for assessing histological activity in asymptomatic chronic active hepatitis. Hepatology **1** (1981) 431–435
3. Sun Y.N., Horng M.H.: Assessing liver tissue with an automatic computer morphometry system. IEEE Engineering in Medicine and Biology **3** (1997) 66–73
4. Lin X.Z., Horng M.H., Sun Y.N., Shien S.C., Chow N.H., Guo X.Z.: Computer morphometry for quantitative measurement of liver fibrosis: Comparison with Knodell's score, colorimetry and conventional description reports. Journal of Gastroenterology and Hepatology **3** (1998) 75–80
5. Horng M.H., Sun Y.N., Lin X.Z.: Texture feature coding method for classification of liver sonography. European Conference of Computer Vision, London, ECCV96 (1996) 209–218
6. Sun Y.N., Horng M.H., Lin X.Z., Wang J.Y.: An ultrasonic image analysis system for liver diagnosis. IEEE Engineering in Medicine and Biology **6** (1996) 93–101

Automatic Computation of Brain and Cerebellum Volumes in Normal Subjects and Chronic Alcoholics

S. L. Hartmann[1], M. H. Parks[2], H. Schlack[2], W. Riddle[3],
R. R. Price[3], P. R. Martin[2], and B. M. Dawant[4]

[1] Department of Biomedical Engineering,
[2] Department of Psychiatry,
[3] Department of Radiology,
[4] Department of Electrical and Computer Engineering, Vanderbilt University,
Nashville, Tennessee, USA
{slh, dawant}@vuse.vanderbilt.edu

Abstract. Automatic volumetric measurements of brain structures and substructures is a prerequisite for longitudinal studies as well as studies aimed at measuring and quantifying differences between populations. This study tests the hypothesis that a fully automatic, atlas–based method can be used for the computation of the volume encompassed by the dura, the volume of the brain, and the volume of the cerebellum from which indices of atrophy are estimated. The method has been tested on normal volunteers and alcoholic patients. It has been validated both by comparing contours obtained manually and automatically and by repeating the measurements on serial acquisitions. Results demonstrate that the method is both robust and accurate, even in the presence of large morphological differences due to severe atrophy caused by chronic alcoholism.

1 Introduction

A number of atlas–based methods have been proposed in the recent past to label and segment structures and substructures in medical images [1]. These techniques involve the segmentation of a reference volume and its non–rigid registration to the volume to be segmented. Possible approaches include the use of landmarks in which the deformation is computed based on control points and interpolated through the remainder of the volume. But, the automatic or semi–automatic identification of these control points remains challenging. Other techniques attempt to maximize intensity similarity on a voxel–by–voxel basis. These methods have the advantage of being fully automatic but they may be affected by large morphological differences between brain volumes. Results reported in the literature typically involve normal subjects or patients with pathologies that do not drastically alter the shape of the brain, such as schizophrenia or epilepsy. In these applications, small deformations are sufficient to warp one brain onto the other. In contrast, the study presented herein involves chronic alcoholics with

A. Kuba et al. (Eds.): IPMI'99, LNCS 1613, pp. 430–435, 1999.

very severe brain atrophy. Severe atrophy considerably reduces the size of the cerebellum and enlarges the sulci and the ventricles. This decreases the similarity between the atlas and the subject volumes, thus challenging deformation algorithms. This work tests and evaluates the robustness of an automatic method for the computation of pre–atrophy brain volumes and the post–atrophy brain and cerebellum volumes.

2   Methods

2.1   Data Sets

Seven normal volunteers and seven patients with a history of alcoholism were used in theis study. Multiple 3–D magnetic resonance (MR) image volumes were obtained of each subject. Normal subjects were scanned three times within a period of three weeks (n=5) or within a period of 5 months (n=2). Alcoholic subjects were admitted to a detoxification program, and the first scan was obtained within 5 days of abstinence. The second scan was obtained within one month, followed by a third scan at approximately 3 months after the first scan. An additional image volume obtained with the same imaging parameters was used as an atlas. All image volumes were acquired with a General Electric 1.5 Tesla Signa MR scanner using a spoiled gradient echo pulse sequence. Each volume consists of 124 sagittal slices, and each slice has dimensions of 256×256 pixels. Voxel dimensions were $.94 \times .94 \times 1.3$ mm^3.

2.2   Image Registration

The registration algorithm consists of two major steps. First, a seven–parameter (three rotation angles, three translation vectors, and one scaling factor) transformation that brings the two volumes into global correspondence is computed. Next, the volumes are deformed using a non–rigid transformation to bring these two volumes into local correspondence. Both of these steps are fully automatic. Because the method used in step (2) is also used to compute the transformation in step (1) the local transformation method is described first. All the algorithms used in this study were written in IDL (Interactive Data Language, Research Systems, Inc.) and executed on a Sun Ultra 1 workstation (Sun Microsystems, Mountain View, CA).

Local Registration: Recently, Thirion [2] presented the problem of image matching in terms of demons (by analogy with Maxwell's demons). This is a general framework in which object boundaries in one image are viewed as semi–permeable membranes. The other image, considered as a deformable grid, diffuses through these interfaces driven by the action of effectors (the demons) situated within the membranes. Various kinds of demons can be designed to apply this paradigm to specific applications. In the particular case of deformations based on voxel–by–voxel intensity similarity the demons paradigm is similar to optical flow methods. It is an independent implementation of this approach that has been used in this study [3]. This algorithm results in a deformation field (i.e., a displacement vector for every voxel in the volume) that can be used to warp one image onto the other. Global Registration: Prior to applying the deformation algorithm, the images to be matched are brought into approximate correspondence using a seven–degrees–of–freedom transformation. Displacement vectors computed as described in the previous section were used to identify a set of points in the first image and a corresponding set of points in the second image. These homologous points are then used to compute the global transformation. Typically, the global transformation computed with this approach is not as accurate as one computed with other methods, such as mutual information. However, it has the advantage of being fast and is sufficiently accurate to serve as a reliable starting point for the deformation algorithm.

2.3   Segmentation

The atrophy indices of interest require pre– and post–atrophy brain volumes as well as cerebellum volume. Pre–atrophy brain volumes are difficult to obtain, so instead, the intra–dural volume was used as the reference to which brain volumes are compared. The intra–dural volume in the atlas was determined by careful manual delineation. Contours were outlined in each slice of the sagittal volume, and a binary mask of the intra–dural volume was created. This same method was repeated to obtain a binary volume of the cerebellum (both hemispheres) in the atlas volume. The region was segmented to include the entire cerebellum region, and individual folia were not followed. Note that the first volume also included the cerebellum. In order to segment the intra–dural region and the cerebellum in subject volumes, the atlas was first registered to each volume. The deformation field was then applied to the binary atlas volumes to create intra–dural and cerebellum masks in each individual volume.

2.4   Volume Measurements

The intra–dural brain volume of each subject is determined simply by the volume of the mask created by projecting the atlas mask onto each individual volume. The brain volume (white and gray matter) is obtained by thresholding the intra–dural image to eliminate cerebrospinal fluid. The threshold value was manually chosen in the atlas volume. In order to compensate for inter–scan intensity variations, this threshold level was automatically adjusted to the proper value for subject volume using a histogram equalization technique. This threshold was then applied to the segmented intra–dural images, and a brain volume was determined. The cerebellum volumes were computed in the same manner as the brain volumes, using a separate intensity threshold.

3   Results

Figure 1 illustrates qualitatively the type of results that were obtained. The left panel shows one slice in the atlas volume. The right panel shows the slice with the same index in one of the patient volumes. Observe the large amount of atrophy (enlarged sulci and ventricles and atrophied cerebellum) visible in the patient volume. The middle row shows the slice with the same index in the volume obtained by warping the normal brain volume onto the atrophied brain volume. After deformation, the ventricles in the normal brain volume have been dramatically enlarged, the thickness of the corpus callosum has been reduced, sulci have been enlarged, and the overall shape of the head has been modified, but the integrity of the cortical structures has been preserved. Figure 2 illus-

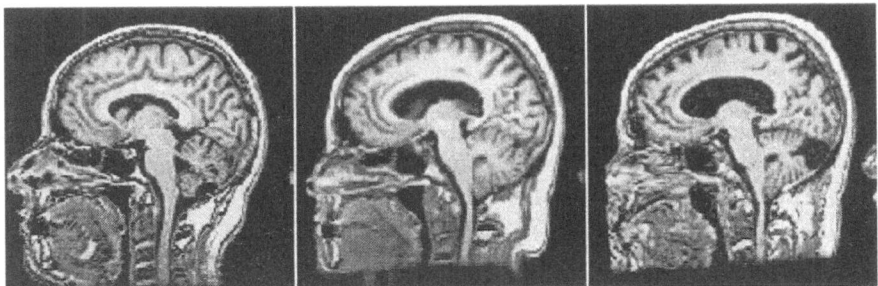

Fig. 1. Results of the elastic registration algorithm

trates representative results for the automatic segmentation of the cerebellum. This figure shows one slice in each of three alcoholic subject volumes with the cerebellar contours obtained with the automatic technique overlaid in white. Observe the ability of the algorithm to produce accurate results even when the shape and orientation of the cerebellum varies greatly from one volume to the other. To evaluate our results quantitatively we differentiate between repeata-

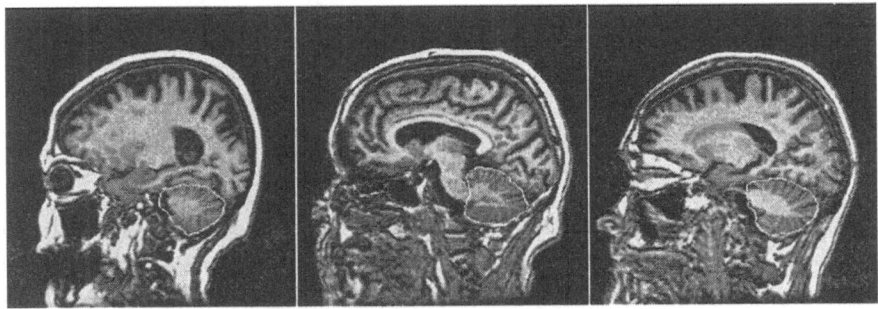

Fig. 2. Automatic cerebellum segmentation results for three alcoholic subjects

bility and accuracy. The data set used in this study includes three acquisitions per subjects (both for the normal and the alcoholic volunteers). This permits the evaluation of the consistency and repeatability of our measurements. Indeed, changes are not expected in the volume encompassed by the dura in either the normal or the patient population and only minor changes (if any) are expected in the brain and cerebellar volumes for the normal population. Changes related to abstinence may be observed both in the brain and the cerebellum volumes for the patient population. Consistent values for structures that are not expected to change in serial scans of the same subject are thus good indicators of the reliability of our measurements. Accuracy has been assessed by comparing the results obtained automatically to results obtained by manual delineation.

3.1   Repeatability

Figure 3 shows the intra–dural volumes obtained for both the normal and the patient population. For each subject the figure shows the volume computed for each acquisition. Space restrictions preclude the inclusion of similar figures for the cerebellar volumes but results were comparable.

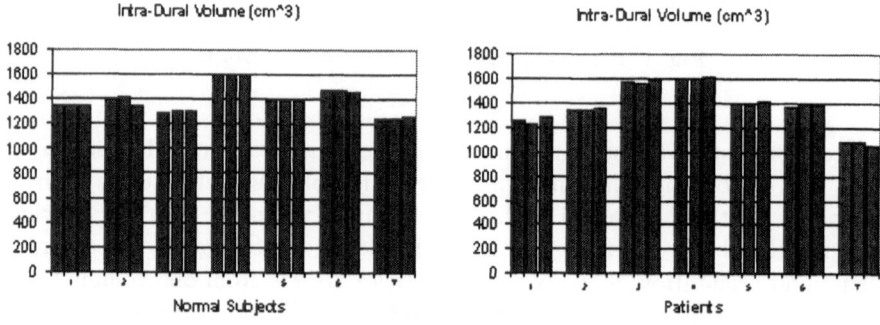

Fig. 3. Intra–dural volumes, determined automatically, for each normal and alcoholic subject used in this study

3.2   Accuracy

For each and every volume, four slices were segmented manually (two for the brain and two for the cerebellum). These slices were chosen by determining the range on which the structures were visible in the image volumes and randomly selecting two slices per structure within this range. Ranges, and therefore selected slices, were different for the cerebellum and for the brain. The similarity between contours obtained manually and contours obtained automatically were computed using a similarity index S derived from the kappa statistic [4]. This index varies between 0 and 1 (1 indicates perfect agreement between two contours while 0 indicates no overlap) and is sensitive to both differences in size and structure orientation. This strategy resulted in 84 brain and cerebellum contours for the normal population and 84 contours for the alcoholic subjects. The mean similarity indices for the normal subjects were 0.98 for the intra–dural volume and 0.95 for the cerebellar volume. These indices were 0.97 and 0.94 for the alcoholic subjects.

4   Discussion

This study demonstrates that fully automatic, robust, and accurate segmentation of the whole brain and cerebellum can be accomplished using atlas–based methods. To the authors' knowledge, this is the first time that results have been reported on a study involving atlas–based segmentation of brains with pathologies that alter brain morphology to the extent observed in this data set. Intra–dural volumes demonstrate the excellent repeatability of the results. Accuracy was tested by comparing contours delineated manually and contours delineated automatically. Arguably, manually delineated contours are not the ultimate gold standard. But, in this case the contours were drawn by the same rater on the atlas and on each individual slice used for the evaluation. The entire atlas was also delineated twice and similarity indices of 0.98 and 0.96 were observed for the intra–dural and cerebellum volumes, respectively. The average similarity indices we have observed between manual and automatic delineation on the slice selected for evaluation are therefore comparable to the intra–rater variability. Thus, results obtained on this data set support the hypothesis that automatic delineation is as reliable and accurate as manual delineation when the manual segmentation is performed by a single individual.

Acknowledgment

This work was supported in part by NIH grant R01 AA 10583.

References

1. Maintz, J.B., Viergever, M.A.: A survey of medical image registration. Medical Image Analysis **2** (1998) 1–36
2. Thirion, J–P.: Image matching as a diffusion process: an analogy with Maxwell's demons. Medical Image Analysis **2** (1998) 243–260
3. Hartmann, S.L.: Automatic segmentation of medical images using optical flow based atlas deformation. Master's Thesis, Department of Biomedical Engineering, Vanderbilt University (1998)
4. Zijdenbos, A., Dawant, B.M., and Margolin, R.: Morphometric analysis of white matter lesions in MR images: method and validation. IEEE Transactions on Medical Imaging **13** (1994) 716–724

Reconstruction from Slow Rotation Dynamic SPECT Using a Factor Model

Arkadiusz Sitek, Edward V. R. Di Bella, and Grant T. Gullberg

Department of Radiology, University of Utah, Salt Lake City UT 84108, USA

Abstract. Slow rotation acquisition of dynamic data has several advantages over fast rotation acquisition which is currently the method of choice used for the acquisition of dynamic data in SPECT. Slow rotation is currently not used because of error from inconsistent data. In this work, we develop a method of reconstructing from projections that are inconsistent in time due to being acquired during a slow acquisition. Our method is based on a factor model of physiological data. A series of dynamic images are reconstructed, where each reconstructed image corresponds in time to only one projection. Such an under-determined reconstruction is shown to be possible through utilization of a factor model. Computer simulations are performed using simple phantoms. We found that we are able to accurately reconstruct the dynamic sequence for simple phantoms with temporal behavior corresponding to teboroxime-Tc-99m heart imaging.

1 Introduction

Single Photon Emission Computed Tomography (SPECT) can be used to acquire dynamic data. The acquisition protocol is usually based on the use of a fast camera rotation. Such acquisitions are made only with multiple detector cameras which have the ability to rotate quickly and acquire consecutive, complete sets of tomographic projections. A complete set of tomographic data is acquired over a very short period of time (approximately 10 seconds) and the resulting number of counts in the acquired projections is very low. The tomographic sets are reconstructed to form a series of dynamic images which are very noisy due to low projection counts. The assumption made during reconstruction is that radionuclide distribution remains constant during the acquisition of one set of projections. This approximation may be unreliable, especially in the time just after injection when changes of activity in the object are very fast. In our lab, with a Picker 3000XP, the best temporal resolution with fast rotation was 5.7 seconds. Another important aspect of fast rotation acquisition is the amount of computer time and disk storage needed to process a dynamic study. Each tomographic set of projections must be stored end then reconstructed. For the above reasons, dynamic SPECT with fast rotation is a difficult and computer time consuming method.

There are a variety of methods in PET and SPECT which estimate kinetic parameters directly from projections. They require prior reconstruction of tomographic sets in order to estimate the object boundary [2], or to estimate the

A. Kuba et al. (Eds.): IPMI'99, LNCS 1613, pp. 436–441, 1999.

initial set of factors through SVD analysis of reconstructed dynamic sequences [3].

In this paper we consider a different approach to dynamic SPECT. In this approach the acquisition of the dynamic SPECT data is similar to the standard static acquisition of SPECT data [4]. Only a small number of rotations of the camera is required during the scan. Such an acquisition type creates time inconsistencies in the projections, *i.e.* each projection "sees" different activity in the object.

We propose a reconstruction technique which reconstructs a sequence of dynamic images from these inconsistent projections using a factor model of the physiological images [5,6]. Each reconstructed dynamic image corresponds in time to only 1 projection unlike in the fast rotation case where one dynamic image corresponds to a tomographic set of projections. By using a short time per projection, this method can provide a much better temporal resolution than that obtained with fast rotation. The very important advantage of this method is that it does not require a three or more detector system; it can be used with a two detector or single detector system. Only positivity constraints are put on the temporal or geometrical representation of the factors, and no *a priori* information is used in the reconstruction.

The time activity curves (TACs) can be determined from the sequence of reconstructed images by using region of interest (ROI) measurements or factor analysis of dynamic structures (FADS) [6]. We used the ROI technique for the extraction of TACs which then were used for the evaluation of the reconstruction method presented in this paper.

We present the results of our reconstruction method from a simulation of a simple phantom. A comparison is made between two different types of acquisition protocols and two different reconstruction parameters.

2   Methods

The reconstruction was done by constructing a least squares objective function where forward projection was modeled assuming a factor model of the data:

$$f(\mathbf{C}, \mathbf{F}) = \sum_{j,t=1}^{M,K} \frac{(\sum_{i,p=1}^{N,P} \alpha_{ji}(t) \cdot \mathbf{C}_{ip} \cdot \mathbf{F}_p(t) - \mathbf{P}_j(t))^2}{\mathbf{P}_j(t)} \tag{1}$$

where $\mathbf{F}_p(t)$ is a value of factor p at time t and $\mathbf{C}_{ip}$ is a geometrical definition of the factor; i is a pixel index. The α is a tomographic system matrix, and $\mathbf{P}_j(t)$ is the number of counts measured in bin j at projection (or time when projection was taken) t.

The minimization of (1) will yield the values of $\mathbf{C}$ and $\mathbf{F}$, but these values are not physiologically meaningful since: (a) in general, the number of factors used for the forward projection in (1), P, is different than the number of physiological factors and (b) the results of the minimization, matrices $\mathbf{C}$ and $\mathbf{F}$, are not mathematically unique. In all simulation experiments presented in this paper, the number of factors used in the reconstruction was equal to or higher than the number of physiological factors in the analyzed study. The physiologically meaningful result of this method is the dynamic sequence of images which is a result of $C \cdot F$ multiplication. Although in this paper we consider only a 2D case, this method has straightforward extension to 3D. All equations in this paper are valid for this 3D case. The objective function was minimized by use of the conjugate gradient method. The non-negativity constraints were imposed on C and F by adding to the objective function a term which penalized negative values of these matrices.

Preliminary computer simulations were performed in order to verify the reconstruction method. A simple phantom consisting of 4 squares. These squares corresponded to blood, myocardium, liver, and right ventricle. Their geometrical representation is presented in Fig. 1(a) . In all simulations, uptake of Teboroxime-Tc-99m in the myocardium was simulated using a two compartmental model [7] with wash-out $k_{12} = 0.4 \text{min}^{-1}$, and wash-in $k_{21} = 0.8 \text{min}^{-1}$, and fraction of blood in the tissue $f_v = 0.15$. Simulations were performed in 2D using 64x64 pixel images. Simulations were performed without noise and with Poisson noise added to the projection data. The total number of counts in each sinogram for the simulation with noise was equal to 3.8×10^5. Ten realizations of the noise in the sinograms were performed. The data acquisition was performed assuming two detector heads positioned with a relative angle of 90 deg; 183 projections per head was simulated. Each head made a total of 3 rotations during the acquisition. The projections were generated in a 64 bin matrix. Simulations with noise were performed in 2 modes of acquisition. In the first mode, the time per projection, 6 seconds, was the same for all projections. For the second mode, the time per projection was 2 seconds for the first 61 projections, and it was increased to 6 seconds for the next 61 projections, and the final 61 projections lasted 10 seconds each. The non-uniform time per projection acquisition mode was used to increase the temporal resolution at the beginning of the acquisition when changes in radionuclide distribution were most rapid.

The reconstructed dynamic sequences had 183 images (the same as the number of projections), each of size 64×64 pixels. The TACs for the 4 different components: myocardium, blood, liver, and right ventricle, were extracted from region of interest (ROI) measurements from the reconstructed dynamic sequences. Geometrically, the ROIs were defined as the 8×8 squares positioned in the center of each of the 4 components. The kinetic parameters of the simulated uptake of teboroxime in the heart were also calculated using the RFIT fitting program [8] from the obtained TACs. Parameters (k_{12}, k_{21}, f_v) of the compartmental model, and their standard deviations, were calculated for each ROI. The standard deviations were calculated based on the 10 realizations of noise in the projections.

3   Results

The results of the simulations with noise gave the exact match between the simulated and obtained by the method curves. These results are not presented. Figure 1 shows sinograms of the noisy square phantom. The time per projection was 6 seconds for each projection in sinogram (b) and varied from 2 seconds to 6 seconds to 10 seconds in the three sections of sinogram (c). It is apparent from the sinograms that for the first frames there are rapid changes of activity which become smaller for later time frames. Different times per projection causes the discontinuity of the sinogram seen in Fig. 1(c).

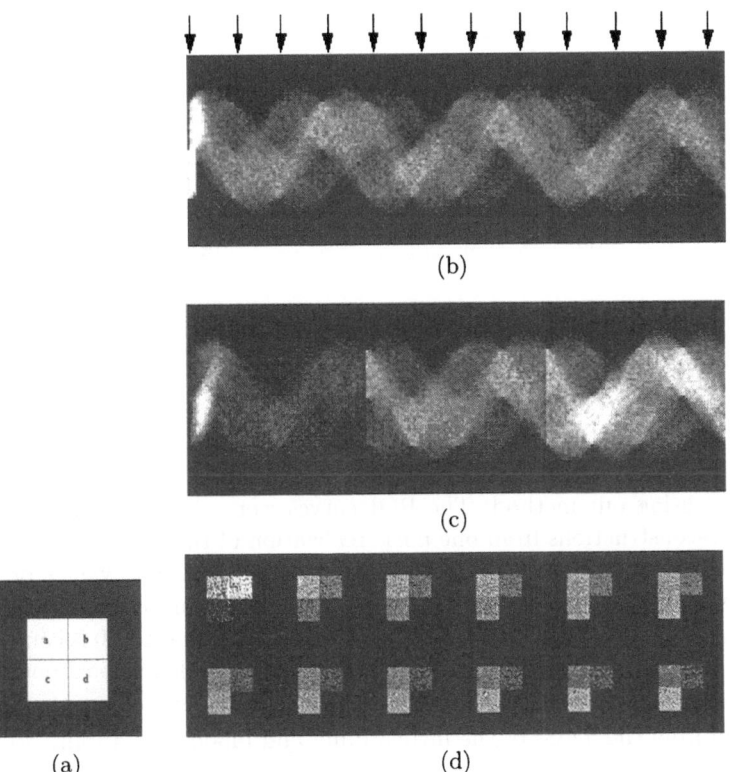

Fig. 1. Simulated object (a). The sinograms for one detector obtained for uniform (b) and non-uniform (c) temporal sampling. The reconstructed images from sinogram (b) are presented in (d). Only 12 out of total 183 reconstructed images. Images in (d) correspond to times marked on the sinogram (b) by arrows

The reconstructions from the sinograms in the Fig. 1(b) is presented in Fig. 1(d). Only a small number of reconstructed images is shown (there were a total of 183 reconstructed images). Images in Fig. 1(d) correspond to projections marked by arrows on the sinogram in Fig. 1(b).

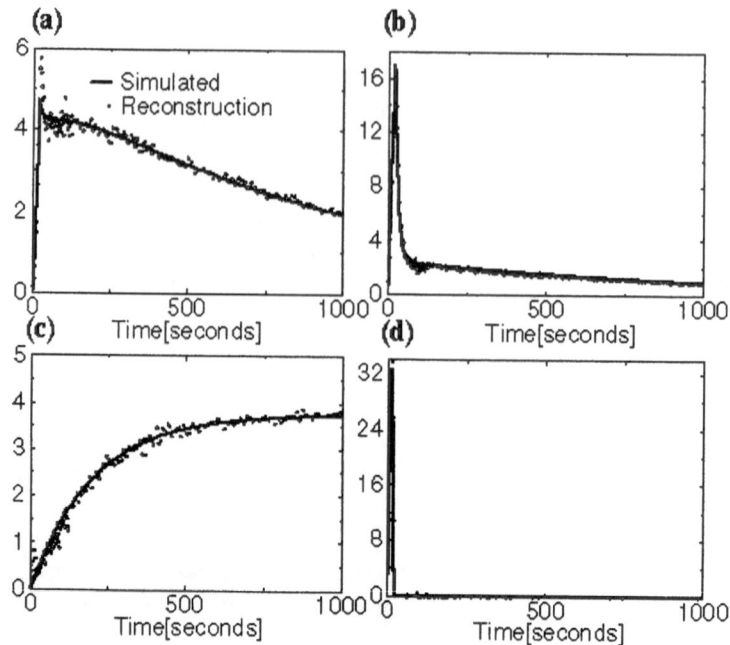

Fig. 2. TAC obtained by ROI measurments from reconstructed series of images. The temporal behavior of the factors corresponded uptake of Teboroxime-Tc-99m in heart. (a) corresponds to myocardium, (b) to blood, (c) to liver, and (d) to right ventricle

Figure 2 shows the comparison between the simulated curves and the TACs obtained using our method. The ROI curves were obtained from dynamic sequence reconstructions from one noise realization of the projection data. Figure 2 presents results for non-uniform temporal sampling. The values of TACs in Fig. 2 were scaled, *i.e.* the values of the TAC for the projections with 2 second duration were multiplied by 3, and values corresponding to 10 second duration were divided by 1.67, so that all projections corresponded to 6 second duration.

Parameters of the kinetic model were calculated for each noise realization of the data from the TACs of the myocardium and blood. The results are summa-

Table 1. Calculated kinetic parameters with standard deviations

		k_{12} [min^{-1}]	k_{21} [min^{-1}]	f_v
Simulated		0.40	0.80	0.15
Uniform	P=4	0.399 ± 0.029	0.802 ± 0.061	0.097 ± 0.023
temporal sampling	P=5	0.392 ± 0.034	0.785 ± 0.059	0.093 ± 0.023
Non-uniform	P=4	0.390 ± 0.017	0.789 ± 0.034	0.128 ± 0.024
temporal sampling	P=5	0.388 ± 0.021	0.780 ± 0.047	0.117 ± 0.029

rized in Table 1. The standard deviation of wash-in and wash-out parameters and bias of f_v was decreased by using non-uniform sampling. There is no visible difference between the reconstructions with $P = 4$ and $P = 5$.

The values of the calculated kinetic parameters agreed with simulated values within the standard deviation. Standard deviations were calculated over multiple noise realizations of the projection data. Use of non-uniform temporal sampling improved the temporal resolution of the dynamic acquisitions and often improved the precision and accuracy of kinetic parameters obtained (Table 1).

In future studies we plan to investigate the use of different methods for minimization of the objective function. We intend to optimize the slow rotation acquisition protocol using computer simulations with a more realistic anatomic phantom. Finally, experimental validation of this method will be performed for teboroxime-Tc-99m heart and MAG3-Tc-99m renal studies in animals and in patients.

4 Acknowledgments

This work was supported by NIH Grant No. RO1 HL 39792.

References

1. Chiao, P. C., Rogers. W. L., Clinthorne, N. H., Fessler, J. A., Hero, A. O.: Model-based estimation with boundary side information or boundary regularization. IEEE Trans. Med. Imag. **13** (1994) 227–234
2. Matthews, J., Bailey, D., Cunningham, V.: The direct calculation of parametric images from dynamic PET data using maximum-likelihood iterative reconstruction. Phys. Med. Biol. **42** (1997) 1155–1173
3. Zeng, G. L., Gullberg, G. T., Huesman, R. H.: Using linear time-invariant system theory to estimate kinetic parameters directly from projection measurements. IEEE Trans. Nuc. Sci. **42** (1995) 2339–2346
4. Limber, M. N., Celler, A., Barney, J. S., Limber, M. A., Borwein, J. M.: Direct reconstruction of functional parameters for dynamic SPECT. IEEE Trans. Nuc. Sci. **42** (1995) 1249–1256
5. Sitek, A., DiBella, E. V. R., Gullberg, G. T.: Direct extraction of tomographic time activity curves from dynamic SPECT projections using factor analysis. J. Nucl. Med. **39** (1998) 144P
6. Wu. H-M., Hoh, C. K., Choi, Y., Schelbert, H. R., Hawkins, R. A., Phelps, M. E., Huang, S-C.: Factor analysis for extraction of blood time-activity curves in dynamic FDG-PET studies. J. Nucl. Med. **36** (1995) 1714–1722
7. Coxson, P. G., Salmeron, E. M., Huesman, R. H., Mazoyer, B. M.: Simulation of compartmental models for kinetic data from a positron emission tomograph. Comput. Methods. Programs. Biomed. **37** (1992) 205–214
8. Huesman, R. H., Mazoyer, B. M.: Kinetic data analysis with a noisy input function. Phys. Med. Biol. **32** (1987) 1569–1579

Spectral Factor Analysis for Multi–isotope Imaging in Nuclear Medicine

I. Buvat[1], S. Hapdey[1], H. Benali[1], A. Todd-Pokropek[1,2], and R. Di Paola[1]

[1] U494 INSERM, CHU Pitié-Salpêtrière, Paris, France
buvat@imed.jussieu.fr
[2] Department of Medical Physics, University College London, London, UK

Abstract. In nuclear medicine, simultaneous dual-isotope imaging is used to determine the distribution of two radiotracers from a single acquisition and for emission/transmission (E/T) imaging in SPECT. However, no general solution to the cross–talk problem caused by scattered and unscattered photons has been found yet and accurate quantification cannot be performed. We describe a *general* method of spectral factor analysis (SFA) for multi–isotope acquisitions. SFA corrects for cross–talk due to unscattered and scattered photons in planar or SPECT imaging involving two or more radiotracers and for E/T scans. A Tc-99m/I-123 phantom study shows that quantitative accuracy is within 10% with SFA, while errors up to 170% are observed using conventional spectral windows.

1 Introduction

In nuclear medicine, simultaneous dual–isotope imaging is used to determine the distribution of two imaging agents labeled with two different isotopes (e.g., [1,2]) and also for simultaneous emission/transmission (E/T) imaging in SPECT, where one radioisotope is used for transmission scanning while the other is used for the emission study [3]. The major problem with simultaneous dual–isotope acquisition procedure is the cross–talk between the two isotopes. Photons emitted by one radioisotope can be detected in the energy window dedicated to the acquisition of photons emitted by the other and conversely. Cross–talk can be caused by unscattered photons if the photopeaks corresponding to the two radioisotopes partially overlap. Cross–talk is also systematically introduced by scattered photons from the highest energy isotope which are detected in the energy window corresponding to the lowest energy isotope. The magnitude of cross–talk varies with the experimental conditions but it is admitted that the resulting images are not trustworthy without some cross–talk correction [4].

There is currently no method accepted as a standard for cross–talk correction. Symmetrical and off-set energy windows are used (e.g., [1,5]) to reduce cross–talk but do not remove it. Subtraction methods involving at least three energy windows have also been proposed (e.g., [5,6]). However, none of these approaches offers a reliable solution when cross–talk is caused by both scattered

A. Kuba et al. (Eds.): IPMI'99, LNCS 1613, pp. 442–447, 1999.

and unscattered photons. In addition, these empirical approaches need substantial changes and specific calibration for each combination of isotopes.

We describe here a general method for the analysis of multi–isotope acquisitions using a spectral factor analysis (SFA). SFA corrects for cross–talk due to both unscattered and scattered photons.

2 Theory

As different radioisotopes can be distinguished by their emission energy spectrum, SFA analyzes the set of spectra detected in the pixels of the planar images (or projections in SPECT), using either a list mode or a multispectral acquisition technique. For the sake of simplicity, we consider here planar imaging (the extension to SPECT is discussed below). A planar acquisition with spectral information consists of a set of E spectral images, each image including photons detected in a small energy interval. $\mathbf{X}_i(e)$ is the number of photons detected in pixel i of image e.

The model assumes that each noise–free spectrum can be written as a linear combination of K spectral components f_k common to all pixels i, i.e.:

$$\mathbf{X}_i(e) = \sum_{k=1}^{K} a_k(i) f_k(e) + \varepsilon_i(e), \tag{1}$$

where $a_k(i)$ is the number of photons in pixel i distributed according to the spectrum f_k and $\varepsilon_i(e)$ represents noise.

For multi–isotope imaging with R isotopes, the spectral components f_k are R scatter–free spectra f_r and $K - R$ scatter spectra. For each isotope r, the $\{a_r(i)\}$ coefficients ($i = 1, \ldots, N$, N is the number of pixels in an image) associated with the scatter–free spectrum f_r give the scatter–free image of isotope r. Solving the model consists in estimating the scatter–free and scatter spectra f_k and the associated $a_k(i)$. This is performed using SFA, derived from the latest developments regarding factor analysis of medical image sequences [7,8]. In the following, we briefly describe the four steps of SFA.

Data preprocessing. First, the spectra corresponding to spatial neighbor pixels are added (e.g., using 4×4 pixel non overlapping ROIs), which is equivalent to a coarse spatial sampling. This reduces the number of spectra to be analyzed and increases the signal–to–noise ratio in each spectrum. Spectra corresponding to irrelevant regions in the images are also discarded, resulting in M spectra $\mathbf{Y}_i$. The model (1) can be written:

$$\mathbf{Y}_i(e) = \sum_{k=1}^{K} a'_k(i) f_k(e) + \varepsilon'_i(e), \tag{2}$$

where the $\{a'_k(i)\}_{i=1,\ldots,M}$ is the image (with coarse sampling) associated with the spectrum f_k and $\varepsilon'_i(e)$ represents noise.

Orthogonal analysis. This stage filters the spectra $\mathbf{Y}_i$, to estimate their noise–free components Y_i assuming these components belong to a low dimensional space S (typically < 5D). S is estimated using an orthogonal decomposition adapted to the Poisson nature of the set of spectra $\{\mathbf{Y}_i\}_{i=1,\ldots,M}$, namely a correspondence analysis (CA). CA yields an orthogonal spectral basis from which a Q–dimensional space S, spanned by the Q eigenvectors associated with the largest Q eigenvalues of the covariance matrix decomposed by CA, is obtained [9].

Oblique analysis. The oblique analysis estimates the spectra f_k underlying the model (1) assuming they belong to the subspace S. It is also assumed that the dimension Q of S is equal to the number K of spectra underlying the physical model. To estimate the f_k, a priori knowledge pertaining to the spectra f_k and to the images a'_k must be used [7]. We know that $f_k(e) \geq 0$ and $a'_k(i) \geq 0$ since they represent numbers of photons. In addition, for each scatter–free spectrum $f_r(e) = 0$ for some energy channels where there is no photopeak. Using this information, the R scatter–free spectra f_r are first located in S using the target apex–seeking (TAS) method [10]. Next, the $K - R$ scatter spectra f_k are estimated iteratively by minimizing the number of negative $f_k(e)$ and $a'_k(i)$ values while taking into account the confidence interval around each estimated $f_k(e)$ or $a'_k(i)$ [8].

Oblique projection. An oblique projection finally determines the coefficients $a_k(i)$ of equation (1) given the original spectra $\mathbf{X}_i$ and the estimated spectra f_k [8]. The set of coefficients $\{a_r(i)\}_{i=1,\ldots,N}$ corresponding to the scatter–free spectrum f_r gives the scatter–free image of the isotope r.

3   Material and Methods

The phantom (Fig. 1) consisted of 2 series of 9 overlapping Petri dishes ($?$=8.6cm, 1.3 cm thick), including various mixtures of I–123 (emission energy of 159 keV) and Tc–99m (emission energy of 140 keV) in water (Table 1).

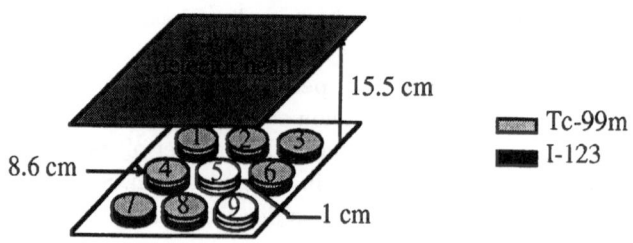

Fig. 1. Phantom used for the acquisition

A planar view of the phantom gave an image of 9 dishes with variable mixtures of Tc–99m and I–123. The total Tc–99m and I–123 activities were 23.1 and 24.8 GBq respectively. A 20 min acquisition (6.45 million counts) was performed on a Elscint Helix gamma camera, equipped with a low energy high resolution collimator, using 32 spectral images (3.5 keV wide each) with a matrix 256×256 (pixel size = 1.47 mm) between 63 and 175 keV.

Table 1. Percentages of Tc–99m and I–123 activity in each dish of the phantom

dish number	1	2	3	4	5	6	7	8	9
percentage of Tc–99m	36	32	22.6	15	0	68.3	83.5	89.7	0
percentage of I–123	64	68	77.4	85	0	31.7	16.5	10.3	0

The resulting 32 images were processed using SFA: 8×8 pixel grouping, TAS of the Tc–99m photopeak assuming it was zero between 63 and 126 keV and between 154 and 175 keV and TAS of the I–123 photopeak assuming it was zero between 63 and 143.5 keV. A scatter spectrum was estimated using non–negativity constraints only. The SFA cross–talk free images were compared to the Tc–99m and I–123 images obtained using "optimal" energy windows [11]: a 15% window centered on 140 keV (129.5–150.5 keV) for Tc–99m and a 154–175 keV window for I–123 (called WIN images below).

The Tc–99m and I–123 images were analyzed by drawing circular ROIs inside each dish (?=4.5 cm). The mean number of counts inside each ROI was calculated. Using the Tc-99m (resp. I–123) image, the dish with the largest mean number of counts N_{Tcmax} (resp. N_{Imax}) was identified and, for each dish d, the ratio of the mean number of counts N_{Tc-d} (resp. N_{I-d}) in the dish d to N_{Tcmax} (resp. N_{Imax}) was determined. These ratios N_{Tc-d}/N_{Tcmax} and N_{I-d}/N_{Imax} represent the activity ratios (AR) between different regions in the Tc–99m and I–123 images. In each dish d, the AR N_{Tc-d}/N_{I-d} was also determined. All AR were compared to their true values theoretically derived given the real activity in the dishes and the attenuation effect. As this was planar imaging, no absolute quantitation was attempted.

4   Results

The spectra (Fig. 2) estimated using SFA and the location of the spectral windows used for WIN as defined above show that, when using WIN, cross–talk in the Tc–99m window is due to scattered photons and unscattered I–123 photons and that some Tc–99m unscattered photons are outside the Tc–99m window. On the other hand, cross–talk in the I–123 image is mostly due to scattered photons. WIN I–123 window also rejects many I–123 unscattered photons.

Figs. 3a–b show the Tc–99m and I–123 AR measured in the different dishes for the estimated Tc–99m and I–123 images. Using WIN Tc–99m image, errors up to 81% (ROI 3) and 170% (ROI 4) were observed for low N_{Tc-d}/N_{Tcmax} values (22.5 and 11.0% respectively). With the SFA Tc–99m image, the largest errors observed for N_{Tc-d}/N_{Tcmax} AR were 4.4% and 5.8% for ROIs 6 and 8 where the true AR were 73.2% and 87.8% respectively.

The differences in performance between the methods where less obvious for the I–123 images, with errors between 1.5% (ROI 6) and 9.7% (ROI 5) for WIN,

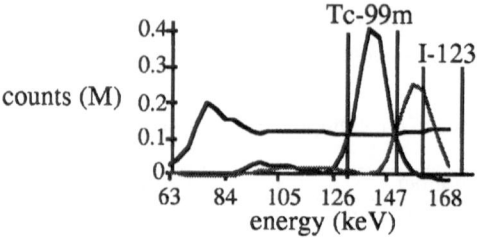

Fig. 2. Spectra estimated using SFA and spectral windows used in WIN

and between 0.8% (ROI 9) and 9.3% (ROI 7) for SFA. The I–123 AR measured in cold dishes 5 and 9 were < 1.5% with SFA and they were between 4.5 and 11.8% with WIN.

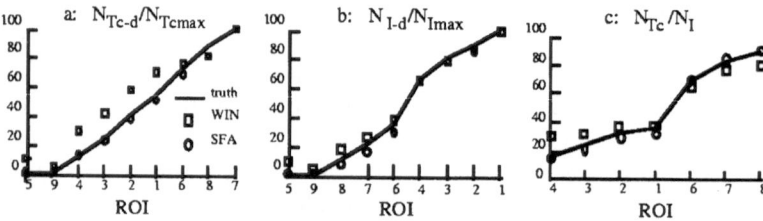

Fig. 3. Relative quantitation results from the WIN and SFA Tc–99m and I–123 images

Fig. 3c shows the estimated N_{Tc-d}/N_{I-d} AR, the WIN images yielded an overestimation of the AR for the lowest AR and an underestimation for the highest AR, with errors between +13.9% (ROI 4) and -9% (ROI 8). SFA images gave errors between -1.5% (ROI 7) and +4.4% (ROI 1).

5   Discussion and Conclusion

Simultaneous dual–isotope studies are currently hindered by cross–talk problems, for which there are no satisfactory solutions yet [4]. The SFA method offers a general solution, since it can be used a priori for any radioisotope combination, both for studies involving two radiopharmaceuticals and for E/T studies. SFA is a data driven approach and the severity of cross–talk does not have to be known a priori. However, as the linear model underlying SFA is quite general, a priori knowledge must be used to find the solution appropriate to the physics of the problem. This a priori knowledge relates to the energy range in which the photopeaks should be zero and does not have to be extremely precise: a change of few keV in the definition of this energy range (up to 10 in our example) did not affect the results. SFA corrects for cross–talk due to scattered and unscattered photons. SFA takes advantage of the Poisson nature of the data when filtering the noise (in the orthogonal analysis) and when estimating the model components (in the oblique analysis). The method permits a quantitative interpretation of the results, which is of paramount importance for E/T imaging. SFA model is not stationary, i.e. it does not intrinsically assume that the scatter spectrum has the same shape in every pixel. However, estimating at least 4 spectra is needed to make the analysis non stationary. In our example, accurate results were obtained when assuming scatter stationarity (i.e. considering 3 factors only).

The challenging Tc–99m/I–123 phantom we considered showed that SFA outperformed the method using energy windows, which is the only alternative proposed so far for this couple of radioisotopes.

Although we gave evidence that SFA could offer a solution to the cross–talk problem, further investigations involving other combinations of radioisotopes, in emission/emission or E/T studies should now be conducted. So far, only planar images have been processed, but SPECT data can be dealt with similarly using a single SFA of the spectra corresponding to all projections, before reconstruction.

References

1. Devous, M.D., Payne, J.K., Lowe, J.L.: Dual–isotope brain SPECT imaging with Technetium–99m and Iodine–123: clinical validation using Xenon–133 SPECT. J. Nucl. Med. **33** (1992) 1919–1924
2. Schoeder, H., Topp, H., Friedrich, M., Jatzkewitz, A., Roser, M.: Thallium and indium antimyosin dual–isotope single–photon emission tomography in acute myocardial infarction to identify patients at further ischaemic risk. Eur. J. Nucl. Med. **21** (1994) 415–422
3. Bailey, D.L.: Transmission scanning in emission tomography. Eur. J. Nucl. Med. **25** (1998) 774–787
4. Links, J.M.: Simultaneous dual–radionuclide imaging: are the images trustworthy? Eur. J. Nucl. Med. **23** (1996) 1289–1291
5. Ivanovic, M., Weber, D.A., Loncaric, S., Franceschi, D.: Feasability of dual radionuclide brain imaging with I–123 and Tc–99m. Med. Phys. **21** (1994) 667–674
6. Moore, S.C., English, R.J., Syravanh, C., Tow, D.E., Zimmerman, R. E., Chan, K.H., Kijewski, M.F.: Simultaneous Tc–99m/Tl–201 imaging using energy–based estimation of the spatial distribution of contaminant photons. IEEE Trans. Nucl. Sci. **42** (1995) 1189-1195
7. Benali, H., Buvat, I., Frouin, F., Bazin, J.P., Di Paola, R.: Foundations of factor analysis of medical image sequences. Image and Vision Computing **12** (1994) 375–385
8. Buvat, I., Benali, H., Di Paola, R.: Statistical distribution of factors and factor images in factor analysis of medical image sequences. Phys. Med. Biol. **43** (1998) 421–434
9. Benali, H., Buvat, I., Frouin, F., Bazin, J.P., Di Paola, R.: A statistical model for the determination of the optimal metric in Factor Analysis of Medical Image Sequences (FAMIS). Phys. Med. Biol. **38** (1993) 1065–1080
10. Buvat, I., Benali, H., Frouin, F., Bazin, J.P., Di Paola, R.: Target apex–seeking in factor analysis of medical image sequences. Phys. Med. Biol. **38** (1993) 123–138
11. Hindié, E., Mellière, D., Jeanguillaume, C., Perlemuter, L., Chéhadé, F., Galle, P.: Parathyroid imaging using simultaneous double–window recording of Technetium–99m–sestamibi and Iodine–123. J. Nucl. Med. **39** (1998) 1100–1105

Structural Group Analysis of Functional Maps

Olivier Coulon[1,2], Jean-Francois Mangin[2], Jean-Baptiste Poline[2],
Vincent Frouin[2], and Isabelle Bloch[1]

[1] TSI Department, Ecole Nationale Supérieure des Télécommunications, 46, rue
Barrault, 75631 Paris Cedex 13, France
coulon@ima.enst.fr
[2] Service Hospitalier Frédéric Joliot, CEA, 91401 Orsay Cedex, France
mangin@shfj.cea.fr

Abstract. We present here a new method for cerebral activation detection. This method is performed on individual activation maps of any
sort and aims at performing a multi-subject group analysis while preserving individual information and overcoming problems induced by spatial
normalisation. The analysis is made through a multi-scale object-based
description of individual maps. It is these structural descriptions which
are compared, rather than the images themselves. The comparison is
made through a graph, on which a labelling process is performed. The
label field on the graph is modelled by a Markov random field, which
allows us to introduce high-level rules of data interrogation.

1 Introduction

Understanding the neural substratum of human brain function is a growing field
of research. Due to the very noisy nature of functional images, brain activation
detection has essentially been approached so far in terms of statistical analysis
[1,2] using a common anatomical reference. Although they have been validated
in a wide range of applications, these analyses lead to some problems in terms of
localisation and/or detection with regard to anatomy. In particular, the spatial
normalisation performed to compare images from different subjects matches normally only gross features. Moreover, anatomical information is poorly handled,
and after a statistical analysis, it is generally difficult to estimate from the group
result the areas activated in individual subjects. This knowledge should help the
study of inter-subject functional and anatomical variability and would improve
localisation with regard to anatomy. We propose here a new method based on a
description of individual activation maps in terms of structure. This is followed
by the comparison of these descriptions across subjects, rather than comparing directly the images at a voxel level in a stereotactic space. The method is
designed to overcome, as far as possible, the problems induced by spatial normalisation [7]. After detection over a group of subjects, the method allows an
easy way to get back to the individual structures, and more generally permits
high level interrogation, and in the future more informed analysis, of functional
data sets.

A. Kuba et al. (Eds.): IPMI'99, LNCS 1613, pp. 448–453, 1999.
© Springer-Verlag Berlin Heidelberg 1999

2   Methods

The method presented here is applicable to any kind of individual "activation map": e.g. PET or fMRI difference images, t-maps, etc. It is divided into the three following steps. First, each individual map involved in the study is described by its scale-space primal sketch. Second, a graph is built that matches all the primal sketches. Finally, a labelling process is performed on the graph, which aims to identify the objects representing functional activations and those representing noise.

2.1   The Scale-Space Primal Sketch

The scale-space primal sketch is a representation, based on well-known properties of linear scale-space allowing the description of the 1st order structure of an image [4]. We present its structure very briefly. For more precise details, we invite the reader to refer to [3], or to [5] for the particular 3-dimensional case applied to activation maps. This hierarchical multiscale description makes explicit the behavior of objects (*grey-level blobs*) through the scales of a linear scale-space. It is composed of multiscale objects (*scale-space blobs*) linked by bifurcations representing their relative behavior, as illustrated in a symbolic way in Fig. 1. Measurements are assigned to the scale-space blobs to characterize their geometrical features and lifetime along the scale axis.

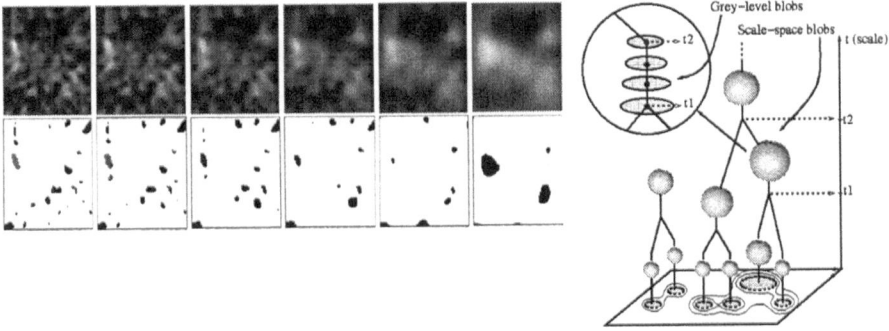

Fig. 1. A slice of different scale levels of an activation map, the corresponding blobs, and a symbolic representation of the scale-space primal sketch

2.2   The Comparison Graph

We want to create a comparison graph such that it contains the primal sketches of all the subjects involved in the analysis, and such that it makes explicit all potential repetitions of an object across subjects, while being exhaustive, but without taking any decision about their validity. To compare different primal sketches we normalise them with usual procedures [6]. A longer term aim is to build the spatial referential using subjects individual anatomy and a high-level description of this anatomy, in terms of landmarks and identified structures [10]. The comparison graph should be a convenient framework for this purpose. The first criterion to link two blobs belonging to two different primal sketches is the overlap of their spatial and scale support. If it is fulfilled, we create a direct link $[b_1 - b_2]_{out1}$ between the two scale-space blobs b_1 and b_2 (Fig. 2). Since we want

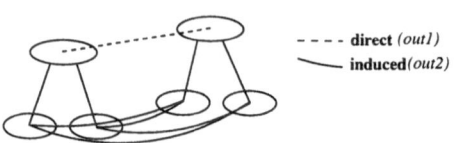

- - - - **direct** (*out1*)
——— **induced**(*out2*)

Fig. 2. A *direct* link induces additional links at finer scales

to introduce some flexibility in the position of activations, to overcome potential normalisation problems, we have to allow close blobs to be linked even if they have no spacial overlap. We therefore use the fact that a direct link might not represent exactly an activation but may suggest the presence of an activation at a finer scale. We then define *induced* links (*out2* links) as follows. If b_1 and b_2 are two blobs having no direct link between them, they have an induced link $[b_1 - b_2]_{out2}$ if they are "under" (in their primal sketches) two blobs c_1 and c_2 having a direct link $[c_1 - c_2]_{out1}$, and if they have a scale overlap (Fig. 2). Allowing blobs without spatial overlap to be linked is a key feature of the process, since it provides greater flexibility for overcoming spatial normalisation limitations.

2.3   The Detection Model: Use of a Markovian Random Field

Activation detection is performed using a labelling process that uses the inter-subject comparison graph previously described. Our aim is to associate a positive label to each activation in the graph, and a null label to the structures of non-interest. An activation (i.e. a positive label) is associated to a spatial localisation, and can therefore have one occurrence in each of the individual primal sketches. The basic model we use to perform the detection is the following:
1. a blob representing an activation is likely to have high measurements;
2. two blobs representing the same activation must be linked in the graph and have the same positive label;
3. two blobs representing the same activation are likely to have spatial supports close to each other;
4. an activation should have only zero or one occurrence per subject.
Given the local aspect of the dependencies that are defined within the graph, we model the label field as a Markov random field and, through a classical *maximum a posteriori* process, the optimal labelling is done by minimising a

Gibbs distribution related energy [8]. For more details, the reader should refer to [9]. The energy is defined with potential functions on cliques of different order in the graph. Each potential function models either one or two rules in the above-specified model. Rule (1.) is modelled using a potential function defined over 1st order cliques (blobs). When a blob has a positive label, the higher the associated measurements are, the lower the potential is, following a piecewise linear function. Rule (4.) is modelled using a function V_{ps}, defined on each primal sketch, and linearly increasing with the number of occurences of each positive label in the primal sketch. Rules (2.) and (3.) are modelled by an inter primal sketch 2nd order clique potential function. On such a clique, when the two blobs have the same positive label, the associated potential is a function that decreases with a measurement of similarity between the two blobs. This similarity function is the second way, in the whole process, to overcome problems induced by spatial normalisation. At the moment, we use an overlapping function for $out1$ links, and an Euclidean distance function for $out2$ links. The aim, in the long term, is to have an individual anatomy-related similarity function which somehow would provide an improvement to spatial normalisation.

The total energy function is then minimised using a stochastic algorithm, the Gibbs sampler with annealing [8], which is shown to provide good convergence. After minimisation, the process produces a set of positive labels, each one representing an activation and having an occurrence in a number of primal sketches. We therefore know the occurrence, or the absence of occurrence, of each activation for any subject. This occurrence can then be mapped on the individual anatomy of the subject for localisation considerations.

3   Results

The process presented here has been tested on a PET motor protocol, including 10 subjects and 12 images per subject. For each subject, an individual statistical t-map was first computed using the SPM software [1], contrasting a periodic auditory-cued right hand movement and a rest condition. A primal sketch was then built from each of the individual maps, and the 10 primal sketches were compared using the labelling process. A group analysis was also performed using SPM software , and used as a reference to validate our results. Numerous activations were found at a very significant level in the group map in the expected brain regions.

After our labelling process, several observations arise.

- All high-significance expected activations were detected, although given the functional variability it is difficult to compare a pure group analysis with a method that considers individual information.

- Two false positive were detected, but they were both outside the brain and caused by border effects (easily eliminated).

- A classical threshold on the individual maps yielded poor results for every map being, either too selective, or too noisy. This shows a crucial advantage of our method; the detection is processed for each subject taking into account not only the intensity in the map but also the knowledge of other subjects maps.

- The relevance of each detected positive label was correlated with its associated local energy. This was further confirmed by simulations. In particular, when a positive label corresponds to no real activation, its local energy is high enough to discriminate it from labels associated with real activations.

- Localisation accuracy is lowered by the lack of an automatic scale selection method to represent each detected scale-space blob. Furthermore, experiments

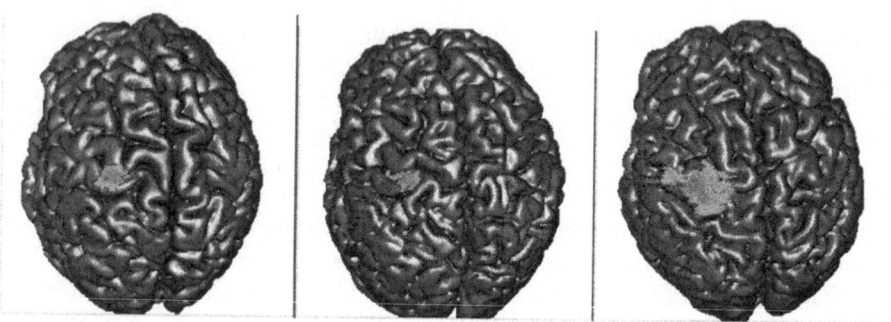

Fig. 3. individual mapping of the primary motor activation on 3D rendering of subject anatomy

with simulated activation maps including two different objects showed a detection rate of 100% (no false negative) for a localisation variability up to twice the size of the objects, which shows a good resistance to inter-subject variability. Simulations on a very large number of noise images are currently being run to assess a precise evaluation of the error rate.

4   Conclusion

We have presented here a new method to analyse brain functional images that considers functional activation detection at a structural level, and permits a way of getting back to individual results after detection over a group of subjects. It uses the power and comprehensiveness of multiscale methods to describe image structure by looking at their whole scale-space without any *a priori* information concerning scales of interest and without any "coarse-to-fine" strategy. A major difference from classical methods is the comparison at an object level, which permits us to introduce higher level criteria for the analysis and is a way to overcome inter-subject variability effects. The process has proved to be able to detect efficiently expected activations with a PET dataset. It is promising for functional MRI studies, since fMRI provides more reliable individual maps than PET. Further research still has to be undertaken to solve outstanding questions, particularly concerning the choice of the optimal scale used to represent (as opposed to detect) a scale-space blob, since the extent of the reported activations depends on this scale. Secondly, a precise evaluation of the data-driven potential functions still has to be properly investigated from the distribution of measurements associated with the blobs. We showed that the spurious effects of spatial normalisation could be reduced by means of the comparison graph and of an appropriate definition of similarity between blobs from different subjects. Although it is difficult to relate the proposed analysis to standard statistical analyses, it is worth noting that there is some analogy with analyses using random effect linear models. Specifically, activation detection is performed using a subject by subject variability rather than on a scan by scan variability. Finally, we would like to point out the fact that using a Markovian model for the detection allows the user of such a system to interrogate the data in ways that can be designed according to the experimental question. It is very easy to define new potential functions in which one can introduce, for instance, a priori information about a precise expected location, or about the search for a network of activations instead of isolated ones. Thus, the system can explore multi-subject functional data sets in a higher level manner than has been achieved so far.

References

1. Friston, K.J., Holmes, A.P., Poline, J.B., Worsley, K.J., Frith, C.D., Frackowiak, R.S.J.: Statistical parametric maps in functional imaging: a general linear approach. Human Brain Mapping **2** (1995) 189–210
2. Worsley, K.J., Marrett, S., Neelin, P., Vandal, A.C., Friston, K.J., Evans, A.C.: A unified statistical approach for determining significant signals in images of cerebral activation. Human Brain Mapping **4** (1996) 58–73
3. Lindeberg, T., Eklundh, J.O.: Scale-space primal sketch: construction and experiments. Image and Vision Computing **10**:1 (1992) 3–18
4. Koenderink, J.J.: The structure of images. Biological Cybernetics **50** (1984) 363–370
5. Coulon, O., Bloch, I., Frouin, V., Mangin, J.F.: Multiscale measures in linear scale-space for characterizing cerebral functional activations in 3D PET difference images. ScaleSpace'97, LNCS **1252** (1997) 188–199
6. Ashburner, J., Friston, K.J.: Human Brain Function, chapt. 3 (1997) 43–58, Academic Press
7. Lester, H., Arridge S.R.: A survey of hierarchical non-linear medical image registration. Pattern Recognition **32**:1 (1999) 129-149
8. Geman S., Geman, D.: Stochastic relaxation, Gibbs distributions, and the bayesian restoration of images. IEEE Trans. on Pattern Analysis and Machine Intelligence, **6**:6 (1984) 721–741
9. Coulon, O.: Analyse multi-échelle de cartes d'activations fonctionnelles cérébrales. PhD Thesis (1998), Ecole Nationale Supérieure des Télécommunications, TSI Department, ENST-98E019.
10. Mangin, J.F., Frouin, V., Bloch, I., Régis, J., Lopez-Krahe, J.: From 3D magnetic resonance images to structural representations of the cortex topography using topology preserving deformations. Journal of Mathematical Imaging and Vision, **5**:4 (1995) 297–318

Incorporating an Image Distortion Model in Non–rigid Alignment of EPI with Conventional MRI

Colin Studholme[1], R. Todd Constable[1], and James S. Duncan[1]

Departments of Diagnostic Radiology and Electrical Engineering,
Yale University New Haven CT 06520-8042 U.S.A.

Abstract. This paper addresses the problem of accurately mapping echo planar image (EPI) data acquired for functional MRI studies to conventional T_1 weighted anatomical MRI. In particular here we examine the correction of spin echo image distortion resulting from magnetic field inhomogeneity. To do this we must account for both geometric and intensity distortions within the EPI data. This approach combines ideas on multi-modality registration criteria, non-rigid registration and models of geometric and intensity distortion in MR image formation. Specifically the relationship between the geometric and intensity distortion in spin echo EPI imaging is used to constrain the geometric correction estimate and replaces the arbitrary smoothing energy term in non-rigid registration.

1 Introduction

The interpretation of functional magnetic resonance images (FMRI) is heavily dependent on their precise anatomical location. It is common for functional imaging studies to include an additional conventional T_1 acquisition to provide anatomical context. Current multi-modality registration methods enable many types of functional image data to be accurately aligned with anatomical data [14,9]. These methods generally account for differences in patient positioning and imaged field with a global rigid or affine geometric transformation. In practice echo planar image (EPI) data used in functional imaging can exhibit severe localised geometric distortion. This is particularly apparent in acquisitions through the brain where bone or air boundaries with soft tissues result in significant magnetic field inhomogeneities. Errors such as these can lead to mis-placing of functional signals by many millimeters, resulting in the possible displacement of a response into a neighbouring gyri [5].

Current approaches to accurate mapping of this data to anatomical MRI involve a correction of these EPI artifacts using field mapping acquisitions [13,7,6,8] prior to rigid alignment with anatomical MRI. This requires considerable additional imaging time and may introduce errors arising for example from flow effects [7]. In this paper we propose the use of a direct non-rigid registration but employing geometric constraints derived from a model of spin echo imaging

A. Kuba et al. (Eds.): IPMI'99, LNCS 1613, pp. 454–459, 1999.

distortion. The key step here is to use the link between geometric errors and the resulting localised intensity distortion in spin echo EPI. This allows us to define a direct global intensity criteria expressing the quality of the geometric match between EPI and anatomical MRI without the need for additional smoothing terms on the estimated warp.

2   Distortion in Spin Echo Anatomical and EPI Imaging

During the spin echo imaging process magnetic field gradients are imposed on the patient tissues. Any variation from the assumed linear gradient results in phase or frequency shifts in the recorded k-space signal. For conventional anatomical T_1 spin echo imaging there is a displacement error due to local magnetic field inhomogeneity $\Delta B_o(x, y, z)$ in the phase (y), frequency (x) and slice encode (z) directions. Briefly, from [7] and by substitution (see [1]), these displacements from (x, y, z) to (x_A, y_A, z_A) are described by,

$$x_A = x + \frac{\Delta B_o(x, y, z)}{G_{xA}}, \tag{1}$$

$$y_A = y, \tag{2}$$

and

$$z_A = z + \frac{\Delta B_o(x, y, z)}{G_{zA}}, \tag{3}$$

where G_{xA}, G_{yA} and G_{zA} are the imaging gradients imposed in the respective axes. The resulting y (phase encode) axis has no distortion, while the x (frequency encode) and z (slice encode) have magnetic field related displacement errors. For typical imaging sequences these may result [7] in pixel shifts of only $0.1mm$.

For spin echo EPI functional imaging the displacements take a slightly different the form [7],

$$x_F = x + \frac{\Delta B_o(x, y, z)}{G_{xF}}, \tag{4}$$

$$y_F = y + \frac{\Delta B_o(x, y, z)(2\tau_{ramp} + NT)}{G_{yF}\tau_{ramp}}. \tag{5}$$

and

$$z_F = z + \frac{\Delta B_o(x, y, z)}{G_{zF}}. \tag{6}$$

Now, in the phase encode y axis, the resulting displacement is scaled by a factor $(2\tau_{ramp} + NT)/\tau_{ramp}$ compared to the other axes. The factor N from the imaging matrix results in a significant displacement, and for typical imaging parameters [7] we have the possibility of shifts of one or more pixels.

2.1   Intensity Distortion

Considering the general case of 3D spin echo imaging, the change in coordinate system from true point locations (x, y, z) to displaced points at (x_F, y_F, z_F) result in a change in signal strength governed by the Jacobian of the distortion transformation [1]. So, if we have an estimate of the geometric correction mapping between the correct anatomical space to the distorted EPI space: $T_e : (x, y, z) \mapsto (x_F, y_F, z_F)$, the estimate of the corresponding corrected EPI image intensity value $f_e(x, y, z)$ from the distorted measured values $f_m(x_F, y_F, z_F)$ is given by [1],

$$f_e(x, y, z) = f_m(T_e(x, y, z))/J(x, y, z). \tag{7}$$

This relationship is the key to introducing geometrical constraints into the intensity based correction criteria. Effectively it can be seen as a form of signal conservation in the distortion process. As the image is compressed locally, signal from many voxels is mapped to fewer voxels. Conversely, where the image is expanded, signal from one voxel is mapped to many voxels.

2.2   Relative Distortion

If we assume that the rigid body rotations between the axes of the two scans will be small (say less than 5 degrees). Then the phase, frequency encode and slice select directions in the EPI and anatomical MR are closely aligned. If the frequency and slice select gradients are similar ($G_{xF} \approx G_{xA}$ and $G_{zF} \approx G_{zA}$) then the resulting distortions will be small so that $x_F \approx x_A$ and $z_F \approx z_A$. This leaves displacement in the phase encode y axis. In a conventional spin echo scan, the displacement due to the field inhomogeneity (2) is negligible. In EPI imaging, the acquisition of multiple phase encode steps, with a single excitation pulse, results in significant displacements along the phase encode axis.

3   Correction Criteria Using Signal Conservation Model

Entropy based multi-modality registration criteria [11,3] provide a powerful approach to spatially aligning one image with another where there is some spatial correspondence of structure delineated by the two images. The key problem with non-rigid registration is the need to introduce constraints on the smoothness of the geometric transformation. This prevents unconstrained motion in regions of the image where there are no corresponding structures, particularly in the multi-modality case. The nature of the smoothing approach depends on the application [4,2]. A common approach to smoothing the geometric transformation is to include an energy term, such as Tikhonov regularlisation [12] which leads to the optimisation of a cost function which is a combination of the intensity similarity and the smoothness energy.

The basic idea behind our correction approach is to use a global similarity measure between the EPI image $f_e(T(x, y, z))$ with estimated correction transformation $T_e(x, y, z)$ and a conventional anatomical acquisition $g(x, y, z)$, as a measure of geometric and intensity correction.

Using the Jacobian term to modify the EPI intensities will result in bright regions of the image being more sensitive to local changes in the transformation estimate than darker regions. To avoid this we take logarithms of equation (7) and derive a correction criteria between Log corrected EPI $f' = \ln(f)$ image values,

$$f'_e(x, y, z) = f'_m(T_e(x, y, z)) - J'_e(x, y, z), \tag{8}$$

and the original anatomical MR values $g()$. We maximise an entropy based registration criteria [10] derived from mutual information [3,11] which provides a form of image overlap invariance,

$$\arg\max_{T_c} \left\{ \frac{H(g) + H(T_e(f'_e))}{H(g, T_e(f'_e))} \right\}. \tag{9}$$

The terms $H(g)$ and $H(f'_e)$ are the marginal entropies of values in the anatomical and EPI images respectively and $H(g, f'_e)$ is the joint entropy. All entropies are evaluated from values in the overlap of the two modalities.

4   Experimental Registration Results

The transformation estimate between the two images is controlled by a combination of the local warp to account for distortion and the six rigid transformation parameters determining patient positioning,

$$T_e(x, y, z) = T_{patient}(x, y, z) + T_{\Delta B_0}(x, y, z). \tag{10}$$

In EPI field mapping techniques the measured displacement field is commonly approximated by a low order polynomial (eg [7,8]). Here we use a cubic B-spline to parameterise the local warp over the image volume. Registration was initiated by first running a rigid registration to form a good starting estimate. From this estimate, a two step process was applied iteratively, consisting of a simple gradient ascent with respect to the local B-spline parameters followed by a global rigid re-registration. Spline grid points with an isotropic spacing of 15mm were used. Tri-linear interpolation was used to estimate intermediate values in the EPI image for voxel locations in the anatomical spin echo image. A discrete histogram of 64×64 intensity bins was used to estimate the marginal and joint entropies in (9).

The registration algorithm was applied to correcting spin echo EPI to MRI for a volunteer image set. Examples of the quality of the correction are provided by the coronal slices in Fig. 1. Here the downward displacement of the temporal lobes is recovered while in the medial portion of the brain, displacement in the opposite direction in the same slice is also recovered.

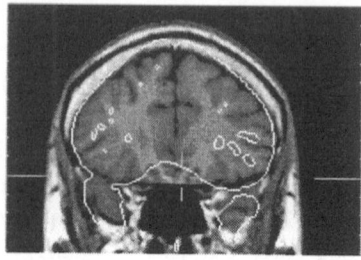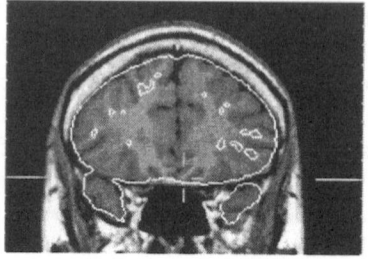

Fig. 1. Example coronal slices through the spin echo MR volume toward the front of the patient with an iso-intensity contour from spin echo EPI overlayed to illustrate spatial alignment. Initial global rigid registration estimate (left) and estimate with non-rigid registration (right)

A second set of anatomical and functional images were acquired and for these a set of t-maps indicating activation was then calculated. The alignment algorithm was applied to correct one frame of spin echo EPI from this sequence onto to a high resolution anatomical scan. This transformation was then used to map the t-map data back to the anatomical reference. Figure 2 illustrates the effect of the local geometric correction on the location of t-map activations.

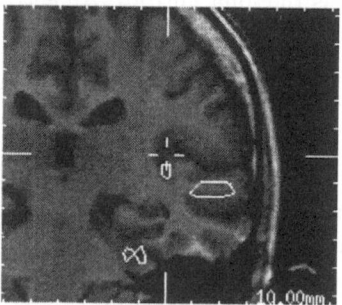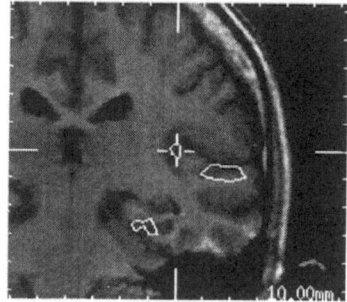

Fig. 2. Example correction on a functional imaging study. Coronal slices through the spin echo T_1 MR anatomical image volume with t-map activation displayed as contour. Global rigid only registration (left) and local warp with signal conservation term (right) showing displacement of activation into gray matter

5   Discussion

In this paper we have begun to address the general problem of precisely aligning functional MRI scans with conventional anatomical acquisitions. We have concentrated here on spin echo imaging acquisitions. We have used knowledge of the image formation and distortion processes in the two MRI scans to impose constraints on the correction estimate. In particular we have modified a common entropy based alignment criteria using knowledge of signal conservation to enforce geometric constraints on the correction warp. It is interesting to note that the causes of distortions are commonly related to material boundaries within the patient (for example soft-tissue boundaries with bone in the orbits and around the petrous bone [7]) which are themselves visible within the MRI acquisitions. These boundaries therefore inherently provide local image constraints on the alignment close to where distortions are occurring.

Overall the initial results with this approach indicate that combining MR distortion models with multi-modality registration techniques can produce precise mapping of functional information to anatomical images, and provide a viable alternative to field mapping techniques.

References

1. Chang, H., and Fitzpatrick, J.M.: A technique for accurate MR imaging in the presence of field inhomogeneities. IEEE Trans. Med. Imaging **11** (1992) 319–329
2. Christensen, G.E., Rabbitt, R.D., and Miller, M.I.: Deformable templates using large deformation kinematics. IEEE Transactions on Image Processing **5** (1996) 1435–1447
3. Collignon, A., Maes, F., Delaere, D., Vandermeulen, D., Suetens, P., and Marchal, G.: Automated multimodality image registration using information theory. In Bizais Y., Barillot C, and Di Paola R., editors, Proceedings of Information Processing in Medical Imaging, Brest, Kluwer Academic Publishers (1995) 263–274
4. Collins, D.L., Evans, A.C., Holmes, C., and Peters, T.M.: Automatic 3D segmentation of neuro-anatomical structures from MRI. In Bizais Y., Barillot C., and Di Paola R., editors, Proceedings of Information Processing in Medical Imaging, Brest, France, Kluwer Academic Publishers (1995) 139–152
5. Farzaneh, F., Reidener, S.J., and Pelc, N.J.: Analysis of T_2 limitations and off-resonance effects on spatial resolution and artifacts in echo-planar imaging. Magnetic Resonance in Medicine **14** (1990) 123–139
6. Jesmanowicz, A., and Hyde, J.S.: Real-time two-shot EPI auto shim overall shimming polynomials. In Proceedings of the Society of Magnetic Resonance (1995) page 618
7. Jezzard, P., and Balaban, R.S.: Correction of geometric distortion in echo planar images from B_o field variations. Magnetic Resonance in Medicine **34** (1995) 65–73
8. Reber, P.J., Wong, E.C., Buxton, R.B., and Frank, L.R.: Correction of off resonance-related distortion in echo planar imaging using EPI-based field maps. Magnetic Resonance in Medicine **39** (1998) 328–330
9. Studholme, C., Hawkes, D.J., and Hill, D. L. G.: Robust fully automated 3D registration of MR and PET images of the brain using multiresolution voxel similarity measures. Medical Physics **24** (1997) 25–35
10. Studholme, C., Hill, D.L.G., and Hawkes, D.J.: An overlap invariant entropy measure of 3D medical image alignment. Pattern Recognition **32** (1999) 71–86
11. Viola, P.A. and Wells, W.M.: Alignment by maximisation of mutual information. In Proceedings of the 5th International Conference on Computer Vision (1995) 15–23
12. Wahba, G.: Spline Models for Observational Data. Society for Industrial and Applied Mathemeatics, Philadelpiha, 1990
13. Weisskoff, R.M. and Davis, T.L.: Correcting gross distortion on echo planar images. In Proceedings of the Society of Magnetic Resonance (1992) 4515
14. West, J., Fitzpatrick, J.M., and et al.: Comparison and evaluation of retrospective intermodality registration techniques. Journal of Computer Assisted Tomography **21** (1997) 554–566

The Distribution of Target Registration Error in Rigid-Body, Point-Based Registration

Jay B. West and J. Michael Fitzpatrick

Department of Computer Science, Vanderbilt University, Nashville, TN 37235, USA

Abstract. Point-based registration is performed by matching a set of homologous points in two spaces. It is common to use such techniques as an aid to navigation during neurosurgical procedures. For many years, statistics concerning Target Registration Error (TRE) have been studied qualitatively using numerical simulations. We present here an expression that gives a good approximation to the distribution of TRE for any given target and configuration of fiducial points.

1 Introduction

The point-based registration problem is as follows: given a set of homologous points in two spaces, find a transformation that brings the points into approximate alignment. In many cases the appropriate transformations are rigid, consisting of translations and rotations. Medical applications abound in neurosurgery, for example, where the head can be treated as a rigid body [3,11,6,15,10,22,16]. The points, which we will call *fiducial* points, may be anatomical landmarks or may be produced artificially by means of attached markers. In the case that we address here, the spaces are three dimensional and may consist, for example, of two MR volumes, a CT volume and an MR volume or PET volume, or, in the case of image-guided neurosurgical applications, an image volume and the physical space of the operating room itself. The rigid-body, point-based image registration problem is typically defined to be the problem of finding the translation vector and rotation matrix that produces the least-squares fit of the corresponding fiducial points. The appropriate translation vector is simply the mean displacement between the two point sets. The problem of determining the rotation matrix can be easily reduced to the "Orthogonal Procrustes problem" [12,20]. Peter Schönemann published the first solution to that problem in 1966 [20]. His solution was rediscovered independently in 1983 by Golub and van Loan [9] and again in 1987 by Arun *et al.* [1]. These latter solutions, unlike the former, employ the method of Singular Value Decomposition (SVD), but they can easily be shown to be equivalent to Schönemann's solution [13].

The solution is unique, but can be expected to yield an imperfect registration in the presence of errors in locating the points. Maurer *et al.* [18,16] suggested three useful measures of error for analyzing the accuracy of point-based registration methods.

A. Kuba et al. (Eds.): IPMI'99, LNCS 1613, pp. 460–465, 1999.

1. *Fiducial localization error (FLE)*, which is the error in locating the fiducial points.
2. *Fiducial registration error (FRE)*, which is the root-mean-square distance between corresponding fiducial points after registration.
3. *Target registration error (TRE)*, which is the distance between corresponding points other than the fiducial points after registration.

The term "target" is used to suggest that the points are directly associated with the reason for the registration. In medical applications they are typically points within, or on the boundary of, lesions to be resected during surgery or regions of functional activity to be examined for diagnostic purposes.

Much work has been done [5,14,11,6,18,16,17,4] using numerical simulations to investigate the properties of FRE and TRE. Unknown to many of those performing these simulations, Sibson [21] gave in 1979 an approximation to the distribution of FRE. In 1998 Fitzpatrick *et al.* derived an equation which allows calculation of an approximation to the root mean square value of TRE [8,7], and agrees with the published simulations. In what follows, however, we give for the first time an approximation to the *distribution* of TRE, rather than just its expected value.

2   The Model

We make a simplifying assumption in this work: that the fiducial localization error in one space is identically zero. This assumption does not generally hold in real registration problems, but the derivation may easily be extended to the case in which FLE is nonzero in both spaces.

Let N be the number of fiducials and K be the spatial dimension. In general, we may write X as the N-by-K matrix whose rows correspond to the position vectors of the fiducial points in one space, and Y as the N-by-K matrix representing the fiducials in the other space. The registration problem is to find a K-by-K orthogonal matrix, R, and a 1-by-K translation vector, t, so that the points $x_i R + t$ are in optimal alignment with the corresponding points y_i in Y. By "optimal alignment", we mean that rms(FRE) is minimized, *i.e.*, R and t are chosen to minimize

$$tr((Y - XR - t)^t (Y - XR - t)). \tag{1}$$

In this work, we assume that X is related to Y by a rigid-body transformation representing a re-orientation of the rigid body to which the points are attached, and a N-by-K matrix F of perturbations representing the fiducial localization error. We assume that the elements of F are independent, zero-mean normal variables with equal variance, *i.e.*, that the FLE has the same distribution at each fiducial point and in each of the coordinate directions at every point. This assumption allows the use of a closed-form solution for the registration problem itself, and as pointed out by Sibson [21], permits us to neglect the rigid body transformation relating X and Y, as FRE and TRE are independent of this re-orientation. We note that, under these assumptions, the variance of each element of F is equal to $\langle \mathrm{FLE}^2 \rangle / K$.

We thus simplify the problem to that of registering X to $Y = X + F$. As the choice of origin for X is arbitrary, we choose the centroid of X to be the origin.

3   The Distribution for the Case $K = 3$

Choosing coordinate axes coincident with the principal axes of the fiducial configuration, and with the fiducials' centroid as the origin, it may be shown [2][1] that

$$\mathrm{TRE}^2(x, y, z) \sim \frac{\langle \mathrm{FLE}^2 \rangle}{3}(k_1 \chi_1^2 + k_2 \chi_1^2 + k_3 \chi_1^2), \tag{2}$$

where

$$k_1 = \left(1/N + \frac{x^2 z^2}{(x^2 + y^2)(\Lambda_{22}^2 + \Lambda_{33}^2)} + \frac{y^2 z^2}{(x^2 + y^2)(\Lambda_{11}^2 + \Lambda_{33}^2)} + \frac{x^2 + y^2}{\Lambda_{11}^2 + \Lambda_{22}^2} \right),$$

$$k_2 = \left(1/N + \frac{y^2(x^2 + y^2 + z^2)}{(x^2 + y^2)(\Lambda_{22}^2 + \Lambda_{33}^2)} + \frac{x^2(x^2 + y^2 + z^2)}{(x^2 + y^2)(\Lambda_{11}^2 + \Lambda_{33}^2)} \right),$$

$$k_3 = 1/N.$$

This equation provides an approximation to the true distribution of TRE^2. By taking the expected value of Eq. 2, noting that the expected value of each χ_1^2 variable is 1, we have that

$$\langle \mathrm{TRE}^2(x, y, z) \rangle = \frac{\langle \mathrm{FLE}^2 \rangle}{3}(k_1 + k_2 + k_3) = \langle \mathrm{FLE}^2 \rangle \left(\frac{1}{N} + \frac{1}{3} \sum_{i=1}^{3} \sum_{j \neq i}^{3} \frac{r_i^2}{\Lambda_{ii}^2 + \Lambda_{jj}^2} \right). \tag{3}$$

This is in agreement with the expression derived in [8,7], and, as shown there, exhibits the $1/\sqrt{N}$ dependence observed by Hill [11], Evans [6], and Maurer [17], and the ellipsoidal spatial dependence observed recently by Maurer [17] and by Darabi [4].

4   Comparison with Simulations

As we do not have access to very large numbers ("large" being of the order of tens of thousands) of patient datasets, we must rely on numerical simulations to check the correctness of the result given in Eq. 2. We chose four values of N for which to perform the comparison: $N = 3, 4, 10, 20$. We used the same model

---

[1] This technical report is available on the World Wide Web as **http://cswww.vuse.vanderbilt.edu/~jayw/tre_dist.ps** or **tre_dist.pdf**

to simulate FLE and thus generate values of TRE as in our previous work [8,7], generating fiducials within a cube of side 200 mm, targets within a cube of side 400 mm, and FLE in each direction as a normal variable whose variance was 3.33 mm. Using this fairly large value of FLE allows us to be conservative with the statements we make concerning the quality of the approximation to TRE^2, as the difference between the TRE^2 distribution given in (2) and the true distribution will tend to grow with increasing FLE.

For each perturbation and registration iteration in the simulation, we output a value of TRE. We generated an equal number of TRE values using Eq. 2 with a random number generator [19] employed to produce samples of the chi-squared variables. For each value of N, we produced 1,000,000 simulated TRE values and the same number of values based on Eq. 2, which we will call "generated" values. We compared the two distributions using the Kolmogorov-Smirnov test [19]. For the cases $N = 3$ and 4, the K-S test showed a significant difference ($p \leq 0.01$) between the distributions. For $N = 10$ and 20, the test showed that the difference between the distributions was not significant ($p \leq 0.05$).

To explore the differences between the true and approximate distribution, we next performed ten runs each of 1,000,000 iterations for the simulator and generator. In the tables that follow, we show the percentage difference, 100(generated − simulated)/simulated, in rms value, median, and 95th percentile values between the simulated and generated value for each value of N. For all the tabulated values, the difference between the simulated and generated value was significant (two-tailed t-test, $P < 0.01$).

Table 1. Simulated vs Generated rms TRE values (mm)

N	Simulated (± sd)	Generated (± sd)	% difference
3	6.8701 (0.0026)	6.8681 (0.0037)	-0.0291
4	4.6866 (0.0026)	4.6845 (0.0019)	-0.0448
10	1.8552 (0.0009)	1.8547 (0.0008)	-0.0270
20	1.3812 (0.0008)	1.3809 (0.0007)	-0.0217

Table 2. Simulated vs Generated median TRE values (mm)

N	Simulated (± sd)	Generated (± sd)	% difference
3	5.7220 (0.0030)	5.7358 (0.0028)	0.2412
4	3.6902 (0.0031)	3.7195 (0.0023)	0.7940
10	1.5834 (0.0006)	1.5845 (0.0010)	0.0695
20	1.1763 (0.0009)	1.1780 (0.0011)	0.1445

Table 3. Simulated vs Generated 95th percentile TRE values (mm)

N	Simulated ($\pm$ sd)	Generated ($\pm$ sd)	% difference
3	11.8465 (0.0069)	11.8167 (0.0116)	-0.0298
4	8.4374 (0.0035)	8.3835 (0.0072)	-0.0539
10	3.1189 (0.0033)	3.1163 (0.0013)	-0.0036
20	2.3270 (0.0008)	2.3236 (0.0014)	-0.0034

5   Discussion

We can see from Tables 1, 2, and 3 that the distribution given in Eq. 2 is a good approximation to the actual distribution of TRE, for the fiducial configurations and targets which we used. The generated values do not match the simulated ones exactly: they tend to overestimate the median and underestimate the 95th percentile. However, we note that for our configurations, a conservative estimate of TRE may be generated by simply increasing the generated value by 1% at the 95th percentile: in all cases, this gives a value which is above the 99% upper confidence bound of the mean simulated value. This shows that the results given by Eq. 2 are close enough to the exact values to be of use to those who wish to gain a conservative, but fairly accurate, estimate of TRE in clinical practice.

6   Conclusion

We have derived an approximation to the distribution of TRE, and proved via numerical simulations that the result is close enough to the exact one to be of use for clinical estimation of expected values and confidence intervals for TRE.

References

1. K. S. Arun, T. S. Huang, and S. D. Blostein: Least-squares fitting of two 3-D point sets, IEEE Trans. Pattern Anal. Mach. Intell. **9** (1987) 698-700
2. West J. B. and J. M. Fitzpatrick: The distribution of target registration error in rigid-body, point-based registration, Tech. Rep. CS99-01, Department of Computer Science, Vanderbilt University (1999)
3. P. Clarysse, D. Gibon, J. Rousseau, S. Blond, C. Vasseur, and X. Marchandise: A computer-assisted system for 3-D frameless localization in stereotaxic MRI, IEEE Trans. Med. Imaging **10** (1991) 523-529
4. K. Darabi, P. Grunert, and A. Perneczky: Accuracy of intraoperative navigation using skin markers. In: Computer Assisted Radiology and Surgery 1997, Springer-Verlag, Berlin (1997) 920-924
5. A. C. Evans, S. Marrett, D. L. Collins, and T. M. Peters: Anatomical-functional correlative analysis of the human brain using three dimensional imaging systems, Medical Imaging III: Image Processing, vol. Proc. SPIE 1092 (1989) 264-274
6. A. C. Evans, T. M. Peters, D. L. Collins, P. Neelin, and C. Gabe: Image registration based on discrete anatomic structures. In: Interactive Image-Guided Neurosurgery, American Association of Neurological Surgeons, Park Ridge, IL (1993)

7. J. M. Fitzpatrick, J. West, and C. R. Maurer, Jr.: Predicting error in rigid-body, point-based registration, IEEE Trans. Med. Imaging **17** (1998) 694-702
8. J. M. Fitzpatrick, J. B. West, and C. R. Maurer, Jr.: Derivation of expected registration error for rigid-body, point-based image registration, Medical Imaging 1998: Image Processing, vol. Proc. SPIE 3338-01 (1998) 16-27
9. G. Golub and C. van Loan: Matrix Computations. Johns Hopkins University Press, Baltimore, Maryland (1983)
10. D. L. G. Hill, D. J. Hawkes, M. J. Gleeson, T. C. S. Cox, A. J. Strong, W.-L. Wong, C. F. Ruff, N. D. Kitchen, D. G. T. Thomas, J. E. Crossman, C. Studholme, A. J. Gandhe, S. E. M. Green, and G. P. Robinson: Accurate frameless registration of MR and CT images of the head: Applications in surgery and radiotherapy planning, Radiology **191** (1994) 447-454
11. D. L. G. Hill, D. J. Hawkes, Z. Hussain, S. E. M. Green, C. F. Ruff, and G. P. Robinson: Accurate combination of CT and MR data of the head: Validation and applications in surgical and therapy planning. In: 3D Advanced Image Processing in Medicine 1992
12. J. R. Hurley and R. B. Cattell: The Procrustes program: Producing direct rotation to test a hypothesized factor structure, Behav. Sci. **7** (1962) 258-262
13. V. R. Mandava: Three Dimensional Multimodal Image Registration Using Implanted Markers, PhD thesis, Vanderbilt University, Nashville, TN (1991)
14. V. R. Mandava, J. M. Fitzpatrick, C. R. Maurer, Jr., R. J. Maciunas, and G. S. Allen: Registration of multimodal volume head images via attached markers, Medical Imaging VI: Image Processing, vol. Proc. SPIE 1652 (1992) 271-282
15. C. R. Maurer, Jr. and J. M. Fitzpatrick: A review of medical image registration. In: Interactive Image-Guided Neurosurgery American Association of Neurological Surgeons, Park Ridge, IL (1993)
16. C. R. Maurer, Jr., J. M. Fitzpatrick, M. Y. Wang, R. L. Galloway, Jr., R. J. Maciunas, and G. S. Allen: Registration of head volume images using implantable fiducial markers, Tech. Rep. CS-96-03, Department of Computer Science, Vanderbilt University (1996)
17. C. R. Maurer, Jr., J. M. Fitzpatrick, M. Y. Wang, R. L. Galloway, Jr., R. J. Maciunas, and G. S. Allen: Registration of head volume images using implantable fiducial markers, IEEE Trans. Med. Imaging **16** (1997) 447-462
18. C. R. Maurer, Jr., J. J. McCrory, and J. M. Fitzpatrick: Estimation of accuracy in localizing externally attached markers in multimodal volume head images, Medical Imaging 1993: Image Processing, vol. Proc. SPIE 1898 (1993) 43-54
19. W. H. Press, B. P. Flannery, S. A. Teukolsky, and W. T. Vetterling: Numerical Recipes in C, Cambridge University Press, New York (1990)
20. P. H. Schönemann: A generalized solution of the orthogonal Procrustes problem, Psychometrika **31** (1966) 1-10
21. R. Sibson: Studies in the robustness of multidimensional scaling: Perturbational analysis of classical scaling, J. R. Statist. Soc. B **41** (1979) 217-229
22. J. B. West, J. M. Fitzpatrick, M. Y. Wang, B. M. Dawant, C. R. Maurer, Jr., R. M. Kessler, R. J. Maciunas, C. Barillot, D. Lemoine, A. Collignon, F. Maes, P. Suetens, D. Vandermeulen, P. A. van den Elsen, S. Napel, T. S. Sumanaweera, B. Harkness, P. F. Hemler, D. L. G. Hill, D. J. Hawkes, C. Studholme, J. B. A. Maintz, M. A. Viergever, G. Malandain, X. Pennec, M. E. Noz, G. Q. Maguire, Jr., M. Pollack, C. A. Pelizzari, R. A. Robb, D. Hanson, and R. P. Woods: Comparison and evaluation of retrospective intermodality brain image registration techniques, J. Comput. Assist. Tomogr. **21** (1997) 554-566

A Fast Mutual Information Method for Multi-modal Registration

Xu Meihe, Rajagopalan Srinivasan, and Wieslaw L. Nowinski

Biomedical Lab, Kent Ridge Digital Labs, 21 Heng Mui Keng Terrace,
Singapore 119613
{xumeihe, srini, wieslaw}@krdl.org.sg

Abstract. This paper describes a fast Mutual Information (MI) method for registering volumetric medical images. The new technique originates from the method designed by Viola [1] wherein registration is achieved by iteratively adjusting the relative position and orientation until the MI between two volumetric images is maximized. In this iterative process if n number of samples are used then there are $O(n^2)$ exponential calculations per iteration. The method proposed in this paper reduces the number of exponential computations by using an index table for estimating the Gaussian density functions (GDF). The index table is optimally pre-computed using automatic segmentation based on zero-crossing of wavelet transform. Thus a majority of exponential computations is reduced to index-intensity comparisons. The table lookup process is speeded up using a search mechanism based on probability priority. The proposed method has been successfully used to register both normal and pathological MRI and CT datasets. Experimental results show that this approach yields identical results in a fraction of time taken by the original method. The speedup increases with the number of samples used. For example, with 50 samples the speedup is 2.73 and for 100 samples it increases to 5.5.

1 Introduction

A variety of volume registration methods is described in [6]. Most of them either involve user-based homologus feature selection or tedious preprocessing such as segmentation of surfaces or tissue layers. Over the last few years, approaches based on "similarity metrics" have begun to appear and MI is one of them. MI methods assume little about the functional relationship between the intensities of the two images and do not require any segmentation. Hence they are popular and useful. MI methods have been used to solve different types of registration problems in [3,7,8].

MI is expressed as an expectation of the negative logarithm of the probability density. In [3] the joint and marginal distributions are estimated by normalizing the joint and marginal histograms of the overlapping parts of both images. Calculation of histograms in each iteration is prohibitively expensive. In [1] the Parzen window method is used on a set of samples drawn from the overlapping

A. Kuba et al. (Eds.): IPMI'99, LNCS 1613, pp. 466–471, 1999.
© Springer-Verlag Berlin Heidelberg 1999

parts of the two images to estimate the image intensity distribution. This approach did improve the speed performance. However, if n number of samples are used then there are $O(n^2)$ exponential calculations per iteration for the estimation of GDF. This paper presents an approach which speeds up the method of [1] using the following strategies.

- Estimation of GDF is simplified using a lookup table which is built in the pre-processing stage. Thus a large number of exponential computations are reduced to mere index-intensity comparisons.
- To optimize the construction of lookup table and hence pre-processing time, the GDF is computed and stored for only a few *relevant intensities*. The *relevant intensities* are identified using segmentation based on an automatic thresholding method [4] that uses the zero-crossing of the wavelet transform [5]. MI methods do not require any pre-segmentation. However, the thresholding method used here is low-cost, automatic and does not require a priori information or expert guidance.
- To speed up the table retrieval, a search scheme based on *probability priority* is used.

The remaining sections are organized as follows. In Sect. 2, an overview of the method is given. Section 3 addresses the proposed method. Section 4 has implementation details and Sect. 5 provides the conclusion.

2   MI Method

Given a reference volume with intensities $u(p)$ and a test volume with intensities $v(p)$, Mutual information I is defined in terms of entropy and is a function of the transformation T:

$$I(u(p, v(T(p))) \equiv h(u(p)) + h(v(T(p))) - h(u(p), v(T(p))),$$

where $h(.)$ is the entropy of a random variable. We try to seek a transformation T that maximizes the mutual information between these two volumetric images. In order to seek a maximum of the MI, an approximation to its derivative can be given as follows:

$$\frac{d\hat{I}}{d\tau} = \frac{1}{N_B} \sum_{s_i \epsilon B} \sum_{s_j \epsilon A} (v_i - v_j)^T [W_v(v_i, v_j)\psi_v^{-1} - W_w(w_i, w_j)\psi_{vv}^{-1}]\frac{d}{d\tau}(v_i - v_j),$$

where A and B are the two sample sets N_B is the number of samples in B, $u_i \equiv u(P_i), v_i \equiv v(T(P_i))$, and $w_i = [u_i, v_i]^T$. τ is the parameter (rotation vector and translation components) of transformation. When the optimization is involved, we prefer to represent the rotation vector with fewer optimization parameters in the absence of any constraints. The derivatives of intensities with respect to rotation vector can be inferred from its antisymmetric matrix operator [10]. The weighting factors are defined as:

$$W_\alpha(s_i, s_j) \equiv \frac{G_{\psi_\alpha}(s_i - s_j)}{\sum_{p_k \epsilon A} G_{\psi_\alpha}(s_i - s_k)}.$$

G is the GDF with the covariance ψ. When s is a vector, ψ is the covariance matrix (assumed to be diagonal). A stochastic gradient descent scheme is used to optimize the parameters of the transformation. The registration is performed in a coarse-to-fine manner on a hierarchy of data volumes that had been generated by wavelet decomposition.

3   Speedup of MI method

In the process of searching for the transformation by the stochastic gradient descent, a large number of exponential calculations are involved at each iteration. For example, even for relatively small sample sizes ($N_A = N_B = 50$), there are at least 5000 exponential computations in each iteration. The gradient of the MI has to be updated at each iteration and hence is computationally intensive. This can be circumvented by creating an index table before the iterative process. The index table stores the values of the GDFs. However, if the exponential computations for all possible intensity values are performed, it requires considerable pre-processing time. A possible solution to this bottleneck is to store the GDFs of only a few *relevant intensities*. This could be done by mapping all the intensities onto a smaller range. Such ad-hoc mapping would result in inaccuracies and information loss. We employ an automatic approach based on zero-crossing of the wavelet transform [4] for selecting the thresholds. Thresholds are located to the left/right of the positive/negative crossover of zero-crossing in a convolved histogram. The representative *relevant intensities* is chosen as the maximum point between the positive and negative crossovers. To ensure the validity of the thresholds and *relevant intensities* across multi-levels, a coarse-to-fine adjustment of the thresholds which takes advantage of multi-scale information is given by a minimum distance criterion. The index table stores the result of the GDFs for these *relevant intensities* only. In majority of cases, this table can be used directly to get the GDF. In other words, a large number of exponent components are reduced to mere comparisons during the table retrieval process.

Given a sample intensity u_i or v_i, it is also important to efficiently retrieve the corresponding GDF value from the index table. Generally it is impossible, on the average, to complete the search of n items in fewer than $\lg n$ comparisons by *binary search*. From the histogram analysis of the intensities, it is apparent that one or more samples occur more often than the others. This nature of distribution can be exploited by using a search method that compares the sample with items based on the priority of the item's probability of occurence. This *probability priority search* method is preferable since it locates a given item quickly. During the segmentation in the pre-processing phase, the probabilities of each item can be approximated by the area under each segment curve in the histogram.

4   Implementation and Results

The proposed method was implemented on an *SGI/O2* workstation. We investigated the performance of our registration scheme by aligning 3D MR with CT images. For the results shown in Table 1 and Table 2, MR data served as the

Table 1. Comparison of results between original and proposed scheme

scheme	Rotn vector (rad. measure)			Transl. vector (mm)		
	rx	ry	rz	tx	ty	tz
original	-0.0652	0.0321	-0.0118	5.873	-0.325	120.82
proposed	-0.0647	0.0326	-0.0122	5.924	-0.317	120.01

Table 2. Timing comparison for two schemes

scheme	Pre pro time (sec)	samples No. ($N_A = N_B$)	Time(sec) per itern.	Total Time for 6000 itern
original	0.985	50	0.0172	104.18
		80	0.0487	293.18
		100	0.0746	448.58
proposed 15x15 table	1.011	50	0.0062	38.21
		80	0.0103	62.81
		100	0.0134	81.41
proposed 256x256 table	1.328	50	0.0063	39.12
		80	0.0105	64.32
		100	0.0137	83.53

reference and CT as the test data. The automatic threshold scheme partitioned the intensity interval $[0, 4096]$ into 15 segments. The pre-processing produced a 15×15 table. Table 1 provides a comparison between the two schemes. The results of the proposed scheme are basically identical to that of the original method. Table 2 compares the average computation time of the two methods, which includes the pre-processing time and time for each iteration, on average. Fig. 1 shows the time taken by the two methods for different number of samples. It can be seen that the speedup of the proposed approach increases with increasing number of samples. Fig. 2 shows some examples of the final configuration of the MR-CT registration obtained using the proposed approach.

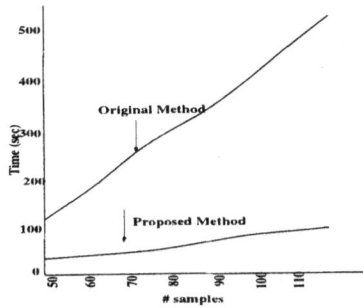

Fig. 1. Graph of samples number vs time (iteration No.=6000)

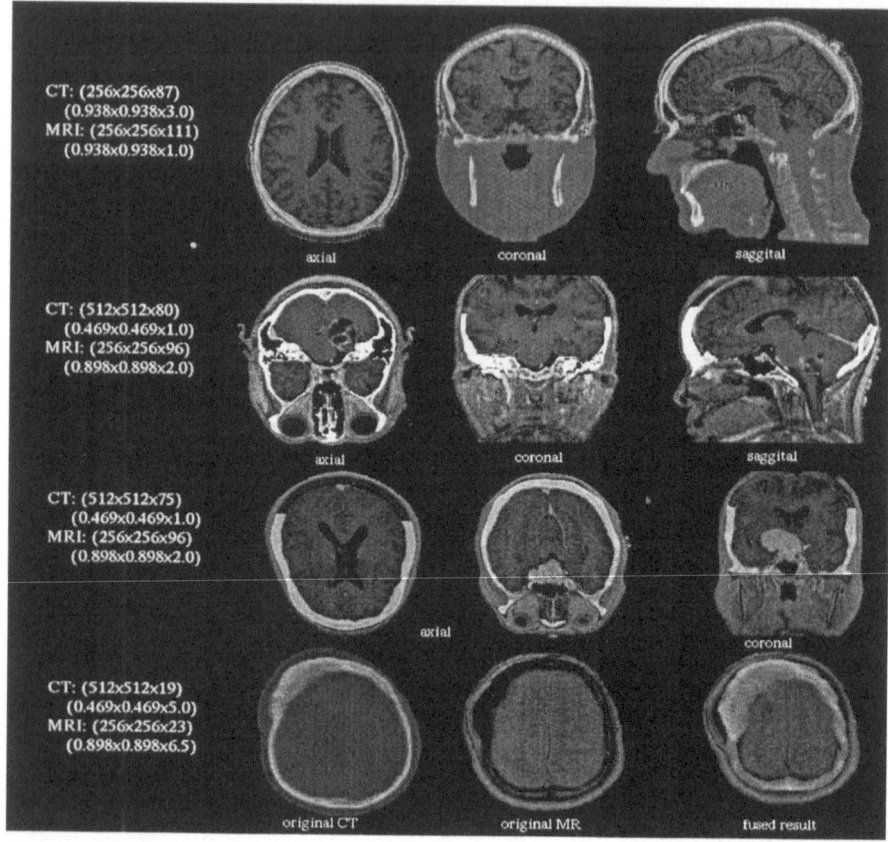

CT: (256x256x87)
   (0.938x0.938x3.0)
MRI: (256x256x111)
   (0.938x0.938x1.0)

CT: (512x512x80)
   (0.469x0.469x1.0)
MRI: (256x256x96)
   (0.898x0.898x2.0)

CT: (512x512x75)
   (0.469x0.469x1.0)
MRI: (256x256x96)
   (0.898x0.898x2.0)

CT: (512x512x19)
   (0.469x0.469x5.0)
MRI: (256x256x23)
   (0.898x0.898x6.5)

Fig. 2. Qualitative results of the proposed MI algorithm. The normal dataset used in the first row corresponds to the one used in Table 1 and 2. Last three rows correspond to pathological cases

5   Conclusion

We have presented a fast MI method for registering multi-modal data. The proposed method provides identical results in a fraction of the time required by the original method. We are in the process of integrating this algorithm into the VIVIAN [9] neurosurgery planning system and this would help us to clinically validate the results.

Acknowledgments

The authors would like to thank the funding agency - National Science and Technology board and the Institution - Kent Ridge Digital Labs for their magnanimous support during the course of this work.

References

1. Viola P.: Alignment by maximization of Mutual Information. PhD dissertation, MIT (1995)
2. Viola P., William M.W.: Alignment by maximization of Mutual Information. Proc. 5th Intl. conference on Computer Vision (1995) 16–23
3. Maes F., Collignon A., Vandermeulen D., Marchal G., Suetens P.: Multimodality image registration by maximization of Mutual Information. IEEE Trans. Medical Imaging **16-2** (1997) 187–198
4. Olivo, J.C. : Automatic threshold selection using the wavelet transform. Graphical Models and Image Processing **56-3** (1994) 205–218
5. Mallat S.: Zero-crossing of a wavelet transform. IEEE Trans. Information Theory **37-4** (1991) 1019–1033
6. Maintz A.J.B., Viergever M.A.: A survey of medical image registration. Medical Image Analysis **2-1** (1998) 1–36
7. Delia P.M., Theodore R.J, Plantec M.B. : Registration of functional magnetic resonance imagery using mutual information. SPIE Medical Imaging (1997) 621–630
8. Gaens T., Maes F., Vandermeulen K., Suetens P.: Non-rigid multimodal image registration using mutual information. MICCAI '98 proceedings (1998) 1099–1106
9. Luis S., Kockro R.A., Chua G.G: Multimodal volume-based tumor neurosurgery planning in the Virtual Workbench. MICCAI '98 proceedings (1998) 1007-1015
10. Ayache, N.: Artificial vision for mobile robots-Stereo-vision and multisensor perception. MIT Press (1991)

Voxel Similarity Measures for 3D Serial MR Brain Image Registration

Mark Holden[1], Derek L. G. Hill[1], Erika R. E. Denton[2],
Jo M. Jarosz[2], Tim C. S. Cox[3], and David J. Hawkes[1]

[1] Radiological Sciences and Biomedical Engineering. The Guy's, King's and St
Thomas' School of Medicine, King's College London, London SE1 9RT, U.K.
Derek.Hill@kcl.ac.uk
[2] Radiology and Neuroimaging Depts, King's College Hospital, London SE5 9RS
[3] Institute of Neurology, UCL, Queen's Square, London WC1N 3BG

Abstract. We investigated 7 different similarity measures for rigid body
registration of serial MR brain scans. To assess their accuracy we used a
set of 33 clinical 3D serial MR images, manually segmented by a radiologist to remove deformable extra-dural tissue, and also simulated brain
model data. For each measure we determined the consistency of registration transformations for both sets of segmented and unsegmented data.
The difference images produced by registration with and without segmentation were visually inspected by two radiologists in a blinded study.
We have shown that of the measures tested, those based on joint entropy
produced the best consistency and seemed least sensitive to the presence
of extra-dural tissue. For this data the difference in accuracy of these
joint entropy measures, with or without brain segmentation, was within
the threshold of visually detectable change in the difference images.

1 Introduction

In this paper, we report the results of a systematic comparison of seven similarity
measures for serial MR registration. We assess the accuracy of the measures using
simulated MR brain images [2], and quantify consistency using images from a
clinical study [3]. We compare the performance of the measures on the clinical
data with, and without segmentation of extra-dural tissue. We interpret these
results in the context of a blinded visual assessment study.

2 Methods

Our clinical data is from five growth hormone deficient adults undergoing therapy
and six normal subjects [3]. Each subject was scanned 3 times at 3 monthly
intervals. An additional normal subject was scanned twice on the same day,
for assessing observer sensitivity to synthetic misregistration. All images were
axial T1 weighted 3D spoiled gradient echo with 1x1x1.8mm voxels, including
head and brain stem. A phantom was scanned to measure scaling errors [3,7].
The clinical images were manually scalp segmented by a radiologist to eliminate
deformable extra-dural tissue, using Analyze (Mayo Clinic, Rochester, MN, US).

A. Kuba et al. (Eds.): IPMI'99, LNCS 1613, pp. 472–477, 1999.

Simulated MR Brain Image with Added Noise and Distortion Simulated data was based on the McGill full anatomical MR brain model image [2]. Two noiseless images were used, 1 with 40% RF inhomogeneity intensity distortion and 1 without. Noise in a modulus MR image is Rician distributed [4]. To simulate Rician noise a numerical complex random variable was added to each voxel of the noiseless (real) image and then the modulus was taken to produce a magnitude image. The random variable was constructed from 2 Gaussian distributed ones for the real and imaginary parts. The simulated Rician noise was parameterised by measuring the mean and standard deviation of intensities of an artefact free region of a clinical scan corresponding to air [6].

Similarity Measures and Registration Algorithm The ideal similarity measure would have one optimum at the point of registration. Viola states that for images that differ only by Gaussian noise, the χ^2 measure is optimal; with a linear intensity transformation the Pearson product moment measure is optimal, and where the intensity transformation is unknown joint entropy is likely to be optimal [11]. Two important properties of serial MR images that effect similarity measures are: intensity distortion (due to RF inhomogeneity and motion artefact) and deformation of extra-cranial tissue (approximately 20% of typical brain scans). We have implemented 3 measures used by other researchers in serial MR: (1) mean squared difference in intensities (chi) χ^2 [5]; (2) Pearson product-moment cross correlation (ncc) [8]; (3) ratio image uniformity (riu) [12]. We have also implemented 4 measures proposed for other medical image matching applications: (4) mutual information (mi) [9]; (5) normalised mutual information (nmi) [10]; (6) entropy of the difference image (edi) [1]; (7) pattern intensity, radius 1, $\sigma = 10$, (pi) [13]. The measures can be put into two groups: (a) those based on entropy: mi, nmi, edi and (b) those based on correlation: chi, ncc, pi, riu. Our algorithm optimises the measures using a multi-resolution strategy similar to Studholme [10].

Consistency of Two Transformations For two rigid-body transformations $\mathbf{T}_1$ and $\mathbf{T}_2$ in homogeneous form, $\mathbf{T}_2\mathbf{T}_1$ is the result of first applying $\mathbf{T}_1$ then $\mathbf{T}_2$. Given two transformation estimates $\mathbf{T}_a$ and $\mathbf{T}_b$, mapping points, $p(i)$, from image 1 to image 2, the difference between these transformations is the mean voxel displacement $\langle dp \rangle = \frac{1}{N_0} \sum_{\forall i \in I_0} | \Delta(p(i)) |$ in the brain region I_0 containing N_0 voxels. The RMS analogue is: $dp_{rms} = \frac{1}{N_0} \sqrt{(\sum_{\forall i \in I_0} | \Delta(p(i)) |^2)}$.

Consistency of 3 Transformations For N images there are $P(N, 2) = \frac{N!}{(N-2)!}$ possible transformations. So for 3 images there are 6 different transformations between image pairs. If we consider 3 transformations $\mathbf{T}_{12}, \mathbf{T}_{23}, \mathbf{T}_{31}$ between image pairs ($\mathbf{T}_{12}$ transforms image 1 into image 2) then in the absence of error, $\mathbf{T}_{31}\mathbf{T}_{23}\mathbf{T}_{12}$ is the identity $\mathbf{I}$. Registration solutions, inevitably, have some error so: $\mathbf{T}_{31}\mathbf{T}_{23}\mathbf{T}_{12} = \mathbf{I} + \Delta\mathbf{T}$, i.e. $\Delta\mathbf{T} = \mathbf{I} - \mathbf{T}_{31}\mathbf{T}_{23}\mathbf{T}_{12}$ is the error (internal inconsistency). Applying the error transformation to each voxel location, $p(i)$, and taking the modulus, the mean error over the image is: $\frac{1}{N_0} \sum_{\forall i \in I_0} | \Delta \mathbf{T}(p(i)) |$.

Registration of Clinical Data and Measurement of Consistency All registration was rigid body (6 degrees of freedom) and 5 resolution levels. The search interval ranged from 4mm or degrees to 0.01mm or degrees. For all 11 subjects, the first image (baseline) was registered to the second, the second to the third and the third to the first, giving 33 transformations for unsegmented images and 33 for images where the target was segmented. A set of 66 registrations was performed with each similarity measure. The consistency of 33 transformation estimates obtained without segmentation and 33 with segmentation was calculated. The triangular (internal) consistency for 11 measurements with segmentation and 11 without were also determined. Each consistency measurement was expressed as the mean, RMS, and maximum brain voxel shift (μm).

Assessment of Difference Images from Clinical Data Three sets of difference images, derived from different groups of subjects, were used during assessment: the first was used to train radiologists, the second to test their abilities at detecting misregistration, and the third for assessment of misregistration differences between data registered with or without prior segmentation. For training, difference images were created with varying amounts of misregistration [3,7]. For testing radiologist's ability to detect misregistration the two consecutive scans of the normal subject were used to eliminate the possibility of any anatomical change in subject or scanner calibration. The second image was registered to the first by maximising normalised mutual information [10] and transformed into the coordinate frame of the first by sinc interpolation (radius 6). The first image was then subtracted from the aligned second one to produce a difference image which corresponded to no added misregistration. Ten increasing amounts of misregistration were added synthetically by calculating successively scaled down versions of the original 6D transformation (corresponding to mean voxel shifts $50 - 500\mu$m in 50μm steps). Difference images for the clinical study were produced by registering the second and third images to the first by maximising normalised mutual information (as above). For each subject the second and third images were then transformed into the coordinate frame of the first (as above) and the first image was subtracted to produce two difference images ($2 - 1$ and $3 - 1$) from registration with segmented data and two from registration with unsegmented data. Radiologists were trained to recognise different amounts of misregistration using the training set. Then they rated the misregistration of each randomised difference image on a 7 point scale.

Registration of Simulated Data We used the noiseless brain model image and the noiseless brain model with 40% RF inhomogeneity from McGill University [2] to create four image pairs: (a) 2 identical images; (b) 2 images with added noise; (c) 1 noiseless image with RF inhomogeneity and one without; (d) 2 images with added noise 1 with, 1 without RF inhomogeneity.

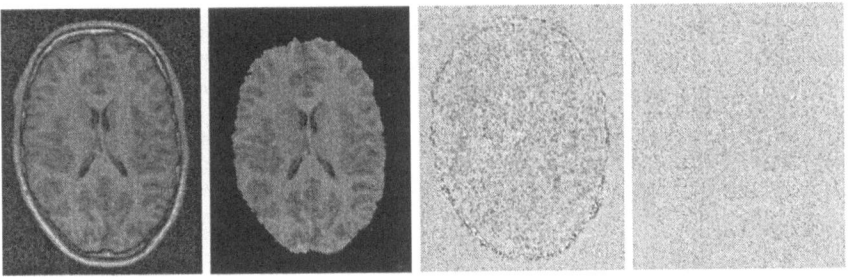

Fig. 1. Axial planes through clinical images: non-segmented (left), segmented, difference, McGill with simulated Rician noise (right)

3 Results

Three sets of results are given: (1) Consistency measurements for transformation estimates from registration of clinical data (segmented and not segmented) for the 7 measures. (2) Scores from radiologists' visual assessment of clinical difference images (segmented and not segmented). (3) Consistency measurements of the transformation estimates obtained from registration of the simulated data with the 7 measures. All consistency measurements correspond to the mean, RMS, and maximum voxel displacements over the segmented brain region and are given in μm, rounded to the nearest μm.

Registration Consistency for the 7 Similarity Measures The mean / standard deviation of 33 measurements of the mean voxel shift (μm) for registration solutions with and without segmentation of clinical data were: 122/46 (mi), 121/48 (nmi), 164/74 (ncc), 175/76 (chi), 8429/5316 (edi), 700/1503 (pi), 880/609 (riu). The smallest mean/standard deviation of 33 measurements of the maximum voxel shift were 223/96 (mi), 222/96 (nmi). Table 1 shows averaged consistency measurements for $T_{31}T_{23}T_{12}$ with each of the 7 measures, for segmented and unsegmented data.

Visual Assessment of Difference Images Assessed misregistration was correlated with the added misregistration. For observer A the Spearman rank correlation coefficient (ρ) was 0.96 for observer B, ρ was 0.79. Inter-observer agreement was also tested and ρ was 0.85. These results suggest that radiologists are sensitive to misregistration in difference images corresponding to a mean, RMS and maximum voxel shift, over the brain, of: 195, 199, 299 μm respectively. There was no perceived difference in perceived misregistration with and without segmentation using the nmi measure (p=0.35).

Registration Consistency with Simulated Images Registration accuracy was measured by comparing the transformation estimate with the identity using

6 different starting estimates. The mean/standard deviation of voxel shift for
the 6 starting transformations for the four image pairs was (μm): (a) less than
10/3 for all measures; (b) 127/2 (chi), 135/3 (edi), 121/2 (mi), 126/2 (ncc),
137/3 (nmi), 343/23 (pi), 416/74 (riu); (c) 8/2 (chi); 39/14 (edi); 51/1 (mi);
25/5 (ncc); 43/6 (nmi); 12/1 (pi); 30/7 (riu). There was a failure for riu which
was omitted; (d) 203/3 (chi); 253/2 (edi); 163/5 (mi); 133/2 (ncc); 194/7 (nmi);
391/26 (pi); 402/57 (riu).

Table 1. Mean (standard deviation) of 11 consistency measurements ($\mathbf{T}_{31}\mathbf{T}_{23}\mathbf{T}_{12}$).
Registration without prior segmentation (left) and with prior segmentation (right)

measure	unsegmented data			segmented data		
	mean	RMS	max	mean	RMS	max
chi	91 (28)	96 (31)	165 (55)	99 (31)	104 (33)	169 (62)
edi	1757 (1148)	1780 (1198)	2160 (2072)	66 (35)	69 (36)	117 (55)
mi	88 (23)	94 (26)	168 (53)	78 (29)	82 (31)	139 (59)
ncc	87 (37)	93 (40)	168 (73)	97 (25)	101 (27)	168 (63)
nmi	86 (32)	92 (35)	162 (70)	78 (29)	81 (30)	133 (57)
pi	1565 (2204)	1690 (2391)	3348 (4809)	145 (94)	154 (100)	278 (181)
riu	1221 (553)	1276 (549)	2100 (748)	258 (92)	276 (101)	531 (224)

4   Discussion and Conclusion

Table 1 shows that 4 of the 7 measures produced transformation estimates that
were consistent to within 331 μm whether or not the data was pre-segmented
and also had the best internal consistency ($\mathbf{T}_{31}\mathbf{T}_{23}\mathbf{T}_{12}$) for non-segmented data.
For the joint entropy measures the mean of the maximum inconsistency between
registrations with and without segmentation was 223 μm. The results from visual assessment of synthetically misregistered data indicated that the threshold
for detecting misregistration corresponded to a mean and maximum inconsistency of about 200 and 300 μm respectively. These inconsistencies are larger
than the averaged measured mean and maximum inconsistency suggesting that
these inconsistencies are too small to be reliably detected by the visual inspection of difference images. For non-segmented data, there was little difference in
the internal consistency of transformation estimates for those measures based
on correlation (chi and ncc) and for those based on joint entropy (mi and nmi).
However, registration results with and without prior segmentation were more
self-consistent for those based on joint entropy. Results with the simulated images suggested that image noise had a significant effect on registration accuracy.
However, the highest resolution matching was done with images at the original
resolution without any filtering to reduce the impact of noise. It is possible that
low pass filtering with intensity thresholding might improve performance of some
measures. Our results show that the similarity measures based on mutual information are the most suitable for rigid body registration of serial MR images of
the head. Using our optimisation strategy we achieve registration solutions with

and without extra-dural tissue segmentation that are consistent to within the threshold of observer discernibility (i.e. 200-300 μm). Our results apply under the conditions of typical scalp deformations and small scale anatomical change.

Acknowledgements

We thank Philips Medical Systems, EasyVision Advanced Development for funding, the McConnell Brain Imaging Centre, MNI, McGill University for use of the simulated brain data and Dr. D. Russell-Jones for the clinical data.

References

1. Buzug T. M., Weese J., Fassnacht C., and Lorenz C.: Using an Entropy Similarity Measure to Enhance the Quality of DSA Images with an Algorithm Based on Template Matching. VBC'96, SPIE Proc. **1808** (1996)
2. D.L. Collins, A.P. Zijdenbos, V. Kollokian, J.G. Sled, N.J. Kabani, C.J. Holmes, A.C. Evans: Design and Construction of a Realistic Digital Brain Phantom. IEEE Transactions on Medical Imaging **17 (3)** (1998) 463–468.
3. E.R.E. Denton, M. Holden, J.M. Jarosz, C. Studholme, T.C.S. Cox, D.L.G Hill: The identification of cerebral volume changes in treated growth hormone deficient patients using serial 3-D MR image processing. Radiology **209P (SS)** (1998) 1492
4. Gudbjartsson H. and Patz, S.: The Rician Distribution of Noisy MRI data. Magnetic Resonance in Medicine **34** (1995) 910–914
5. Hajnal J. V., Saeed N., Soar E. J., Oatridge A., Young, I.R. and Bydder, G. M.: A Registration and Interpolation Procedure for Subvoxel Matching of Serially Acquired MR Images. JCAT **19 (2)** (1995) 289–296
6. Henkelman, R. M.: Measurement of Signal Intensities in the Presence of Noise in MR Images. Medical Physics **12 (2)** (1985) 232–233
7. M. Holden, E. R. E. Denton, J. M. Jarosz, T. C. S. Cox, D. J. Hawkes, D. L. G. Hill: Detecting small anatomical change with 3D serial MR subtraction images. SPIE, Medical Imaging **3661** (1999)
8. Lemieux L, Wieshmann U.C., et al.: The detection and significance of subtle changes in mixed-signal brain lesions by serial MRI scan matching and spatial normalisation. Medical Image Analysis **2 (3)** (1998) 227–242
9. Maes, F. and Collignon, A. and Vandermeulen, D. and Marchal, G. and Suetens, P.: Multimodality image registration using mutual information. IEEE Trans. on Medical Imaging **16 (2)** (1997) 187–198
10. Studholme C, Hawkes DJ, Hill DLG: An Overlap Invariant Entropy Measure of 3D Medical Image Alignment. Pattern Recognition **32 (1)** (1999) 71–86
11. Viola P.: Alignment by Maximization of Mutual Information. Ph.D. Thesis Massachusetts Institute of Technology (1995)
12. Woods R.P., Grafton S.T., Holmes C.J., Cherry S.R., and Mazziotta J. C.: Automated Image Registration: 1. General Methods and Intrasubject, Intramodality Validation. JCAT **22 (1)** (1998) 139–152
13. Weese J., Penney G.P., Desmedt P., Buzug T.M., Hill D.L.G. and Hawkes D.J.: Voxel-Based 2-D/3-D Registration of Fluoroscopy Images and CT Scans for Image-Guided Surgery. IEEE Trans. on Info. Tech. in Biomedicine **1 (4)** (1997) 284–293

Radial Basis Function Interpolation for Freehand 3D Ultrasound

Robert Rohling[1], Andrew Gee[1], Laurence Berman[2], and Graham Treece[1]

[1] University of Cambridge, Department of Engineering, Trumpington Street,
Cambridge CB2 1PZ, UK
{rnr20, ahg, gmt11}@eng.cam.ac.uk
[2] University of Cambridge, Department of Radiology, Addenbrooke's Hospital,
Cambridge CB2 2QQ, UK
lb@radiol.cam.ac.uk

Abstract. Freehand 3D ultrasound imaging produces a set of irregularly spaced B-scans, which are typically reconstructed on a regular grid for visualisation and data analysis. Most standard reconstruction algorithms are designed to minimise computational requirements and do not exploit the underlying shape of the data. We investigate whether approximation with splines holds any promise as a better reconstruction method. A radial basis function approximation method is implemented and compared with three standard methods. While the radial basis approach is computationally expensive, it produces accurate reconstructions without the kind of visible artifacts common with the standard methods.

1 Introduction

In freehand 3D ultrasound, a position sensor is attached to a conventional ultrasound probe and a set of 2D B-scans are acquired, along with their relative locations. This allows the irregularly spaced B-scans to be reconstructed into a regular 3D voxel array for visualisation. The reconstruction step is important: any loss of image quality, or the introduction of artifacts, should be avoided.

The literature reveals several reconstruction methods, which are all rather simple because they were designed to minimise the time and memory requirements. The most common methods are voxel nearest neighbour (VNN), pixel nearest neighbour (PNN) and distance-weighted (DW) interpolation.

VNN interpolation is easy to understand: each voxel is assigned the value of the nearest B-scan pixel [6]. There are no parameters to set. In common with the other reconstruction techniques, reconstruction artifacts can be observed in slices through the voxel array, since the interpolated image is a collage of projections from the intersected B-scans. Registration errors, including tissue motion and sensor errors, contribute to slight misalignment of the B-scans. This results in mismatches among the neighbouring pieces of the collage. The lines of intersection between the pieces then become visible – see Fig. 1(a).

The two-stage **PNN** algorithm is the most popular reconstruction method [4]. In the first stage (bin-filling), the algorithm runs through each pixel in every B-scan and fills the nearest voxel with the value of that pixel. Multiple contributions

A. Kuba et al. (Eds.): IPMI'99, LNCS 1613, pp. 478–483, 1999.

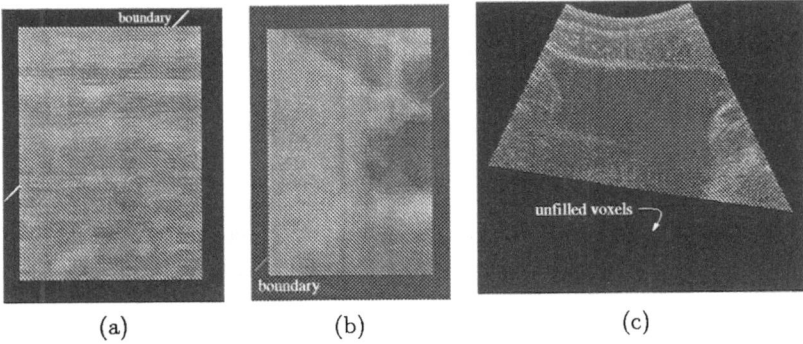

Fig. 1. Reconstruction artifacts. In (a), VNN interpolation is used to reconstruct an examination of a neck muscle. In (b), PNN interpolation is used for an examination of the thyroid. In (c), DW interpolation is used for an examination of the bladder

to the same voxel are usually averaged. The parameters to set at this stage are the weights on the multiple contributions. The second stage (hole-filling) fills any remaining gaps in the voxel array. A variety of hole-filling methods have been used, including averaging of filled voxels in a local neighbourhood [4]. The parameters to set at this stage are the weights of the voxels used to fill the gaps. Artifacts can be generated by this two stage process: a slice passing through both first stage and second stage filled voxels may show the boundary between the bin-filled regions and the smoothed hole-filled regions — see Fig. 1(b).

Like VNN, **DW** interpolation proceeds voxel by voxel. Instead of using the nearest pixel, each voxel is assigned the weighted average of some set of pixels from nearby B-scans. The parameters to choose are the weight function and the size and shape of the neighbourhood. The simplest approach employs a spherical neighbourhood of radius r_{max} around each voxel [1]. All pixels in the sphere are weighted by the inverse distance to the voxel and then averaged. If r_{max} is too small, gaps may result, as in Fig. 1(c). Yet if r_{max} is too large, the voxel array will be highly smoothed, since the effect of the weighting is quickly swamped by the larger number of data points falling into the larger local neighbourhood.

2   Radial Basis Function Interpolation

There have been no previously published attempts at functional interpolation of freehand 3D ultrasound data, since there are severe computational demands to overcome. After surveying recent advancements in trivariate interpolation of large data sets, a method was discovered that ideally suits the freehand 3D ultrasound reconstruction problem. This method was developed by researchers at the University of Illinois for interpolation of multivariate geographical data sets [3]. They dubbed the method "completely regularized splines with tension".

Consider a set of pixel values p_j $(j = 1 \ldots N)$ located at positions $\mathbf{x}_j = (x_j, y_j, z_j)$ with respect to the voxel array. The goal is to find a spline $S(\mathbf{x})$ that passes as close as possible to the data points and is as smooth as possible. These two requirements can be combined in such a way that $S(\mathbf{x})$ fulfills

$$\sum_{j=1}^{N} |p_j - S(\mathbf{x}_j)|^2 + wI(S) = \text{minimum}. \tag{1}$$

The first component is the deviation of the spline from the data points, and the second is a smoothness function $I(S)$. The weight w determines the relative cost of the two components. The solution can be expressed as

$$S(\mathbf{x}) = T(\mathbf{x}) + \sum_{j=1}^{N} a_j \mathbf{R}(\mathbf{x}, \mathbf{x}_j) \tag{2}$$

where $T(\mathbf{x})$ is the trend function, a_j are scalar coefficients, and $\mathbf{R}(\mathbf{x}, \mathbf{x}_j)$ is an RBF (radial basis function) whose form depends on the choice of $I(S)$.

For the 2D case, if $I(S)$ is chosen to minimise the cost of the second derivatives, the familiar thin plate spline results. If the same $I(S)$ is used for the 3D case, the first derivatives of the RBF become divergent at the data points. By choosing a more general $I(S)$, we obtain an analytic expression for the RBF with regular derivatives of all orders [2]. This results in $T(\mathbf{x}) = a_0$, a constant, and

$$\mathbf{R}(\mathbf{x}, \mathbf{x}_j) = \frac{\phi^3}{4\pi} \left[\frac{1}{\phi r} \text{erf} \left(\frac{\phi r}{2} \right) - \frac{1}{\sqrt{\pi}} \right] \tag{3}$$

where $r = |\mathbf{x} - \mathbf{x}_j|$ is the distance from $\mathbf{x}$ to $\mathbf{x}_j$, and erf is the error function. The parameter ϕ is a generalised tension parameter, controlling the distance over which the point influences the resulting hypersurface. The multiplicative constant $\phi^3/4\pi$ can be omitted, since it can be combined with the coefficients a_j. The spline coefficients can then be found by solving the set of linear equations

$$a_0 + \sum_{j=1}^{N} a_j \left[\mathbf{R}(\mathbf{x}, \mathbf{x}_j) + \delta_{ij} w \right] = p_i \quad \text{for} \quad i = 1 \ldots m \quad \text{and} \quad \sum_{j=1}^{N} a_j = 0 \tag{4}$$

where δ_{ij} is the Kronecker delta function. There are two parameters to set: ϕ controls the tension, and w controls the level of approximation. The goal of tuning the parameters is to find the optimal balance between the requirements of obtaining small deviations from the data points and avoiding overshoots.

For computational efficiency, the RBF interpolant cannot be calculated using all the data points of an ultrasound examination at once: the input data must be divided into manageable **segments**. Individual interpolating functions are then calculated for each segment. To ensure smooth connections among the RBF's of neighbouring segments, overlapping **windows** are used. A window is established around each segment in such a way that it encompasses not only all the data points in the segment but also a sufficient number of neighbouring data points. All data points in the window are then used to calculate the RBF's for that segment. Since the windows overlap each other, the RBF for each segment will closely match the neighbouring RBF's. Full details of a novel windowing technique suitable for use with freehand 3D ultrasound data can be found in [5].

3   Comparison of Reconstruction Methods

A fan-shaped sweep of a human bladder was performed *in vivo* with a 3.75 MHz curvilinear array probe (0.34 mm wide pixels). Since the true anatomical function is unknown, the reconstruction methods were tested by artificially removing data from the examination, and then evaluating their ability to predict the intensity values in the gaps. First, a B-scan near the middle of the sweep was selected. The voxel array (with voxels equal in size to the pixels) was aligned with this B-scan so that pixels fell exactly onto voxels. A percentage of the pixels were then removed randomly from the B-scan, creating gaps of various sizes. The rest of the pixels and all other B-scans were used in the interpolation to fill the voxel array. The values of the removed (original) pixels could then be compared with the values of the voxels aligned with them, and an average error computed:

$$V = \frac{1}{M} \sum_{i=1}^{M} |p_i - c_i| \tag{5}$$

where p_i is the original pixel that was removed from the reconstruction, c_i is the interpolated value of the voxel aligned with p_i and M is the number of removed pixels. A low value of V indicates a good ability to interpolate over the gaps.

The tests were performed with eight different percentages of removed data: 0%, 25%, 50%, 75%, 100%, 300%, 500% and 700%. For the 25% to 100% tests, pixels were removed only from the selected B-scan n. The 300% test removed all of B-scan n and all of B-scans $n-1$ and $n+1$. The 500% and 700% tests removed B-scans $n\pm2$ and $n\pm3$ as well. The 0% test was included because a reconstruction method may not replicate the original data points. For the 0% test alone, V was calculated over all pixels of the selected B-scan. The eight tests were repeated for ten different B-scans to give mean and variance estimates of V.

Typical algorithms were implemented in each of the conventional reconstruction categories and compared with the new RBF method. The hole-filling stage of the PNN algorithm used the average of the filled voxels in a $3 \times 3 \times 3$ neighbourhood. The remaining unfilled voxels were then filled by averaging originally filled voxels in a $5 \times 5 \times 5$ neighbourhood and so on, until all voxels were filled. This is similar to the method described in [4]. The DW method was implemented with an inverse distance weight within a spherical neighbourhood. r_{max} was set to the smallest value which avoided gaps in the reconstructions. The RBF method used the windowing technique described in [5]. Each segment contained at most 30 data points. The tension and approximation parameters were tuned manually by viewing a slice of the voxel array. A low tension ($\phi = 25$) combined with a small amount of smoothing ($w = 0.1$) gave optimal results. These values fall within the range typically used for geographic data interpolation [3].

4   Results

The results are tabulated in Table 1: examples of the interpolated images can be found in [5]. A second experiment with different data produced similar results [5].

Table 1. Interpolation error V. μ is the mean of V and σ is the standard deviation. † means that the assertion $\mu > \mu_{RBF}$ is statistically significant for a confidence level of 0.05. ⋆ means that the assertion $\mu < \mu_{RBF}$ is statistically significant for a confidence level of 0.05. The assertions are tested with the paired-sample t-test statistical method

Test	VNN		PNN		DW		RBF	
	μ	σ	μ	σ	μ	σ	μ	σ
0%	0.00⋆	0.00	0.00⋆	0.00	0.00⋆	0.00	0.96	0.03
25%	5.60†	0.39	5.01†	0.22	5.37†	0.09	3.57	0.25
50%	5.50†	0.40	5.08†	0.25	5.32†	0.09	3.85	0.31
75%	5.27†	0.50	5.19†	0.35	5.24†	0.10	4.13	0.40
100%	4.13	0.38	5.25†	0.40	5.11†	0.14	4.29	0.37
300%	6.92	0.40	7.03†	0.15	6.85†	0.12	6.69	0.19
500%	8.50†	0.23	7.80†	0.14	7.62⋆	0.11	7.73	0.16
700%	9.37†	0.26	8.36	0.18	8.07⋆	0.09	8.37	0.16

The VNN method produced sharp, detailed reconstructions. At 25%, 50% and 75%, the nearest neighbours of the voxels came mainly from the remaining pixels of the selected B-scan. Therefore, the interpolated image appeared as a patchwork of irregularly shaped pieces and relatively large values of V result. For the 100% to 700% tests, the interpolated image was formed from the projection of pixels from the nearest B-scans. The join lines between the portions of the projected data were indiscernible, suggesting that registration errors were small and the images varied slowly from one B-scan to the next.

The PNN method produced more blurred reconstructions. At 25%, 50% and 75%, the gaps were filled mainly by averaging the remaining pixels in the original B-scan. The interpolated image appeared as a patchwork again, with relatively large values of V. The mean of V increases progressively for the 100% to 700% tests. The reconstructions exhibited significant artifacts, especially for the 500% and 700% tests. Visible boundaries were evident between portions filled, for example, using a $7 \times 7 \times 7$ neighbourhood, and portions filled using a $9 \times 9 \times 9$ neighbourhood, because they involve different amounts of smoothing.

The DW reconstructions also exhibited artifacts. At 25%, 50% and 75%, the reconstructions comprised voxels filled by the original data (weighted by infinity), along with voxels in the gaps that were calculated from a weighted average of neighbouring pixels. The interpolated image was therefore a combination of the original pixels and smoothed data in the gaps. Apart from progressive blurring as more data was removed, no other artifacts were apparent.

The RBF technique performed marginally better than the others. At 25%, 50% and 75%, the mean of V is considerably lower than the other methods and the resulting interpolated data appeared the most detailed and least artificial. This demonstrates the ability of a functional method to use the shape of the underlying data to interpolate across the gaps. Yet at percentages of 100% and greater, the RBF is not always significantly better than the other methods. One of the reasons for this is that the underlying shape of the anatomical data is lost when the gaps become too large. Another problem is that the RBF approaches the trend term of the interpolation function in the largest gaps. In general, the RBF method produced no visible artifacts in the interpolated data, apart from progressive blurring as the percentage of removed data increased.

The performance of the RBF was largely unchanged for tensions ϕ in the range 10 to 25 and smoothing w in the range 0.01 to 0.1. A potential improvement lies in the use of anisotropic tension [2], which should be high within the B-scans to avoid overshoots, and low orthogonal to the B-scans to fill the gaps. This would reduce the blurring in the gaps between B-scans.

The major disadvantage of the RBF technique is its considerable computational expense. However, the segmentation of the voxel array means the RBF method is amenable to parallel processing. Since many modern ultrasound machines already have the capacity for parallel processing (the Toshiba Powervision 7000 used for these examinations contains more than 60 Pentium processors), a practical implementation of the RBF method is not infeasible.

5   Conclusions

The RBF method performs better than the traditional reconstruction techniques, though not remarkably so. However, many opportunities exist to exploit the unique properties of the RBF method. For example, derivatives can be calculated directly from the RBF's. Accurate derivatives are often required in applications such as visualisation, registration and segmentation. A functional representation can also be useful for data compression and filtering. Also, since an approximating function in general misses the data points, the distance it misses them by can be considered the predictive error. A large predictive error may be indicative of image misalignment, so determining which regions have large predictive errors can be useful for investigations into registration errors.

References

1. Barry, C.D., Allott, C.P., John, N.W., Mellor, P.M., Arundel, P.A., Thomson, D.S., Waterton, J.C.: Three-dimensional freehand ultrasound: image reconstruction and volume analysis. Ultrasound Med. Biol. **23** (1997) 1209–1224
2. Mitášová, H., Mitáš, L.: Interpolation by regularized splines with tension: I. theory and implementation. Mathematical Geology **25** (1993) 641–655
3. Mitášová H., Mitáš, L., Brown, W.M., Gerdes, D.P., Kosinovsky, I., Baker, T.: Modelling spatially and temporally distributed phenomena: new methods and tools for GRASS GIS. Int. J. Geograph. Info. Systems **9** (1995) 433–446
4. Nelson, T.R., Pretorius, D.H.: Interactive acquisition, analysis and visualization of sonographic volume data. Int. J. Imaging Sys. Techn. **8** (1997) 26–37
5. Rohling, R.N., Gee, A.H., Berman, L.: Radial basis function interpolation for 3-D ultrasound. Technical report CUED/F-INFENG/TR 327, University of Cambridge, Department of Engineering, July 1998
6. Sherebrin, S., Fenster, A., Rankin, R., Spence, D.: Freehand three-dimensional ultrasound: implementation and applications. In van Metter, R.L., Beutel, J. editors, Proc. Medical Imaging 1996, SPIE 2708 (1996) 296–303

Nonlinear Smoothing of MR Images Using Approximate Entropy – A Local Measure of Signal Intensity Irregularity

Geoffrey J. M. Parker[1], Julia A. Schnabel[2], and Gareth J. Barker[1]

[1] NMR Research Unit, Institute of Neurology, University College London, Queen
Square, London, WC1N 3BG, UK
g.parker@ion.ucl.ac.uk
[2] Dept. of Computer Science, University College London, Gower Street, London, UK
Now at: Images Sciences Institute, University Hospital Utrecht, The Netherlands

Abstract. Approximate entropy ($ApEn$) is a computable measure of
sequential irregularity that is applicable to sequences of numbers of finite
length. As such, it may be used to determine how random a sequence of
numbers is. We exploit this property to determine the relevance of image
information; to determine whether a spatial signal intensity distribution
varies in a regular fashion — and is therefore likely to be an image feature
or image texture, or is highly random — and likely to be noise. We
present an outline of two possible methodologies for creating an $ApEn$-
based noise filter: a modified median filter and a modified anisotropic
diffusion scheme. We show that both approaches lead to effective noise
reduction in MR images, with improved information-retaining properties
when compared with their conventional counterparts.

1 Introduction

Nonlinear geometric schemes provide elegant methods for smoothing digital images. Anisotropic diffusion [1] and its subsequent developments (see e.g. [2,3]) use the magnitude of local intensity gradients to determine object edges to be preserved in preference to less significant gradients (assumed to be noise or structures of little interest), which are smoothed. An alternative method for identifying significant image information may be to determine whether the local spatial intensity distribution is ordered or random. We have investigated the use of approximate entropy ($ApEn$) [4,5,6], a finite computable measure of sequential irregularity which is applicable to short sequences of numbers to determine local pixel intensity regularity. We investigate using $ApEn$ to determine whether spatially fluctuating signal contains a degree of regularity — and is therefore likely to be an image feature or texture, or is highly random — and likely to be noise. From this, we construct effective noise reduction filters, which retain improved levels of detail when compared with existing methods.

A. Kuba et al. (Eds.): IPMI'99, LNCS 1613, pp. 484–489, 1999.
© Springer-Verlag Berlin Heidelberg 1999

2   Theory and Application

To summarise the mathematical definition of *ApEn* [4,5,6]: given an array of size N and an integer m, under the conditions $0 < m \leq N$, a sequence of real numbers $u := (u(1), u(2), \ldots, u(N))$, and a real number r (where $r \geq 0$), let the distance between two sub-sequences $x(i) = (u(i), u(i+1), \ldots, u(i+m-1))$ and $x(j) = (u(j), u(j+1), \ldots, u(j+m-1))$, be defined as $d(x(i), x(j)) = max_{p=1,2,\ldots,m}(|u(i+p-1) - u(j+p-1)|)$. Then let $C_i^m(r) = \{$number of $j \leq (N - m + 1)$ such that $d(x(i), x(j)) \leq r\}/(N - m + 1)$. Now define

$$\Phi^m(r) = \frac{1}{N - m + 1} \sum_{i=1}^{N-m+1} \log C_i^m(r), \qquad (1)$$

$$ApEn(m, r, N)(u) = \Phi^m(r) - \Phi^{m+1}(r). \qquad (2)$$

$ApEn(m, r, N)(u)$ may be interpreted as a measure of the maximum frequency at which number sequences within u of length m occur compared with sequences of length $m+1$. High values of *ApEn* imply randomness; low values imply order.

We hypothesise that *ApEn* may be used to distinguish useful image information (edges, textures) from noise. We modify median and anisotropic diffusion schemes using the *ApEn* value derived from a local neighbourhood in a weighting function for existing smoothing schemes. We reduce smoothing when *ApEn* is low and allow smoothing when it is high.

All *ApEn* calculations use the following parameters: $N = 25$ (a 5×5 neighbourhood), $m = 1; r = 0$. As the above definition of *ApEn* is for 1D sequences, we treat the intensities within the neighbourhood as a 1D raster array of size N for *ApEn* calculation. To minimise directional bias, the mean *ApEn* is calculated from two 1D arrays, with data entered up/down and then left/right.

2.1   *ApEn* Median Filter

The transformation of an image, k, with pixel intensity $I_k(x, y)$ to the modified median-filtered image with intensity $I_{k+1}(x, y)$ is given by

$$I_{k+1}(x, y) = ApEn_k(x, y)_{local} M(x, y)_{local} + \{1 - ApEn_k(x, y)_{local}\} I_k(x, y), \qquad (3)$$

where $ApEn_k(x, y)_{local} = ApEn(m, r, N)(u)$ calculated within the $\sqrt{N} \times \sqrt{N}$ neighbourhood centred at (x, y) of the kth image and normalised over the whole of the kth image; $M(x, y)_{local}$ is the median intensity within the neighbourhood.

Figures 1(a–d) show a comparison of the effects of the conventional and *ApEn*-modified median filter. The modified filter produces sharper edges and better preservation of detail due to *ApEn* being low (so restricting smoothing) in regions dominated by structural information (e.g. tissue interfaces) and high (so allowing smoothing) in regions of relatively constant mean intensity corrupted by random noise (Fig. 1(b)).

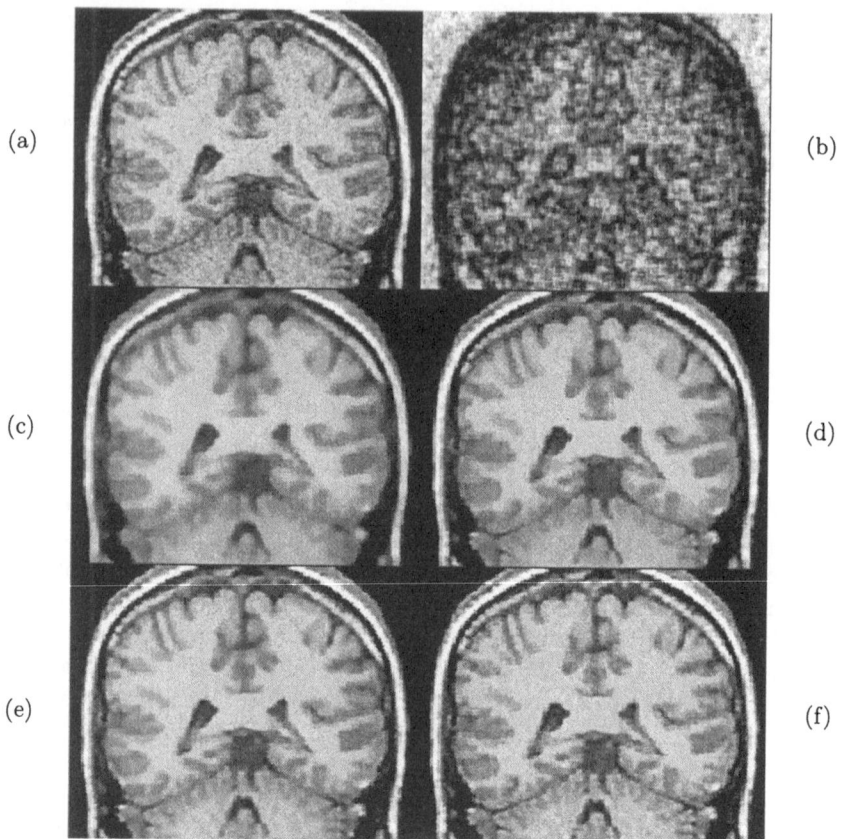

Fig. 1. (a) MR image with added Gaussian noise (SD=5). (b) *ApEn* distribution. (c–f) image (a) after application of: (c) median filter (5 × 5 mask; 1 iteration); (d) *ApEn*-modulated median filter (5 × 5 mask; 3 iterations); (e) anisotropic diffusion (2 iterations); (f) *ApEn*-modulated anisotropic diffusion (3 iterations). Mean noise reductions: (c) 71 %; (d) 74 %; (e) 58 %; (f) 62 %

2.2 *ApEn* Anisotropic Diffusion

A formulation of the 2D edge-affected anisotropic diffusion scheme is [1]

$$\frac{\partial I(x,y,t)}{\partial t} = div[g(\|\nabla I\|)\nabla I]\,, \tag{4}$$

$$g(\|\nabla I\|) = e^{-\left(\frac{\|\nabla I\|}{K}\right)^2}\,. \tag{5}$$

where t is an artificial time parameter, ∇I is the local intensity gradient, $g(\|\nabla I\|)$ is an 'edge-stopping' function, and K, the Canny noise estimator [7], is set to 85 %. This is applied as an explicit Euler forward scheme [8], with a regularising scale of 0.8 [2] and a time step of 0.25. We modify (5) by introducing

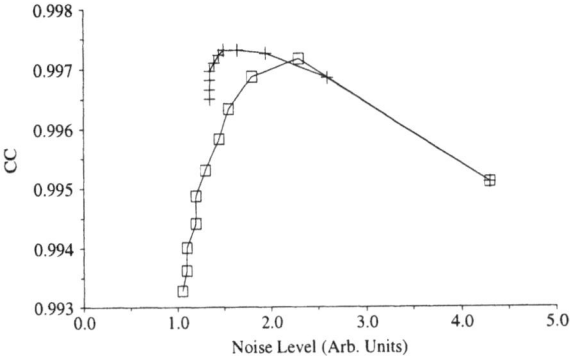

Fig. 2. Correlation coefficient (*CC*) as a function of noise levels (arbitrary units). *Squares*: anisotropic diffusion. *Crosses*: *ApEn*-modified anisotropic diffusion

$ApEn(x,y)_{local}$ as a modulating term (a similar approach to [9]), to give G:

$$G(\|\nabla I\|, ApEn(x,y)_{local}) = e^{-\left(\frac{\|\nabla I\|}{K}\right)^2} ApEn(x,y)_{local}{}^{b}, \qquad (6)$$

where b is determined empirically. We use $b = 1$, causing G to be reduced at low *ApEn* values (ordered case) relative to high *ApEn* values (disordered case).

Figures 1 (e) and (f) show a comparison of standard and *ApEn*-modified anisotropic diffusion (the differences are less than in Figs. 1(c) and (d), as anisotropic diffusion filters generally out-perform median filters). The unmodified filter reduces noise more than the modified scheme for a given number of iterations, due to the retarding effect of the *ApEn* modulation, but retains less detail for a given noise reduction. Further differences are seen by examining how useful image information is preserved through iterative filtering after the application of Gaussian noise. We do this by calculating the correlation coefficient between the filtered images and the original noise-free image [10] (Fig. 2). The *ApEn*-modified scheme retains more information for a given noise reduction, up to what appears to be a stopping point (from experiments to date). The unmodified scheme progresses to further noise reduction at the expense of information in the image as a whole.

ApEn reduces the smoothing occurring to textural features which, although they do not possess well-defined edges, may represent important image information (Fig. 3). More uniform regions experience approximately the same degree of smoothing by both the modified and unmodified schemes.

3   Conclusions

We have estimated *ApEn* within small image neighbourhoods, and shown differences between regions dominated by structural information and by noise (Fig. 1(b)). *ApEn* is then used to reduce noise by modulating the effects of existing

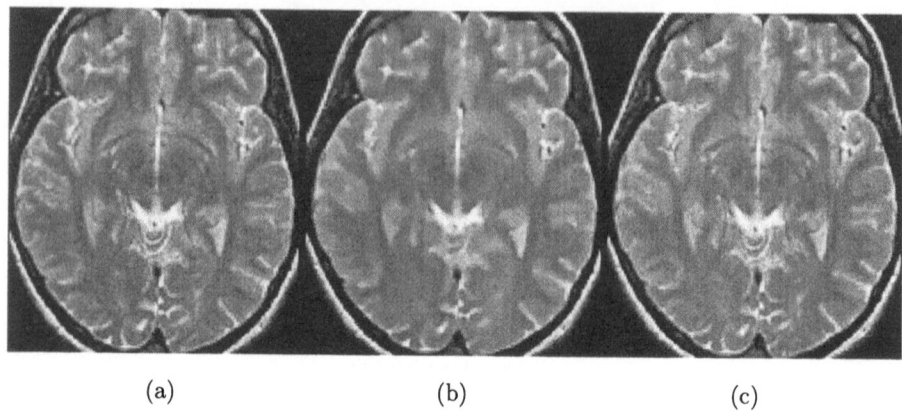

(a)   (b)   (c)

Fig. 3. (a) Original image. (b) Smoothed with anisotropic diffusion filter (5 iterations). (c) Smoothed with modified anisotropic diffusion filter (5 iterations)

schemes. The modified schemes are weighted towards removing spatially random signal (noise), whilst retaining more orderly information.

$ApEn$ differs from conventional concepts of entropy [11] as its calculation includes steps concerning the relationship between neighbouring (or higher order distances, dependent upon the choice of m) intensity values, and how often these relationships occur, rather that relying upon a statistical description of the histogram of all values within the region of interest. It is this point that also makes it distinct from measures such as intensity variance. We have made preliminary comparisons with filters based on the local 2D autocorrelation (adapted from [12]) of pixel values, and found that the information retaining properties of using $ApEn$ are superior (data not shown).

The diffusion time (or number of iterations) required for a given noise reduction is increased by $ApEn$ modulation, due to its retarding effect (see (3) and (6)). We normalise $ApEn(x, y)$ over the whole image, so with $b = 1$ (see (6)), the smoothing at each step is less than or equal to that possible with the unmodified schemes, and the stability of the original scheme [8] is not compromised. Less image information is lost for a given noise reduction when incorporating $ApEn$.

The parameters used to calculate $ApEn$, and for weighting the modulation (see (3) and (6)), were chosen for effectiveness of noise suppression, feature preservation, and ease of computation. The time for computation of $ApEn$ scales as $\approx 2m(N - m + 1)^2$. We used small N, allowing relatively quick computation and spatially localised neighbourhoods. However, there is a statistical advantage in larger N [6], implying increased accuracy in calculated values of $ApEn$. The effects of using alternative values of b, m, N, and r are left to future work.

The current pseudo-2D local $ApEn$ calculation may potentially be developed to a true 2D (and any other dimensionality) vector calculation of $ApEn$, as suggested by Singer and Pincus [13]. However, initial experiments (data not shown here) suggest that our pseudo-2D approach is effectively rotation-invariant, justifying the application of 1D *ApEn* calculations in a 2D setting.

We have presented a novel framework for noise reduction in medical images. We have applied our techniques to many medical and synthetic images (not shown here) and have found that they consistently out-perform the unmodified schemes. The techniques presented may have application to a range of MRI techniques including quantitative studies such as functional MRI, perfusion imaging, and diffusion tensor imaging, each of which typically suffers from low signal-to-noise ratios. The capability of *ApEn* to distinguish noise from image structure may also make it a suitable candidate for texture preserving filtering tasks.

Acknowledgments

GJMP and GJB are funded by the Multiple Sclerosis Society of Great Britain and Northern Ireland. JAS received support from Leverhulme Trust grant F/134/BZ and Netherlands Science Organisation (NWO) project 612–21–001. Thanks to Simon Arridge of the Computer Science Dept., UCL for discussions, and Val Stevenson and Sam Free, both of the Institute of Neurology, for images.

References

1. Perona, P., Malik, J.: Scale space and edge detection using anisotropic diffusion. IEEE Trans. Pattern Anal. Machine Intell. **12** (1990) 629–639
2. Catté, F., Lions, P.-L., Morel, J-M., Coll, T.: Image selective smoothing and edge detection by nonlinear diffusion. Siam. J. Numer. Anal. **29** (1992) 182–193
3. Gerig, G., Kübler, O., Kikinis, R., Jolesz, F.A.: Nonlinear anisotropic filtering of MRI data. IEEE Trans. Med. Imag. **11** (1992) 221–232
4. Pincus, S.M., Huang, W-M.: Approximate entropy: statistical properties and applications. Commun. Statist. Theory Meth. **21** (1992) 3061–3077
5. Pincus, S.M., Kalman, R.E.: Not all (possibly) "random" sequences are created equal. Proc. Natl. Acad. Sci. USA. **94** (1997) 3513–3518
6. Pincus, S.M., Singer, B.H.: Randomness and degrees of irregularity. Proc. Natl. Acad. Sci. USA. **93** (1996) 2083–2088
7. Canny, J.: A computational approach to edge detection. Pattern Anal. Machine Intell. **8** (1986) 679–698
8. Niessen, W.J., Ter Har Romeny, B.M., Florack, L.M.J., Viergever, M.A.: A general framework for geometry-driven evolution equations. Int. J. Comput. Vision. **21** (1997) 187–205
9. Bajla, I., Srámek, M.: Nonlinear filtering and fast ray tracing of 3-D image data. IEEE Engineering in Medicine and Biology **March/April** (1998) 73–80
10. Sanchez-Ortiz, G.I., Rueckert, D., Burger, P.: Knowledge-based tensor anisotropic diffusion of cardiac MR images. MedIA **3** (1999)
11. Gonzalez, R.G., Woods, R.E.: Digital image processing. Addison–Wesley (1993)
12. Chatfield, C.: The analysis of time series. 4th edn. Chapman and Hall, London New York (1989)
13. Singer, B.H., Pincus, S.: Irregular arrays and randomization. Proc. Natl. Acad. Sci. USA. **95** (1998) 1363–1386

New Variants of a Method of MRI Scale Normalization

László G. Nyúl[1,2] and Jayaram K. Udupa[1]

[1] Medical Image Processing Group, Department of Radiology,
University of Pennsylvania, Philadelphia, PA 19104–6021, USA
{nyul, jay}@mipg.upenn.edu
[2] Department of Applied Informatics, József Attila University,
P.O.Box 652, H–6701 Szeged, Hungary

Abstract. One of the major drawbacks of Magnetic Resonance Imaging (MRI) has been the lack of a standard and quantifiable interpretation of image intensities. This causes many difficulties in image display and analysis. We have devised a two-step method wherein all images can be transformed in such a way that for the same protocol and body region, in the transformed images similar intensities will have similar tissue meaning. Normalized images can be displayed with fixed windows without the need of per case adjustment. More importantly, extraction of quantitative information about healthy organs or about abnormities, such as tumors, can considerably be simplified. This paper introduces and compares new variants of this normalization method that can help to overcome some of the problems with the original method.

1 Introduction

A variety of MRI protocols (for example pulse sequences) are currently available that allow the setting up of different contrasts among the different tissues within the same organ system. Unfortunately, one of the major difficulties with the MRI techniques has been that intensities do not have a fixed meaning, not even within the same protocol for the same body region obtained on the same scanner for the same patient. This implies that MR images cannot be displayed at preset windows; one always has to adjust the window settings per case. The lack of a meaning for intensities also poses problems in image segmentation and quantification. What we need is that for protocols that are the same or "close" to each other, the resulting images should also be "close".

Attempts have been made to calibrate MR signal characteristics at the time of acquisition using phantoms. Postprocessing techniques that are applied to the image data that do not have any special acquisition requirements are however more attractive. There does not seem to have been any serious attempt to address this problem in the past.

The method described in [1] offers a simple way of transforming the images so that there is a significant gain in similarity of the resulting images. It is a

A. Kuba et al. (Eds.): IPMI'99, LNCS 1613, pp. 490–495, 1999.

two-step method consisting of a training step (executed only once for each protocol and body region) and a transformation step (executed on each image). This new transformation results in standard scales for different protocols and body regions. Intensities in the transformed images have meanings, and standard window settings can be determined for different tissues. However, the original, mode-based method is often not appropriate if the application is image segmentation, where we need more accurate meaning on the normalized scale even for relatively small ranges. This paper introduces and compares new variants of this normalization method that can help to overcome some of the problems with the original method.

2   Methods

Overview of the Normalization Method. We consider an image as a 3-dimensional array of volume elements (voxels) with intensity values assigned to each voxel. We assume that all "valid" intensities are positive integers and the value 0 means "no measured data". We denote the minimum and maximum occuring intensities in an image by m_1 and m_2, respectively.

It is desirable to cut off the "tails" of the histogram of the image because they often cause problems. Usually the high intensity tail corresponds to artifacts and outlier intensities. With this in mind, let pc_1 and pc_2 denote the minimum and maximum percentile values that are used to select a range of intensity of interest (IOI). Let the actual intensity values corresponding to pc_1 and pc_2 in the histogram be p_1 and p_2.

Based on over 20 body region/protocol combinations, we have observed mainly two types of histograms among MR images: unimodal and bimodal. In case of bimodal histograms, we can usually use the mode (μ) that corresponds to the main foreground object in the image as a histogram landmark. With unimodal histograms the mode usually corresponds to the background so we need to select some other landmark. This may be for example the shoulder of the hump of the background intensities. Since most of the protocols we studied produce bimodal histograms we will describe this case in more detail.

Our overall approach is as follows. Let the minimum and the maximum intensities on the standard scale for the IOI be s_1 and s_2, respectively. In the training step, the landmarks (p_{1j}, p_{2j}, μ_j) obtained from each of a set of images are mapped to the normalized scale by mapping the intensities from $[p_{1j}, p_{2j}]$ onto $[s_1, s_2]$ linearly. Then the mean (μ_s) of these mapped μ_js is computed. In the transformation step, for any given image, the actual second mode μ_i obtained from its histogram is matched to μ_s by doing two separate linear mappings: the first from $[p_{1i}, \mu_i]$ to $[s_1, \mu_s]$ and the second from $[\mu_i, p_{2i}]$ to $[\mu_s, s_2]$.

Choosing the Standardization Parameters. Although, once the training step is done, the corresponding transformation step is fully determined, there are several possibilities to tailor the normalization to the specific needs of an application. For example, s_1 should not be 0 if the values below p_1 need to be distinguished from "nothing" (i.e., value 0). Further, $s_2 - s_1$ should be large enough not to merge neighboring intensities after the transformation. When $pc_1 > 0$ and/or $pc_2 < 100$, the values in $[m_{1i}, p_{1i}]$ and $[p_{2i}, m_{2i}]$ may be mapped to $[s'_{1i}, s_1]$ and $[s_2, s'_{2i}]$, respectively, where s'_{1i} and s'_{2i} are determined by applying the mapping in the two linear sections corresponding to $[p_{1i}, \mu_i]$ to $[s_1, \mu_s]$ and $[\mu_i, p_{2i}]$ to $[\mu_s, s_2]$. We refer to this scale as "open". When all intensities in $[m_1, p_1]$ and $[p_2, m_2]$ are mapped to s_1 and s_2, respectively, we refer to the scale as "closed".

Choosing the Landmarks. The choice of the actual landmark is also an important factor. The mode-based method described above works fine for several MR protocols and several body regions but there are cases (and applications) wherein this simple method is not appropriate. As an example, consider the shape of the gray matter (GM), white matter (WM), and CSF distributions in fast spin-echo (FSE) proton density (PD) brain images. Their relative locations vary among studies and even among studies of the same patient. Figure 1 shows some histogram shapes all of which were found in histograms of patient studies. We recall here that in FSE PD images, GM regions are brighter than WM regions. The weakness of the mode-based method is that sometimes the mode (the peak location) corresponds to GM intensity (Figs. 1a, 1b), and in other cases, it corresponds to WM intenstity (Figs. 1d, 1e), or it may also correspond to intensities that lie between real GM and WM (Fig. 1c). Therefore, when we match the mode to a fixed location on the normalized scale, we may match GM in some cases and WM in the others. Because of this "switching" behavior, the mode-based method is often not appropriate if the application is image segmentation, where we need more accurate meaning on the normalized scale even for relatively small ranges. In order to eliminate the "switching" behavior, one approach is to choose the median of the main body of the histogram as a landmark to match. We do this on the reduced histogram (i.e., after removing the background and the noise (high percentile)). This landmark remains consistent even in cases where the histogram has two similar peaks (Figs. 1a, 1e) or asymmetric shape (Figs. 1b, 1d). We may also use more histogram landmarks, such as quartiles and deciles, to better define the standard histogram.

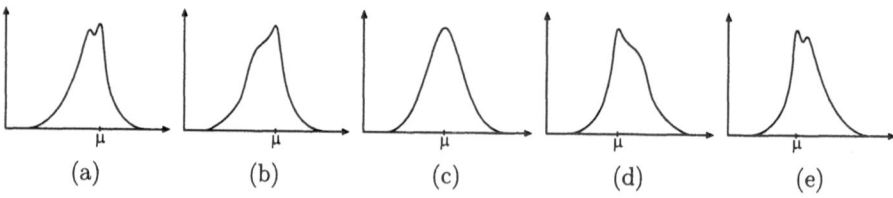

(a)   (b)   (c)   (d)   (e)

Fig. 1. Shapes of brain MRI histograms. For clarity, only the main body of the histogram (corresponding to the brain) is shown

3   Evaluation

For the validation of the method for each protocol and body region we need to consider the following variations in image data: (i) intra-patient (time-to-time) variation, (ii) inter-patient variation, (iii) variations among different machines of the same manufacturer, and (iv) variations among machines of different types. The following sections describe the methods of evaluation that we used to examine how different kinds of variations are affected by the different variants of the normalization. For all tests $s_1 = 1$, $s_2 = 4095$, $pc_1 = 0$, and $pc_2 = 99.8$ were used with "closed" and "open" scale, mode- and median-based variants, using linear segment-by-segment mapping. The training was done by using 10 different patient studies of the particular protocol and body region.

3.1   Qualitative Comparison

We conducted qualitative comparisons for the following MRI protocols: FSE PD, FSE T2, spin-echo (SE) PD, SE T2, T1 with Gadolinium enhancement (T1E), and SPGR. 30 studies each of FSE PD, FSE T2 and T1E, and 10 studies each of SE PD, SE T2 and SPGR were transformed using the corresponding "trained" parameters. Two ways of visual comparisons were made: by displaying at fixed gray level window settings before and after transformation, and by displaying the binary images obtained at fixed threshold ranges. For lack of space, only the former is illustrated below.

Images in the first row of Fig. 2 show a slice from each of three different patient studies. They are displayed at the same gray level window that was actually set up for the first image. This window is not appropriate for the other two data sets because they have quite different intensity ranges. In the second row, the same slices are displayed, after normalization with the open-scale median-based method, at a fixed "standard" brain window that we devised after examining a few normalized images. The structures are well portrayed and the contrast is more similar than that of the originals.

3.2   Quantitative Comparison

Two types of quantitative tests on data sets of brain obtained from three protocols FSE PD, FSE T2, T1E were conducted.

Test 1: Intra-patient Variation. We used the same training data sets and parameter configurations as for qualitative comparison. The test method for all three protocols was the same. Two scans acquired at different time instances were randomly selected for 15 patients. The time distance between the two scans of the same patient varied between 1 and 6 years. For each patient, we registered the first scan to the second via a rigid transformation based on intensity value correlations. Because these patients had Multiple Sclerosis (MS), the lesions were segmented [2,3] and removed for the purpose of comparison. Without this step

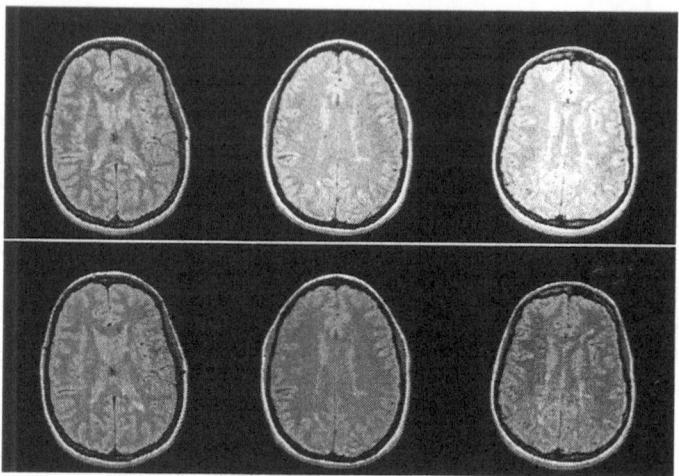

Fig. 2. Images displayed at fixed gray level windows. Original FSE PD images from different patients (first row), and after normalizing with the open-scale median-based method (second row)

the difference between the images due to the disease whould have perhaps distorted the results. The similarity of a pair of these registered, lesion-removed images was measured by the mean squared intensity difference (normalized to the original range of the images) NMSD. This similarity measure was computed for every pair of images before and after normalization for the different parameter configurations. Table 1 shows that the mean value of the NMSD after transformation is smaller than that before transformation. It also shows that using the median-based normalization the mean of NMSD is further reduced. The mean values of NMSD for the pairs of studies were compared using the paired t-test. The results show that the change in the means of NMSD is statistically significant (mostly $p < 0.01$) for all three pairs: before and after mode-based, before and after median-based, between mode- and median-based.

Table 1. Mean and standard deviation of NMSD before and after normalization with the closed-scale mode-based and with the open-scale median-based method

	FSE PD		FSE T2		T1E	
	mean	sd	mean	sd	mean	sd
before	0.0199	0.0177	0.0217	0.0182	0.0110	0.0074
after mode-based	0.0078	0.0102	0.0080	0.0080	0.0085	0.0072
after median-based	0.0039	0.0058	0.0036	0.0051	0.0019	0.0017

Test 2: Inter-patient Variation. For this comparison we randomly selected 12 FSE PD and 12 FSE T2 data sets from our database. All images were previously segmented into WM, GM, CSF, and MS lesion (LS) regions. We calculated the

statistics over the population of images for each of these regions separately. The normalization parameters were the same as those for the other comparisons. For each of these regions in each image i in each of these protocols, we calculated the normalized mean intensity (NMI) by dividing the mean intensity in the region by $m_{2i} - m_{1i}$. This was repeated for each set of the transformed images wherein normalization was done by dividing the mean intensity in the region by $s_2 - s_1$. The coefficient of variation of the NMI values before and after normalizations are shown in Table 2. The table indicates that the intensities on the normalized scale have more consistent tissue meaning than those on the original scale and that the median-based normalization outperforms the mode-based method in achieving similar tissue meaning of intensities.

Table 2. Coefficient of variation, expressed in %, of the NMI of different tissues in FSE PD and T2 images

	WM		GM		CSF		LS	
	PD	T2	PD	T2	PD	T2	PD	T2
before	14.61	14.83	51.23	51.81	46.77	46.85	31.54	31.61
after mode-based	2.55	2.13	1.95	2.18	3.24	5.46	3.20	5.01
after median-based	1.59	2.53	1.26	1.85	2.97	5.11	2.51	5.04

4   Concluding Remarks

The proposed intensity scale normalization methods produce more similar intensity meanings than the original images based on both qualitative and quantitative measures. Using the open-scale variant, it is possible to set better intensity of interest ranges while still being able to distinguish relevant information at the ends of the scale. Intensity values in the transformed images have more consistent meanings, tissues have better defined ranges on the median-based normalized scale than those on the mode-based normalized scale. Quantitative tests showed that the normalized mean squared difference between two different scans of the same subject is reduced if the new median-based and open-scale variants are used, and that this change is statistically significant. They also showed that the inter-patient variation of the intensities within different tissues also decreases.

References

1. Nyúl, L., Udupa, J.: On standardizing the MR image intensity scale. Radiology **209(P)** (1998) 581–582
2. Samarasekera, S., Udupa, J., Miki, Y., Grossman, R.: A new computer-assisted method for the quantification of enhancing lesions in multiple sclerosis. J. Comput. Assist. Tomogr. **21** (1997) 145–151
3. Udupa, J., Wei, L., Samarasekera, S., Miki, Y., van Buchem, M., Grossman, R.: Multiple sclerosis lesion quantification using fuzzy-connectedness principles. IEEE Trans. Med. Imaging **16** (1997) 598–609

Method for Estimating the Intensity Mapping between MRI Images

Alexei M. C. Machado[1,3], Mario F. M. Campos[1], and James C. Gee[2]

[1] DCC – Universidade Federal de Minas Gerais
Caixa Postal 702, Belo Horizonte, MG, 30161-970, Brazil
{alexei, mario}@dcc.ufmg.br
[2] Department of Radiology - University of Pennsylvania
3400 Spruce Street, Philadelphia, PA, 19104, USA
gee@rad.upenn.edu
[3] DCC – Pontifícia Universidade Católica de Minas Gerais
Av. Dom Jose Gaspar, 500, Belo Horizonte, MG, 30535-610, Brazil

Abstract. A method is presented for determining the intensity mapping between MRI images that may have been acquired using different sequences or instruments. The method can be applied to fully elastic matching and produces spatially localized probability functions that are capable of representing in an efficient way strong intensity distortions due, for instance, to the shading effect in MRI.

1 Introduction

In image matching, the correspondence between the images is evaluated using a similarity measure which quantifies the plausibility of observing an arbitrary feature f_T in one image when feature f_R is seen in the second image. In this work, we present a measure designed for intensity values as they appear on MRI images that may have been acquired using different sequences or scanners. The measure takes into account partial volume voxels, adapts to spatially varying intensity degradations, and is estimated jointly with the unknown mapping that warps the two images into spatial register.

Various similarity measures that utilize statistical properties of the registered images have been proposed recently and used with great success to rigidly register multi-modal images of the same scene [1,2,3]. Maintz *et al.* [4] have made a preliminary attempt to extend the mutual information measure to non-rigid registration by using the alignment result from optimizing the measure as a first estimate to the elastic correction of small deformations. In related work, Gee and co-workers [5] developed a non-rigid matching technique capable of handling large-valued deformations, in which the intensity mapping between the images is represented as a conditional probability density that is determined simultaneously with the calculation of the unknown spatial transformation. Different approaches to estimating this conditional density have been further investigated in [6] and these are extended in the current work wherein a formal model is constructed that explicitly considers partial volume and position-dependent effects.

A. Kuba et al. (Eds.): IPMI'99, LNCS 1613, pp. 496–501, 1999.

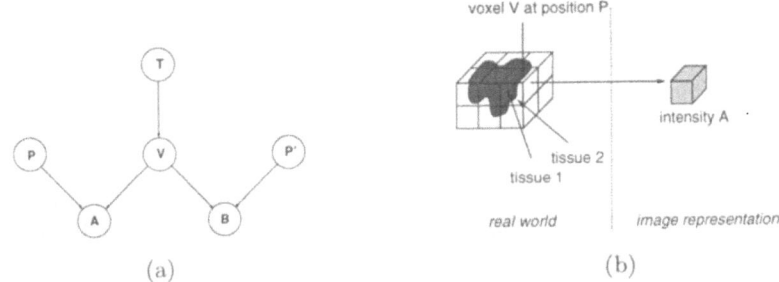

Fig. 1. (a) A causal network for the observation model. (b) A voxel V with intensity A at position P, composed of more than one tissue T

2   Methods

The relationship between the variables of the intensity mapping problem in image matching can be better understood when they are displayed as a causal model [7]. The model in Fig. 1a specifies that the intensity of each voxel in the image depends on the tissue composition within the voxel and on the voxel's position within the scanner volume. This model shows that the same voxel composed of a fixed combination V of different tissue types may produce different intensities A and B when placed in different locations or scanners P and P', respectively. Fig. 1b illustrates the problem of partial volume tissue composition, in which a single voxel V at position P may be composed of more than one tissue type T. In this case, the intensity A assigned to the voxel will be a weighted average of its component tissue intensities, whose values are a function of position within the imaging volume.

Since the intensity variable A is influenced by the voxel's partial volume mixture V of tissue types and the position P at which the voxel is placed, the probability that it assumes a value a is *conditioned* on the values of V and P. This quantitative information is denoted as $P(a|v, \mathbf{p})$, also known as an *observation or sensor model*. We can state the same for intensity observations in the second image for the matching problem, where $P(b|v, \mathbf{p}')$ is the conditional probability that a tissue mixture v produces intensity b at position $\mathbf{p}'$. The goal of this work is to determine the conditional probability relating our observation models so that it can be used to guide the matching process.

The relationship between tissue type and partial volume composition is represented in the causal model graph by an arrow that conditions the probability of V given a pure tissue type T. Since the proportion of tissue types in an arbitrary voxel can assume any relative combination, the variable V takes on as many discrete values. The closer this number is to the number of intensity values displayed in the images, the more accurate our representation will be of the partial volume mixtures. The conditional probability matrix $P(v|t)$ and the prior $P(t)$ can be estimated using the intensity histograms obtained from a labeled atlas.

During the matching process, for each voxel located at $\mathbf{p}'$ of known intensity b in image B, the aim is to find its corresponding voxel in image A. To do so, it is necessary to determine how likely it is for a voxel with intensity a placed at position $\mathbf{p}$ to contain the same tissue mixture that the original voxel in B is composed of. The problem can be stated as the determination of the probability $P(a|\mathbf{p}, b, \mathbf{p}')$ that a voxel in image A induces intensity a given that it is placed at position $\mathbf{p}$ and corresponds to intensity b at position $\mathbf{p}'$ in the second image B. Conditioning $P(a|\mathbf{p}, b, \mathbf{p}')$ on the exhaustive set of partial volume mixture values, we have that

$$P(a|\mathbf{p}, b, \mathbf{p}') = \sum_k [P(a|\mathbf{p}, b, \mathbf{p}', v_k)P(v_k|\mathbf{p}, b, \mathbf{p}')].$$

In addition to the dependencies between the variables, the causal model in Fig. 1 also represents the conditional independent relationships between them: given that tissue mixture value v is known, the information about variables B and P' do not contribute to our belief about the value of A. In other words, A is *conditionally independent* of B and P' given that V is known: $P(a|\mathbf{p}, b, \mathbf{p}', v) = P(a|v, \mathbf{p})$. Moreover, since A is unknown, it causes the variable V to be independent of P: $P(v|\mathbf{p}, b, \mathbf{p}') = P(v|b, \mathbf{p}')$. From these independent relationships, it follows that

$$P(a|\mathbf{p}, b, \mathbf{p}') = \sum_k [P(a|v_k, \mathbf{p})P(v_k|b, \mathbf{p}')]. \tag{1}$$

Using Bayes's formula, we have that

$$P(v_k|b, \mathbf{p}') = P(b, \mathbf{p}'|v_k)P(v_k)/P(b, \mathbf{p}'),$$

which together with (1) leads to

$$P(a|\mathbf{p}, b, \mathbf{p}') = \frac{1}{P(b, \mathbf{p}')} \sum_k [P(a|\mathbf{p}, v_k)P(b, \mathbf{p}'|v_k)P(v_k)]. \tag{2}$$

Using the definition of conditional probability, we have that

$$P(b, \mathbf{p}'|v) = P(b|v, \mathbf{p}')P(\mathbf{p}'|v), \tag{3}$$

where $P(\mathbf{p}'|v) = P(\mathbf{p}')$ since P' is independent of V when variable B is unknown. From (2) and (3) it follows that

$$P(a|\mathbf{p}, b, \mathbf{p}') = \frac{P(\mathbf{p}')}{P(b, \mathbf{p}')} \sum_k [P(a|\mathbf{p}, v_k)P(b|\mathbf{p}', v_k)P(v_k)]. \tag{4}$$

Finally, conditioning $P(v_k)$ on the exhaustive set of mixture values, (4) becomes

$$P(a|\mathbf{p}, b, \mathbf{p}') = \frac{P(\mathbf{p}')}{P(b, \mathbf{p}')} \sum_k [P(a|\mathbf{p}, v_k)P(b|\mathbf{p}', v_k) \sum_i [P(v_k|t_i)P(t_i)]]. \tag{5}$$

We see that $P(a|\mathbf{p}, b, \mathbf{p}')$ is an average of the product of the observation models for each partial volume tissue mixture, weighted by its *a priori* probability.

In order to use (5) for MRI image matching, the models $P(a|\mathbf{p}, v)$ and $P(b|\mathbf{p}', v)$ are considered to be Gaussian. Specifically, the probability that a tissue mixture v_k imaged at position $\mathbf{p}$ produces intensity a is described by a Gaussian distribution with mean $\mu_{Ak\mathbf{p}}$ and variance σ_A^2. This model is appropriate for MRI images, but should be replaced with the relevant distribution in other imaging situations. Since our probabilities are represented in practice by tables, our method is applicable to any class of distributions. Assuming discrete Gaussian distributions for the observation models, $P(a|\mathbf{p}, b, \mathbf{p}')$ becomes

$$\frac{P(\mathbf{p}')}{P(b, \mathbf{p}')} \sum_k \left[\frac{\exp -\frac{(a-\mu_{Ak\mathbf{p}})^2}{2\sigma_A^2}}{\sum_{i=0}^{M-1} \exp -\frac{(i-\mu_{Ak\mathbf{p}})^2}{2\sigma_A^2}} \frac{\exp -\frac{(b-\mu_{Bk\mathbf{p}'})^2}{2\sigma_B^2}}{\sum_{i=0}^{M-1} \exp -\frac{(i-\mu_{Bk\mathbf{p}'})^2}{2\sigma_B^2}} \sum_i [P(v_k|t_i)P(t_i)] \right] \tag{6}$$

where M is the number of intensity values.

Since the variance can be assumed spatially constant and is easily determined from the image background, the only unknowns to be computed are the mean values $\mu_{Ak\mathbf{p}}$ and $\mu_{Bk\mathbf{p}'}$. These values can be determined with the aid of labeled images. Taking observation model A as an example, the value of $\mu_{Ak\mathbf{p}}$ for each position $\mathbf{p}$ and tissue mixture v_k can be approximated by considering the intensity values that each tissue assumes in the neighborhood of position $\mathbf{p}$. Based on the tissue histogram computed for the region around position $\mathbf{p}$ and on a prior distribution model for the tissue types with respect to the particular acquisition protocol, the expected distribution of partial volume tissue mixtures for the region can be determined. The tissue mixture distribution H_V and the intensity histogram H_I are then matched to determine the mean intensity of the mixture in the region around $\mathbf{p}$. The purpose is to determine a function $F(v_k)$ that will indicate the corresponding intensity for each value v_k, so that

$$\frac{\int_{-\infty}^{F(v_k)} H_I(x)dx}{\int_{-\infty}^{+\infty} H_I(x)dx} = \frac{\int_{-\infty}^{v_k} H_V(x)dx}{\int_{-\infty}^{+\infty} H_V(x)dx}. \tag{7}$$

To compute the local tissue mixture mean intensities and the probability $P(a|\mathbf{p}, b, \mathbf{p}')$, a prior model for the tissue mixtures is required. Since a single image does not provide sufficient information to infer the partial volume tissue composition of any voxel, the global intensity histogram for a labeled atlas is used to estimate the prior distribution. The idea stems from the fact that in the process of labeling the atlas into its major tissue components the expert assigns a partial volume voxel to the pure tissue type that is most representative of the voxel's contents. This then is reflected in the variance of the intensity histogram, from which a probability distribution can be obtained. In this work, the distribution was approximated by a Gaussian model, although other models can be used as well. The method has proven to be robust to this assumption in the case when both images are acquired with the same protocol. Based on the prior model Π for tissue mixtures and the tissue histogram H_T, the histogram H_V in (7) can be computed as $H_V(v) = \sum_i H_T(t_i)\Pi(t_i, v)$, where the case for a normally distributed prior with means μ_i and variances σ_i^2 for each tissue t_i implies that $\Pi(t_i, v) = (1/\sqrt{2\pi\sigma^2}) \exp -(v - \mu_i)^2/2\sigma_i^2$.

3   Experimental Results

The set of MRI images used as the input to the algorithms was extracted from the Harvard Atlas [8]. The atlas was reformatted into 8-bit 256×123 horizontal slices. All voxels not classified as gray matter, white matter, or cerebrospinal fluid were given the gray-level value 0. In order to demonstrate the method's robustness to intensity distortions, a second volume was created by applying to the atlas a multiplicative low-frequency sinusoidal signal with an amplitude of 0.2.

(a)   (b)

Fig. 2. (a) Horizontal slice 124 of the Harvard Atlas. (b) Horizontal slice 129 of the noisy version of the atlas

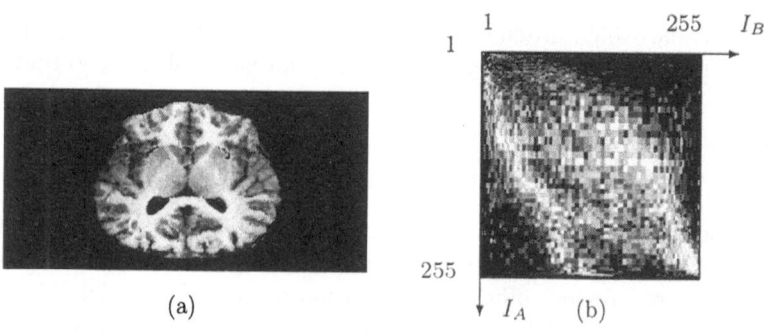

(a) I_A (b)

Fig. 3. (a) Result of warping slice 124 (image A) to match slice 129 (image B). (b) Inferred global probability map $P(I_B|I_A)$

The method was evaluated using slice 124 (image A) of the original atlas and slice 129 of the noisy version of the atlas (image B)—see Fig. 2. The result of deforming slice 124 of image A to match noisy slice 129 of image B is shown in Fig. 3a, with the inferred global probability map $P(I_B|I_A)$ depicted in Fig. 3b.

The probabilities are displayed in gray scale so that the largest in each column appears white. The grid dimensions are proportional to the contribution of each intensity value in the image histograms. As can be seen, the deformed image is similar to the target image B but correctly exhibits the distribution of intensity values found in image A.

4   Conclusion

A method is presented for determining the intensity mapping between MRI images that may have been acquired using different sequences or scanners. The mapping is estimated directly from the image data, explicitly models partial volume voxels and spatially varying intensity degradations, and is computed jointly with the unknown spatial transformation in an iterative matching algorithm. The importance of the method is two-fold: it is a tool to model the instruments used in the acquisition step so that more effective data processing techniques can be developed. For the important problem of image matching, the method makes possible a principled approach to likelihood modeling or the construction of similarity metrics. A poor model of the intensity mapping for the image pair to be registered may lead to false matches, regardless of the prior constraints employed and will bias all subsequent morphological analyses.

References

1. Woods, R.P., Grafton, S.T., Holmes, C.J., Cherry, S.R., Mazziotta, J.C.: Automated image registration: I General methods and intra-subject intra-modality validation. Journal of Computer Assisted Tomography **22** (1998) 141-154
2. Viola, P.: Alignment by maximization of mutual information. International Journal of Computer Vision **24**(2) (1997) 137-154
3. Maes, F., Collignon, A., Vandermeulen, D., Marchal, G., Seutens, P.: Multimodality image registration by maximization of mutual information. IEEE Transactions on Medical Imaging **16**(2) (1997) 187-198
4. Maintz, J., Meijering, E., Viergever, M.: General multimodal elastic registration based on mutual information. In: Proc. SPIE Medical Imaging 1998: Image Processing. Bellingham (1998)
5. Gee, J.C., Haynor, D.R., Reivich, M., Bajcsy, R.K.: Finite element approach to warping of brain images. In: Proc. SPIE Medical Imaging 1994: Image Processing. Bellingham (1994)
6. Machado, A.M.C., Gee, J.C., Campos, M.F.M.: Likelihood modeling for image warping. To appear: Proc. SPIE Medical Imaging 1999: Image Processing. Bellingham (1999)
7. Pearl, J.: Probabilistic Reasoning in Intelligent Systems: Networks of Plausible Inference. Morgan Kaufman (1991)
8. Shenton, M., Kikinis, R., Jolesz, F., Pollak, S., LeMay, M., Wible, C., Hokama, H., Martin, J., Metcalf, D., Coleman, M., McCarley, R.: Abnormalities of the left temporal lobe and thought disorder in schizophrenia: A quantitative magnetic resonance imaging study. N. Eng. J. Med. **327** (1992) 604-612

Author Index

Subject Index

Lecture Notes in Computer Science

For information about Vols. 1–1548
please contact your bookseller or Springer-Verlag